NURSING LEADERSHIP AND MANAGEMENT

First Canadian Edition

Patricia Kelly

University of Texas, Austin

Heather Crawford

Executive Director Professional and Nursing Practice

Peace Country Health Region

Grande Prairie, Alberta

NELSON / EDUCATION

NELSON / EDUCATION

**Nursing Leadership and Management,
First Canadian Edition**

by Patricia Kelly and Heather Crawford

**Associate Vice President,
Editorial Director:**
Evelyn Veitch

Senior Acquisitions Editor:
Kevin Smulan

Marketing Manager:
William De Villiers

Senior Developmental Editor:
Rebecca Ryoji

**Photo Researcher/Permissions
Coordinator:**
Daniela Glass

Production Service:
Gunjan Chandola,
ICC Macmillan Inc.

Copy Editor:
Mariko Obokata

Proofreader:
Barbara Storey

Indexer:
Maura Brown

**Senior Manufacturing
Coordinator:**
Charmaine Lee-Wah

Design Director:
Ken Phipps

Managing Designer:
Katherine Strain

Cover Design:
Johanna Liburd

Cover Image:
Jupiterimages

Compositor:
ICC Macmillan Inc.

Printer:
Edwards Brothers

**Library and Archives Canada
Cataloguing in Publication Data**

Kelly, Patricia, 1941–
  Nursing leadership and management / Patricia Kelly, Heather Crawford. — 1st Canadian ed.

Includes bibliographical references and index.
ISBN 978-0-17-610335-4

  1. Nursing services— Administration—Textbooks. 2. Leadership—Textbooks. I. Crawford, Heather, 1950– II. Title.

RT89.K45 2007   362.17'3068
C2007-906682-8

NOTICE TO THE READER

This book is dedicated to my husband, Maurice; my loving dad and mom, John and Joan Trantom; to my wonderful son and daughter, Brent and Ashley; to my stepson and stepdaughter, Greg and Michelle; to my incredible granddaughter, Eden; to my mentors, Dr. John Horne and Virginia Sinnott; to my special friend, Anne-Marie; to Tom, Gayle, Nabil, and Lynne; and to my nursing friends and colleagues, Joan Doran, Vicki Pennick, Sandra Trubyk, and Sharon Schwindt, who have supported me throughout this book and during our many years together as nurses.

CONTENTS

CHAPTER 5

Population-Based Health Care Practice 93

CHAPTER 6

Personal and Interdisciplinary Communication 112

CHAPTER 7

Politics and Consumer Partnerships   129

UNIT III
PLANNING CARE

CHAPTER 8

Nursing Leadership and Management   142

CHAPTER 9

Strategic Planning and Organizing Client Care   170

CHAPTER 10

Effective Team Building   188

CHAPTER 13

Delegation of Nursing Care   237

UNIT IV

MANAGING CARE

CHAPTER 14

First-Line Unit Management   249

CHAPTER 15

Change and Conflict Resolution   266

CHAPTER 16

Power   284

UNIT V
EVALUATION

CHAPTER 17

Managing Performance and Outcomes Using an Organizational Quality Improvement Model   295

CHAPTER 18

Decision Making   316

UNIT VI

OTHER PROFESSIONAL CONSIDERATIONS

CHAPTER 19

Legal Aspects of Client Care   338

CHAPTER 20

Ethics and the Profession of Nursing   353

CHAPTER 21

Collective Bargaining   372

UNIT VII

PREPARATION FOR ENTRY-LEVEL NURSING PRACTICE

CHAPTER 22

Career Planning and Development: Creating Your Path to the Future   385

CONTRIBUTORS

John P. Angkaw, RN, BScN, MEd(c)
Public Health Nurse
Region of Peel Public Health—Alcohol, Drugs and Addictions
Brampton, Ontario
Chapter 6: Personal and Interdisciplinary Communication
Chapter 13: Delegation of Nursing Care

Heather Crawford, BScN, MEd, CHE
Doctoral Student, McMaster University
Executive Director Professional and Nursing Practice
Peace Country Health Region
Grande Prairie, Alberta
Chapter 1: Canada's Health Care Environment
Chapter 2: Basic Clinical Health Care Economics
Chapter 4: Nursing and Health Care Informatics
Chapter 7: Politics and Consumer Partnerships
Chapter 9: Strategic Planning and Organizing Client Care
Chapter 10: Effective Team Building
Chapter 11: Budget Concepts for Client Care
Chapter 12: Effective Staffing
Chapter 14: First-Line Unit Management
Chapter 15: Change and Conflict Resolution
Chapter 17: Managing Performance and Outcomes Using an Organizational
    Quality Improvement Model
Chapter 19: Legal Aspects of Client Care
Chapter 21: Collective Bargaining

Amy Curzon, RN
The Sheridan Institute of Technology and Advanced Learning
Brampton, Ontario
Chapter 6: Personal and Interdisciplinary Communication

Eric Doucette, RN
Professional Practice Leader
Brant Community Healthcare System
Brantford, Ontario
Chapter 8: Nursing Leadership and Management
Chapter 18: Decision Making

Pat Frederickson
Former Executive Director/Registrar
College of Licensed Practical Nurses of Alberta
Chapter 7: Politics and Consumer Partnerships

Rita McGregor
Former Director of Professional Practice
College of Licensed Practical Nurses of Alberta
Chapter 7: Politics and Consumer Partnerships

Ined Parmar, RN, BScN, MA GNC (C)
Professor
The Sheridan Institute of Technology and Advanced Learning
Brampton, Ontario
Chapter 18: Decision Making

Victoria E Pennick, RN, MHSc
Senior Clinical Research Project Manager
Managing Editor, Cochrane Back Group
Institute for Work & Health
Toronto, Ontario
Chapter 3: Evidence-Based Practice
Chapter 5: Population-Based Health Care Practice

Sandra Trubyk, MSA, BN, BA
Coordinator and Professor
School of Community and Liberal Studies
The Sheridan Institute of Technology and Advanced Learning
Brampton, Ontario
Chapter 16: Power

Janice Waddell RN, PhD
Associate Professor
Associate Director, School of Nursing
Ryerson University
Toronto, Ontario
Chapter 22: Career Planning and Development: Creating Your Path to the Future

Nancy Walton, PhD
Associate Professor, School of Nursing, Faculty of Community Services
Chair, Research Ethics Board
Ryerson University
Toronto, Ontario
Chapter 20: Ethics and the Profession of Nursing

PREFACE

Nursing Leadership and Management is designed to help students and beginning nurses develop the knowledge and skills to lead and manage nursing care delivery in the 21st century. Every nurse today must lead and manage nursing care delivery, and the need for nurse leaders and nurse managers has never been greater. The nursing shortage is pressuring health care organizations to require nurses to do more with less and to adapt quickly to change.

Today's nurses need to have the competencies required for the 21st century, which calls for changes to nursing, medical, and other health care curricula. Some recommendations for the health care profession highlight the need for nurses to be educated in a broader way, including education in the areas of interdisciplinary teamwork, population-based health care, evidence-based practice, informatics, ethics, quality improvement, culture, and change, to name just a few.

This text addresses many of these topics, along with others, to prepare the beginning nurse leader and manager to successfully function in the modern health care system. Many of the chapters are written by nursing faculty. Others are written by clinical nurses who are specialists in their fields. These contributors are from various areas of Canada, thus providing a broad view of nursing leadership and management.

ORGANIZATION

Nursing Leadership and Management consists of 22 chapters grouped into seven units. These seven units will provide beginning nurse leaders and managers with the expertise needed to succeed in today's health care environment. They are arranged as follows:

- **Unit I** presents the changing health care environment and basic clinical economics.
- **Unit II** outlines a new health care model, emphasizing the role of evidence-based health care, nursing and health care informatics, population-based health care practice, interdisciplinary and personal communication, and politics and consumer partnerships in health care today.
- **Unit III** discusses planning care through leadership and management, strategic planning and organizing client care, effective team building, budget concepts for client care, the allocation of human resources for effective staffing, and delegation of client care.
- **Unit IV** discusses organizing and coordinating care. It presents first-line client care management, change and conflict resolution, and power.
- **Unit V** covers evaluation of care, including managing outcomes using an organizational performance improvement model, and decision making.
- **Unit VI** presents other professional considerations, such as legal aspects of client care, ethical dimensions of client care, and collective bargaining.
- **Unit VII** presents preparation for entry-level nursing practice. It discusses career planning, your first job, and integrating personal and professional needs.

An appendix outlines how to prepare for the Canadian Registered Nurse Examinations (CRNE) and the Canadian Practical Nurse Registration Examinations (CPRNE). The textbook uses graphics and photographs to engage readers and enhance their learning. Photographs provide visual reinforcement of concepts such as teamwork and the changes occurring in health care settings today while adding visual interest. Figures and tables depict concepts and activities described in the text.

FEATURES

Each chapter includes several pedagogical features that provide the reader with a consistent format for learning and an assortment of resources for understanding and applying the knowledge presented. These features include the following:

- Objectives state each chapter's learning goals.
- An introduction to each chapter briefly describes the purpose and scope of the chapter.
- A bulleted list of key concepts at the end of each chapter assists the reader in remembering and using the material presented.
- Review questions and review activities encourage students to think critically by applying chapter content to real-world situations and reinforcing key leadership and management skills. Exercises are numbered in each chapter to facilitate using them as assignments or activities.
- Key terms appear in bold type in each chapter and are designed to encourage the understanding of new terms presented in the chapter.
- References are the key to finding the sources of the material presented in each chapter.
- Suggested readings help the reader to find additional information concerning the topics covered in each chapter.

Special features are used throughout the text to emphasize key points and to provide specific types of information:

- An opening quote by a nursing or health care theorist provides a professional perspective on the chapter's topic.
- An opening scenario with thought-provoking questions introduces each chapter and establishes the background for the reader's approach to the chapter.
- Critical Thinking sections encourage serious consideration and personal reflection on important topics.
- Interviews with staff nurses, nurse practitioners, nursing managers and leaders, nursing administrators, nursing risk managers, nursing faculty, doctors, clients, and a hospital administrator are sprinkled throughout the chapters to illustrate various points of view. Interviews with Dr. Ginette L. Rodger, Dr. Lynn Nagle, Dr. Tim Porter-O'Grady, and other nursing leaders are included in some chapters.
- Literature applications illustrate the applicability of current literature for practice.
- Case studies provide real-world illustrations of the chapter's topic.
- Web exercises guide the reader to the Internet and provide Internet addresses for the latest information related to the chapter content.

ACKNOWLEDGMENTS

Many people must work together to produce any book. A comprehensive book such as this requires even greater effort and the coordination of many people with various areas of expertise. I would like to thank all the contributors for their time and effort and for sharing their knowledge gained through years of experience in both the clinical and academic setting. I thank them all for being responsive, making the necessary revisions, and sounding happy to hear from me whenever I e-mailed or called them. I also thank the reviewers for their time spent critically reviewing the manuscript and providing the valuable comments that have added to this text.

I would like to acknowledge and sincerely thank the team at Nelson Education Ltd. who have worked to make this first Canadian edition a reality. Rebecca Ryoji, senior developmental editor, Higher Education, is a great individual who has worked tirelessly and brought knowledge, guidance, humour, and attention to help keep me motivated and on track throughout the project. Thanks also to the production team: Mariko Obokata, copy editor; Daniela Glass, permissions co-ordinator; Gunjan Chandola, project manager; Barbara Storey, proofreader; Maura Brown, indexer.

A special huge thank you goes to my husband and best friend, Maurice, supporting me through each stage of the project. I could not have done this project without his help!

ABOUT THE AUTHOR

Heather Crawford earned a bachelor of science degree in nursing from the University of Toronto School of Nursing; a master's degree in education from Brock University in St. Catharines, Ontario; and a Certified Health Executive (CHE) designation from the Canadian College of Health Service Executives. She is currently pursuing her doctoral studies in nursing at McMaster University. Heather has held progressively responsible positions as a health care administrator in both community hospitals and academic tertiary/quaternary acute care institutions. She was director of surgical, obstetrical and gynecological nursing at the Wellesley Hospital in Toronto; vice president of St. Joseph's Hospital in Brantford, Ontario; nursing director of critical care, cardiac sciences, and internal medicine at the Royal Alexandra Hospital in Edmonton, Alberta; and vice president and chief nursing officer of the Health Sciences Centre in Winnipeg, Manitoba. In addition, she held the position of director of practice and policy at the College of Nurses of Ontario.

Heather has taught at The Mack Centre, School of Nursing, Niagara College; George Brown College of Applied Arts and Technology; Mohawk College, Hamilton, Ontario; Ryerson University, Toronto; University of Alberta; and the Sheridan College Institute of Technology and Advanced Learning. Heather has taught fundamentals of nursing, adult medical-surgical nursing, obstetrical nursing, nursing leadership and management, nursing issues and trends, and legal aspects of nursing. She has taught nursing conferences on quality improvement and scope of practice in Alberta, Manitoba, and Nova Scotia. Heather is a member of the College of Nurses of Ontario, the Registered Nurses Association of Ontario, the Canadian Nurses Association, and the Canadian College of Health Service Executives. She is registered with the College and Association of Registered Nurses of Alberta.

Heather has served on the board of directors of Mount Carmel Clinic, Winnipeg, Manitoba, and Cancer Care Manitoba. She also was a member of the board of directors at St. Joseph's Hospital and the St. Joseph's Hospital Foundation in Brantford, Ontario.

Over the course of her career, Heather has been registered as an RN in three provinces: Ontario, Alberta, and Manitoba. Heather can be reached at hcmq@sympatico.ca.

HOW TO USE THIS BOOK

Quote A nursing or health care theorist quote presents a professional's perspective regarding the topic at hand; read this quote as you begin each new chapter and see whether your opinion matches or differs, or whether you are in need of further information.

Chapter Objectives These goals indicate the performance-based, measurable objectives that are targeted for mastery upon completion of the chapter.

Opening Scenario This mini case study with related critical thinking questions should be read prior to delving into the chapter; it sets the tone for the material to come and helps you identify your knowledge base and perspective.

Case Study These short cases with related questions present a beginning clinical nursing management situation calling for judgment, decision making, or analysis in solving an open-ended problem. Familiarize yourself with the types of situations and settings you will later encounter in practice, and challenge yourself to devise solutions that will result in the best outcomes for all parties, within the boundaries of legal and ethical nursing practice.

Literature Application Study these key findings from nursing and health care research, theory, and literature, and ask yourself how they will influence your practice. Do you see ways in which your nursing could be affected by these literature findings and research results? Do you agree with the conclusions drawn by the author?

Critical Thinking Ethical, legal, delegation, and performance improvement considerations are highlighted in these boxes. Before beginning a new chapter, page through and read the Critical Thinking sections and jot down your comments or reactions, then see whether your perspective changes after you complete the chapter.

Real World Interviews Real world interviews with well-known nursing leaders, such as Dr. Ginette L. Rodger, Dr. Lynn Nagle, Dr. Tim Porter O'Grady, and others are included as well as interviews with nurses, doctors, hospital administrators, staff, clients, and family members. As you read these, ask yourself whether you had ever considered that individual's point of view on the given topic. How would knowing another person's perspective affect the care you deliver?

Key Concepts This bulleted list serves as a review and study tool for you as you complete each chapter.

Key Terms Study this list prior to reading the chapter, then again as you complete a chapter, to test your true understanding of the terms and concepts covered. Make a study list of terms you need to focus on to thoroughly appreciate the material of the chapter.

Review Questions These questions will challenge your comprehension of objectives and concepts presented in the chapter and will demonstrate your mastery of the chapter content, build critical thinking skills, and achieve integration of the concepts.

Review Activities These thought-provoking activities at the close of a chapter invite you to approach a problem or scenario critically and apply the knowledge you have gained.

Exploring the Web Internet activities encourage you to use your computer and reasoning skills to search the Web for additional information on quality and nursing leadership and management.

References Evidence-based research, theory, and general literature, as well as nursing, medical, and health care sources, are included in these lists; refer to them as you read the chapter and verify your research.

Suggested Readings These entries invite you to pursue additional topics, articles, and information in related resources.

Photos, Tables, and Figures These items illustrate key concepts.

CHAPTER 1

Canada's Health Care Environment

Patricia Kelly, RN, MSN
Adapted by: Heather Crawford, BScN, MEd, CHE

Our health care system defines us as communities, as a society, and as a nation. What Canadians are prepared to do, and more importantly, what we are not prepared to do for each other when we are sick, vulnerable, and most in need, says a great deal about Canada, our basic values, and the values that we want to hand on to future generations of Canadians. (Margaret Somerville, AM, FRSC, DCL Founding Director, McGill Centre for Medicine, Ethics, and Law, McGill University, Montreal, Quebec)

OBJECTIVES

Upon completion of this chapter, the reader should be able to:

1. Identify how health care is organized and funded in Canada.
2. Review the movement toward population health and disease management.
3. Discuss health care variation and evidence-based practice.
4. Review the Canadian Adverse Events Study and the Institute of Medicine's Committee on Health Care Reports.
5. Identify recent changes and current forces and trends influencing the development of caring, multidisciplinary nursing and health care delivery in Canada.

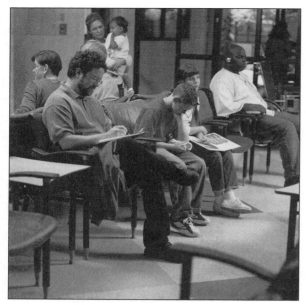

We've been here almost four hours already.

You have just moved back to the province, and have seen a couple of old friends. They tell you they had to take their four-year-old son to the Emergency Department three days ago because he had a cut on his forehead. Although their son is all right now, they are worried about the length of time they waited in the Emergency Department before being treated, their lack of a family physician, and the attitude of the health professionals they met. This scene occurs over and over again in today's health care environment as Canadians struggle to find a way to ensure access to cost-effective, quality care for themselves and their families.

What are your thoughts about this situation?

What advice do you have for the family?

How can you contribute to improving access to health care for your friends and for the community?

In order to manage and lead effectively, it is imperative that every health care professional have a working knowledge and understanding of Canada's health care system. Too many nurses comment on the system, without really knowing its history.

Health care delivery in Canada is a combination of public and private initiatives organized to provide citizens with access to cost-effective, quality health care. Canadians are living longer, and are generally in better health than previous generations. However, challenges in the health sector remain, including the reform of our health care system. Recent surveys indicate that most Canadians believe that they are in very good to excellent health. Life expectancy, as well as health-adjusted life expectancy, has increased; the infant death rate has

dropped; many infectious diseases have been practically eliminated; and medical techniques have continued to evolve (Canada. Statistics Canada, 2006, p. 159).

Although Canadians are healthier today than they were in the past, a number of problems persist. Heart disease, cancer, mental health problems, HIV/AIDS, asthma, obesity, and diabetes continue to affect many Canadians. Ongoing threats to public health are posed by new infectious disease strains, such as severe acute respiratory syndrome (SARS), the West Nile virus, and infection from Clostridium difficile bacteria (Canada. Statistics Canada, 2006, p. 159). National newspapers and other publications regularly report on health problems in the Aboriginal community. First Nations adults, depending on their age group, are two to eight times more likely to have diabetes than the general Canadian population (Health Council of Canada [HCC], 2007, p. 14). The incidence of diabetes is also increasing in First Nations children and adolescents. First Nations people have higher than average rates for the risk factors of smoking, alcohol use, obesity, and physical inactivity (HCC, 2007). The need for access, quality, and cost-effectiveness has driven various initiatives to improve health care in the past and present.

Present-day nursing's role in quality health care began to develop in Canada in the aftermath of Florence Nightingale's efforts in London. Her emphasis on cleanliness, fresh air, regular client observation, and monitoring of mortality rates, though familiar today, was radical in the management of client care at that time. Nightingale illustrated mortality rates with a coxcomb diagram (Figure 1-1).

Nightingale used these coxcomb diagrams to dramatize the number of preventable deaths in the Crimean war campaign. The light blue wedges on the coxcomb measured from the centre of the circle represent the deaths from preventable diseases. Although Nightingale managed clients and their environment closely, she also emphasized health promotion and disease prevention. She paid close attention to physicians and government policymakers, recognizing their influence on her freedom to practise (Simms, Price, & Ervin, 2000). Nightingale's ideas spread from England to Canada in the 1870s. The Nightingale model of nursing reflected the social environment of the era. Today's nurse can improve the quality of client care by understanding and dealing with many of these same issues affecting today's health care system and the nursing profession. However, today's nurses practise in an information model within a global context.

In this chapter, we discuss how Canadian health care is organized, funded, and accredited. We introduce the topics of population health and disease management. We then explore clinical variation and malpractice. We also

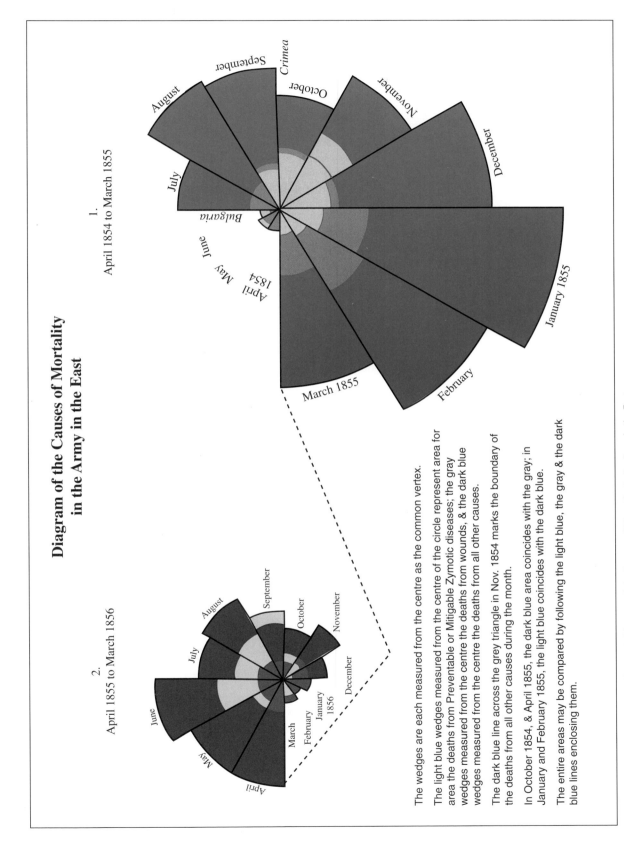

**Diagram of the Causes of Mortality
in the Army in the East**

1.
April 1854 to March 1855

2.
April 1855 to March 1856

The wedges are each measured from the centre as the common vertex.

The light blue wedges measured from the centre of the circle represent area for area the deaths from Preventable or Mitigable Zymotic diseases; the gray wedges measured from the centre the deaths from wounds, & the dark blue wedges measured from the centre the deaths from all other causes.

The dark blue line across the grey triangle in Nov. 1854 marks the boundary of the deaths from all other causes during the month.

In October 1854, & April 1855, the dark blue area coincides with the gray; in January and February 1855, the light blue coincides with the dark blue.

The entire areas may be compared by following the light blue, the gray & the dark blue lines enclosing them.

Figure 1-1 Florence Nightingale's Coxcomb Diagram of the Causes of Mortality in the Army in the East

Source: By permission of the Houghton Library, Harvard University. EC85.N5647.858n.

review the Canadian Adverse Events Study and two Institute of Medicine Committee on Health Care reports from the United States, which address the important issue of client safety. Finally, we discuss recent changes and the current trends and forces affecting health care and the development of caring, multidisciplinary nursing.

ORGANIZATION OF HEALTH CARE

Canada's health care system has evolved over the past five decades, and is based on a combination of political, social, and economic influences. Its goal is to provide Canadians with reasonable access to medically necessary insured services, without the need to pay. The Canadian provinces are constitutionally responsible for the administration and delivery of health services (Constitution Act, 1867). In other words, the provinces decide how much money will be spent on health services, where these services will be delivered, where hospitals will be located, and how many doctors will be needed. The Canadian Constitution gives the federal government responsibility for health care in the Yukon, Nunavut, and the Northwest Territories; and for the health care of Aboriginal people who live on reserve; members of the armed forces and veterans; the Royal Canadian Mounted Police (RCMP); and inmates of federal institutions. The Yukon, Nunavut, and Northwest Territories have assumed responsibility for health care, even though they do not have formal constitutional powers over health care because they do not have the status of a province. This system, which gives all Canadians access to health care, has undergone many changes since universal health care was implemented in 1968 (Canada. Statistics Canada, 2006, p. 160).

In 1947, Saskatchewan was the first province to introduce public, universal *hospital* insurance. By 1957, the Government of Canada introduced legislation to share in the cost of these services. By 1961, all provinces and two territories had public insurance that provided access to hospital services. In 1962, Saskatchewan again led the way by providing insurance for *physician* services, in addition to the hospital services previously provided. The Canadian Government again shared the cost of physician services in 1968. By 1972, all provinces and territories had extended their insurance plans to include both physician and hospital services.

In 1977, under the Federal-Provincial Fiscal Arrangements and Established Programs Financing Act, 1977 (EPF), cost sharing was replaced with block funding, which was a combination of cash payments and tax points. According to this new funding arrangement, provincial and territorial governments had the flexibility to invest health care funding according to their needs and priorities. Federal transfers for postsecondary education were included in the EPF transfer, in addition to funding for medical and hospital services.

New federal legislation, called the Canada Health Act, was passed in 1984. The Canada Health Act was based on five principles:

1. *Universality* — All residents of Canada must be entitled to public health insurance coverage.
2. *Comprehensiveness* — All medically necessary services provided by hospitals and doctors must be covered.
3. *Accessibility* — Reasonable access by insured people to medically necessary hospital and physician services must be unimpeded by financial or other barriers.
4. *Portability* — People must remain covered while temporarily absent from their province.
5. *Public administration* — Health plans must be administered by a nonprofit, public authority.

Two provisions in the Canada Health Act covered cost sharing. The first provision stipulated that there could not be extra billing for medical services by doctors who work under the terms of the health insurance plan of the province or territory. The second provision stated that no user charges would be required for insured health services by hospitals or other providers under the provincial or territorial health care plan.[1]

The federal cash and tax transfers that supported health care and postsecondary education were combined with federal transfers that supported social services and social assistance to form one block funding mechanism known as the Canada Health and Social Transfer (CHST). This change came about as a result of federal legislation that was passed in 1995, but did not come into force until the beginning of fiscal year 1996–97. Some provinces receive equalization payments from the federal government, which allow those provinces to provide reasonably comparable levels of service at reasonably comparable levels of taxation. In addition, Canada's three territories receive additional federal financial support through Territorial Formula Financing, to assist them to provide public services.[2]

In 2003, the first ministers (the prime minister of Canada plus the provincial and territorial premiers) agreed on the Accord on Health Care Renewal, which provided for changes to support access, quality, and long-term sustainability of the health care system. Reforms targeted primary health care renewal, coverage for both short-term acute home care and the cost of prescribed drugs that reach high or catastrophic levels, enhanced access to diagnostic and medical equipment, and better accountability from governments. Under the Accord, the federal government cash transfers in support of health care were increased, and, effective April 2004, the CHST cash and tax transfers were split into the Canada Health Transfer for health, and the Canada Social Transfer for postsecondary education, social services, and social assistance.[3]

In 2004, further reforms were announced by the first ministers in "*A 10-Year Plan to Strengthen Health Care.*" This plan focused on improving access to quality care and reducing wait times. Other key reforms included health human resources; Aboriginal health; home care; primary health care; prescription drug coverage and elements of a national pharmaceutical strategy; health care services in the North; medical equipment; prevention, promotion, and public health; and enhanced reporting on progress made on these reforms. To support this plan, the federal government again increased health care cash transfers and applied an escalator as of 2006–07 to provide predictable growth in federal funding.[4]

TYPES OF HEALTH CARE SERVICES

Health care can be categorized into four levels (Table 1-1): health promotion, disease and injury prevention (protection), diagnosis and treatment of existing health

TABLE 1-1	TYPES OF HEALTH CARE SERVICES	
Type of Care	**Description**	**Examples**
Health Promotion	*Goal:* To improve or maintain health status *Explanation:* General health promotion and protection against specific illnesses or disability	Lifestyle modification for health (e.g., smoking cessation, nutrition counselling) Promotion of a safe environment (e.g., sanitation, protection from toxic agents) Population Health
Disease and Injury Prevention	*Goal:* To protect from the spread of disease, to alleviate disease, and to prevent further disability through early intervention *Explanation:* Early detection and intervention	Screening and immunization
Diagnosis and Treatment of Existing Health Problems	*Goal:* To maintain and/or improve the level of health functioning of the client *Explanation:* Includes primary, secondary, and tertiary care (i.e., first, second, and third levels of encounter with the health system)	*Primary care:* the first contact entry to the health care system (e.g., a physician or a nurse practitioner who provides health promotion, illness prevention) *Secondary care:* a specialized medical service or hospital to which the client is referred by the primary care physician (e.g., for detection and early intervention) *Tertiary care:* A specialized, highly technical care related to diagnosing and treating complicated or unusual health problems (e.g., regional or provincial hospitals equipped with high-tech equipment and services)
Rehabilitation	*Goal:* To minimize effects and to prevent permanent disability from a chronic or irreversible condition *Explanation:* Restorative and rehabilitative activities to obtain a client's optimal level of functioning	Education and retraining Provision of direct care Environmental modifications (e.g., advising on necessity of wheelchair accessibility for a person who has experienced a cardiovascular accident [i.e., a stroke]) Continuing Care

problems (i.e., primary, secondary, and tertiary care), and rehabilitation.

HEALTH CARE PROFESSIONALS IN CANADA

Health care professionals in Canada include a wide range of regulated and unregulated care providers. Regulated providers include, but are not limited to, physicians, nurses, physiotherapists, occupational therapists, and dentists. Family members, friends, community volunteers, and non-regulated workers make up the second category. In 2000, more than 1.5 million Canadians worked in health and social services (Canada. Statistics Canada, 2006, p. 160).

In 2004, of the total regulated nursing workforce of 315,139, of which 246,575 (78.2 percent) were registered nurses (RNs), 63,443 (20.1 percent) were licensed practical nurses (LPNs), and 5,121 (1.6 percent) were registered psychiatric nurses (RPNs) (Canadian Institute for Health Information [CIHI], 2005). Most of Canada's registered nurses and licensed practical nurses worked in hospitals, with increasing numbers working in community health. The number of RNs in Canada increased by 3.4 percent from 2000 to 2004.[5]

In 2004, the average age of regulated nurses was 44.6 years, an increase from 44.5 years in 2003. Nurses aged 50 to 54 in 2004 were the largest group, accounting for 17.4 percent of the entire regulated nursing workforce (CIHI, 2005, p. 2). Physicians were the second largest group of regulated health care professionals. In 2000, more than 57,800 physicians worked in clinical and non-clinical practices in Canada, an increase of 5.3 percent from 1996. During this four-year period, the increase in the number of specialists was higher than the increase in the number of family physicians.

Similar to nurses, the average age of physicians in Canada has been rising at a faster rate than some other professions (Canada. Statistics Canada, 2006, p. 161). Despite the increased number of physicians, more than 3.6 million Canadians, or 14 percent of the population, did not have a family physician in 2003. Of these, more than 1.2 million people were unable to find a family physician, and the other 2.4 million had not looked for one (Canada. Statistics Canada, 2006, p. 161).

These subcultures of health professions affect client care delivered in various settings. Table 1-2 lists the generalized characteristics of three of these subcultures of health professionals identified by Byers (1997). These dynamic characteristics are constantly changing the culture of the health care organization and the way these groups work with each other to provide quality health care.

HEALTH CARE SPENDING

Canada spent approximately $142 billion on health care in 2005, or an average of $4,411 per person. After the effects of inflation have been taken into account, this amount was nearly three times more than the health care spending in 1975.[6] Ten percent of the gross domestic product was dedicated to health care spending in 2005, a level first reached in 1992 (Canada. Statistics Canada, 2006, p. 161). In 2005, 69.6 percent of total health care expenses in Canada, or $98.8 billion, was paid for from taxes. The rest of the funding, $43.2 billion, or 30.4 percent of total health care spending, came from the private sector, which generally funded services such as dental care, vision care, chiropractic care, and medication.[7] Private health services are those services we pay for directly ourselves or services that are covered through private insurance plans or employee benefit plans.

Hospitals accounted for 30 percent of the total health care expenditures in 2003. In 2004, hospital spending was followed closely by retail drug sales and physician services (Canada. Statistics Canada, 2006, p. 161). In 2005, $7.8 billion was spent on public health.[8] Canada spent approximately 10.4 percent of its economic output (i.e., gross domestic product) on health care in 2005.

According to the most recent international data, from 2002, Canada was the fifth-highest spender on health care among universal-access countries in the Organisation for Economic Co-operation and Development (OECD) (see Figure 1-2.). This comparison of health spending did not account for the effects of populations of different ages. Estimates indicated that Canada spent more on health care than all OECD nations with universal-access health care systems, with the exception of Iceland and Switzerland. Both age-adjusted and non-adjusted statistics suggested that the Canadian health care program did not suffer from a lack of funding (Esmail & Walker, 2005, p. 15). The United States was not included in the survey because it does not have a universal-access health care system; in 2003, the United States spent 15 percent of its gross domestic product (GDP) on health care.[9]

TABLE 1-2	GENERALIZED CHARACTERISTICS OF THREE SUBCULTURES OF HEALTH PROFESSIONALS		
Characteristics	**Nursing**	**Medicine**	**Health Care Administration**
Major task	Client care; client safety	Diagnosis and treatment of disease; client safety	Organizational continuity; quality of care; quality of work life; client safety; managing change and stability
Membership	Historically female, white, middle-class; humanistic	Historically male, white, middle- and upper-class; scientific	Historically male-dominant;* rational
Leading role strength	Comforter; nurturer; health educator	Lifesaver and problem-solver; miracle worker	Keeper of the house; protector
Role centrality	Coordinator of health services	Gatekeeper of health services	Proprietor of health services; holder of the purse strings
Relationships with other professional groups	Collaborative ethic	Autonomy; directing the team	Negotiating; seeks cooperation
Model of authority within profession	Hierarchy	Collegiality; equality	Hierarchy
Perspective	Client-centered; clinical unit/area	Client- and practice-centered	Hospital's business and government relations
Conflict management	Interpersonal approach	Use leverage available (e.g., resources and authority) to maintain control	Structural and rational approach
Core dilemmas in era of health care reform	Degree of proactivity within context of high uncertainty; traditional vs. new role initiatives	Choice of organizational and network affiliations, and the conditions and extent of affiliation; the future destiny of medical specialists	Options for investing strategic resources during an era of high future uncertainty
Major threats (current)	Decrease in job security; constraints on staffing levels and other resources; (undesirable) changes in role; nursing shortage	Health economics; changes in role; losses in authority and income; malpractice	Organizational survival; job security (restructuring; regionalization; rationalization)

*The management of Catholic hospitals, typically run by orders of Catholic sisters, is a notable exception to the generalizations about health care administrators.

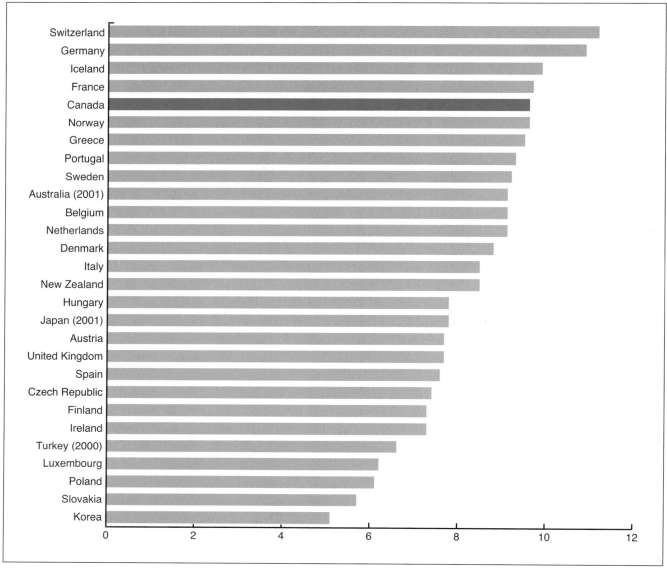

Figure 1-2 Unadjusted Total Expenditure (%GDP) on Health, 2002

Source: Adapted from OECD (2004). OECD Health Data 2004: *A Comparative Analysis of 30 Countries,* 3rd ed. CD-ROM. Paris: OECD. Reprinted with Permission.

APPROACHES TO HEALTH CARE IN CANADA

Population health, integrated health care delivery, and disease management have begun to develop as an approach to health care in Canada.

POPULATION HEALTH

Population health is an approach to health care that focuses on the determinants of health in order to help reduce inequities among different groups in the population, particularly the people who are the most vulnerable. The determinants of health include a range of factors that explain why a person is or is not healthy, such as income, social status, education, employment and working conditions, healthy child development and nutrition, to name a few (Raphael, 2004). This broader approach to health examines not only the health of individuals but also the health of the population, factors that affect health overall, and trends in the health of different groups of people within our society. The ultimate goal is to improve the health of the entire population (see Figure 1-3).

This deceptively simple story speaks to the complex set of factors or conditions that determine the level of health of every Canadian

Why is Jason in the hospital?

Because he has a bad infection in his leg.

But why does he have an infection?

Because he has a cut on his leg and it got infected.

But why does he have a cut on his leg?

Because he was playing in the junk yard next to his apartment building and there was some sharp, jagged steel there that he fell on.

But why was he playing in a junk yard?

Because his neighbourhood is kind of run down. A lot of kids play there and there is no one to supervise them.

But why does he live in that neighbourhood?

Because his parents can't afford a nicer place to live.

But why can't his parents afford a nicer place to live?

Because his Dad is unemployed and his Mom is sick.

But why is his Dad unemployed?

Because he doesn't have much education and he can't find a job.

But why . . .?

— from Toward a Healthy Future: Second Report on the Health of Canadians

Figure 1-3 Determinants of Health: What Makes Canadians Healthy or Unhealthy?

Source: Public Health Agency of Canada, Population Health. What determines health. Retrieved from http://www.phac-aspc.gc.ca/ph-sp/phdd/determinants/index.html, March 25, 2007. Reproduced with the permission of the Minister of Public Works and Government Services Canada, 2007.

In 1974, the Canadian minister of health, Marc Lalonde, published a seminal report on the determinants of health. In the decades since the Lalonde Report, Canadians have continued to focus on population health, as demonstrated by such reports as Achieving Health for All: A Framework for Health Promotion, in 1986, by then federal minister of health, Jake Epp (the report was known familiarly as the Epp Report), the Ontario government's 1999 report, Early Years Study, and the work conducted by the Canadian Institute for Advanced Research. This population health approach has been endorsed in the recommendations of all recent Canadian reports on health care, including Canada Health Action: Building on the Legacy (National Forum on Health, 1997); Quebec's Emerging Solutions, known familiarly as the Clair Report (Quebec. Commission d'étude sur les services de santé et les services sociaux, 2000); Saskatchewan's Caring for Medicare: Sustaining a Quality System, known familiarly as the Fyke Report (Saskatchewan. Commission on Medicare, 2001); Alberta's A Framework for Reform, known familiarly as the Mazankowski Report (Premier's Advisory Council on Health, 2001); Reforming Health Protection and Promotion in Canada, known familiarly as

the Kirby Report (Canada. Parliament. Senate. Standing Committee on Social Affairs, Science and Technology, 2002); and Building on Values: The Future of Health Care in Canada (Commission on the Future of Health Care in Canada, 2002).

In 1999, the Canadian Institute for Health Information (CIHI) launched the Canadian Population Health Initiative (CPHI) to expand the public's knowledge of population health. From 2004 to 2007, CPHI had three key areas of focus: healthy weights, environment and health, and healthy transitions to adulthood. CPHI increases population health understanding in these areas by concentrating on the following four complementary functions: building an improved understanding of the factors affecting population health; improving the health of Canadians through new policy development; forming collaborative networks with groups and individuals to improve understanding of the determinants of health; and disseminating information on population health issues.[10]

These social determinants of health contribute significantly to whether individuals stay healthy or become ill. They also determine whether a person possesses the physical, social, and personal resources to identify and achieve

TABLE 1-3	EVIDENCE-BASED STUDIES: WHAT THEY SHOW

- Positive association between income and health (Wilkins, Berthelot, & Ng, 2002)
- Relationship between job strain and coronary heart disease (CHD) especially among blue-collar workers and men (Theorell, 2001)
- Coordinated or integrated service delivery is more effective, efficient, and less costly than single-focus initiatives (Browne et al., 2001)
- Evidence that occupational injuries, the degree of awareness of the dangers in the workplace, and installation of home safety features are associated with limited literacy (Health Canada, 2003)
- Homelessness and health (Hwang, 2001)

TABLE 1-4	FEATURES OF THE NEW ROLE OF HEALTH CARE MANAGEMENT IN A POPULATION HEALTH SYSTEM

- Emphasis on the continuum of care
- Emphasis on maintaining and promoting wellness
- Accountability for the health of defined populations
- Differentiation based on ability to add value
- Success achieved by increasing the number of individuals served and keeping people healthy
- Goal is to provide care at the most appropriate level
- Integrated health delivery system
- Managers operate service areas across organizational borders
- Managers actively pursue quality and continuous improvement

personal aspirations, satisfy needs, and cope with the environment (Raphael, 2004, p. 1). Table 1-3 summarizes some of the findings from evidence-based studies. Table 1-4 identifies some of the features of the new role of health care management in a population health system.

Populations do not become healthier as the result of large investments in clinical care after illness has begun. Populations become healthier when we invest in preventing illness and keeping people healthy. The overall health of Canadians should be measured by considering a number of indicators from a population health perspective. These measures address some of the key determinants of health and allow the health of Canada's populations to be compared to other populations around the world. Based on the United Nations Human Development Index of income per capita, literacy, and life expectancy, Canada scores very high;

however, the United Nation's Human Poverty Index (HPI) shows a different picture. The HPI measures relative deprivation in terms of standard of living, education, and longevity. According to this measure, Canada is in 11th place behind the Scandinavian countries, Germany, France, Japan, and Spain. On this index, Canada is not doing as well as it should (Commission on the Future of Health Care in Canada, 2002, p. 10).

Life expectancy at birth is one of the most established and widely available summary measures of health status. In 2003, the life expectancy at birth in Canada was 79.9 years, almost two years higher than the OECD average, and fifth among all OECD countries. Canada's infant mortality rate decreased from a rate of 27.3 deaths per 1,000 live births in 1960 to 5.3 deaths per 1,000 in 2003 (Commission on the Future of Health Care in Canada, 2002, p. 11).

Another key consideration in addressing the performance of any health care system is equity. Equity addresses questions such as whether some groups in our society have better access to health care or better health outcomes than others (Goddard & Smith, 2001). Significant disparities exist between people who live in Atlantic Canada and the rest of the country, and those who live in the northern part of Canada versus the south. For example, one study demonstrated that the inhabitants of the Nunavik region in Quebec live an average of 15.8 years less than those who live in Richmond, British Columbia (Commission on the Future of Health Care in Canada, 2002, p. 16).

If our society really wants to increase the health of Canadians, perhaps resources would be better directed toward strengthening the determinants of health: health care system influences (e.g., access to medical care and health care costs); individual influences (e.g., the impact of lifestyle and genetics); interpersonal, social, and work influences (e.g., job satisfaction and social supports); community influences (e.g., the availability of services and programs); and environmental influences (e.g., air quality and water quality) (Donatelle & Davis, 1998). A society that spends so much on medical care that it cannot or will not spend adequately on other health-enhancing activities may actually be reducing the health of its population (Evans & Stoddard, 1990).

PUBLIC HEALTH

The **public health system** plays a different role. It is responsible for helping protect Canadians from injury and disease and for helping Canadians to stay healthy. Experts in the field of public health suggest that there are three responsibilities of a public health system:

1. Health Emergencies — to prevent, discover, and respond to outbreaks of infectious disease, such as SARS or influenza; to work with national security agencies to respond to disasters, bioterrorism, and other threats to Canada's health security
2. Chronic Disease and Injury Prevention — to help to prevent and manage chronic diseases, such as diabetes, cancer, and mental illness; to help to prevent injuries
3. Health Promotion — to promote good health; to contribute to government policies that affect our health, such as policies on poverty, housing, and the environment.[11]

See Table 1-5 for a list of the many individuals involved in public health services.

In 2003, the prime minister appointed a minister of state for public health. The immediate priority of the new minister was to oversee the creation of the Public Health Agency of Canada, whose mandate was to focus on emergency preparedness and response, infectious and chronic disease prevention and control, and injury prevention, supported by a collaborative, national network.[12]

The National Collaborating Centre for Public Health will provide national focal points for key priority areas in public health, building on established regional expertise. The centre will speed up the development and implementation of new research findings and best practices in

TABLE 1-5	WHO DELIVERS PUBLIC HEALTH SERVICES?

The public health system, like the health care system, involves doctors, nurses and a wide range of health professionals. But it involves many more people too, including:

- Provincial and territorial chief medical officers of health
- Local chief public health officers
- Community leaders
- Teachers and school principals
- Families
- Employers
- Aboriginal communities
- Multicultural communities
- Social organizations
- Sports and recreation clubs

Source: Public Health Agency of Canada. Who delivers public health services? Retrieved from http://www.phac-aspc.gc.ca/about_apropos/federal_strategy_e.html, July 16, 2006. Reproduced with the permission of the Minister of Public Works and Government Services Canada, 2007.

TABLE 1-6	SIX NATIONAL COLLABORATING CENTRES FOR PUBLIC HEALTH

1. National Collaborating Centre for Determinants of Health (Atlantic)
2. National Collaborating Centre for Public Policy and Risk Assessment (Quebec)
3. National Collaborating Centre for Infrastructure, Info-Structure and New Tools Development (Ontario)
4. The National Collaborating Centre for Infectious Diseases (Manitoba)
5. The National Collaborating Centre for Environmental Health (British Columbia)
6. The National Collaborating Centre for Aboriginal Health (British Columbia)

Source: Public Health Agency of Canada. National Collaborating Centre program — A brief overview. Retrieved from http://www.phac-aspc.gc.ca/php-psp/pdf/brief_overview.pdf, March 25, 2007. Reproduced with the permission of the Minister of Public Works and Government Services Canada, 2007.

public health practice. See Table 1-6 for the six centres that have been identified.

In addition to the six National Collaborating Centres for Public Health, the establishment of a new Pan-Canadian Public Health Network is underway. The Network will serve to collaborate on public health issues and to facilitate national approaches to public health policy and planning. It will also work with the six National Collaborating Centres for Public Health to foster linkages among provinces, territories, academia, and non-governmental organizations, and to help translate knowledge into practice at all levels of the public health system across Canada.[13]

The Canadian Public Health Association (CPHA) is a national, independent, not-for-profit, voluntary association that represents public health in Canada and provides linkages to the international public health community. The mission of CPHA is to advocate for the improvement and maintenance of personal and community health according to the public health principles of disease prevention, health promotion and protection, and healthy public policy.[14] See Table 1-7 to learn the goals of the CPHA.

PRIMARY HEALTH CARE

Primary health care refers to basic, everyday health care: visiting a family doctor or nurse practitioner, talking to a dietician or pharmacist, or calling a toll-free health advice line to talk to a health professional. It is usually the first encounter with a health care provider. Primary health care is about preventing people from becoming ill or being injured, managing chronic conditions and making the most effective use of health provider expertise. In addition, primary health care relates to improving both the quality of health care and access to health care services. Primary health care has five guiding principles:

1. Equitable access to health and health services

2. Public participation
3. Appropriate technology
4. Intersectoral collaboration
5. Reorientation of the health system to promote health and prevent disease and injury

For example, in Ontario, the Sault Ste. Marie Group Health Centre's congestive heart failure program reduced hospital re-admissions by 44 percent in two years. Primary health care is not a new concept. A number of well-established primary health care centres across Canada have been in operation for many years—for example, the North East Community Health Centre in Edmonton, Alberta.

Countries around the world agreed to the importance of primary health care in 1978, when the World Health Organization (WHO) held an international conference on primary health care, which concluded with the Alma Ata Declaration, the first international declaration underlining the importance of primary health care. This approach was accepted by member countries of the WHO as the key to achieving the goal of "Health for All by the Year 2000." Four international conferences have been held since Alma Ata: in Adelaide, Australia (1988); Sundsvall, Sweden (1991); Jakarta, Indonesia (1997); and Mexico City, Mexico (1999). The theme of the most recent conference was on bridging the equity gap and strengthening the "art and science" of health promotion and the political skills and actions needed for health promotion to ensure healthy public policy. Although none of the 13 institutes of the Canadian Institute for Health Research (CIHR) has been dedicated to health promotion research per se, one is called the Institute for Population and Public Health.

The first ministers of Canada met in 2000, and agreed that improving primary health care was crucial to the renewal and long-term sustainability of the health

TABLE 1-7	GOALS OF THE CPHA

CPHA achieves its mission through the following nine goals:

1. Acting in partnership with a range of disciplines including health, environment, agriculture, transportation, other health-oriented groups and individuals in developing and expressing a public health viewpoint on personal and community health issues;

2. Providing an effective liaison and partnership between CPHA's Provincial/Territorial Branches/Associations;

3. Providing an effective liaison and network both nationally and internationally in collaboration with various disciplines, agencies, and organizations;

4. Encouraging and facilitating measures for disease prevention, health promotion and protection, and healthy public policy;

5. Initiating, encouraging, and participating in research directed at the fields of disease prevention, health promotion, and healthy public policy;

6. Designing, developing, and implementing public health policies, programs, and activities;

7. Facilitating the development of public health goals for Canada;

8. Identifying public health issues and advocating for policy change;

9. Identifying literacy as a major factor in achieving equitable access to health services

Source: Canadian Public Health Association. About CPHA: Goals. Retrieved from http://www.cpha.ca/english/inside/about/about.htm, August 2, 2006. Copyright CPHA. All rights reserved.

care system. As a result, the federal government invested $800 million in the Primary Health Care Transition Fund to support the provinces and territories in their plans to improve and expand primary health care delivery in Canada. Following the release of the Romanow Report in 2002, the first ministers continued their focus on primary health care. The 2003 Health Care Renewal Accord identified primary health care as a priority and placed particular focus on increasing access and building primary health care teams.

INTEGRATED HEALTH CARE DELIVERY SYSTEMS

An **integrated delivery system** is a network of health care organizations that provides or arranges to provide a coordinated continuum of services to a defined population and is willing to be held clinically and fiscally accountable for the outcomes and the health status of the population served (Shortell, 1996).

A coordinated continuum of health care services includes prevention, wellness, and health promotion services, as well as acute, restorative, and maintenance care to serve the needs of a population of clients in a specific geographic area. These services are delivered by a network of organized, community-oriented health and social service systems focused on broad aspects of health care and chronic disease management. This network can include hospitals and nursing homes, as well as schools, public health departments, and social and community health organizations that provide service and education programs to address smoking cessation, exercise, and other illness prevention and health promotion initiatives.

A type of integrated delivery system used in Canada is called **regionalization**. Nine provinces have some form of regionalization in place. There are four main features in Canadian regionalization:

1. The regions are predominantly defined by geography; that is, they occupy specific areas within the province and receive their mandate and authority from the provincial government.

2. The authority, which had previously been held by individual organizations or agencies, is consolidated at the regional level into one authority.

3. The regions are now responsible for a full range of health services, from community health to mental health to long-term care to acute care to health promotion (Lewis & Kouri, 2004).

4. The provincial governments transferred their health care responsibility to the regional health authorities.

Regionalization is different in Ontario, where a regional cancer care network exists, regions are in place for such clinical services as obstetrics, and planning bodies are geographically defined (i.e., Local Health Integration Networks).

Regionalization was recommended by the provincial task forces and commissions of the 1980s, which were charged with creating a new direction for health care. Because fragmentation was a concern, the solution was thought to be the consolidation of organizations and boards, and their integration into a more responsive and participatory system. The Health Services Restructuring Commission, chaired by Duncan Sinclair, was established in 1996 for a period of four years. Its mandate was to find solutions to such issues as rising costs, resistance to change, and lack of accountability (Sinclair, Rochon, & Leatt, 2005). The expected results were fewer "turf" battles, increased collaboration, and rationalization of services. The outcomes would include cost savings, increased efficiency, equity, increased consumer participation, increased accountability, and an emphasis on health promotion and prevention (Lewis & Kouri, 2004). See Table 1-8 for a summary of the potential impact of regionalization on attaining health system goals.

Regionalization in Canada's health care delivery has seen little stability. Most regions have restructured at least once since they were originally formed. See Table 1-9 for the changes in regionalization, by province, from the time of implementation to 2003.

In September of 2004, the Ontario minister of health announced the government's three-year health transformation agenda, which included the formation of Local Health Integration Networks (LHINs). The intent of these LHINs was to ensure that health care in Ontario would be more client-focused, results-driven, integrated, and sustainable (Sunnak, 2005). The LHINs are responsible for planning, integrating, and funding local health services, including hospitals, community care access centres, home care, long-term care, mental health, community health centres, and addiction and community support services. In Ontario, 16 district health councils were disbanded in March 2005 to make way for 14 LHINs. In June 2005, the province announced the appointment of 14 new chief executive officers, nine of whom were registered nurses, and 42 board members, including chairs and directors (Sunnak, 2005). At the time of this writing, the LHINs were not yet fully operational.

TABLE 1-8	POTENTIAL IMPACT OF REGIONALIZATION ON HEALTH SYSTEM GOAL ATTAINMENT

1a GOAL: Aligning Needs and Resources; Potential Impact of Regionalization: High

Factors Increasing Potential Impact	Factors Decreasing Potential Impact	Current Canadian Circumstances
Province genuinely committed to needs-based resource allocation and population health mandate	Province only rhetorically committed to needs-based and population health approach and more traditional in practice	Restrictions on reallocation vary from some to significant
RHA supports and prioritizes population health mandate	RHA uncommitted to mandate	Provinces struggling with population health mandate and accountability
RHA has authority to reallocate resources	Provincial funding rules rigid	RHAs struggling with population health mandate and accountability
Good needs-assessment protocols	Constrained RHA autonomy to reallocate resources	Needs assessments generally done but of varying quality
Good performance measurement and reporting mechanisms	Province focuses on utilization targets, not impact or distribution	Information systems still developing
Disadvantaged populations have effective voice and influence	Provincial government allows interest groups to end-run regions and have directions and decisions reversed	Performance measurement and reporting in early stages
Elites support a needs-based allocation of resources	RHAs responsive to interest groups and agenda derailed	Some provincial governments more prone to end-runs and intervention in RHA affairs than others
Evidence-based policy and practice	Provider resistance	
Adequate information base re: interventions as well as needs	Poor needs-assessment protocols	
	Poor performance measurement and reporting mechanisms	

(Continued)

TABLE 1-8	POTENTIAL IMPACT OF REGIONALIZATION ON HEALTH SYSTEM GOAL ATTAINMENT (CONTINUED)

1b GOAL: Integration of Services; Potential Impact of Regionalization: High

Factors Increasing Potential Impact	Factors Decreasing Potential Impact	Current Canadian Circumstances
Wide scope of services falling within RHA mandate	Important services (MDs, drugs) outside purview of RHAs	Generally wide range of services under RHA authority
Consolidation of authority over various programs and sectors	Vestigial program autonomy (affiliation agreements, competitive and narrowly focused program boards)	MDs and drugs not included in RHA mandates
Provincial funding formulae aligned with goal	Provincial funding formulae misaligned with goal	Regions have privately owned facilities and affiliation agreements
RHA autonomy to reallocate resources	Constrained RHA autonomy to reallocate resources	Provincial funding often comes with conditions such as utilization targets
Organizational charts that promote integrated planning and management	Organizational charts that promote "silo" thinking	Issues with provider contracts and morale
	Historical program territoriality	
	Resistance of providers	

1c GOAL: Service Quality and Evidence-Based Practice; Potential Impact of Regionalization: Low

Factors Increasing Potential Impact	Factors Decreasing Potential Impact	Current Canadian Circumstances
Rewarded by provincial funding and payment mechanisms	Perverse incentives in provincial funding and payment mechanisms	Payment mechanisms generally indifferent to evidence-based performance
Provincial health quality (HQ) and evidence-based practice (EBP) activities/resources	Absence of provincial HQ and EBP leadership	Two provinces (Sask and Ab) have established a quality council; others, e.g., Manitoba, planning to do so
An academic community committed to EBP	Lack of emphasis in academic programs	Several provinces have centres that promote EBP but impact limited
Good information and performance measurement systems	Lack of interest in HQ and EBP among opinion leaders and providers	Academic programs vary in commitment to EBP
Provider culture well disposed to HQ and EBP	Poorly developed information and performance measurement systems	Provider culture ambivalent toward HQ and EBP
RHA authority to allocate resources	Provincially set utilization targets as a condition of funding	Some RHAs have invested considerably in EBP, and QI initiatives
RHA control over number and distribution of MDs	Excess capacity in some sectors	Information systems in early stages
	Excess funding that papers over substandard practice	Fee-for-service generally rewards volume over efficiency
	Public opposition to changes in access, service configuration	Generally restricted ability to reallocate resources at RHA level
	Provider opposition	RHAs have limited authority to create or close programs and facilities
		RHAs generally have little control over number and distribution of MDs, though increasing in some provinces

(Continued)

1d GOAL: Health Promotion and Prevention; Potential Impact of Regionalization: Moderate

Factors Increasing Potential Impact	Factors Decreasing Potential Impact	Current Canadian Circumstances
Provincial and RHA commitment to these activities	Public preoccupation with acute and medical care	Public health on radar screen because of SARS, West Nile, flu epidemics
Explicit and high-profile mandate to pursue these activities	Weak provincial commitment	Some RHAs very active in community development
Strong RHA leadership and buy-in from significant provider constituencies	Weak RHA commitment	Many RHAs have pursued intersectoral partnerships and programs
Accountability for performance in these areas	Lack of provider interest	
Mechanisms to ensure voices of the dispossessed are heard	Impatience with long-term time frame for achievement of goals	
	Lack of public and media interest	

1e GOAL: Improved Accountability; Potential Impact of Regionalization: Moderate

Factors Increasing Potential Impact	Factors Decreasing Potential Impact	Current Canadian Circumstances
Substantial authority and autonomy truly devolved to RHA	RHA has little authority and autonomy	Devolution to RHAs incomplete and some power has been reconsolidated at the provincial level in recent years
Sufficient RHA authority over the programs under its jurisdiction (i.e., clear and widespread consolidation of authority)	Public regards only provincial government as accountable	Government assumes ownership of major decisions even if RHA initiates them
Non-partisan board structures and behaviour	RHA boards partisan in nature	Consolidation of authority from local to the regional level has been partial
Public confident in RHA and views it as legitimate decision-making body with a mandate to change	Provincial government responds to end-runs and overrules RHA decisions	Elections terminated in Sask, Alta, Quebec; exist in PEI since 1999 and initiated in NB in 2004
Provincial government resistance to end-runs	RHAs attempt to offload tough decisions on government	Performance reporting to public still in embryo
RHAs willing to make and take responsibility for tough decisions	Opposition makes RHA-level decisions a constant political issue	Health remains a high-profile political issue among public
Opposition recognizes the devolution and legislative debate is altered	Poor information and reporting mechanisms	Public holds provincial government accountable to greater extent than RHA
Media create sense of legitimacy of RHA as decision-maker		Legislative debate for the most part traditional, partisan
Good information used and available for prioritizing		Media focuses on government behaviour more than RHAs
Good reporting mechanisms in place		

(Continued)

TABLE 1-8	POTENTIAL IMPACT OF REGIONALIZATION ON HEALTH SYSTEM GOAL ATTAINMENT (CONTINUED)

1f GOAL: Increased Public Participation; Potential Impact of Regionalization: Moderate

Factors Increasing Potential Impact	Factors Decreasing Potential Impact	Current Canadian Circumstances
Explicit and high-profile mandate to pursue these activities	Weak RHA commitment	Some RHAs very active in experimenting with public participation
Tradition of civic engagement in various sectors	Lack of public and media interest	Does not appear in most performance agreements and indicator sets
Public believes its participation will be valued and valuable	Not included in performance agreements and indicator sets	
Included in performance agreements and indicators as important measure		

Source: Lewis, S., & Kouri, S. (2004). Regionalization: Making sense of the Canadian experience. *Healthcare Papers, 5*(1), 17–19. Reprinted with Permission.

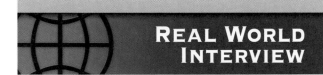

REAL WORLD INTERVIEW

Our first priority will be to introduce ourselves to our communities and establish new relationships with health-care organizations and community members. This will be a necessary step to accomplish what we need to do.

RNAO member Georgina Thompson,
newly appointed Chair of the South East LHIN

Source: Sunnak, A. (2005). LHINs: Bringing it all back home Ontario's shift to integrated health services. *Registered Nurse Journal,* 17(4), 15. Reprinted with Permission.

HORIZONTAL AND VERTICAL INTEGRATION

Health care networks can be horizontally or vertically integrated. **Horizontal integration** occurs when a health care system contains several organizations of one type, such as hospitals. Health care networks can also be vertically integrated. **Vertical integration** occurs when different stages of health care are linked and delivered by one agency.

DISEASE MANAGEMENT

Research demonstrates that **disease management** is a cost-effective approach both to improve service quality and integration and to promote consumer empowerment and quality of life. A number of disease management programs and research studies are conducted across Canada.

The Chronic Disease Self-Management Program (CDSMP) was developed at the Stanford Patient Education Research Center under the direction of Kate Lorig, R.N.; Virginia Gonzalez, M.P.H.; and Diana Laurent, M.P.H. The CDSMP is based on the assumption that people who live with chronic conditions have similar problems and concerns, and have to deal with their disease and the impact it has on their lives and their psychological health. People with no health care background in chronic conditions, but who have been instructed about those conditions, can teach the chronic disease self-management program more effectively than health professionals. Studies have determined that the way the content is taught is far more important than the subject matter that is taught. In a five-year research project, the CDSMP was evaluated in a randomized study including more than 1,000 subjects. The people who took part in the program were found to have improved their healthful behaviours, improved their health status, and decreased their stays in hospital.[15]

| TABLE 1-9 | CHANGES IN REGIONALIZATION FROM TIME OF IMPLEMENTATION TO 2003, BY PROVINCE | | |

Province	Established	Restructured	Selected Changes
British Columbia	1997	2001	There are now five RHAs (covering 16 Health Service Delivery Areas) and 1 Provincial Health Service Authority. Board members are appointed. Before restructuring, there were 11 Regional Health Boards, 34 Community Health Councils and seven Community Health Services Societies
Alberta	1994	2002 and 2003	As of April 2003, there are nine RHAs and all members are appointed. Before that there were 17 RHAs. In 2002, Alberta moved from an all-appointed board member structure to one that was two-thirds elected and one-third appointed. It reverted to an entirely appointed structure in 2003
Saskatchewan	1992	2002	There are 12 regional health authorities and board members are appointed. Before that there were 32 health districts whose boards were initially all appointed. From 1995 to 2002, two-thirds of board members were elected and one-third appointed
Manitoba	1997–1998	2002	There are 11 RHAs with appointed board members. Before restructuring, there were 12 RHAs
Quebec	1989–1992	2001, and 2003–04	There are 18 RHAs whose roles have been in transition since November 2003. Before 2001, board members were elected by a representative caucus of stakeholders and CEOs were appointed by the RHA board. Since then, board members and regional CEOs have been appointed by the province, and CEOs are accountable jointly to the Deputy Minister and the regional board. In 2003, Quebec initiated a reorganization of its regional structures, which is currently in progress
Nova Scotia	1996	2001	There are nine District Health Authorities, with appointed boards. Before restructuring, there were four RHAs
New Brunswick	1992	2002	There are 8 RHAs, which had previously been Hospital Corporations Board members are appointed. Since 2004, boards will consist of eight elected and seven appointed members
Prince Edward Island	1993–1994	2002	There are four RHAs, with mixed elected and appointed members, and a Provincial Health Services Authority responsible for secondary and tertiary acute care services. Before restructuring, there were five RHAs
Newfoundland	1994	—	There are six institutional health boards, four health and community services boards, two integrated boards, a Nursing Home Board, and a Cancer Treatment and Research Board. Board members are appointed

Source: Lewis, S., & Kouri, S. (2004). Regionalization: Making sense of the Canadian experience. *Healthcare Papers, 5*(1), 21. Reprinted with Permission.

In Canada, the Chronic Disease Self-Management Program was implemented in 1998, by the University of Victoria—Centre on Aging, as a pilot program in the Yukon, and subsequently became a permanent government-funded program. In 2000, the Centre on Aging implemented the program in the Vancouver and Richmond health regions, where it also became a permanent program. In 2001, Health Canada provided a grant to the

Centre on Aging to implement a 28-month project, The Diabetes Self-Management Program. From 2003 to 2006, the Centre on Aging received a grant from the British Columbia Ministry of Health to implement the program in British Columbia. In March 2006, the Centre on Aging received funds to implement the program at the same level for the next three years.[16]

Other disease management programs in Canada include, but are not limited to, the Cardiovascular Program in Nova Scotia; the Northern Diabetes Health Network in Ontario; arthritis, falls, fractures, and osteoporosis programs in various locations; and the Western GTA (Greater Toronto Area) Stroke Network.

The Western GTA Stroke Network includes a consortium of hospitals and Community Care Access Centres that work with the Heart and Stroke Foundation of Ontario, the Ministry of Health and Long-Term Care, and LHINs to implement a coordinated approach to stroke care throughout the Western GTA. As a result of the collaboration, stroke outcomes are anticipated to improve and quality of life enhanced through awareness, education, and prevention measures.

The Kahnawake Schools Diabetes Prevention Program, in a First Nations community near Montreal, has reduced incidence rates of diabetes to almost the Canadian average (Health Council of Canada [HCC], 2007).

The Island Lake Regional Renal Health Program in northern Manitoba has been a catalyst for change in the prevention of diabetes and other chronic health conditions. This innovative program brought care to the community, avoided disruption caused by long periods away from home, and allowed the community to focus its efforts on managing the disease and keeping healthy (HCC, 2007).

ACCREDITATION

The Canadian Council on Health Services Accreditation (CCHSA) is the current national organization that assists health service organizations across Canada to examine and improve the quality of care and service they provide to clients. CCHSA is currently updating its accreditation program by building on the strengths of the Achieving Improved Measurement (AIM) program. This upgraded accreditation program will be phased in starting in 2009. Program components include quality dimensions, self assessments, on-site surveys, and a survey report, as well as standards related to leadership and governance, human resources, information management, the environment, and high-risk areas, such as medication management. The new program has eight dimensions of quality, including population focus, accessibility, safety, work life, client-centred services, continuity of services,

efficiency, and effectiveness (Canadian Council on Health Services Accreditation, 2007). The accreditation program is based on national standards developed and updated by experts in the field, through peer review and knowledge exchange.

Accreditation is a two-part process, consisting of self-assessment and peer review. The self-assessment component is completed to determine whether the organization complies with national standards. Areas examined include client care and delivery of service, information management practices, human resources development and management, the organization's governance, and the management of the environment. Peer review is completed by individuals (surveyors) external to the organization, who perform the accreditation survey, using the same national standards, to independently evaluate the organization. During their on-site visit, the surveyors meet with a variety of individuals, from direct care providers, clients, and their families, to board members and administrative staff from the organization, to discuss their expectations, perceptions, and experiences.[17]

Following the accreditation process, initial findings from the survey are provided to the organization in a verbal presentation to the organization. Within a few months, the organization receives a formal written evaluative report. The focus of the report is the organization's strengths and the areas requiring improvement. Recommendations are also made to assist the organization to develop plans for improvement and/or to maintain its strengths. See Table 1-10 for a list of the health services programs covered by the CCHSA accreditation program.

All CCHSA clients are currently accredited using the Achieving Improved Measurement (AIM) program and standards. This system ensures consistency in the accreditation process. It also enables organizations to compare their accreditation results over time and to share information on good practices. In 2006, CCHSA introduced new standards on Child Welfare, Hospice Palliative and End-of-Life Care, Biomedical Laboratory Services, and supplementary criteria for Telehealth.[18]

HEALTH CARE VARIATION AND EVIDENCE-BASED PRACTICE

Research on variation in medical care practice first began to be reported in the 1970s (Wennberg & Gittelsohn, 1973). Depending on what part of the country you lived in, client outcomes and costs varied significantly for the same health care condition. Studies on unnecessary surgery (Leape, 1987) and the occurrence of preventable

TABLE 1-10	**CCHSA ACCREDITATION PROGRAM COVERAGE**

The CCHSA accreditation program covers a diversity of health care and service areas:

- Acute Care
- Acquired Brain Injury
- Ambulatory Care
- Assisted Reproductive Technology Clinical Services
- Assisted Reproductive Technology Laboratory Services
- Biomedical Laboratory, Blood Banks and Transfusion Services
- Canadian Forces Health Services
- Cancer Care
- Child Welfare Services
- Cognitive, Behavioural, or Psychosocial Developmental Disabilities
- Community Health Services
- Critical Care
- First Nations and Inuit Addictions Services
- First Nations and Inuit Community Health Services
- Home Care
- Hospice Palliative and End-of-Life Care
- Long-Term Care
- Maternal/Child
- Mental Health
- Rehabilitation
- Specific Standard Requirements for Biomedical Laboratory Services
- Specific Standard Requirements for Blood Bank and Transfusion Services
- Substance Abuse and Gambling

Source: Canadian College on Health Services Accreditation. Accreditation program. Retrieved from http://www.cchsa.ca/ default.aspx?page=36&cat=27. April 1, 2007. © CCHSA 2007.

complications in clients (Adams, Fraser, & Abrams, 1973) led to more research into variations in physician practice patterns. Nursing and physician clinicians, as well as clients, began to consider which health care practices led to good health care outcomes. Previously, few studies had addressed the effect of various interventions on client outcomes. In 1992, the Institute for Clinical Evaluative Sciences started to guide decision making and suggest future research in Ontario by providing unbiased, evidence-based knowledge and recommendations related to care delivery, drug therapy, treatment modalities, health technology, and patterns of service utilization.[19]

VARIATION IN CLIENT OUTCOMES

Many variables affect client outcomes, including the severity of the client's illness. As mentioned earlier, health care outcome findings must be adjusted to allow for these variables. The process of statistically altering client data to reflect significant client variables is called **risk adjustment.** One of the difficulties of data on groups of client outcomes is the variable conditions of different clients in a group, even for clients admitted for the same diagnosis. For example, the conditions of each of two diabetic clients can be very different. One client can be a new diabetic client with few complications. The other client can be a more seriously ill diabetic client with many complications. These variations make it very difficult to identify the impact of a health care treatment on a single client's outcomes when all clients are grouped and compared. When the difficulties in gathering data based on valid and reliable client record review by trained reviewers are added to this situation, the difficulties in using risk adjustment on data become clear (Wolper, 1999). If, after reviewing client records, all client record reviewers do not extract identical data, the data compilation figures from the record reviewers will be quite different, significantly affecting the accurate measurement of client outcomes.

CANADIAN HEALTH SERVICES RESEARCH FOUNDATION

The Canadian Health Services Research Foundation (CHSRF) is an independent, not-for-profit corporation established with funds from the federal government and its agencies. It promotes and funds management and policy research in health services and nursing in order to increase the quality, relevance, and usefulness of this research for health system policymakers and managers. The CHSRF also collaborates with these health system decision-makers to support and enhance their use of research evidence when addressing health management and policy challenges. CHSRF projects always involve researchers, managers, and policymakers from academia and Canada's health system.

The priorities identified for research from 2004 to 2007 include managing for quality and safety; management of the health care workplace; primary health care; and nursing leadership, organization, and policy.[20]

In 2003, the CHSRF received $25 million, a 13-year grant for the Executive Training for Research Application (EXTRA) program, to develop the capacity of health service executives and their organizations to use research.[21] EXTRA is an intensive training program

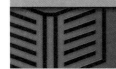

LITERATURE APPLICATION

Citation: Priest, A. (2006). What's ailing our nurses? A discussion of the major issues affecting nursing human resources in Canada. Ottawa: Canadian Health Services Research Foundation.

Discussion: In 2005, the Canadian Health Services Research Foundation commissioned a review of six major research documents on Canadian nursing human resource issues. These research documents included:

1. Nursing Sector Study Corporation. (2005). *Building the future: An integrated strategy for nursing human resources in Canada.* Ottawa: Nursing Sector Study Corporation.
2. Canadian Medical Association/Canadian Nursing Association. (2005). *Toward a Pan-Canadian framing network for health human resources.* Ottawa: Canadian Medical Association/Canadian Nursing Association.
3. El-Jardali, F., & Fooks, C. (2005). *An environmental scan of current views on health human resources in Canada: Identified problems, proposed solutions, and gap Analysis.* Toronto: Health Council of Canada.
4. Maslove, L. (2005). *Key and current health policy issues in Canada.* Ottawa: Canadian Policy Research Networks.
5. Maslove, L., & Fooks, C. (2004). *Our health, our future: Creating quality workplaces for Canadian nurses: A progress report on implementing the final report of the Canadian Nursing Advisory Committee.* Ottawa: Canadian Policy Research Network.
6. Baumann, A., O'Brien-Pallas, L., Armstrong-Stassen, M., Blythe, J., Bourbonnais, R., Cameron, S., Irvine Doran, D., Kerr, M., McGillis Hall, L., Vézina, M., Butt, M., & Ryan, L. (2001). *Commitment and care: The benefits of a healthy workplace for nurses, their patients and the system.*

The key messages included the following: the nursing shortage demands immediate action; clients' and nurses' welfares are closely aligned; the main focus needs to be the retention of existing nurses rather than boosting the number of education seats available; an improved work environment is key to retaining and attracting new nurses; of the many ways to address the crisis, practical policy and practice solutions have been identified, but few have been implemented; and overcoming barriers requires cooperation between professional associations and different levels of government with a dedicated political will.[22]

Implications for Practice: Nurses need to be cognizant of current research initiatives and evidence in order to be part of the solution.

Source: Priest, A. (2006). What's ailing our nurses? A discussion of the major issues affecting nursing human resources in Canada. Ottawa: Canadian Health Services Research Foundation. Reprinted with Permission.

designed to assist health leaders to become better decision-makers by teaching them how to find, assess, and interpret research-based evidence.[23]

CANADIAN ADVERSE EVENTS STUDY

International jurisdictions, such as the United States, the United Kingdom, and Australia, recognize that health care safety concerns are real, and their systems are prone to error. The 1999 U.S. Institute of Medicine report, "To Err is Human," was an important stimulus for action, when it estimated that between 44,000 and 98,000 U.S. citizens die each year as a result of medical errors. This study and similar studies in Australia and the United Kingdom have provided the evidence base that is key to maintaining the momentum to move forward in addressing the issue of client safety. Canada recently completed its first national study on adverse events in acute care hospitals. The study found that in 2000, of approximately 2.5 million adult hospital admissions, nearly 7.5 percent (185,000) resulted in an adverse event. Of these, approximately 38 percent (70,000) were considered to be preventable. In total, the researchers estimated that, in 2000, between 9,000 and 24,000 clients experienced an adverse event that was preventable, and later died. These results indicate that the incidence of health system error in Canada is comparable with other industrialized countries (Baker, Norton, Flintoft, Blais, Brown, Cox, J., et al., 2004).

As a result of the increased focus on client safety in Canada, the Canadian government budgeted $50 million from 2002 to 2007 for the creation of the Canadian Patient Safety Institute. In addition, many health care organizations have initiated efforts to improve client safety (Baker, Norton, Flintoft, Blais, Brown, Cox, J., et al., 2004). An independent national nonprofit agency, the Institute for Safe Medication Practices Canada (ISMP Canada), is committed to promoting medication safety in all health care settings.

NEW CANADIAN COUNCIL ON HEALTH SERVICES ACCREDITATION PATIENT SAFETY STANDARD

The Canadian Council on Health Services Accreditation has always focused on client safety, and has identified several ways to incorporate client safety into its accreditation

---

TABLE 1-11   **NATIONAL EFFORTS RELATED TO CLIENT SAFETY**

1. Policy statements related to client safety from the Canadian Nurses Association, the Canadian Healthcare Association and the Canadian College of Health Service Executives

2. Saskatchewan client safety initiatives built upon the recommendations from the Fyke Report (2001)

3. Canada's first Health Quality Council (2002)

4. Saskatchewan has Quality Care Coordinators for each regional health authority

5. Manitoba Health implemented a policy mandating reporting of critical incidents and other events in Manitoba health care organizations (2003)

6. Manitoba Institute for Patient Safety and Quality Care and a Provincial Patient Safety Council created in 2003

7. Health Services Utilization and Outcomes Commission in Alberta assumed responsibility for assessing client safety in the province

8. Calgary Health Region created the Quality Improvement Health Information portfolio to provide leadership, infrastructure, and support to clinical and non-clinical teams throughout the Region

9. Alberta government supported the development of an electronic health record that will contribute to improved safety and quality of care

10. Nova Scotia government established a formal provincial Health Care Safety Working Group to create a comprehensive plan to support districts with their safety initiatives

11. Ontario government announced two client safety initiatives: the development of a province-wide Patient Safety Team and a Safe Medication Support Service (2002)

Source: Bonney, E., & Baker, G. R. (2004). Current strategies to improve patient safety in Canada: An overview of federal and provincial initiatives. *Healthcare Quarterly, 7*(2), 36–41. Reproduced with Permission.

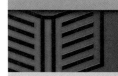

LITERATURE APPLICATION

Citation: Baker, G. R., Norton, P. G., Flintoft, V., Blais, R., Brown, A., Cox, J., Etchells, E., Ghali, W. A., Hébert, P., Majumdar, S. R., O'Beirne, M., Palacios-Derflingher, L., Reid, R. J., Sheps, S., & Tamblyn, R. The Canadian Adverse Events Study: The incidence of adverse events among hospital patients in Canada. *Canadian Medical Association Journal, 170*(11), 1678–1686.

Background: Research into adverse events (AEs) has highlighted the need to improve client safety. AEs are unintended injuries or complications that arise from health care management and result in death, disability, or a prolonged hospital stay. The incidence of AEs among clients in Canadian acute care hospitals was estimated by the authors.

Methods: One teaching hospital, one large community hospital, and two small community hospitals in each of five provinces (British Columbia, Alberta, Ontario, Quebec, and Nova Scotia) were randomly selected. From each hospital, for the fiscal year 2000, a random sample of charts was reviewed for non-psychiatric, non-obstetric adult clients. Trained reviewers screened all eligible charts, and physicians reviewed the positively screened charts to identify AEs and determine their preventability.

Results: At least one screening criterion was identified in 1,527 (40.8 percent) of 3,745 charts. The physician reviewers identified AEs in 255 charts. After adjustment for the sampling strategy, the AE rate was 7.5 per 100 hospital admissions (95% confidence interval [CI] 5.7– 9.3). Among the clients with AEs, events judged to be preventable occurred in 36.9 percent (95% CI 32.0%–41.8%), and death occurred in 20.8 percent (95% CI 7.8%–33.8%). Physician reviewers estimated that 1,521 additional hospital days were associated with AEs. Although men and women experienced equal rates of AEs, clients who had AEs were significantly older than those who did not (mean age [and standard deviation] 64.9 [16.7] v. 62.0 [18.4] years; $p = 0.016$).

Interpretation: The overall incidence rate of AEs of 7.5 percent in this study suggests that, of the almost 2.5 million annual hospital admissions in Canada similar to the type studied, about 185,000 are associated with an AE, and close to 70,000 of these are potentially preventable.

Source: "RESEARCH: The Canadian Adverse Events Study: The incidence of adverse events among hospital patients in Canada." Reprinted from CMAJ, 25 May 2004; 170(11), Page(s) 1678–1686 by permission of the publisher. © 2004 Canadian Medical Association.

programs, including a sentinel event policy; a database to track the use of indicators by organizations, including indicators relating to client safety; and the tracking of trends in quality improvement, including client safety initiatives (Bonney & Baker, 2004, p. 37). Following a lengthy process of literature review, consultations with experts, and many meetings with the CCHSA's Patient Safety Advisory Committee, six Patient Safety Goals and a number of related Required Organization Practices (ROPs) were prioritized for 2005. All accredited organizations must comply with these goals and practices (Murphy & Greco, 2004). A full listing of CCHSA's Patient Safety Goals and all Required Organizational Practices can be found on the CCHSA website at www.cchsa.ca. The Canadian College of Health Service Executives has also written a position statement on the health executive's role in client safety. Examples of national efforts related to client safety can be found in Table 1-11.

INSTITUTE OF MEDICINE COMMITTEE ON HEALTH CARE QUALITY REPORTS

In 1999, the Institute of Medicine (IOM) released a report titled *To Err Is Human: Building a Safer Health System.* The report concluded that more people die annually from medication mistakes than from highway accidents, breast cancer, or AIDS (Kohn, Corrigan, & Donaldson, 1999). A second IOM committee report released in 2001, *Crossing the Quality Chasm: A New Health System for the 21st Century* (Kohn, Corrigan, & Donaldson, 2001), recommends that "all health care organizations, professional groups, and private and public purchasers should adopt as their own the explicit purpose of reducing the burden of illness, injury, and disability, and improving the health and functioning of the people of the United States." Health providers should pursue six major areas for improvement of health care (Maddox, 2001) see Table 1-12.

The second IOM report identified four major areas to target for change in the health care environment: information technology, payment, clinical knowledge, and the professional workforce (Kohn, Corrigan, & Donaldson, 2001).

QUALITY HEALTH CARE

It is useful to consider a basic framework for quality health care. Donabedian (1966) conceptualized such a framework (Bull, 1997). This framework is composed of the elements of structure, process, and outcome.

TABLE 1-12   MAJOR AREAS TO BE PURSUED IN HEALTH CARE—THE SECOND IOM REPORT

Health care should be:

- Effective—providing services based on scientific knowledge to all who could benefit and refraining from providing services to those not likely to benefit (avoiding overuse and under use).

- Client-centred—providing care that is respectful of and responsive to individual client preferences, needs, and values and ensuring that client values guide all clinical decisions.

- Timely—reducing waits and sometimes harmful delays for both those who receive and those who give care.

- Efficient—avoiding waste, in particular waste of equipment, supplies, ideas, and energy.

- Safe—avoiding injuries to clients from care intended to help them.

- Equitable—providing care that does not vary in quality because of personal characteristics, such as gender, ethnicity, geographic location, and socioeconomic data.

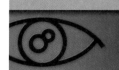

CRITICAL THINKING

Nurses who work in large health care settings can sometimes feel lost and may wonder how they and their system can deliver quality in the midst of rapid change. What can nurses do to ensure safe, high-quality care? Thinking about the following may be useful:

What can I do at my level to manage care and support and to contribute to the quality of health care in my organization and community? How can I work well with other people in my nursing unit, in the organization, and in the community? Where can I find "best evidence" clinical practice guidelines to apply to client care in my organization and community? How much do I control care or anything else at a beginning level? I want to be optimistic, yet realistic!

STRUCTURE, PROCESS, OUTCOME

Using Donabedian's framework, a health care organization that wishes to develop quality will organize or structure itself for quality. Quality client care does not just happen. It must be planned. Quality is the result of assessing client needs and delivering care to meet those needs. Donabedian's framework has three elements: structure, process, and outcome.

Structure elements of quality lay a foundation for quality health care by identifying which structures must be in place in a health care system to deliver quality. Structure elements consist of such things as a well-constructed hospital, quality client care standards, quality staffing policies, environmental standards, and the like.

Process is the next element of the quality framework. **Process elements of quality** build on the structure elements and take quality a step further. Process elements identify which nursing and health care interventions must be in place to deliver quality. Process elements are such things as managing the health care process, utilizing clinical practice guidelines and standards for nursing and medical interventions, administering medications, and the like.

Finally, an outcome element completes the quality framework. **Outcome elements of quality** are the end results of quality care. Outcome elements review the status of clients after health care has been delivered. Outcomes reflect the presence of structure and process elements of quality. Outcomes ask whether the client is better as a result of health care. If a quality hospital (structure) and quality standards (process) are in place, clients should experience good health (outcome). See Table 1-13 for examples of structure, process, and outcome quality performance measures in three domains of activity: clinical care, financial management, and human resources management.

For quality to occur, monitors of all three elements of Donabedian's framework—structure, process, and outcome—should be in place. Today, many people who review quality focus initially on outcome evaluation. Quality outcomes are considered to be at least partially reflective of having quality structures and quality processes in place. For example, if a client is breathing better after health care interventions for an asthma attack, this

TABLE 1-13   EXAMPLES OF PERFORMANCE MEASURES BY CATEGORY

Domain of Activity

	Clinical Care	Financial Management	Human Resources Management
Structure	*Effectiveness* ■ Percentage of active physicians who have credentials ■ CCHSA accreditation ■ Number of residencies and filled positions ■ Presence of council for quality improvement planning	*Effectiveness* ■ Qualifications of administrators in finance department ■ Use of preadmission criteria ■ Presence of an integrated financial and clinical information system	*Effectiveness* ■ Ability to attract desired registered nurses and other health professionals ■ Size (or growth) of active physician staff ■ Salary and benefits compared to other organizations ■ Quality of in-house staff education
Process	*Effectiveness* ■ Rate of medication error ■ Rate of nosocomial infection ■ Rate of post-surgical wound infection ■ Rate of normal tissue removed *Productivity* ■ Ratio of total client days to total full-time equivalent (FTE) nurses ■ Ratio of total admissions to total FTE staff ■ Ratio of physician visits to total FTE physicians *Efficiency* ■ Average cost per client day ■ Total cost per client day	*Effectiveness* ■ Days in accounts receivable ■ Use of generic drugs and drug formulary ■ Market share ■ Size (or growth) of shared service arrangements *Productivity* ■ Ratio of collection to bad debt ■ Ratio of total admissions to FTE in finance department ■ Ratio of new capital to fundraising staff *Efficiency* ■ Cost per collection ■ Debt/equity ratio	*Effectiveness* ■ Grievances ■ Promotions ■ Organizational climate *Productivity* ■ Ratio of line staff to managers *Efficiency* ■ Cost of recruiting
Outcome	*Effectiveness* ■ Case-severity-adjusted mortality ■ Client satisfaction ■ Client functional health status	*Effectivenes* ■ Return on investments ■ Operating margins ■ Size (or growth) of government grants for teaching and research ■ Bond rating	*Effectiveness* ■ Turnover rate ■ Absenteeism ■ Staff satisfaction

quality outcome may be a reflection of quality structures (e.g., good equipment and medications) and quality processes (e.g., nursing and medical interventions). Of course, the client's overall initial health status and other factors also affect the outcome. When outcomes are not good, nurses and other health care leaders must examine the structure and process elements critically. Change in these elements may be needed to improve health care quality. See Chapter 17 for examples of other indicators of the quality of nursing care.

THE 3M HEALTH CARE QUALITY TEAM AWARDS

In 1994, the Canadian College of Health Service Executives and 3M Health Care launched the 3M Health Care Quality Team Awards to recognize innovation in health services by linking the concepts of quality and teams. These awards are presented annually to recognize teams who are using quality frameworks to create measurable outcomes within their programs and services, in addition to demonstrating enhancements in client care.

OUTCOME MEASUREMENTS

Outcomes can be measured to indicate an individual's clinical state, such as the severity of an illness, the course of an illness, and the effect of interventions on the individual's clinical state. Outcome measures involving a client's functional status evaluate a client's ability to perform activities of daily living (ADLs). These measures assess physical health in terms of function, mental and social health, the cost of care, health care access, and general health perceptions. The measures distinguish the concepts of physical and mental health, and identify five indicator categories of clinical status: functioning, physical symptoms, emotional status, client/family evaluation, and perceptions about quality of life. Selected quality-of-life measures include quality-adjusted life years (QALY), quality-adjusted life expectancy (QALE), and quality-adjusted healthy life years (QUALY) (Drummond, Stoddart, & Torrance, 1994).

A 2001 study by McGillis Hall et al. suggested that a higher proportion of registered nurses and registered practical nurses on inpatient medical surgical and obstetrical units in Ontario teaching hospitals was associated with better health and quality outcomes for the clients at the time of hospital discharges, and with lower rates of medication errors and wound infections.[24]

RECENT CHANGES IN HEALTH CARE

Several changes have taken place recently in health care. A major current issue in Canada is how to balance the demands of rights under the Canadian Charter of Rights and Freedoms (in the first part of Constitution Act, 1982) and the realities of economic pressure and public demands. One of the most recent reports commissioned to examine these issues was *Building on Values: The Future of Health Care in Canada*. This report of the Commission on the Future of Health Care in Canada was prompted by increased public dissatisfaction, escalating health care costs, and evidence of systems failure (e.g., access and quality of care issues). The report contained 47 costed recommendations. See Table 1-14 for 11 critical areas of focus from

TABLE 1-14	ELEVEN CRITICAL AREAS OF FOCUS

1. Sustaining service, needs and resources, new governance
2. Sustaining Medicare; expanding the Canada Health Act to include accountability
3. More comprehensive use of information management and technology
4. Investing in health care providers—role changes and supply, demand, and distribution of health personnel
5. Primary health care and prevention—focus on wellness and health promotion
6. Improving access and ensuring quality—reducing waiting times and improving access to local and global resources, multicultural services
7. Rural and remote communities—again, access to quality care services
8. Home care services—home care, community mental health and palliative care services under the jurisdiction of Canada Health Act to ensure funding
9. Prescription drugs—a national drug agency to monitor costs and safety
10. Aboriginal health—health disparities, consolidate funding
11. Globalization—international alliances

Source: Commission on the Future of Health Care in Canada. (2002). *Building on values: The future of health care in Canada.* Saskatoon: Commission on the Future of Health Care in Canada. Commissioner: Roy J. Romanow, pp. xxiii–xxxiv. Reproduced with the permission of the Minister of Public Works and Government Services Canada, 2007.

the recommendations. See Table 1-15 for a summary of the federal commissions related to health care.

PRIVACY LEGISLATION IN CANADA

Canada has two federal privacy laws: the Privacy Act and the Personal Information Protection and Electronic Documents Act. Through the Privacy Act, which took effect in 1983, individuals are given the right to access and request correction of their personal information that is held by federal government organizations.

Individuals are protected by the Personal Information Protection and Electronic Documents Act (PIPEDA), which sets out ground rules for how private sector organizations collect, use, or disclose personal information. Individuals have the right to access and request correction of their personal information that organizations may have collected. This right not only applies to private sector organizations but also to personal information collected, used, or disclosed by the service industry.

Each province and territory has privacy legislation governing the collection, use, and disclosure of personal information held by government agencies. These acts provide individuals with a general right to access and correct their personal information.[25]

CANADIAN COLLEGE OF HEALTH SERVICE EXECUTIVES

Health care executives and managers in Canada face many challenges in today's health care environment,

TABLE 1-15	FEDERAL COMMISSIONS ON HEALTH CARE

Commission on the Future of Health Care in Canada (Romanow Commission, 2001 to 2002).

Standing Senate Committee on Social Affairs, Science and Technology Study on the State of the Health Care System in Canada (Kirby Committee, 1999 to 2002)

National Forum on Health (1994 to 1997)

Health Services Review '79 (1979 to 1980)

A New Perspective on the Health of Canadians (Lalonde Report, 1973 to 1974)

Royal Commission on Health Services (Hall Commission, 1961 to 1964)

Source: Health Care System. Commissions and inquiries: Federal commissions on health care. Health Canada. Retrieved from http://www. hc-sc.gc.ca/hcs-sss/com/index_e.html, August 2, 2006. Reproduced with the permission of the Minister of Public Works and Government Services Canada.

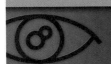

CRITICAL THINKING

You work in a large health care organization. One of your clients is not following her health care regime. You wonder what thought processes this client is using to justify continuing an activity that presents risks to her health.

How can you best assist this client in your health care organization and community? What kinds of structures, processes, and outcomes will your organization want to develop to improve care to this client and to the population of clients that your organization serves? How can you work in the community to enhance this population's choices for diet, exercise, or lifestyle?

TABLE 1-16	CCHSE COMPETENCIES*

Leadership

- Vision
- Team building
- Flexibility in leadership style
- Flexibility in managing change
- Stress Management
- Commitment to consumer
- Commitment to organization
- Commitment to stakeholders
- Commitment to health service management profession

Communication

- Verbal communication
- Listening
- Written communication

Lifelong Learning

- Self-directed learning
- Teaching/mentoring

Consumer/Community Responsiveness and Public Relations

- Public relations
- Responsiveness

Political and Health Environment Awareness

- Political awareness and sensitivity
- Health environment (trends/issues) awareness

Conceptual Skills

- Analysis and synthesis
- Problem-solving
- Systems thinking

Results Management

- Planning
- Implementation
- Monitoring/evaluating

Resource Management

- Human resources
- Financial resources
- Capital/material assets
- Information dissemination

Compliance to Standards

- Accreditation
- Ethical standards
- Legal standards

*Adapted from: Canadian College of Health Service Executives: General Managerial Competencies; (1984 revised 2002)

Source: MacKinnon et al. (2004). Management competencies for Canadian health executives: Views from the field. *Healthcare Management Forum, 17*(4), 16. Reprinted with Permission.

including the need for accountability, health human resource shortages, increasing consumer demands, and balancing budgets. In order to successfully manage these areas, health care executives need to master a variety of managerial competencies. As part of the Certified Health Executive (CHE) designation, individuals are evaluated on Canadian College of Health Service Executives competencies, which are defined as "the skills and knowledge that Canadian health service executives have identified as critical to providing efficient and effective delivery of health services" (MacKinnon, Chow, Kennedy, Persaud, Metge, & Sketris, 2004). See Table 1-16 for the nine general categories of these competencies.

OTHER FORCES INFLUENCING HEALTH CARE

Shortell and Kaluzny (2000) identify nine major forces influencing health care: capitation; payment of clinicians based on performance using clinical practice guidelines; new technology; the aging population; genetic engineering; increasing cultural diversity; new diseases; information management; and the globalization of the world economy continue to shape health care in the new millennium (see Table 1-17). These changes,

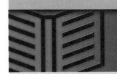

LITERATURE APPLICATION

Citation: Soukup, S. M. (2000). Preface to section on evidence-based nursing practice. *Nursing Clinics of North America, 35*(2), xvii–xviii.

Discussion: Author discusses a nurse's response to queries as to whether she has integrated evidence-based practice. The nurse responds, "Yes, I practise state-of-the-art nursing. My education and professional practice experiences have prepared me to care for more than 700 chronically ill clients annually, in the past five years. These clients have an average reported expected pain rating of 6.9 (using a scale of 1 to 10, with 10 being severe pain), and my pain management interventions have kept these clients, during my hours of care, at a reported actual pain rating of 4. Also, as a team member, these clients have not had any known pressure ulcers, skin tears, or catheter-related infections. On two occasions, for clients who were dying, I created a humanizing environment for these clients and their families when they were rapidly transferred from the critical care unit. My documentation has met organizational standards during monthly peer reviews; I have provided leadership for emergencies with positive outcomes; and physician and client satisfaction rating for clinical practice on our unit is 9.5 on a scale of 10, with 10 being the highest. Our unit-based team has not had a needle-stick-related or back-related injury during the past two years."

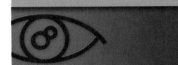

CRITICAL THINKING

Are hospitals in your area rated? What kinds of ratings are given to hospitals? Review the criteria and evaluation system used to rate the hospitals. Is it valid and reliable? Are the criteria important to quality and client satisfaction? Will you choose a hospital for your own family's care using a rating system like this?

as well as the emergence of terrorism and bioterrorism, continue to call for ongoing changes in the education of health care professionals.

TRENDS IN CANADIAN HEALTH CARE

Canadians' needs for health care quality and access continue to develop. Nurses who work in health care today continue the tradition of nursing caring and excellence that began with Florence Nightingale, who served clients in her time by meeting their needs. Today's nurse will

prosper by continuing this commitment to a personal ethic of social responsibility, service, and caring. Caring is the core of nursing practice because it renders technical, curative procedures tolerable and safe, by helping clients and families weather their illness and sustain or regain familiar life worlds (Benner, 2000).

NURSING ROLE

Nursing has come a long way in the past 100 years. Six characteristics are commonly used to assess whether a job is a profession: maintaining quality education of the practitioner, following a code of ethics, receiving compensation commensurate with the work, being organized to promote a needed service, having autonomy in practice, and being recognized by the government with licensure (Pinkerton, 2001). Nursing is recognized as a profession in most circles today, though nurse–physician work relationships continue to evolve. In the late 1990s, some nurses still reported "knowing the right thing to do and having no support or authority to carry it out" (Aroskar, 1998). Development of the nurse–physician relationship must be part of improving the health care delivery system, particularly because when nurses and physicians work together, client care improves (Baggs & Ryan, 1990).

INTERDISCIPLINARY NURSING

Fooks (2005) suggests that one of the challenges we will face in the future is an interdisciplinary care environment. This challenge has arisen as a result of the

TABLE 1-17	NINE FORCES INFLUENCING HEALTH CARE DELIVERY AND THEIR IMPLICATIONS FOR MANAGEMENT

External Force	**Management Implication**
1. Capitated payments, expenditure targets, or global budgets for providing care to defined populations	■ Need for increased efficiency and productivity ■ Redesign of client care delivery ■ Development of strategic alliances that add value ■ Increased growth of networks, systems, and physician groups
2. Increased accountability for performance	■ Information systems that link financial and clinical data across episodes of illness and "pathways of wellness" ■ Effective implementation of clinical practice guidelines ■ Ability to demonstrate continuous improvements of all functions and processes
3. Technological advances in the biological and clinical sciences	■ Expansion of the continuum of care ■ Need for new treatment sites to accommodate new treatment modalities ■ Increased capacity to manage care across organizational boundaries ■ Need to confront new ethical dilemmas
4. Aging of the population	■ Increased demand for primary care, wellness, and health promotion services among the 65- to 75-year-old age group ■ Increased demand for chronic care management among those older than age 75 ■ Challenge of managing ethical issues associated with prolongation of life
5. Increased ethnic or cultural diversity of the population	■ Greater difficulty in understanding and meeting client expectations ■ Challenge of managing an increasingly diverse health services workforce
6. Changes in the supply and education of health professionals	■ Need for creative approaches in meeting the population's need for disease prevention, health promotion, and chronic care management services ■ Need to compensate for shortages in some categories of health professionals (i.e., physical therapy, pharmacy, and some areas of nursing) ■ Need to develop effective teams of caregivers across multiple treatment sites
7. Social morbidity (e.g., AIDS, drugs, violence, "new surprises")	■ Ability to deal with unpredictable increases in demand ■ Need for increased social support systems and chronic care management ■ Need to work effectively with community agencies
8. Information technology	■ Training the health care workforce in new information technologies ■ Increased ability to coordinate care across sites ■ Challenge of managing an increased pace of change due to more rapid information transfer ■ Challenge of dealing with confidentiality issues associated with new information technologies
9. Globalization and expansion of the world economy	■ Need to manage cross-national and cross-cultural tertiary and quaternary client care referrals ■ Increasing the productivity of the Canadian labour force ■ Managing global strategic alliances, particularly in the areas of biotechnology and new technology development

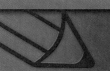

CASE STUDY 1-1

Mrs. Williams comes to your unit from the Emergency Department (ED). Her admitting diagnosis is asthma. Her husband tells you she was really frightened and could not breathe when she came to the ED. They ask you how long she will be in the hospital and what will happen next. You give them a copy of your unit's asthma clinical practice guideline and review it with them.

How can you try to ensure a smooth transition home?

How will you work with your health care organization and the community you serve to ensure that Mrs. Williams and other asthma clients in the community are not admitted with asthma again soon? What kind of teaching will Mrs. Williams need to prevent future attacks?

reorganization and expansion of the ways primary health care is delivered to Canadians. Teamwork with many different professionals will be required in order for the client to have a seamless process within the integrated continuum of care. Education needs to change in order for health professionals to recognize and understand each others' roles and collaborate effectively in the future. The future demands inter- and intra-disciplinary education. The health needs of the future will require a professional nurse who can demonstrate caring and competency, and can practice in an interdisciplinary fashion, planning for the changing health care delivery system. Interdisciplinary practice brings nurses to the table with a more equal footing and diminishes the notion that the team needs a captain to function. When each discipline brings its unique talents to the job of providing care for a client and the client's family, interdisciplinary practice removes the gatekeeper and allows clients access to all caregivers based on the expertise needed. Success in interdisciplinary practice will depend on each profession maintaining the highest standards, including expectations of advanced education, a certification process, and requirements for continuing education to maintain competency (Carroll-Johnson, 2001). The health care of the future will increasingly be outcome-focused, evidence-based, wellness-oriented, population-based, technology-intensive, and highly cost-aware. Nursing must be ready to meet this challenge.

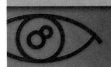

CRITICAL THINKING

Go to the website for The Integrated Pan-Canadian Healthy Living Strategy, 2005 (http://www.phac-aspc.gc.ca/hl-vs-strat/pdf/hls_e.pdf).

What did you find?

How is your province doing on the Healthy Living Strategy indicators?

How could you work with leaders in your community and province to improve your province's performance?

KEY CONCEPTS

- The Canadian system of health care has developed within a political context. Our health care system may be highly sophisticated, but it does not deliver the same level of health care, access, and cost-effective quality to all its citizens.

- Various groups deliver Canadian health care in a variety of settings.

- Canadian health care is paid for by the public and private sectors.

- Health care can be categorized into four levels: health promotion, disease and injury prevention (protection), diagnosis and treatment of existing health problems (including primary, secondary, and tertiary care), and rehabilitation.

- The Canadian Council on Health Services Accreditation is the national organization that accredits health care organizations.

- Donabedian developed a framework for quality. He identified structure, process, and outcome elements of quality. When outcomes are not good, nurses must review the structure and process of health care.

- The Canadian College of Health Service Executives and the 3M Health Care Quality Team Awards provide a framework for the delivery of quality health care.

- Efforts to improve health care must address the multiple determinants of health in Canada.

- Canadian College of Health Service Executives identified nine competencies for the 21st century for health care providers. Nursing and other health care professions will have to adapt to a fast-changing environment in the future.

- Various forces are affecting health care in the new millennium.

- Caring, multidisciplinary nursing practice promises to be an important part of nursing's future role in health care.

KEY TERMS

disease management	process elements of quality
horizontal integration	public health
integrated delivery system	regionalization
outcome elements of quality	risk adjustment
population elements of quality	structure elements of quality
primary health care	vertical integration

REVIEW QUESTIONS

1. Which of the following is the national organization that accredits health care organizations?
   A. Canadian Nurses Association
   B. Canadian College of Health Service Executives
   C. Canadian Institutes of Health Research
   D. Canadian Council on Health Services Accreditation

2. Which of the following is the largest expenditure related to health care in Canada?
   A. hospitals and institutions
   B. physicians
   C. pharmaceuticals
   D. nurses

3. Who identified a structure, process, and outcome framework for quality health care?
   A. Titler
   B. Elazar
   C. Wennberg
   D. Donabedian

4. Which of the following is the name of a national award for quality health care?
   A. Hill Burton
   B. 3M Health Care Quality Team Award
   C. Foundation for Accountability
   D. National Committee on Quality Assurance

REVIEW ACTIVITIES

1. You have just graduated from your nursing education program and have begun working on a new client care unit. Your nurse manager asks you to serve on the team to develop and improve the unit. Give examples of the three elements of quality that you will consider. Consider structure, process, and outcome examples in your answer. How will you monitor the effects of your improvements?

2. Your uncle is a director of quality improvement at a local manufacturing company. He comments on some of his company's activities to improve quality. What can you tell him about the quality improvement activities in the client care unit on which you have recently provided clinical care?

3. Review the Canadian College of Health Service Executives management competencies. Consider how you can improve your own knowledge level in any of the competency areas in which you do not feel comfortable.

EXPLORING THE WEB

- What sites would you recommend to clients and families seeking information about self-help, hospital accreditation, research, and clinical practice guidelines; for example, the Canadian Council on Health Services Accreditation, the Canadian Institutes for Health Research, and the Quality Healthcare Network?

  http://www.hc-sc.gc.ca/hcs-sss/hhr-rhs/collabor/self-auto/index_e.html

  http://www.cchsa.ca

  http://www.cihr.ca

  http://mdm.ca/cpgsnew/cpgs/gccpg-e.htm

- Go to the sites for the CCHSE and 3M Health Care Quality Team Awards and the Canadian Adverse Events Study. What information did you find there?

  http://www.cchse.org/default_awards.asp?active_page_id=931

  http://www.hc-sc.gc.ca/hcs-sss/qual/patient_securit/adverse-indesirable/index_e.html

- Where can you find statistics on health care spending?

  http://www.cihi.ca

- Search the Internet and check these websites: Medicare, Canadian Institute for Health Information, Canadian Nurses Association, Canadian Cancer Society, Heart and Stroke Foundation, Canadian Diabetes Association, Delmar Learning. What did you find?

  http://www.canadianeconomy.gc.ca/English/economy/1957medicare.html

  http://www.cihi.ca

  http://www.cna-nurses.ca

  http://www.cancer.ca

  http://ww2.heartandstroke.ca/Page.asp?PageID=24

  http://www.diabetes.ca

  http://www.delmarlearning.com

- Where can you find information related to diabetes in the Canadian population?

  http://www.healthcouncilcanada.ca/docs/rpts/2007/HCC_DiabetesRpt.pdf

- Go to PubMed. What did you find there? Can you access nursing and medical journals? Would you recommend this site to clients?

  http://www.ncbi.nlm.nih.gov/entrez/query.fcgi?DB=pubmed

- What are some helpful sites for nurses?

  http://www.nursingindex.com/

  http://www.anac.on.ca/

  http://www.cna-nurses.ca/

- Where could you go for information on the eHealth Internet Code of Ethics?

  http://www.ihealthcoalition.org/ethics/ethics.html

- What are some sites to check on The Personal Information Protection and Electronic Documents Act?

  http://www.privcom.gc.ca/legislation/02_06_01_e.asp

REFERENCES

Adams, D. F., Fraser, D. B., & Abrams, H. L. (1973). The complications of coronary arteriography. *Circulation, 48*(3), 609–618.

Alberta. Premier's Advisory Council on Health. (2001). *A framework for reform: Report of the premier's advisory council on health.* Edmonton: Premier's Advisory Council on Health. Chair: Donald Mazankowski.

Aroskar, M. (1998). Ethical working relationships in patient care. *Nursing Clinics of North America, 33*(2), 313–323.

Baggs, J. G., & Ryan, S. A. (1990). ICU nurse-physician collaboration and nursing satisfaction. *Nursing Economic$, 8*(6), 386–392.

Baker, R. Norton, P., Flintoft, V., Blais, R., Brown, A., Cox, J., et al. (2004). The Canadian adverse events study: The incidence of adverse events among hospital patients in Canada. *Canadian Medical Association Journal, 170*(11), 1678–1686.

Benner, P. (2000). The wisdom of our practice. *American Journal of Nursing, 100*(10), 99–103.

Bonney, E., & Baker, G. R. (2004) Current strategies to improve patient safety in Canada: An overview of federal and provincial initiatives. *Healthcare Quarterly, 7*(2), 36–41.

Browne, G., Roberts, J., Burne, C., Gafni, A., Weir, R. and Majumdar, B. (2001). The costs and effects of addressing the needs of vulnerable populations: Results of 10 years of research. *Canadian Journal of Nursing Research, 33*, 65–76.

Bull, M. J. (1997). Lessons from the past: Visions for the future of quality care. In C. G. Meisenheimer, *Improving quality* (2nd ed., pp. 3–16). Gaithersburg, MD: Aspen.

Byers, S. A. (1997). *The executive nurse—leadership for new health care transitions.* Clifton Park, NY: Delmar Learning.

Canada. Parliament. Senate. Standing Committee on Social Affairs, Science and Technology. (2002). *Reforming health protection and promotion in Canada: Time to act.* Ottawa: Standing Committee on Social Affairs, Science and Technology. Chair: Michael Kirby.

Canada. Statistics Canada. (2006). *Canada year book 2006.* Ottawa: Statistics Canada.

Canadian Council on Health Services Accreditation. (2007). "Strengthening the accreditation program: an overview of the new program". Version 4. retrieved from http://www.cchsa.ca/upload/files/pdf/New%20Accreditation%20Program/Strengthening%20Accred%20Program%20(01-11-07)-e.pdf, July 12, 2007.

Canadian Institute for Health Information. (2005). *Workforce trends of licensed practical nurses in Canada, 2004.* Ottawa: Canadian Institute for Health Information.

Carroll-Johnson, R. (2001). Redefining interdisciplinary practice. *Oncology Nursing Forum, 28*(4), 619.

Commission on the Future of Health Care in Canada. (2002). *Building on values: The future of health care in Canada*. Saskatoon: Commission on the Future of Health Care in Canada. Commissioner: Roy J. Romanow.

Constitution Act (1867). formerly the British North America Act (1867). Retrieved from http://www.solon.org/Constitutions/ Canada/English/ca_1867.html, July 31, 2007.

Donabedian, A. (1966). Evaluating the quality of medical care. *Milbank Memorial Fund Quarterly, 44*, 194–196.

Donatelle, R., & Davis, L. G. (1998). *Access to health* (8th ed.). Needham Heights, MA: Allyn & Bacon.

Drummond, M. F., Stoddart, F. L., & Torrance, G. W. (1994). *Methods for the economic evaluation of health care programmes*. Oxford, England: Oxford University Press.

Elazar, D. (1966). *American federalism: A view from the states*. New York: Crowell.

Esmail, N., & Walker, M. (2005) *How good is Canadian health care? 2005 report: An international comparison of health care systems*. (2005 Critical Issues Bulletin) Vancouver: The Fraser Institute

Evans, R., & Stoddard, G. (1990). Consuming health care, producing health. *Social Science and Medicine, 31*(12), 1347–1363.

Fooks, C. (2005). Health human resources planning in an interdisciplinary health care environment: To dream the impossible dream? *Canadian Journal of Nursing Leadership, 18*(3), 26–29.

Fottler, M. D., Blair, J. D., Whitehead, C. J., Laus, M. D., & Savage, G. T. (1989). Assessing key stakeholders: Who matters to hospitals and why? *Hospital and Health Services Administration, 34*(4), 525–546.

Goddard, M., & Smith, P. (2001). Equity of access to health care services: Theory and evidence from the UK. *Social Science & Medicine, 53*, 1149–1162.

Health Canada. (2000). Part one introduction: Challenges. *Quest for Quality in Canadian Health Care, Continuous Quality Improvement*. Retrieved from http://www.hc-sc.gc.ca/hcs-sss/pubs/ care-soins/2000-qual/intro_e.html, July 15, 2006.

Health Canada. (2003). *How does literacy affect the health of Canadians?* Retrieved from http://www.phac-aspc.gc.ca/ ph-sp/phdd/literacy/literacy.html.

Health Council of Canada. (2007). *Why health care renewal matters: Lessons from diabetes*. Retrieved from www.healthcouncilcanada.ca.

Hwang, S. (2001). Homelessness and health. *Canadian Medical Association Journal, 164*(2), 229–233.

Kohn, L., Corrigan, J., & Donaldson, M. (Eds.). (1999). *To err is human: Building a safer health system*. Washington, DC: Committee on Quality of Care in America, Institute of Medicine, National Academy Press.

Kohn, L., Corrigan, J., & Donaldson, M. (Eds.). (2001). *Crossing the quality chasm: A new health system for the 21st century*. Washington, DC: Committee on Quality of Care in America, Institute of Medicine, National Academy Press.

Lando, M. (2000). The framework for a successful merger. *Healthcare Executive, 15*(3), 6–11.

Leape, L. (1987). Unnecessary surgery. *Health Services Research, 24*(3), 351–407.

Lewis, S., & Kouri, D. (2004). Regionalization: Making sense of the Canadian experience. *Healthcare Papers, 5*(1), 12–31.

MacKinnon, N. J., Chow, C., Kennedy, P. L., Persaud, D. D., Metge, C. J., Sketris, I. (2004). Management competencies for Canadian health executives: Views from the field. *Healthcare Management Forum, 17*(4), 15–20.

Maddox, P. (2001). Update on national quality of care initiatives. *Nursing Economic$, 19*(3), 121–124.

Morrissey, J. (2001). Slow down: HIPAA ahead. *Modern Healthcare, 31*(1), 30.

Murphy, T., & Greco, P. (2004). Leadership's role in patient/client safety: Are we doing enough? An accreditation perspective. *Healthcare Management Forum, 17*(14): 34–35.

National Forum on Health. (1997). *Canada health action: Building on the legacy*. Ottawa: National Forum on Health.

Pinkerton, S. (2001). The future of professionalism in nursing. *Nursing Economic$, 18*(3), 130–131.

Quebec. Commission d'étude sur les services de santé et les services sociaux. (2000). *Emerging solutions: Report and recommendations*. Quebec: Commission d'étude sur les services de santé et les services sociaux. Chair: Michel Clair.

Raphael, D. (Ed.). (2004). *Social determinants of health: Canadian perspectives*. Toronto: Canadian Scholars Press Inc.

Saskatchewan. Commission on Medicare. (2001). *Caring for Medicare: Sustaining a quality system: Final report of the Commission on Medicare*. Regina: Standing Committee on Health Care. Chair: Ken Fyke.

Shortell, S. M. (1996). *Remaking health care in America: Building organized delivery systems*. San Francisco: Jossey-Bass.

Shortell, S. M., & Kaluzny, A. D. (2000). *Health care management* (4th ed.). Clifton Park, NY: Delmar Learning.

Simms, L. M., Price, S. A., & Ervin, N. E. (2000). *Professional practice of nursing administration* (3rd ed.). Clifton Park, NY: Delmar Learning.

Sinclair, D., Rochon, M. & Leatt, P. (2005). *Riding the third rail: The story of Ontario's health services restructuring commission 1996–2000*. Montreal: Institute for Research on Public Policy.

Soukup, S. M. (2000). The Center for Advanced Nursing Practice evidence-based practice model: Promoting the scholarship of practice. *Nursing Clinics of North America, 35*(2), 301–309.

Sunnak, A. (2005). LHINs: Bringing it all back home: Ontario's shift to integrated health services. *Registered Nurse Journal, 17*(4), 13–16.

Theorell, T. (2001). Stress and health: From a work perspective. In J. Dunham (Ed.), *Stress in the workplace: Past, present and future*. London: WHURR Publishers.

Wilkins, R., Berthelot, J.-M., & Ng, E. (2002). Trends in mortality by neighbourhood income in urban Canada from 1971 to 1996. *Health Reports (StatsCan), Supplement* 13, 1–28.

Wolper, I. F. (1999). *Health care administration: Planning, implementing, and managing organized delivery systems* (3rd ed.). Gaithersburg, MD: Aspen.

SUGGESTED READINGS

Agency for Healthcare Research and Quality. (2003). The effect of health care working conditions on patient safety. Retrieved from ww.ahrq.gov/clinic/epcsums/worksum.htm.

Alidina, S., Ardal, S., Lee, P., Raskin, L., Shennan, A., Young, L. M. (2006). Regionalization reigns—but is care being delivered accordingly? An evaluation of perinatal care delivery in a regionalized child health network. *Healthcare Management Forum, 19*(2), 22–26.

American Nurses Association. (1995). *Nursing's social policy statement.* Washington, DC: American Nurses Publishing.

Baldridge National Quality Program. (2000). *Health care criteria for performance excellence.* Gaithersburg, MD: Baldridge National Quality Program.

Beach, C. M., Chaykowski, R. P., & Sweetman, A. (Eds.). (2006). *Health services restructuring in Canada: New evidence and new directions.* Montreal: Institute for Research on Public Policy.

Bellack, J. P., & O'Neil, E. H. (2000). Recreating nursing practice for a new century: Recommendations and implications of the Pew Health Professions Commission's final report. *Nursing and Health Care Perspectives, 21*(1), 14–21.

Berman, S. (2000). The AMA clinical quality improvement focus on addressing patient safety. *Joint Commission Journal on Quality Improvement, 26*(7), 428–433.

Berwick, D. M. (1994). Eleven worthy aims for clinical leadership of health system reform. *Journal of the American Medical Association, 272,* 797–802.

Canadian Institute for Health Information. (2004). *Health care in Canada.* Ottawa: Canadian Institute for Health Information.

Casebeer, A., Reay, T., Golden-Biddle, K., Pablo, A., Wiebe, E., Hinings, B. (2006). Experiences of regionalization: Assessing multiple stakeholder perspectives across time. *Healthcare Quarterly, 9*(2), 32–43.

Chodos, H., & MacLeod, J. J. (2004). Romanow and Kirby on the public/private divide in healthcare: Demystifying the debate. *Healthcare Papers, 4*(4), 10–25.

Davidson, A. (2005). Advancing the population health agenda. *Healthcare Management Forum, 18*(4), 17–21.

Dienemann, J. A. (Ed.). (1998). *Nursing administration: Managing patient care* (2nd ed.). Upper Saddle River, NJ: Prentice Hall Health.

Drummond, H., & Stoddart, G. (1995). Assessment of health producing measures across different sectors. *Health Policy, 33,* 219–231.

Ellwood, P. M. (1998). Outcomes management: A technology of patient experience. *New England Journal of Medicine, 318,* 1549–1556.

Ferguson, S. L. (1999). Institute for Nursing Leadership: A new program to enhance the leadership capacity of all nurses. *Nursing Outlook, 47*(2), 91–92.

Fos, P. J., & Fine, D. J. (2000). *Designing health care for populations.* San Francisco: Jossey-Bass.

Ginsberg, E. (1996). *Tomorrow's hospital: A look to the twenty-first century.* New Haven, CT: Yale University Press.

Gosfield, A. G., & Reinertsen, J. L. (2006). The 100,000 lives campaign: Crystallizing standards of care for hospitals. *Healthcare Quarterly, 9*(3), 1–7.

Grol, R., & Grimshaw, J. (1999). Evidence-based implementation of evidence-based medicine. *Joint Commission Journal on Quality Improvement, 25*(10), 503–513.

Guadagnoli, E., Epstein, A. M., Zaslavsky, A., Shaul, J. A., Veroff, D., Fowler, F. J., Jr. et al. (2000). Providing consumers with information about the quality of health plans: The consumer assessment of health plans demonstration in Washington State. *Joint Commission Journal on Quality Improvement, 26*(7), 410–420.

Hamer, R. (1999). Goals 2000: For MDs: Managerial competency. For HMOs: Administrative retooling. *Managed Care, 8*(11), 38.

Heller, B. R., Oros, M. T., & Durney-Crowley, J. (2000). The future of nursing education: Ten trends to watch. *Nursing and Health Care Perspectives, 21*(1), 9–13.

Hurley, J. (2004). Regionalization and the allocation of healthcare resources to meet population health needs. *Healthcare Papers, 5*(1), 34–39.

Joint Commission on Accreditation of Healthcare Organizations. Healthcare at the crossroads: Strategies for addressing the evolving nursing crisis. Retrieved from http://www.jointcommission.org/NR/rdonlyres/5C138711-ED76-4D6F-909F-B06E0309F36D/0/health_care_at_the_crossroads.pdf.

Kelly, L. Y., & Joel, L. A. (1999). *Dimensions of professional nursing* (8th ed.). New York: McGraw-Hill.

Lancaster, J. (1999). *Nursing issues in leading and managing change.* St. Louis, MO: Mosby.

Lang, N. M. (1999). Discipline approaches to evidence-based practice: A view from nursing. *Joint Commission Journal on Quality Improvement, 25*(10), 539–544.

Lea, D. H., & Lawson, M. T. (2000). A practice-based genetics curriculum for nurse educators: An innovative approach to integrating human genetics into nursing curricula. *Journal of Nursing, 39*(9), 418–421.

Levine, D. (2005). A healthcare revolution: Quebec's new model of healthcare. *Healthcare Quarterly, 8*(4), 38–46.

Lindeman, C. A. (2000). The future of nursing education. *Journal of Nursing Education, 39*(1), 5–12.

Lohr, K. N., & Carey, T. S. (1999). Assessing "best evidence": Issues in grading the quality of studies for systematic reviews. *Joint Commission Journal on Quality Improvement, 25*(9), 470–479.

Lovern, E. (2001a, January 1). JCAHO's new tell-all: Standards require that patients know about below-par care. *Modern Healthcare, 31*(1), 2, 15.

Lovern, E. (2001b, May 7). Another makeover: JCAHO moves to rewrite many rules to lessen hospitals' regulatory burden. *Modern Healthcare, 31*(19), 5, 16.

Lovern, E. (2001c, May 28). Oh no, not that type of review: JCAHO singling out more hospitals for noncompliance with standards. *Modern Healthcare, 31*(22), 4–5.

McCloskey, J. C., et al. (1996). Nursing management innovations: A need for systematic evaluation. In K. C. Kelly & M. L. Maas (Eds.), *Outcomes of effective management practice* (pp. 3–19). Thousand Oaks, CA: Sage.

McLaughlin, C. P., & Kaluzny, A. D. (1999). *Continuous quality improvement in health care* (2nd ed.). Gaithersburg, MD: Aspen.

Milstead, J. A. (Ed.). (1999). *Health policy and politics: A nurse's guide* (3rd ed.). Gaithersburg, MD: Aspen.

Nelson, E. C. et al. (2000). Using data to improve medical practice by measuring processes and outcomes of care. *Joint Commission Journal on Quality Improvement, 26*(12), 667–685.

Nicklin, W., & McVeety, J. E. (2002). Canadian nurses' perceptions of patient safety in hospitals. *Canadian Journal of Nursing Leadership, 15*(3), 27–29.

Nicklin, W., & Graves, E. (2005). Nursing and patient outcomes: It's time for healthcare leadership to respond. *Healthcare Management Forum, 18*(1), 9–13.

Norton, D., & Kaplan, R. (2001). *The strategy-focused organization: How balanced scorecard companies thrive in the new business environment.* Boston: Harvard Business School Press.

O'Grady, E. (2000). Access to health care: An issue central to nursing. *Nursing Economic$, 18*(2), 88–90.

Pesut, D. J., & Rezmerski, C. J. (2000). Future think. *Nursing Outlook, 48*(1), 9.

Phipps, Shelley. (2003). *The impact of poverty on health: A scan of research literature.* Ottawa: Canadian Institute for Health Information. Retrieved from http://secure.cihi.ca/cihiweb/dispPage.jsp?cw_page=GR_323_E.

Sackett, D. L., Rosenberg, W. M. C., Gray, J. A. M., Haynes, R. B., & Richardson, W. S. (1996). Evidence-based medicine: What it is and what it isn't. *British Medical Journal, 312*(7023), 71–72.

Scobie, K. B., & Russell, G. (2003). Vision 2020, part 1: Profile of the future nurse leader. *Journal of Nursing Administration, 33*(6), 324–330.

Sinclair, D. G. (2002). Speaking with Michael Kirby. *Hospital Quarterly, 5*(4), 32–39.

Sinclair, D. G. (2004). The big thing we haven't done yet. *Healthcare Papers, 4*(4), 69–73.

Spitzer, W. O. (1998). Quality of life. In D. Burley & W. H. W. Inman (Eds.), *Therapeutic risk: Perception, measurement, and management.* New York: Wiley.

Storch, J. L. (2005). Patient safety: Is it just another bandwagon? *Canadian Journal of Nursing Leadership, 18*(2), 39–55.

Strasen, L. (1999). The silent health care revolution: The rising demand for complementary medicine. *Nursing Economic$, 17*(5), 246–256.

Sullivan, E. J. (1999). *Creating nursing's future: Issues, opportunities, and challenges.* St. Louis, MO: Mosby.

Sutherland, R., & Fulton, J. (1994). *Spending smarter and spending less: Policies and partnerships for health care in Canada.* Ottawa: The Health Group.

Taylor, D. W. (2003). 2020. healthcare management in Canada: A new model home next door. *Healthcare Management Forum, 16*(1), 6–10.

Thompson, L. J., & Martin, M. T. (2004). Integration of cancer services of Ontario: The story of getting it done. *Healthcare Quarterly, 7*(3), 42–48.

Tieman, J. (2001). Coming of age: Disease management making a case for itself clinically and financially. *Modern Healthcare, 31*(28), 26–27, 38.

Tieman, J., & Bellandi, D. (2001). HIPAA will be no holiday: Experts say exhaustive rules may require significant cultural and administrative changes. *Modern Healthcare, 31*(1), 3, 15.

Trofino, J. (1997). The courage to change: Reshaping health care delivery. *Nursing Management, 28*(11), 50–53.

Villeneuve, M., & MacDonald, J. (2006). *Toward 2020: Visions for nursing.* Ottawa: Canadian Nurses Association.

Walt, G. (1994). *Health policy: An introduction to process and power.* London and New Jersey: Zed Books.

Weatherill, S. (2004). Public/private pragmatism. *Healthcare Papers, 4*(4), 74–78.

Weeks, W. B., Hamby, L., Stein, A., & Batalden, P. B. (2000). Using the Baldridge Management System framework in health care: The Veterans Health Administration experience. *Joint Commission Journal on Quality Improvement, 26*(7), 379–387.

Wilson, L. M. (1999). Healthy people: A new millennium. Journal of Nursing Administration's Healthcare Law, Ethics, and Regulation, 1(2), 29–32.

Chapter Endnotes

1. Health Canada, "Canada Health Act Overview." Retrieved from http://www.hc-sc.gc.ca/ahc-asc/media/nr-cp/2002/2002_care-soinsbk4_e.html, April 14, 2007.

2. Health Canada, "Health Care System Federal Transfers to Provinces/Territories." Retrieved from http://www.hc-sc.gc.ca/hcs-sss/delivery-prestation/fedrole/pttransfer/index_e.html, April 14, 2007.

3. Health Canada, "Federal Transfers to Provinces/Territories." Retrieved from http://www.hc-sc.gc.ca/hcs-sss/delivery-prestation/fedrole/pttransfer/index_e.html, April 14, 2007.

4. Health Canada, "Canada Health Act: Federal Transfers and Deductions." Retrieved from http://www.hc-sc.gc.ca/hcs-sss/medi-assur/transfer/index_e.html, April 14, 2007.

5. Canadian Nurses Association, "2004 Workplace Profile of Registered Nurses in Canada." Retrieved from http://www.cna-nurses.ca/CNA/documents/pdf/publications/workforce_profile_2004_e.pdf, April 14, 2007.

6. Canadian Institute for Health Information, "What We Spend," p. 5. Retrieved from http://secure.cihi.ca/cihiweb/products/hcic2006_chap1_e.pdf, April 14, 2007

7. Ibid., p. 6.

8. Ibid., p. 9.

9. Ibid., p. 5.

10. Canadian Institute for Health Information, "About the Canadian Population Health Initiative." Retrieved from http://secure.cihi.ca/cihiweb/dispPage.jsp?cw_page=pop_health_e, August 15, 2006.

11. Public Health Agency of Canada, "The Federal Strategy, What are the responsibilities of a public health system." Retrieved from http://www.phac-aspc.gc.ca/about_apropos/federal_strategy_e.html, August 2, 2006.

12. Public Health Agency of Canada, "Frequently Asked Questions: How is the agency different from what Health Canada does now?" Retrieved from http://www.phac-aspc.gc.ca/media/nr-rp/2004/faq_e.html, August 2, 2006.

13. Public Health Agency of Canada, "Frequently Asked Questions, In what way do the National Collaborating Centres add value to the public health system in

Canada?" Retrieved from http://www.phac-aspc.gc.ca/php-psp/pdf/brief_overview.pdf, March 25, 2007.

14. Canadian Public Health Association, "About CPHA: Mission Statement." Retrieved from http://www.cpha.ca/english/inside/about/about.htm, August 2, 2006.

15. Centre for Aging, "Chronic Disease Self-Management Program History." Retrieved from http://www.coag.uvic.ca/cdsmp/cdsmp_history.htm, August 2, 2006.

16. Ibid.

17. Canadian Council on Health Services Accreditation, "Accreditation Process." Retrieved from http://www.cchsa.ca/default.aspx?page=54&cat=27, August 16, 2007.

18. Canadian Council on Health Services Accreditation, "About Accreditation." Retrieved from http://www.cchsa.ca/default.aspx?page=36&cat=27, March 25, 2007.

19. Institute for Clinical Evaluative Sciences, "Our Research." Retrieved from http://www.ices.on.ca/webpage.cfm?site_id=1&org_id=26, August 2, 2006.

20. Canadian Health Services Research Foundation, "What We Fund, Priority Themes." Retrieved from http://www.chsrf.ca/about/fund_e.php, March 25, 2007.

21. Canadian Health Services Research Foundation, "History, Funding, Services and Mission." Retrieved from http://www.chsrf.ca/about/history_e.php, March 25, 2007.

22. Canadian Health Services Research Foundation, 2006, "What's Ailing Our Nurses? A Discussion of the Major Issues Affecting Nursing Human Resources in Canada." Retrieved from http://www.chsrf.ca/research_themes/pdf/what_sailingourNurses-e.pdf, August 2, 2006.

23. Canadian Health Services Research Foundation, "About EXTRA." Retrieved from http://www.chsrf.ca/extra/overview_e.php, August 16, 2007.

24. McGillis Hall, L., Irvine Doran, D., Baker, G. R., Pink, G. H., Sidani, S., O'Brien-Pallas, L., et al. *A study of the impact of nursing staff mix models and organizational change strategies on patient, system and nurse outcomes.* Retrieved from http://www.chsrf.ca/final_research/ogc/pdf/mcgillis_report.pdf, August 2, 2006.

25. Office of the Privacy Commissioner of Canada, "Fact Sheet, Privacy Legislation in Canada." Retrieved from http://www.privcom.gc.ca/fs-fi/02_05_d_15_e.asp, March 25, 2007.

CHAPTER 2

Basic Clinical Health Care Economics

Laura J. Nosek, PhD, RN
Ida M. Androwich, PhD, RNC, FAAN
Adapted by: Heather Crawford, BScN, MEd, CHE

The Institute of Health Economics is based in Edmonton, Alberta. Its mission, as an independent, not-for-profit organization, is to deliver outstanding health economics, health outcomes, and health policy research and related services. Academia, government, and industry are present and at the table.[1]

OBJECTIVES

Upon completion of this chapter, the reader should be able to:

1. Identify three functions of a health care system.
2. Identify the health reforms related to financing, funding, and delivery.
3. Identify four main models of alternative physician remuneration.
4. Describe costing systems in health care.
5. Describe the issues surrounding the public/private debate.

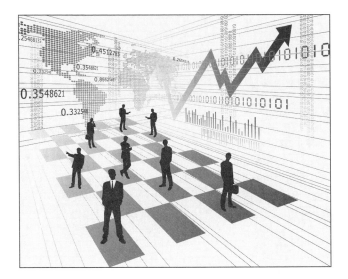

You have been struggling with progressive pain and disability in your knees. You have finally been able to access a physician, who has agreed to be your family doctor. He has suggested numerous remedies to you, but you have already tried most of them. He will set up an appointment with a specialist to determine whether you need a knee replacement. You are becoming progressively discouraged because you will have to wait an estimated seven or eight months before you will get any relief. In the meantime, you are starting to lose your ability to walk independently. However, a private clinic will afford you the ability to get sooner treatment.

What do you think is the problem?

Do you perceive the problem to be the same as the problem perceived by politicians? The economists? The physicians?

When cost is removed from the equation, what drives the decision to provide or not provide health care?

Is that driver a universal value, or is it culturally dependent?

Regardless of how expert, creative, collaborative, and altruistic a health care system may be, it cannot function without money. Over the ages, that money has flowed from varying sources, including philanthropy, volunteerism, fee-for-service, insurance, and government subsidies. Securing the bottom line is basic to achieving the mission of providing health care and is now viewed as the shared responsibility of people around the world.

We once thought that nurses needed only to be educated in the art and the science of providing clinical care to clients. Today, we recognize that nurses must be much more broadly educated. In addition to clinical care expertise, nurses must demonstrate minimal competence in the humanities, management science, and computer science, as well as be skilled in evaluating and applying new knowledge suggested by scientific research.

Canada spends significant dollars on health care on an annual basis, yet morbidity and mortality statistics, in terms of improved health outcomes, lead us to question the value that we receive for our dollars. Researchers commonly focus on life expectancy as an indicator of overall health of a population because it is a relatively reliable measure, especially when making international comparisons. For example, the United States spends considerably more on health care than Canada, but Canadians tend to live longer. In 2003, Canadians' life expectancy at birth was 79.7 years compared to the Americans' life expectancy of 77.2 years. Japan spends less than both countries, but has higher life expectancies: 84.1 years for women and 77.3 years for men.[2]

Florence Nightingale's early search for the "good" versus "mischievous" outcomes of the money spent on health care may have initiated an unspoken commitment to financial stewardship among nurses. It seems fitting, then, that all nurses are required to participate knowledgeably in designing care systems that provide the best possible care at the lowest cost (Chang, Price, & Pfoutz, 2001). Consequently, every nurse today needs to have a basic understanding of clinical health care **economics**— the study of how scarce resources are allocated among possible uses—in order to make appropriate choices among the increasingly scarce resources of the future.

The study of economics is based on three general premises: (1) scarcity—resources exist in finite quantities and consumption demand is typically greater than resource supply; (2) choice—decisions are made about which resources to produce and consume among many options; and (3) preference—individual and societal values and preferences influence the decisions that are made. In a traditional market economy, the sellers sell to the buyers who buy, with each trying to maximize their gains from the transactions. Health care does not fit well in this model. For example, consider the concept of price elasticity, which is related to the price that an individual is willing to pay for a given item. Normally, as the price goes up, the demand goes down. When the purchase is health care, however, the price may be viewed as irrelevant to the decision to purchase. Think of a wristwatch that you might always purchase for $5, but you would likely not buy at $50, and would never consider at $500. Now, imagine that instead of a wristwatch, the item in question is a medication or therapy needed to save your sick child. The consideration of price in the decision-making process is likely quite different. Thus, health care is much less "elastic" with reference to price than many other consumer goods.

Another aspect of health care's difference from the traditional economic model relates to the knowledge of options and payment mechanisms available to the consumer. In a typical market, the buyer is also the payer. In health care, the health care provider (buyer) ordering a hospitalization or treatment is a doctor or nurse. The provider is not the payer, nor is the client (buyer) using the hospital or treatment the payer. The actual **payer** is the third-party reimburser (i.e., the insurance company or government). Consequently, the financial impact of the decision on the provider (buyer) and the client user (buyer) is skewed. Neither of these buyers is the payer.

This chapter presents basic clinical health care economics concepts that are important to the novice nurse entering clinical practice. Included are perspectives on the role cost has played—and will play—in directing health care delivery, the methods for determining the cost of delivering nursing care, and the effect of health care policy on the delivery of nursing care. Recognized nurse experts provide projections for the future impact of economics on clinical nursing.

TRADITIONAL PERSPECTIVE ON THE COST OF HEALTH CARE: HEALTH CARE AS ALTRUISM

The long-standing tradition of health care is to help people achieve their optimal level of health so that they can enjoy their maximum quality of life. **Altruism,** the unselfish concern for the welfare of others, and **ethics,** the doctrine that the general welfare of society is the proper goal of an individual's actions, as opposed to **egoism,** the tendency to be self-centered or to consider only oneself and one's own interests (Agnes, 2000), drove the way health care was viewed and provided. Several early nursing leaders, including Florence Nightingale, Isabel Adams Hampton Robb, and Adelaide Nutting were members of socially prominent families instilled with the value that altruistic service was the expected role of the privileged. Such feelings of dedication to the less fortunate stemmed from medieval infirmaries established by convents and monasteries to care for the aged, orphaned, poor, and disabled. The first hospitals to care for the sick and injured were also charitable institutions established around the 14th century to provide illness care to those who did not have a home or who could not afford home care (Ross-Kerr & Wood, 2003). The people cared for in hospitals were called patients from the Latin *patiens,* meaning "to suffer" (vos Savant, 2001); *client* is used throughout the text to include all individuals who access the health care system as customers.

NEED FOR HEALTH CARE DETERMINED BY PROVIDER

Health care was traditionally delivered from a paternalistic model of governance and control. Health professionals, led by physicians, controlled a vast body of scientific knowledge and skill rendered awesome and mystical by complex scientific language. Command of that scientific knowledge and skill required extensive and expensive education and was not shared with so-called outsiders. The physician determined the type of health care that was needed, independent of the client and even independent of professional colleagues. The physician also decided how much to charge for that care. Decision making about all aspects of health care was the exclusive domain of the professionals.

Less than 40 years ago, no significant difference existed in the provision of health care in Canada and the United States. However, since 1971, the countries have proceeded in dramatically different directions. In order to prevent Canadians from having to incur the costs associated with health care, and to prevent them from being financially disadvantaged, a series of steps took place, which ultimately ended with what we now know as medicare. On the other hand, the United States still has a system of private and public health care, with more than 40 million Americans uninsured.

Esmail and Walker (2005) suggest that, based on comparative evidence, the Canadian health care model is not as good as the models in place in other countries of the Organisation for Economic Co-operation and Development (OECD) (see Table 2-1). They also state that Canada produces longer wait times, is less successful in preventing deaths that are preventable, and costs more than any of the other health systems with comparable objectives. Models that produce better results charge user fees; offer alternative, comprehensive private insurance; and include private hospitals that compete for clients. According to Esmail and Walker (2005), comparatively speaking, Canada underperforms, and needs to consider more successful models in countries that also offer their citizens universal access to health care (see Figure 2-1).

THE RIGHT TO HEALTH CARE AT ANY COST

At the beginning of the 1990s, the cost of providing health care spiralled. Health care expenditures continue to increase annually. In 2005, Canada spent approximately $142 billion on health care, or an average of $4,411 per person. After the effects of inflation are accounted for, this amount is nearly three times more than the health care spending in 1975.[3] Ten per cent of the gross domestic product (GDP) was dedicated to health care spending, a level first reached in 1992 (Canada. Statistics Canada, 2006, p. 161).

As a result of the increased costs, Canada embarked on a road of reform. Processes and organizations were reorganized, reengineered, rationalized, and redesigned. Canadian hospitals were more financially controlled than any other health sector. From 1992 to 1996, hospital expenditures per capita fell 14 percent, and resulted in

TABLE 2-1	PERFORMANCE OF HEALTH SYSTEMS IN OECD COUNTRIES

ExSum Table 1: Performance of Health Systems in OECD Countries

	Mortality Based on Population Statistics			Mortality Closely Related to the Effectiveness of Health Care				
	Healthy Life Expectancy/ Life Expectancy Rank 2001	Infant Mortality Rank 2002	Perinatal Mortality Rank 2002	Mortality Amenable to Health Care Rank 2000	Potential Years of Life Lost Rank 2000	Breast Cancer Mortality Rank 2002	Colorectal Cancer Combined Mortality Rank 2002[1]	Cumulative Rank
Australia	9	15	9	3	6	5	2	1
Sweden	2	2	8	5	2	1	9	2
Japan	1	3	2	2	3	11	4	3
Canada	22	20	12	4	8	10	2	4
Iceland	18	1	1	[12][2]	1	4	7	4
Switzerland	6	12	24	[12][2]	4	9	1	6
France	12	7	18	1	12	6	11	7
Luxembourg	2	18	16	[12][2]	7	6	6	8
Italy	9	13	9	9	9	11	5	9
Norway	6	6	15	7	5	8	14	9
Finland	11	3	3	13	10	2	14	11
Korea	27	23	5	[12][2]	21	3	7	12
Germany	5	10	11	12	11	14	12	13
New Zealand	23	24	13	11	16	13	10	14
Spain	4	5	6	6	14	21	18	15
Austria	15	7	13	14	13	16	17	16
Netherlands	12	15	23	8	15	23	16	17
United Kingdom	20	21	18	18	19	15	13	18
Greece	12	22	25	15	17	17	19	19
Belgium	8	14	20	[12][2]	18	18	20	19
Denmark	19	11	17	10	22	21	25	21
Poland	28	26	22	[12][2]	25	20	22	22
Ireland	20	18	27	17	20	24	21	23
Portugal	24	15	6	16	24	19	23	23
Czech Republic	15	9	4	[12][2]	23	25	24	25
Turkey	15	28	[13][2]	[12][2]	[19][2]	28	28	26
Slovak Republic	25	27	20	[12][2]	26	27	26	27
Hungary	25	25	26	[12][2]	27	26	27	28

Note 1: Combined mortality is the average of male and female mortality percentages.
Note 2: Not all information was available for all nations. Where data was unavailable, the rank of average values has been inserted.

Source: Esmail, N., & Walker, M. (2005). How good is Canadian health care? 2005 report: An international comparison of health care systems. Vancouver: The Fraser Institute, p. 8. Reprinted with Permission.

hospital costs falling 20 percent and hospital costs as a proportion of GDP falling from 3.8 percent to 3.0 percent (Barer, Morgan, & Evans, 2003). As a proportion of gross domestic product, hospital costs in 2002 were back where they had been in the mid-1970s—at just over 3 percent.

O'Neill and Downer (2004) write that the economic burden of health for provinces has reportedly increased from 27 percent of their total expenditures including debt charges in 1975, to 32 percent in 2000. As a result, the cost management challenge is even greater.

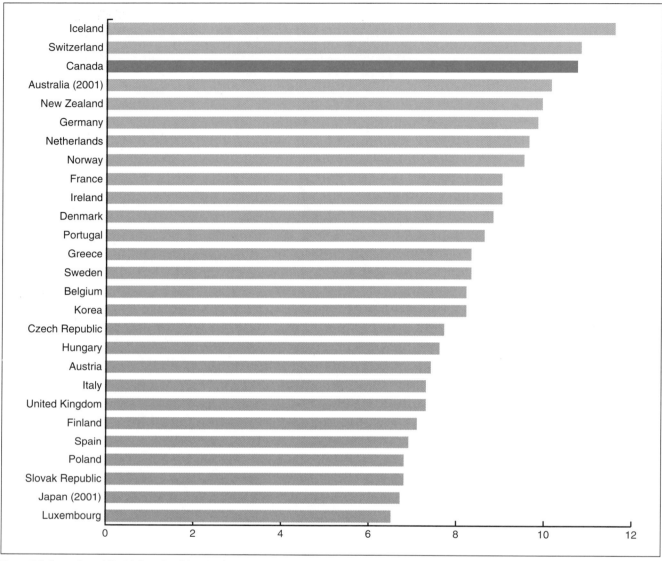

Figure 2-1 Age-adjusted Health Spending (% of GDP) in OECD Countries with Universal Access to Health Care, 2002

Source: Esmail, N., & Walker, M. (2005). How good is Canadian health care? 2005 report: An international comparison of health care systems. Vancouver: The Fraser Institute, p. 4. Reprinted with Permission.

The Canadian media took note of the cutbacks, and began to report on clients being untreated, long waiting lists, and anecdotal reports of catastrophe. Canadians began to lose confidence in their health care system. They were told that costs were escalating, but that quality of care and services was declining. At the same time, a number of provincial royal commissions and inquiries concluded that there was still room for additional rationalization and cost containment within hospital systems (Barer, Morgan, & Evans, 2003).

It didn't take long before questions were being asked about the sustainability of the Canadian health care system. In response to these concerns, a number of additional reports were commissioned.

FEDERAL AND PROVINCIAL REPORTS

The two federal reports were the Romanow Report, *Building on Values, The Future of Health Care in Canada* (Commission on the Future of Health Care in Canada, 2002), and the Kirby Report, *Reforming Health Protection and Promotion in Canada: Time to Act* (Canada. Parliament. Senate. Standing Senate Committee on Social Affairs, Science and Technology, 2002). A number of provincial reports included, from Alberta, *A Framework for Reform*, known familiarly as the Mazankowski Report (Alberta. Premier's Advisory Council on Health, 2001); Saskatchewan's *Caring for Medicare: Sustaining a Quality System*, known familiarly as the Fyke Report (Saskatchewan. Commission on

Medicare, 2001); and from Quebec, *Emerging Solutions*, known familiarly as the Clair Report (Quebec. Commission d'étude sur les services de santé et les services sociaux, 2000). These reports all varied in their recommendations, but together they set the stage for Canada's future. The two federal reports are referenced most frequently. Senator Kirby is attributed to be an advocate of privatization, whereas Romanow is a proponent of the public system.

In the early days, medicare was equated with doctors and hospitals. Although considerable change has occurred over the past 40 years, medicare is still largely organized around hospitals and doctors. Home care, however, is rapidly becoming a critical element of our health system. Not long ago, what are currently day procedures were performed in hospital and required an in-hospital stay of weeks, including convalescence. Today, medication costs are increasing, and they now represent some of the highest costs in the system. Drugs associated with some therapies are not covered by the public system, outside of hospitals, and these costs can be financially devastating for some families. This situation is incompatible with the medicare philosophy (Commission on the Future of Health Care in Canada, 2002).

Canadians want and need a more accountable health care system. Canadians do not accept that things will get better—they want to *know* that things will get better. How? According to Romanow (Commission on the Future of Health Care in Canada, 2002, p. xix), Canadians want to know what is happening with their money—with health care budgets, with hospital beds, with nurses, with doctors, with access, with wait lists, with community care, with diagnostic testing, and whether outcomes are improving. Aboriginal people and some Canadians in rural and remote parts of the country cannot always access medical services where and when they need them (Commission on the Future of Health Care in Canada 2002, p. 220). Also, some medical procedures have unacceptable wait times. These are only a few of the reasons why accountability needs to be addressed.

Accountability

Accountability was a theme of *Looking Back, Looking Forward*, (Ontario Health Services Restructuring Commission, 2000), the Romanow Report (Commission on the Future of Health Care in Canada, (2002), and the First Ministers Health Accord.[4] Shortt and Macdonald (2002) state that public discussions concerning accountability often implied that accountability was synonymous with the collection of quantifiable indicators. However, operationalizing accountability is far more complex than that, and needs to be tailored to individual relationships. According to Brown, Porcellato, and Barnsley (2006), accountability is the catchall word for Canadian health care today. Policymakers, managers, researchers, and providers all refer to accountability in a different way—from the quality of our relationships, to transparency in business dealings, to balanced budgets.

The stakeholders in Canadian health care accountability include the federal government, the provincial governments, the territorial governments, regional health authorities or their equivalents, hospitals, individual providers, physicians, and the public (Shortt & Macdonald, 2002).

Accountability instruments and processes include citizen involvement, through their involvement on boards of health care institutions or regions, or through consultation. Citizens also hold the government accountable through the electoral process. Government ministers are accountable to their legislatures for the operation of their departments. Information that increases the transparency of the government assists to make the government accountable to the people who receive the information. Some governments review the accreditation process as a form of accountability, because an external source confirms the quality of the organization's services. Licensing of professionals, by virtue of their registration, is evidence that they have met the entry-to-practice standards of their profession. Complaints committees of professional bodies will hold the professionals accountable if that is not done by the profession (Shortt & Macdonald, 2002).

In an accountability framework, stakeholder identity predominantly determines the type of relationship. See Table 2-2 for a complete list of accountability instruments associated with accountability processes.

The Province of Ontario introduced Bill 8, the Commitment to the Future of Medicare Act, in November of 2003. This bill was designed to create clear accountability and governance mechanisms between the Ministry of Health and Long-Term Care and health care providers. The hospital boards were made accountable through accountability agreements, and the hospital CEOs were made accountable for the effective and efficient management of the hospitals (Chester, Quigley, & Scott, 2004). Hospitals and the Ministry of Health and Long-Term Care differed in their opinions of Sections 26 and 27 of the bill. Those sections proposed that CEO compensation could be rolled back under certain undefined conditions, a power that was to be used only under exceptional circumstances. The accountability agreements complemented the powers of the minister of health and long-term care that then existed in the Public Hospitals Act. The bill reinforced corporate governance and structures to promote accountability by putting reliance on the accountability chain rather than bypassing it through Sections 26 and 27 (Chester, Quigley, & Scott, 2004) (see Figure 2-2).

Accountability is still a work in progress, which is evolving rapidly, with a growing acceptance of accountability by individuals who have authority. It is important that not just health care demonstrates accountability but

TABLE 2-2	ACCOUNTABILITY INSTRUMENTS ASSOCIATED WITH ACCOUNTABILITY PROCESSES

Process	Instruments
Citizen involvement	consultations board service
Political activity	elections legislature transparency
Constitutional practice	ministerial responsibility public accounts committee
Provision of information	business and strategic plans annual reports access to information
Delegated activity	independent review boards self-governing professions
Review functions	Auditor General and provincial auditors Comptroller General
Managerial functions	program evaluation guideline development report cards performance indicators quality assessment and assurance
Legal contracts	personal service contracts purchase service agreements performance agreements partnerships
Accreditation and credentialing	regional and facility accreditation professional licensing
Complaints procedures	ombudsperson client representatives professional disciplinary committees litigation
Ethical judgments	implicit social standards individual conscience laws

Source: Shortt, S. E. D., & Macdonald, J. K. (2002). Toward an accountability framework for Canadian healthcare. *Healthcare Management Forum, 15*(2), 30. Reprinted with Permission.

all jurisdictions. For an illustration of accountability in the Canadian health care system, see Figure 2-3.

FUNCTIONS OF THE HEALTH CARE SYSTEM

Three functions of the health care system were mentioned briefly in Chapter 1: financing, funding, and delivery.

The **financing** of the system refers to how health care is paid for. Because the Canadian health care system is government-financed, most money is raised in the form of taxes, including income taxes and federal and provincial sales taxes. The federal government transfers funds to the provincial and territorial governments to assist them to fund health care in the provinces and territories. In addition, equalization payments (i.e., cash transfers) are made to the provinces from the federal government in order that the less wealthy Canadian provinces have the ability to deliver government services. These payments

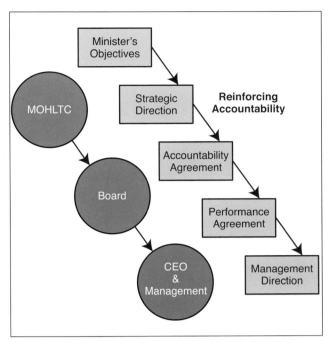

Figure 2-2 Reinforcement of Proper Relationships by Accountability Structures (Bill 8)

Source: Chester, S., Quigley, M., & Scott, G. (2004). Bill 8: Accountability and control. *Healthcare Quarterly, 7*(3), 67. Reprinted with Permission.

are unconditional, which means that the receiving provinces are able to spend the funds on public services according to their own priorities (Hibberd & Smith, 2006, p. 32)

Table 2-3 shows the estimated payments made to the provinces and territories in 2006–07. Some Canadians and/or their employers pay insurance premiums to a private insurer, such as Blue Cross. Canadians can also pay directly out-of-pocket to the health care provider. Figure 2-4 show the financial flows of the Canadian health care system.

The **funding** function of the health care system refers to the way provincial and territorial health plans pay the provider of care. The main form of funding for physicians has been **fee-for-service** (FFS). Physicians are paid separately for each service they provide. Hospitals have been funded on the basis of a global budget, which is a lump-sum payment given to the hospital, based on the number and types of cases they treat (i.e., case mix groups) or their number of client days. Public health is funded by a budget, but home care and nursing home care are funded on a fee-for-service basis or by fees per day (Hibberd and Smith, 2006, p. 33)

The **delivery** function refers to the method used to provide health care to the public. Each delivery method has operated more or less separately. For example, most health facilities have their own boards of directors, and physicians function independently, often as private entities, similar to

businesses. Although hospitals are mostly not-for-profit, some long-term care facilities operate for profit. Client prescriptions are ordered by physicians, but are funded by private insurance or by out-of-pocket expenses.

FINANCE HEALTH REFORM

Neither Kirby nor Romanow suggests changing the basic funding structure that pays for medically necessary hospital and doctor services. User fees and co-payments were still against the principles of the 1984 Canada Health Act. However, finance reform is currently being considered in a number of ways. Some procedures previously covered by health insurance are no longer covered; for example, some provinces no longer cover the cost of circumcision or routine eye exams for a percentage of the population. These de-insured services are no longer considered necessary. Variations also exist in the services that are insured from province to province.

FUNDING HEALTH REFORM

Physician remuneration is the second largest component of public sector health expenditures in Canada. Hospital services are the largest. Recently, according to the 2004 National Physician Survey, about half of family physicians would like to change the way they are compensated. The majority of physicians receive their income from fee-for-service payments. However, the past 10 years has seen a shift towards alternative payment schemes (Devlin, Sarma, & Hogg, 2006). Determining how physicians should be remunerated is not easy. For example, how many minutes should be allocated by a physician to assess a client's condition? How much time does the client think the physician should spend in conversation? Is the social nature of the client's situation important? Does it have an impact on the physical state the client presents? Both the physician and the client have different perspectives and different pieces of information that may affect the treatment being considered. What is the right balance, and how much money should be paid? The client and the government are unable to determine the appropriate quantity and quality of care for a particular condition, and must rely on the physician's advice (Devlin, Sarma, & Hogg, 2006). Physician payment schemes provide a powerful tool to align the preferences of physicians, clients, and insurers (i.e., the government) to produce the best possible health outcomes (Devlin, Sarma, & Hogg, 2006). Figure 2-5 depicts how government choices affect decisions made by physicians, which in turn, influence clients' (patients') choices.

Physician remuneration in Canada has four main models: fee-for-service, capitation, salary, and blended payments. In the fee-for-service (FFS) model, physicians are paid for each unit of service provided to clients. Physicians are able to deliver more services if they reduce the length of time for their consultations. Fee-for-service payments lead to higher use of primary care services than do

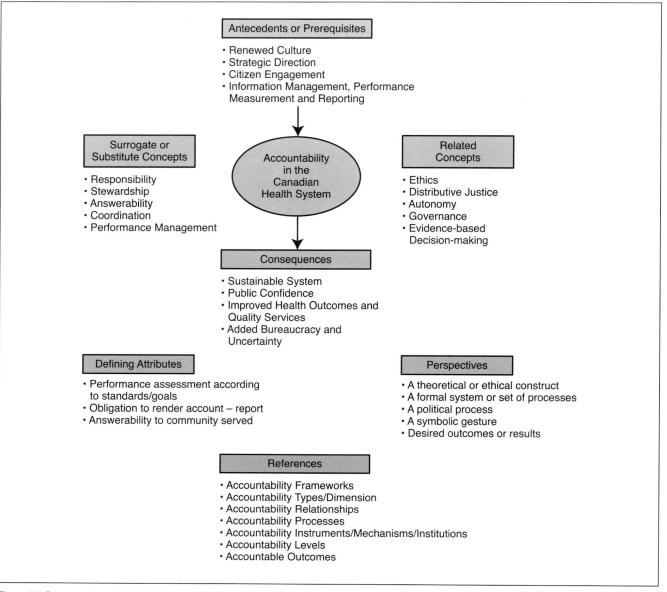

Figure 2-3 Summary: What is Accountability in the Canadian Health System?

Source: Penney, C. (2004). Understanding accountability in the Canadian health system. *Healthcare Management Forum, 17*(2), 10. Reprinted with Permission.

other forms of physician payment. Devlin et al. (2006) state that health care utilization, defined as per-capita consultations, is higher with FFS than with either capitation or a blended payment scheme.

Most provinces fund regions through a global budget. Annually, each region submits a plan that articulates how it will meet the health needs of its residents. The resource requirements and performance evaluation measures are also included. Minor revisions are usually made from year to year. According to Hurley (2004), almost all provinces had declared their intent to develop a needs-based funding formula for allocating the budget to regional health authorities. Ontario, Alberta, Saskatchewan, and British

Columbia have all adopted such a formula for home care and community support services.

Many organizational leaders are aware of the importance of including physicians as managers, or if not as managers, then at least as contributors to their governance activities. However, Harrison and Mitton (2004) believe that **program budgeting and marginal analysis (PBMA)** is a mechanism that can link physicians to organizational decision-making processes. Physicians' knowledge and expertise in client care make their input into organizational processes imperative. These authors highlighted the Alberta experience, particularly in the Calgary Health Region.

TABLE 2-3	ESTIMATED TRANSFER PAYMENTS (CANADA HEALTH TRANSFER, CANADA SOCIAL TRANSFER, AND EQUALIZATION), 2006–2007	
Province or Territory	**Amount Paid (in Billions of Dollars)**	**Amount Paid per Capita (in dollars)**
Nunavut	0.874	28,458
Northwest Territories	0.804	19,244
Yukon	0.554	17,777
Prince Edward Island	0.474	3,428
New Brunswick	2.5	3,290
Nova Scotia	2.7	2,867
Manitoba	3.4	2,861
Newfoundland	1.4	2,687
Quebec	16.7	2,181
British Columbia	7.0	1,619
Ontario	19.4	1,545
Saskatchewan	1.5	1,545
Alberta	5.2	1,544

Source: Department of Finance, Canada, "Federal Transfers to Provinces and Territories." Retrieved from http://www.fin.gc.ca/FEDPROV/mtpe.html, April 15, 2007. Reprinted with permission of the Minister of Public Works and Government Services Canada, 2007.

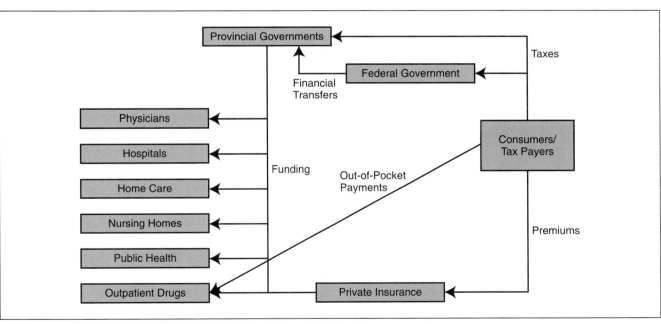

Figure 2-4 Flow of Funds in the Traditional Health Care System in Canada

Source: From Judith M. Hibberd & Donna Lynn Smith, *Nursing Leadership and Management in Canada,* 3rd edition (Figure 2.2 from p. 32). Copyright © Elsevier Canada, a division of Reed Elsevier Canada, Ltd. All rights reserved. Reprinted by permission of Elsevier Canada, 2007.

Harrison and Mitton (2004, p. 22) identify the stages involved in PBMA:

1. Determine the aim and scope of the priority setting exercise.
2. Compile a program budget.
3. Form a stakeholder advisory panel.

4. Determine relevant decision-making criteria and consultation required.
5. Advisory panel identifies options for service growth, resource release for producing the same outcome with fewer resources, or resource release through scaling back or stopping some services.

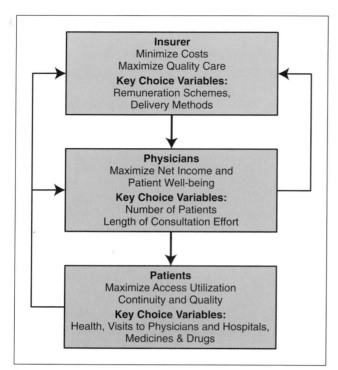

Insurer
Minimize Costs
Maximize Quality Care
Key Choice Variables:
Remuneration Schemes,
Delivery Methods

Physicians
Maximize Net Income and
Patient Well-being
Key Choice Variables:
Number of Patients
Length of Consultation Effort

Patients
Maximize Access Utilization
Continuity and Quality
Key Choice Variables:
Health, Visits to Physicians and Hospitals,
Medicines & Drugs

Figure 2-5 Interactions among the Key Players in the Canadian Health
Care System

Source: Devlin, R.A., Sarma, S. & Hogg, W. (2006). Remunerating primary
care physicians: Emerging directions and policy options for Canada.
Healthcare Quarterly, 9(3), 36. Reprinted with Permission.

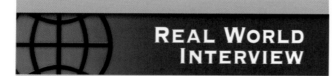

REAL WORLD INTERVIEW

I accompanied my mother to her doctor's appointment.
She asked me to advocate on her behalf because her
physician had told her that she could only present
one issue to ask him about at each visit. On this particular day, she had two issues, and was worried that she
would have to visit the doctor again in the near future.
When I arrived at the physician's office, a sign in the
waiting room confirmed my mother's concern. The sign
stated that only one issue could be discussed with the
doctor per visit. I accompanied my mother into the
doctor's office, and he told us that she would need to
decide which issue was the priority. I was mortified!

Helen Salter, RN

6. Advisory panel recommends funding growth areas
with new resources, decisions to move resources
from one area to another, or to trade-off decisions
to move resources to another service if proof is
demonstrated.

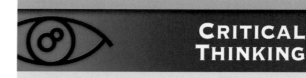

CRITICAL THINKING

Is the physician practice appropriate? Should it be different for the young and elderly?

Given the circumstances in this example, what would
you have done?

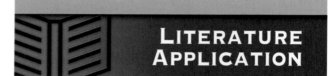

LITERATURE APPLICATION

Citation: Sarre-McGregor, D., & Knoefel, F. D. (2005).
Lessons learned: The implementation of an alternative
funding plan at SCO Health Service in Ottawa. *Healthcare Management Forum, 18*(4), 46–49.

Discussion: The authors describe the Alternative Funding Plan agreement that the physicians of SCO Health
Service, in Ottawa, entered into with the Ministry of
Health and Long-Term Care. The negotiation and process
for establishing the plan are described. Lessons learned
are also outlined.

Implications: Physicians have supported the concept,
and will probably renew the contract when it expires in
2006. Others may wish to take advantage of a similar
scheme, or adapt the process used in this example.

7. Use evidence from a variety of sources to make final
decisions to inform budget planning process.

The PMBA approach was successful in six of the
seven examples cited in the study. The case studies included urban, regional, and rural centres with pediatric,
medical surgical, and acute and chronic care populations. As a result of physician involvement in this budgeting process, the importance of having both medical and
managerial representatives was recognized. If the physicians had not been involved, the participants didn't think
they would have been as successful. Improvement in communication among the medical groups with managers
was noted. This type of budgeting can be used even if the
relationship between the region and the physicians is not
aligned. It was reinforced that if managers ask physicians
for their opinion, the managers must be prepared to listen.

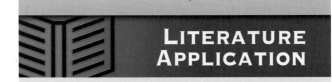

LITERATURE APPLICATION

Citation: O'Neill, M. L., & Downer, P. (2004). Change readiness for SAP in the Canadian healthcare system. *Healthcare Management Forum, 17*(1), 18–25.

Discussion: The study described in this article contributes to the literature that assesses whether the Canadian health care system is ready to embrace the idea of e-business cost management systems. One hundred fifty-four Canadian chief executive officers were surveyed to determine change readiness. A deductive design methodology was used. Although the majority of the CEOs had no e-business cost management system experience, the majority were interested in the concept. Change readiness was found to affect system implementation significantly.

Implications: More information is required as the Canadian health care system considers e-business cost management implementation. The authors recommend that consideration should be given to the development of national performance indicators in this area.

In addition, the physicians were able to learn more about resource allocation, and the impact of shifts in resources on the client population being served. With this type of budgeting, physicians are able to contribute to their health care organizations in a way that allows them to use their clinical expertise, but that doesn't require them to give up their clinical practice.

In this era of increased efficiency, it is important for Canada's health care organizations to understand the costs associated with client care. Many Canadian hospitals are meeting their need for client-specific financial information by using costs based on resource intensity weights (RIWs), which are calculated by the Canadian Institute of Health Information (CIHI), instead of using an in-house case-costing system.

Activity-based costing (ABC) has been recommended as a way to achieve better management accounting information in health care. **Case-costing** systems are a way of operationalizing the ABC concepts. However, because of the expense involved, many hospitals have opted to use the RIW costs. Activity-based costing was developed to improve the way indirect costs were assigned to hospital departments (for example, how does one assign the costs of the human resources department to the emergency department?). The traditional client accounting system allocated the costs of the human resources department

equally to all direct care departments. In activity-based costing, however, the costs of human resources are shared by the direct care departments based on either square footage or the number of employees. The ABC approach, therefore, required increased definition and specificity, such as types and cost of supplies per procedure. The Guidelines for Management Information Systems in Canadian Health Service Organizations (MIS Guidelines) specify the use of simultaneous equations for hospital costing systems because that method meets the theoretical requirement of accounting for the services that indirect departments provide to each other (Borsa & Anis, 2005, p. 21).

Borsa and Anis (2005) compared resource intensity weight costs at St. Paul's Hospital in British Columbia, with case costs for selected client groups, and found that average case costs for surgical clients were 23.9 percent higher than their resource intensity weight costs, whereas the case costs for non-surgical clients were 14.8 percent lower. Average case costs for clients receiving surgical implants were 32.8 percent higher than the resource intensity weight costs. For clients receiving internal defibrillators, average case costs were three times higher.

Borsa and Anis (2005) conclude that the national RIW assignment process in Canada has the potential to provide valuable information for resource benchmarking and provincial funding, but the results of their analysis suggested that further work is needed in order to align the measures with actual resource consumption.

DELIVERY HEALTH REFORM

The main type of reform referred to here is privatization. Much debate and confusion surrounds public–private partnerships in Canada. Romanow didn't recommend any changes to the tax-based funding source for Canada Health Act services. Kirby put forward some ideas concerning user fees and private insurance, but his final report rejected anything other than tax-based methods to fund Canada Health Act services. Marchildon (2004) suggested that the question is really whether private for-profit delivery should replace private not-for-profit or public arm's-length delivery in three situations. The first situation he described relates to contracting out of ancillary services, such as food and laundry services, to existing private, for-profit services. The second context concerns the public–private partnerships (P3s) in the building of new health facilities, which are known in the United Kingdom as private finance initiatives (PFIs). The possibility of private delivery of advanced diagnostic services by First Nations on urban reserves or reserves near large urban centres has raised a third private-delivery issue. Because provincial laws and regulations have no jurisdiction on reserves, the potential to have a parallel private-for-profit alternative to the public system exists. In addition, the legal status of the Canada Health Act on

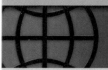

An early focus for interest in public/private partnerships is the "P3" approach to facility construction and operation, and in this area we have had particular success. In the long-term sector, all our new facilities are being built and operated on an award-winning tendering and partnership model. We've opened nearly 300 beds in the past year and are planning another 1.000 beds by 2010. Projects are tendered on equal terms to public, voluntary, and for-profit operators. Operators are full partners in planning and designing their own facilities, instead of taking over buildings designed by the regions or government. They share in the capital costs and then receive standard formula-based operating funding from the region.

The result is that we've built twice as many beds as we could have on the old model. That has enabled us to cut the waiting list for long-term care to less than two months' average turnover, and cut the number of acute care beds blocked by patients awaiting placement by half in the past year. Just as important, we've seen a remarkable leap forward in the design of our facilities and the quality of life for residents. All our new facilities are designed on the aging-in-place model, coordinated with commercial housing, enabling a continuum of service levels and living environments according to need.

With our experience in long-term care, we're looking at the potential for P3s to deliver the same kinds of benefits in other areas.

Sheila Weatherill
President and CEO Capital Health, Edmonton, Alberta

Source: Weatherill, S. (2004). Public/private pragmatism. *Healthcare Papers, 4*(4), 74–78. Reprinted with Permission.

First Nations' territories is also questioned (Marchildon, 2004, p. 67).

Alberta has led the way with privately owned clinics and hospitals, but other provinces have also launched similar services. The April 13, 2006 newsweekly, *Health Edition*, reported that Quebec has decided to implement public–private partnerships to build two new multibillion-dollar hospitals in Montreal, but that the province is scaling down private sector involvement in order to maximize public control. Ontario is also using private capital as part of its $5 billion overhaul of health care infrastructure. Some 29 separate projects have been announced so far using "alternative financing and procurement" arrangements (Health Edition, 2006). Negotiations for P3 contracts can take up to two years to complete.

FUTURE PERSPECTIVE ON THE COST OF HEALTH CARE

Futurists are in demand to guide health care to organize for success. Health care providers have been thrashing in chaos for nearly 20 years, reinventing their structures and processes, right-sizing their enterprises, outsourcing to better focus on their core business, and merging to share scarce or expensive resources. Despite some short-term cost savings and a slowdown in the rise in health care spending, several evolving trends keep the overall cost growing.

The need for highly complex and expensive technology, including microsurgery, continues to develop. New diseases that require expensive or long-term treatment, such as AIDS and Ebola, continue to emerge. With the eradication or successful management of selected diseases, such as tuberculosis, populations are surviving longer. With lengthening survival rates come debilitating diseases of aging.

We look to futurists to help us make decisions about the business we ought to be prepared to provide. Will the Veterans Affairs hospitals go out of business when all the veterans with illness or injuries related to their military service and all the indigent veterans die? Will a few strategically located hospitals provide only an intensive level of care, while acute care is managed on an ambulatory basis without invasive procedures? Will preventive, primary, and restorative care be the purview of advanced nurse practitioners practising in community sites? Will the call for duty no longer be the basis for caring careers (Reverby, 2001)? Will nurses be ordered to care in a society that no longer values caring (Reverby, 1987)?

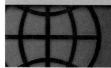

REAL WORLD INTERVIEW

The age of "volume" as a measure of anything is long past. In health care, for so many years, the notion of unparalleled growth and expansion and anything for anyone was common. Subsequent introduction of broader concepts reflecting an understanding of value and sustainability now drive rational thinking about availability and delivery of health services. The issue of "value" now drives all elements of health service from access to delivery and, ultimately, to making a difference. Now we can more clearly enumerate the relationship between inputs and outcomes, process and product. Health services now must be able to establish the connection between what is done and what is achieved. Professions' addictions to what they do now give way to tightening the connection between what is done and what difference it makes. The noise for both nurses and physicians is a closer look by everyone at the "value" of action in the light of the promise it holds. The issue: either deliver, or rethink why you're doing what you're doing. This critical examination and expectation will radically alter the economics and values of health care for the next two decades.

Tim Porter-O'Grady, EdD, PhD, RN, FAAN
Prolific Nurse Author and Speaker on New-Edge Health Care

KEY CONCEPTS

- Health care economics is grounded in past values and culture. Nearly 150 years ago, Florence Nightingale recognized that the resources being used to care for sick people ought to be tracked and analyzed to improve clinical and business outcomes.

- In Canada, the health care system has three main functions: financing, funding, and delivery. Reform is taking place in each of these areas.

- Most physicians wish to be remunerated in a way other than fee-for-service.

- All jurisdictions, including health care, need to demonstrate accountability.

- There is much debate about public–private partnerships.

KEY TERMS

accountability	ethics
altruism	fee-for-service
blended payment schemes	financing
capitation	funding
case-costing	payer
delivery	program budgeting and
economics	marginal analysis
egoism	salary

REVIEW QUESTIONS

1. Economics is the study of
   A. the cost:quality interface.
   B. cost accounting.
   C. the cost of doing business.
   D. how to manage scarce resources.

2. Which of the following nurse leaders was *not* mentioned in this chapter as having a perspective on economics?
   A. Abdellah
   B. Chang
   C. Barton
   D. Henderson

REVIEW ACTIVITIES

1. Interview the chief financial officer of a health care organization to gain an understanding of how various costs are managed. Use the following questions to guide the interview:

   What method is used to measure nursing costs?

   What level of confidence does financial services have in its accuracy, and why?

2. Consult a seasoned member of the medical staff of a health care organization. Ask for a personal perspective on any adjustments in practice that person made relating to cost and quality issues as his or her career unfolded. Compare and contrast what you discover to the experiences of a second medical staff person who has been in

practice for only the past 10 years. What level of passion about the discussion was demonstrated by each intervie-wee? What did they view as their greatest challenge?

3. Explore with a chief nursing officer the most challenging clinical economic issue currently for nursing in the organization and how it is being addressed.

EXPLORING THE WEB

- What sites could you recommend to a colleague interested in tracking health care cost trends over time?

- Go to the site for the Institute of Health Economics: *http://www.ihe.ca*

- Go to the site for The Centre for Health and Policy Studies (CHAPS): *http://www.chaps.ucalgary.ca*

- How does the information differ from the first site?

- Go to the site for the Canadian Institute for Health Information (CIHI): *http://www.cihi.ca*

- What statistics does the site offer?

- Go to a site designed for nurses, such as the Canadian Nurses Association: *http://www.cna-nurses.ca*

- What type of information is available on the site?

- Is it relevant to cost or quality issues?

- Search the following websites for information of interest to nurses:

- *http://www.nurseone-inf-fusion.ca/splash.html*

- *http://www.cna-iic.ca/CNA/documents/pdf/publications/ BG8_Social_Determinants_e.pdf*

- *http://www.rnao.org/Page.asp?PageID=861& SiteNodeID=133*

- *http://www.cadth.ca/*

- *http://www.gaiam.com/*

- *http://www.coachorg.com/*

REFERENCES

Agnes, M. (2000). (Ed.). *Webster's new world collegiate dictionary* (4th ed.). Foster City, CA: IDG Books Worldwide.

Alberta. Premier's Advisory Council on Health. (2001). *A framework for reform: Report of the premier's advisory council on health.* Edmonton: Premier's Advisory Council on Health. Chair: Donald Mazankowski.

Barer, M. L., Morgan, S. G., & Evans, R. G. (2003). Strangulation or rationalization: Costs and access in Canadian hospitals. *Longwoods Review, 1*(4), 10–19.

Borsa, J., & Anis, A. (2005). The cost of hospital care in Canada: A comparison of two alternatives. *Healthcare Management Forum, 18*(1), 19–27.

Brown, A. D., Porcellato, C., & Barnsley, J. (2006). Accountability: Unpacking the suitcase. *Healthcare Quarterly, 9*(3), 72–75.

Canada. Parliament. Senate. Standing Committee on Social Affairs, Science and Technology. (2002). *Reforming health protection and promotion in Canada: Time to act.* Ottawa: Standing Committee on Social Affairs, Science and Technology. Chair: Michael Kirby.

Canada. Statistics Canada. (2006). *Canada year book 2006.* Ottawa: Statistics Canada.

Chang, C., Price, S., & Pfoutz, S. (2001). *Economics and nursing: Critical professional issues.* Philadelphia: F. A. Davis.

Chester, S., Quigley, M., & Scott, G. (2004). Bill 8: Accountability and control. *Healthcare Quarterly, 7*(3), 66–68.

Commission on the Future of Health Care in Canada. *Building on Values: The Future of Health Care in Canada.* Saskatoon: Commission on the Future of Health Care in Canada, 2002. Commissioner: Roy J. Romanow.

Devlin, R. A., Sarma, S., & Hogg, W. (2006). Remunerating primary care physicians: Emerging directions and policy options for Canada. *Healthcare Quarterly, 9*(3), 34–42.

Esmail, N., & Walker, M. (2005). *How good is Canadian health care? 2005 report: An international comparison of health care systems.* Vancouver: The Fraser Institute.

Gillani, A., Jarvi, K., & De Angelis, A. (2005). Fostering a culture of accountability through a performance appraisal system. *Healthcare Management Forum, 18*(1), 35–38.

Griffith, J. (1999). *The well-managed health care organization* (4th ed.). Chicago: Health Administration Press.

Harrison, A., & Mitton, C. (2004). Physician involvement in setting priorities for health regions. *Healthcare Management Forum, 17*(4), 21–27.

Health Edition. (2006) Quebec embracing P3s for new hospital projects. *Health Edition*, March 31.

Hibberd, J. M., & Smith, D. L. (2006). *Nursing leadership and management in Canada* (3rd Ed.). Toronto: Elsevier Mosby.

Hurley, J. (2004). Regionalization and the allocation of healthcare resources to meet population health needs. *Healthcare Papers, 5*(1), 34–39.

Marchildon, G. P. (2004). The public/private debate in the funding, administration and delivery of healthcare in Canada. *Healthcare Papers, 4*(4), 61–68.

O'Neill, M. L., & Downer, P. (2004). Change readiness for SAP in the Canadian healthcare system. *Healthcare Management Forum, 17*(1), 18–25.

Ontario Health Services Restructuring Commission. (2000). *Looking back, looking forward: A legacy report.* Toronto: Ontario Health Services Restructuring Commission.

Penney, C. (2004). Understanding accountability in the Canadian health system. *Healthcare Management Forum, 17*(2), 9–15.

Quebec. Commission d'étude sur les services de santé et les services sociaux. (2000). *Emerging solutions: Report and recommendations.* Quebec: Commission d'étude sur les services de santé et les services sociaux. Chair: Michel Clair.

Reverby (1987) Ordered to care: *The dilemma of American nursing, 1850–1945.* New York: Cambridge.

Reverby, S. (2001). A caring dilemma: Womanhood and nursing in historical perspective. In E. Hein (Ed.), *Nursing issues in the 21st century: Perspectives from the literature.* Philadelphia: Lippincott.

Ross-Kerr, J., & Wood, M. J. (2003). *Canadian nursing issues and perspectives* (4th ed.). Toronto, Philadelphia, London, New York, St. Louis, Sydney: Mosby.

Saskatchewan. Commission on Medicare. (2001). *Caring for Medicare: Sustaining a quality system: Final report of the Commission on Medicare.* Regina: Standing Committee on Health Care. Chair: Ken Fyke.

Shortt, S. E. D., & Macdonald, J. K. (2002). Toward an accountability framework for Canadian healthcare. *Healthcare Management Forum, 15*(2), 24–32.

vos Savant, M. (2001, May 6). Ask Marilyn, *Parade*, 26.

Weatherill, S. (2004). Public/private pragmatism. *Healthcare Papers, 4*(4), 74–78.

SUGGESTED READINGS

Bégin, M. (2004). Public/private boundaries in Canadian healthcare: Some clarification. *Healthcare Papers, 4*(4), 35–40.

Chodos, H., & MacLeod, J. J. (2004). Romanow and Kirby on the public/private divide in healthcare: Demystifying the debate. *Healthcare Papers, 4*(4), 10–25.

Christensen, C., Bohmer, R., & Kenagy, J. (2000, September/October). Will disruptive innovations cure health care? *Harvard Business Review*, 102–112, 199.

Christman, L. (2001). The future of the nursing profession. In E. Hein (Ed.), *Nursing issues in the 21st century: Perspectives from the literature.* Philadelphia: Lippincott.

Copeland, T. (2001, September/October). Cutting costs without drawing blood. *Harvard Business Review*, 155–156, 159–160, 162, 164.

Feldstein, P. (1993). *Health care economics* (5th ed.). Clifton Park, NY: Delmar Learning.

Finkler, S. (2001). *Budgeting concepts for nurse managers* (3rd ed.). Philadelphia: Saunders.

Finkler, S., & Kovner, C. (2000). *Financial management for nurse managers and executives* (2nd ed.). Philadelphia: Saunders.

Friedman, E. (2001). Managed care devils, angels, and the truth in between. In E. Hein (Ed.), *Nursing issues in the 21st century: Perspectives from the literature.* Philadelphia: Lippincott.

Hein, E. (2001). *Nursing issues in the 21st century: Perspectives from the literature.* Philadelphia: Lippincott.

Hoppszallern, S. (2001, January). 2001 benchmarking guide. *Hospitals and Health Networks*, 43–50.

Institute of Medicine. (1990). *Medicare: A strategy for quality assurance.* K. N. Lohr (Ed.). Washington, DC: National Academy Press.

Kenny, N. (2004). Value(s) for money? Assessing Romanow and Kirby. *Healthcare Papers, 4*(4), 28–34.

McCullough, C. (2001). *Creating responsive solutions to healthcare change.* Indianapolis, IN: Sigma Theta Tau International.

McGowan, T. (2004). Does the private sector have a role in Canadian healthcare? *Healthcare Papers, 4*(4), 45–50.

McLean, R. (1997). *Financial management in health care.* Clifton Park, NY: Delmar Learning.

Pink, G. H., Brown, A. D., Daniel, I., Hamlette, M. L., Markel, F., McGillis Hall, L. et al. (2006). Financial benchmarks for Ontario hospitals. *Healthcare Quarterly, 9*(1), 40–45.

Rachlis, M. M. (2005). Medicare: Innovation is the key to sustainability? *Healthcare Management Forum, 18*(1), 28–31.

Rowland, H., & Rowland, B. (1997). *Nursing administration handbook* (4th ed.). Gaithersburg, MD: Aspen.

Sarre-McGregor, D., & Knoefel, F. D. (2005). Lessons learned: The implementation of an alternative funding plan at SCO Health Service in Ottawa. *Healthcare Management Forum, 18*(4), 46–49.

Savage, G., Hoelscher, M., & Walker, E. (1999). International health care: A comparison of the United States, Canada, and Western Europe. In L. Wolper (Ed.), *Health care administration: Planning, implementing, and managing organized delivery systems* (3rd ed). Gaithersburg, MD: Aspen.

Senge, P. M. (2006). *The fifth discipline: The art & practice of the learning organization.* Toronto: Doubleday.

Shamian, J., & Lightstone, E. (1997). Hospital restructuring initiatives in Canada. *Medical Care, 35*(10), 0S62–0S69.

Taylor, W. (2003). 2020 healthcare management in Canada: A new model home next door. *Healthcare Management Forum, 16*(1), 6–10.

Vertesi, L. (2004). Romanow versus Kirby: Resolving the differences. *Healthcare Papers, 4*(4), 41–44.

CHAPTER ENDNOTES

1. Institute of Health Economics, "Mission Statement." Retrieved from http://www.ihe.ca, August, 8, 2006.

2. Statistics Canada, "Life Expectancy for Overall Population." Retrieved from http://www.statcan.ca/english/freepub/82-401-XIE/2002000/considerations/hlt/36ahlt.htm#top, April 14, 2007.

3. Canadian Institute for Health Information, "What We Spend." Retrieved from http://secure.cihi.ca/cihiweb/products/hcic2006_chap1_e.pdf, August 16, 2006.

4. Health Canada, "First Ministers Health Accord." Retrieved from http://www.hc-sc.gc.ca/hcs-sss/delivery-prestation/fptcollab/2003accord/fs-if_1_e.html, July 30, 2007.

UNIT II
A New Health Care Model

CHAPTER
3

Evidence-Based Practice

Rinda Alexander, PhD, RN, CS
Adapted by: Victoria E. Pennick, RN, MHSc

The practice of evidence-based medicine means integrating individual clinical expertise with the best available external clinical evidence from systematic research.
(David L. Sackett, William M. C. Rosenberg, J. A. Muir Gray, R. Brian Haynes, & W. Scott Richardson, 1996)

OBJECTIVES

Upon completion of this chapter, the reader should be able to:

1. Understand the history of evidence-based practice in nursing.
2. Discuss the importance of evidence-based practice.
3. Identify terminology used in research and evidence-based practice.
4. Understand the issues that stimulated the development of an evidence-based practice model for health care delivery.
5. Understand the steps used in evidence-based practice processes.
6. Understand the roles of Canadian organizations in the funding, creation, and dissemination of research to inform evidence-based decision making at the individual, organizational, and policy levels.

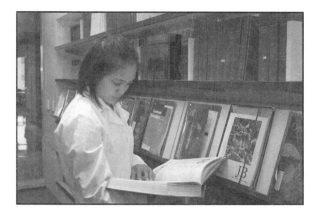

You are at the Nurses' Week luncheon at your institution. Your unit manager and the nursing director to whom she reports stop to chat with you. They say they are concerned about the lack of client-centred care they are observing on some of the units. This variability is affecting client outcomes and was identified as an area for improvement in the client satisfaction section of the recent Hospital Report (OHA Hospital Reports). They have heard about the Registered Nurses' Association of Ontario (RNAO) Nursing Best Practice Guideline on Client-Centred Care and ask you to sit on a task force to see how this guideline can be implemented at the hospital.

This scenario is becoming more common in health care institutions as managers of care explore new ways to improve the quality of care.

What do you know about evidence-based practice?

As the staff nurse, how will you prepare yourself for this task?

As the manager, how will you facilitate the implementation of the Best Practice Guideline?

Many professionals, and society in general, accept the position that nurses are the coordinators of care within institutions. However, as the new health care system continues to evolve, nurses must consider new ways to deliver more effective and efficient interventions. In fact, no greater challenge for nursing exists than ensuring that we have the competencies needed in the 21st century for health care delivery. Nursing leaders and managers are particularly well positioned to ensure that health care organizations have resources and processes in place that enable professional nurses to meet new challenges in the clinical delivery of care. Evidence-based decision making is an important element of quality care in all domains of nursing practice. It is essential to optimize outcomes for clients, improve clinical practice, achieve cost-effective nursing care, and ensure accountability and transparency in decision making (Canadian Nurses Association, 2002). The purpose of this chapter is to discuss the importance of evidence-based practice both to clients and to nursing and to define what constitutes

evidence for clinical practice. Evidence-based decision making is the trend of today. Future trends in health care will require the use of sophisticated evidence-based tools to deliver care and to measure outcomes of care. This trend suggests that nursing must become more comfortable with using a scientific process driven by evidence-based standards and practice guidelines, while also emphasizing continuing quality improvement.

HISTORY OF EVIDENCE-BASED PRACTICE

The evidence-based movement began with medicine. The term **evidence-based medicine** was coined at McMaster University's School of Medicine, in Hamilton, Ontario, during the 1980s. It referred to a clinical learning strategy that had been in use at McMaster University since the 1970s (Evidence-Based Medicine Working Group, 1992). David Sackett, well known in the evidence-based medicine movement, along with his Oxford colleagues, encouraged evidence-based medicine as a way to integrate individual clinical medical experience with external clinical evidence, using a systematic research approach. Sackett and his colleagues defined evidence-based medicine as the "conscientious, explicit, and judicious use of current best evidence in making decisions about the care of individual patients" (1996, p. 71). Evidence-based medicine integrates the clinical expertise of individual clinicians with the best available external clinical evidence from systematic research into the accuracy and precision of diagnostic tests; the clinical examination; and other elements of the therapeutic, rehabilitative, and preventive regimens prescribed for clients.

But health care decision making extends beyond medicine. Before long, the term **evidence-based practice** was coined. It was considered a more encompassing and neutral term that incorporated evidence-based medicine with **evidence-based care**: a blend of the beliefs, values, and attitudes of clients, families, and practitioners, with the most current knowledge of incidence and prevalence of the health care problem at hand and an understanding of the organization and delivery of health care (Silagy & Haines, 1998). Evidence-based clinical decision making should incorporate consideration of the client's clinical state, the clinical setting, and the clinical circumstances (DiCenso, Guyatt, & Ciliska, 2004). In Canada, we have different health care systems in each provincial and territorial jurisdiction, each representing vast areas with scant populations, large urban areas, and the most heterogeneous population in the world. Client expectations and available resources vary widely from setting to setting. Guidelines and care plans, which are based on the best

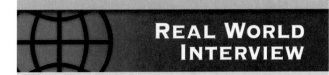

Vicki: Did you ever practise what you would consider to be evidence-based nursing?

Mark: It was my wish to try to grapple with "what should we do" that led me to try to find a way of knowing. I did postgrad training in psychoanalytic theory and practice, which led me to know some things differently, but not in a way that was useful beyond the clinical consultation. I then did a master's in sociology, which again gave me a different way of looking at things and putting things together, but it was only later, when I came across epidemiology and the true concept of fair test that I knew I had found the way of being able to show that something worked or didn't work. So, whilst there were attempts to put some understanding to practice and identify what we should be doing, it was much later that I came across the tools to be able to deal with "here is the language you need to describe it."

Vicki: How did you get involved?

Mark: I started a unit research group and led journal clubs of the inpatient staff and undertook the training of staff in inpatient psychotherapy. None of it was really evidence-based, but used similar tools to evidence-based methods, just without the underpinning of critical appraisal.

Mark Fenton, RN
Cochrane Schizophrenia Review Group

current evidence and developed with local values and resources in mind, help nurses to incorporate evidence into their practice.

IMPORTANCE OF EVIDENCE-BASED PRACTICE

Nothing is more important to clients and professional nurses than evidence-based clinical interventions that can be linked to clinical outcomes and used as a basis for care within the organization. However, until recently, health care organizations have lacked generally agreed-upon standards or processes that are based on evidence.

One strategy to address this lack of standards is the development of evidence-based practice. Generally speaking, nursing, medicine, health care institutions, and health policymakers recognize that evidence-based clinical decision making refers to decisions based on state-of-the-art science reports: a process approach to collecting, reviewing, interpreting, critiquing, and evaluating research and other relevant literature for direct application to client care. We have already discussed that evidence-based clinical decision making should incorporate the best research evidence, taking into consideration the client's clinical state, the clinical setting, and the clinical circumstances. In nursing, **best research evidence** refers to methodologically sound, clinically relevant research on the effectiveness and safety of nursing interventions, the accuracy and precision of nursing assessment measures, the power of prognostic markers, the strength of causal relationships, the cost-effectiveness of nursing interventions, and the meaning of illness or client experiences. Clinical expertise refers to our ability to use clinical skills and past experience to identify the health state of clients or populations, their risks, their preferences and actions, and the potential benefits of interventions; to communicate information to clients and their families; and to provide them with an environment they find comforting and supportive (DiCenso, Guyatt, & Ciliska, 2004).

Applying the best available evidence does not guarantee good decisions, but it is one of the keys to improving outcomes that affect health. Evidence-based practice should be viewed as the highest standard of care, as long as critical thinking and sound clinical judgment support it. Nurses and doctors will always need to search for the best evidence available to support their clinical decisions. Despite the attention paid to evidence-based practice, a large portion of clinical practice is not supported by research. In 1995, Dr David Naylor wrote in *The Lancet*, "Clinical medicine seems to consist of a few things we know, a few things we think we know (but probably don't), and lots of things we don't know at all" (Naylor, 1995, p. 840). It is probably safe to say that nursing is likely in the same position. Institutions of care have a responsibility to provide nurses and other health care professionals with an environment supportive of evidence-based practice.

Demonstrating that outcomes of nursing care are appropriate, effective, efficient, and safe is a major responsibility for nursing. As we consider the art and science of nursing, recognizing the importance of evidence-based practice and stimulating an organizational environment in which evidence-based models of care can flourish will result in improved outcomes of clinical care. Organizations that create a supportive environment for evidence-based practice are more likely to compensate managers and front-line nurses for their participation in academic activities, provide easy access to library resources and computers, include clinical nurse specialists in the staffing mix, use evidence in their management decision making, and adopt evidence-based corporate goals (Udod & Care, 2004).

Nursing practice and its impact are generally not captured in the major administrative databases that inform many funding and human resource decisions. In 1998, the Ontario Ministry of Health and Long-Term Care created the Ontario Nursing Task Force with mandates to examine the impact of health care reform on both the delivery of nursing services and the nursing profession in Ontario and to recommend strategies to ensure and enhance quality of care through effective use of nursing human resources (Joint Provincial Nursing Committee, 2001). As a result, the Ontario government funded the Nursing and Health Outcomes Project (now called the Health Outcomes for Better Information and Care, to reflect the expanded scope of the project), with the goals of identifying nursing-sensitive client outcomes, determining appropriate ways of measuring these outcomes, and identifying databases on which these outcomes could be housed.

The initial outcomes recommended by the Health Outcomes for Better Information and Care project for data collection were functional status, self-care, symptom management, client satisfaction with nursing care, and adverse occurrences. Nurses' job satisfaction was also identified as being an important predictor of client satisfaction and client outcomes. The second phase of the project examined and supported the feasibility of collecting the data in different settings. Front-line nurses found the data collection helped them improve their nursing practice, and nursing executives found value in being able to assess outcomes across clinical settings.

The project is now entering the third phase: a province-wide, standardized collection of client health outcomes, staffing, and quality-of-work-life information, reflecting nursing, pharmacy, physiotherapy, and occupational therapy in acute care, complex continuing care, long-term care, rehabilitation and home care, primary care, mental health, and public health (Ontario Ministry of Health and Long-Term Care, 2002). The results of this project will be an important source of evidence to inform nursing policy and practice. The development of evidence-based guidelines, care plans, and other decision-aid tools will help to transfer the knowledge in a manner that facilitates its use by busy clinicians. Input from the end users will improve the likelihood that these tools will be used.

Evidence-based nursing practice has deep roots. During the Crimean War, Florence Nightingale used her records of nursing interventions (i.e., sanitation, basic hygiene, good nutrition, rest, and a healing environment) and outcomes (i.e., reduced mortality of the wounded soldiers under care from 50 percent to two percent) to prove that more nursing services and supplies were needed (Rafael, 2000). In the 1960s, the Royal College of Nurses

in the United Kingdom assessed the clinical effectiveness of their members and discovered that practice lagged behind the scientific evidence (Estabrooks, Scott-Findlay & Winther, 2004). The 1990s marked the beginning of several evidence-based nursing programs and initiatives. In 1990, Linda O'Brien-Pallas, at the University of Toronto, and Andrea Baumann, at McMaster University, received provincial funding for the forerunner of the Nursing Health Services Research Unit. In 1996, the Joanna Briggs Institute for Evidence Based Nursing & Midwifery was opened in Australia, and the Centre for Evidence Based Nursing was established at University of York in the United Kingdom, followed by the Sarah Cole Hirsch Institute for Best Nursing Practice Based on Evidence in the United States, in 1998. More recently, the School of Nursing at Queen's University in Kingston, Ontario, has become a collaborating centre of the Joanna Briggs Institute. Over the past 20 years, significant work has been accomplished worldwide to implement evidence-based practice into health care organizations.

In the United States, the Agency for Healthcare Research and Quality (AHRQ) has provided stimulus for the evidence-based practice movement by recognizing a need for evidence to guide practice throughout the health care system. In 1997, the AHRQ launched an initiative that established 12 evidence-based practice centres (EPCs). The initiative was renewed in 2002 with 13 EPCs, three of which are located in Canada: at McMaster University, the University of Ottawa, and the University of Alberta. The EPCs develop evidence reports and technology assessments on topics relevant to clinical, social, and behavioural science; economics; and other health care organization and delivery issues. The initiative facilitates the translation of evidence-based research findings into clinical practice by including the input of stakeholders at key decision points along the process.[1]

The Canadian Agency for Drugs and Technologies in Health (CADTH) is a national body that provides Canada's federal, provincial, and territorial health care decision-makers with credible, impartial advice and evidence-based information about the effectiveness and efficiency of drugs and other health technologies. Several provincial governments fund similar health technology assessment initiatives. To ensure the information is relevant and useful to decision-makers, CADTH has established liaison officers, who work with local health care stakeholders to develop strategies that will enable more consistent uptake to practice.[2]

In Ontario, with funding from the Ministry of Health and Long-Term Care, the Registered Nurses' Association of Ontario (RNAO) began the Nursing Best Practice Guidelines (NBPG) project, an initiative to facilitate clinical decisions that were based on the best available evidence. In 2004, Health Canada provided further funding to enable the initiative to disseminate its products across Canada, including translation into French. Currently 30 English guidelines have been prepared, and 12 are available in French. Six *Healthy Work Environments* guidelines have recently been developed to enable nursing leaders and their organizations to create positive work environments for nurses.[3]

ATTRIBUTES OF EVIDENCE-BASED PRACTICE

A new culture that can support evidence-based practice needs to evolve in organizations. Stetler and colleagues (1998) identify three specific actions needed to establish an evidence-based environment within an institution: (1) establish the culture, (2) create a capacity for change, and (3) use the organizational infrastructure to sustain and reinforce change. The authors highlight the need for such activities as defining the meaning of evidence in each agency, beginning to use the term *evidence* in daily practice, and looking for the best evidence when evaluating new goals and new programs. They encourage the use of visible, formal supports for evidence-based practice and the development of systems in the health care agency that support evidence-based practice on an ongoing basis. The authors suggest that the development of these attributes will help make evidence-based practice the usual method of care delivery.

In 1996, Carole Estabrooks conducted a survey of nurses in Alberta to identify the frequency with which they used various sources of information to inform their practice. The respondents most frequently said they used experiential information sources (e.g., client data and personal experience), followed by basic nursing education programs, in-service programs and conferences, policy and procedure manuals, physician sources, intuition, and "what has worked for years." Articles published in nursing research journals ranked fifteenth out of sixteen possible sources. The nurses' reliance on nonscientific knowledge and on their basic nursing education, despite having graduated from their nursing education programs an average of 18 years earlier, is a troubling trend (Estabrooks, 1998). This finding is not appreciably different from what is seen in medicine. Susan Rappolt conducted in-depth interviews with family physicians in three Ontario cities to determine their sources of clinical information. Most participants reported that their first resource was informal consultation with peers. Fifty-four percent turned to readily available and approachable peers, and 24 percent asked only those peers they considered to be experts. The remaining 22 percent searched the literature before, or in conjunction with, consulting expert specialists or innovators (Rappolt, 2002).

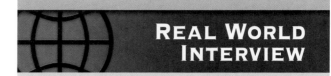

REAL WORLD INTERVIEW

I received a call one day from the nursing director of a long-term care facility. She was looking for someone to help them draft evidence-based care plans that could be used by their multidisciplinary teams in areas such as cognitive impairment, bladder and bowel care, falls prevention, pain management, and skin and wound care. She was aware of the Registered Nurses' Association of Ontario's Nursing Best Practice Guidelines, but needed someone who could search the literature to see if there were more resources available, adapt the information to their setting, and set up educational workshops for staff. There was nobody on staff who had the time to devote to this important work. It had been identified as an area for improvement during their last accreditation.

Vicki Pennick, RN
Managing Editor, Cochrane Back Review Group

Sonia Udod and W. Dean Care at the University of Manitoba conducted a survey to determine which managerial competencies were important to create an environment where evidence-based practice could flourish. Nursing leaders were expected to be role models for evidence-based practice, searching for and appraising the evidence and using it when making their decisions. They were expected to create opportunities for staff to develop networks to facilitate the development of important skills needed in an evidence-based environment, such as computer skills for searching the literature, or critical appraisal skills to assess the quality of what they read. Finally, sharing leadership and decision making among the team and providing psychosocial support to help sustain new behaviours were identified as other important attributes (Udod & Care, 2004).

MISCONCEPTIONS ABOUT EVIDENCE-BASED PRACTICE

Despite the importance and many attributes of evidence-based medicine, physicians have cautioned against relying on external clinical evidence in isolation from clinical expertise: "Evidence based medicine is not 'cookbook' medicine. Because it requires a bottom-up approach that integrates the best external evidence with individual clinical expertise and patients' choice, it cannot result in slavish, cookbook approaches to individual patient care. External clinical evidence can inform, but can never replace, individual clinical expertise, and it is this expertise that decides whether the external evidence applies to the individual patient at all and, if so, how it should be integrated into a clinical decision" (Sackett, Rosenberg, Gray, Haynes, & Richardson, 1996). Nurses and other health care professionals voice similar concerns. Nurses are particularly concerned that evidence-based practice ignores client preferences and values, is atheoretical, uses only quantitative research, and overemphasizes randomized controlled trials and systematic reviews. In an effort to overcome these beliefs, it is incumbent on nursing managers to provide a practice environment that encourages nurses to incorporate the best evidence with their clinical skills, client preferences, and clinical circumstance.

Since not all clinical questions are best answered with a randomized trial, other study designs may offer the best available evidence to answer a particular question. Our nursing knowledge base is built on different theoretical frameworks and sources of information. We have developed theories that identify, analyze, and clarify our moral obligations and values, our interpersonal relationships, and our understanding of client behaviour. Systematic reviews are only a tool for systematically searching, appraising, and synthesizing the literature in an attempt to answer a clinical question. Although the methods used to synthesize results from randomized trials are more advanced, both the Cochrane Collaboration[4] and the Campbell Collaboration[5] are working on systematic review methods that synthesize data from different study designs, including studies of prognosis, non-randomized clinical trials and qualitative research (DiCenso, Guyatt, & Ciliska, 2004; Thomas et al., 2004).

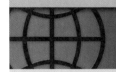

REAL WORLD INTERVIEW

Vicki: How did you end up working with Cochrane?

Mark: My wife took up a new post as a manager of the mental health services in a different part of the UK, which meant we moved with her. As she was managerially responsible for the Psychotherapy Services in that area, I didn't fancy applying to them for work, so looked for alternatives. As we had just had a daughter, I was in the best position to work part-time, doing the nursery drop off and pick up, so found a job with hours to suit, which happened to be in research. Whilst the job was not research-based, just dressed up as such, I eventually found the Cochrane Schizophrenia Group, which offered me a secondment to undertake a review. When that job finished, they offered some short-term project work. We moved again, and I was offered a post at the Centre for Evidence Based Nursing, which I did for 18 months. We moved again, and the Schizophrenia Group offered me a post whilst they were in transition. I've been employed by Cochrane since then.

Vicki: Do you consider the work you do helps to inform clinicians, especially nurses, in evidence-based nursing?

Mark: It's hard to say the work I do as a Trial Search Co-ordinator [librarian] informs nursing directly. However, it has brought me into a sphere of influence, where because of the association I have with Cochrane and evidence, I am asked to peer review project protocols and reports, and sit on national groups, which allows me to apply my training to get "good" research commissioned, and views enshrined in projects that in a few years will be common practice. The systematic reviews I have undertaken outside the duties of my Cochrane position have certainly influenced national and international treatment guidelines and practice. One review has been influential in stopping the practice of clients being physically restrained in accident and emergency departments in some parts of the United States, but has in consequence been partly responsible for people getting horrible doses of sedative drugs as an alternative. I think the work we undertake as a whole is very influential in some areas of nursing, especially those that are more procedure-based, such as wound care, but is still distrusted by many in mental health. Most of the resistance is based on a misunderstanding of research methods, and the argument is reduced to "you can't reduce individuals to a number," or "how do you apply results of research to individuals' type of arguments."

Mark Fenton, RN
Cochrane Schizophrenia Review Group

EVIDENCE: SOURCES, TYPES, AND EVALUATION

Depending on the question, sources of evidence can vary widely. The efficacy of a treatment is best tested with a randomized controlled trial, where the potential for bias is limited by the study design. In contrast, qualitative research is better suited to answering questions that increase our understanding of attitudes, beliefs, and experiences of groups or individuals. Both approaches of scientific enquiry have developed methodological criteria to minimize bias. On the other hand, nursing administrators must make decisions based on evidence that comes from outside the scientific realm. They use **organization evidence** that gives them information about the organization's capacity to execute tasks. This information may be in the form of financial reports, program evaluations, utilization data, and report cards. **Political evidence,** on the other hand, gives a sense of how the various stakeholders may respond to policies; for example, the barriers or facilitators that may have to be managed. This information may be found by conducting environmental scans, holding focus groups, or convening expert panels. In all circumstances, decisions and implementation strategies must be evaluated to determine their effectiveness (Canadian Health Services Research Foundation, 2004).

A growing number of nursing-oriented journals publish scientific literature: Online Journal of Knowledge Synthesis for Nursing, Evidence-Based Nursing, Canadian Journal of Nursing Leadership, Clinical Effectiveness in Nursing, Internet Journal of Advanced Nursing Practice, Canadian Journal of Nursing Research, Clinical Nursing Research, and Worldwide Nursing, to name just a few. Canadian nursing leaders are active participants in many of these journals. In an attempt to assist the busy practitioner in keeping abreast of the literature, Evidence-Based Nursing selects articles from the health-related literature that warrant immediate attention by nurses, appraises them, summarizes them, and adds comments from clinical experts. A growing number of web-based sources are also available. A selection is listed at the end of the chapter. See also Table 3-1 for a list of the funded Canadian nursing research chairs. Research from these programs will be another very important source of evidence for health care decision-makers.

Another way of helping busy clinicians find relevant information is to publish systematic reviews. Since the early work of the McMaster group, methods for review and synthesis of evidence have undergone dramatic advances. Archie Cochrane, a British epidemiologist, was a pioneer in the movement and the impetus behind the development of the Cochrane Collaboration, an international organization that aims to help people make well-informed decisions about health care by preparing, maintaining, and promoting the accessibility of systematic reviews of the effects of health care interventions. The U.K. Cochrane Centre was started in 1992, followed shortly by the Canadian Cochrane Centre, hosted by McMaster University, in 1993.[6] Used initially as a resource to inform medical practice, it wasn't long before nurses became involved in the Cochrane Collaboration as authors, review group co-ordinators, trial search co-ordinators, and editors. Approximately 400 systematic reviews in The Cochrane Library cover a range of nursing interventions, methods in nursing research and economic analyses of a variety of nursing policies and practices.[7]

Some basic methodological differences distinguish the more traditional narrative review from a systematic review. A systematic review uses methods of study selection, appraisal, data extraction, and analysis, which reduce the risk of bias. Systematic reviews typically start with a focused question, develop and execute a comprehensive search strategy, select studies based on explicitly stated inclusion criteria, appraise the methodological quality of the relevant studies, extract and synthesize the data using either a statistical (i.e., a meta-analytical) or qualitative approach, and come to conclusions that are based on the evidence. A narrative review may follow some of the same steps, but it is likely to be answering a broader question, is usually less comprehensive about the literature included, and its results and recommendations may extend beyond the data.[8]

Five steps comprise the evidence-based practice process (although some practitioners may combine some of the steps): (i) ask the clinical question, (ii) search the literature, (iii) critically appraise the potentially relevant literature identified, (iv) decide whether and how to use the information, and (v) evaluate the effects of your decision (Straus & Sackett, 1998). The question and available resources will dictate the extent of the literature search. The decision on how to use the information will be influenced by client preferences and circumstances, by the provider's skill and preference, and by local resources, policies, and practices. Not all inquiries will result in a full systematic review; however, it is always important to evaluate the effects of your decisions and actions. See Table 3-2 for details on the five steps. Table 3-3 gives an overview of research terminology useful in developing skills in evidence-based practice (EBP).

LEVELS OF EVIDENCE

As you may have noticed by now, not all science is equally well designed and equally well carried out, nor are all the published reports equally well written. Busy

TABLE 3-1	CANADIAN NURSING RESEARCH CHAIRS

Name	University	Funding Agency	Area of Research
Dr. Lesley Degner	University of Manitoba	CHSRF/CIHR Chair	Development of Innovative Nursing Interventions to Influence Practice and Policy in Cancer Care, Palliative Care, and Cancer Prevention
Dr. Alba DiCenso	McMaster University	CHSRF/CIHR Chair	Evaluation of Nurse Practitioner/Advanced Practice Nurse Roles and Interventions
Dr. Carole A. Estabrooks	University of Alberta	Canada Research Chairs Program	Canada Research Chair in Knowledge Translation—Tier II
Dr. Nancy Edwards	University of Ottawa	CHSRF/CIHR Chair	Multiple Interventions in Community Health Nursing Care
Dr. Ellen Hodnett	University of Toronto	Heather M. Reisman Chair in Perinatal Nursing Research	Care Throughout the Child-bearing Period
Dr. Nicole Letourneau	University of New Brunswick	Canada Research Chairs Program/Canadian Research Institute for Social Policy (CRISP)	Canada Research Chair in Healthy Child Development.—Tier II
Dr. Janice Lander	University of Alberta	CHSRF/CIHR Chair	Evaluating Innovative Approaches to Nursing Care
Dr. Linda O'Brien-Pallas	University of Toronto	CHSRF/CIHR Chair	Nursing Human Resources for the New Millennium
Dr. Judee E. Onyskiw	University of New Brunswick	Canada Research Chairs Program	Canada Research Chair in Family Violence and Children's Health—Tier II

Source: Canadian Nursing Research Chairs, "Chair Awards." Retrieved from http://64.26.143.46:8765/query.html?qt=nursing+research+chairs& charset=iso-8859-1&rq=0&la=en&style=Standard and http://www.cihr-irsc.gc.ca/e/193.html, August 2006.

clinicians find it impossible to keep abreast of advances in the field by reading all the original research. Fortunately, groups of clinicians and researchers synthesize the information into systematic reviews, clinical guidelines, and quality assessment tools to help us to decide which studies are well conducted. Unfortunately, subjective decisions will always be made in the synthesis of the data in either situation. Therefore, it is incumbent upon the clinician to read and understand a little of the theory behind the science.

When the results of the original studies are unequivocal, and the data can be statistically pooled (e.g., in a meta-analysis), the conclusions in systematic reviews and recommendations for practice in clinical guidelines are likely to be easy to understand. The challenge arises when results from a systematic review may not be statistically or clinically significant, and yet are the best available evidence for use in developing evidence-based clinical guidelines. Since guidelines are in part dependent on the norms and available resources of a jurisdiction, it is not unusual in these circumstances to find different recommendations in different guidelines, based on the same evidence.

A related challenge for health care decision-makers is understanding the grading of the evidence upon which guidelines recommendations are made. Some guideline development groups use alphabetic assignments, others use numeric assignments. Some consider the highest level of evidence to be a well-conducted

TABLE 3-2	**FIVE STEPS IN EVIDENCE-BASED PRACTICE**
1. Define the clinical question	The clinical question may be defined from the perspective of different parties: the client, the clinician, the policymaker, the organization's administrator, or the pharmaceutical industry, to name a few. Each perspective will produce a different question. e.g., What are the effects of the introduction of clinical practice guidelines in nursing (including health visiting), midwifery, and other professions allied to medicine? Are nursing-led inpatient units effective in preparing clients for discharge from hospital compared to usual inpatient care?
2. Search the literature	If you have the time, skills, and resources, you can search the literature yourself. In most cases, it makes more sense to turn to a trained health sciences librarian for assistance. This solution may be problematic for clinicians who are not affiliated with an academic institution or a health care facility with a good library. PubMed (http://www.ncbi.nlm.nih.gov/sites/entrez?db=pubmed), sponsored by the National Library of Medicine and the National Institutes of Health in the United States, is a large, freely accessible database of medical, nursing, and allied health journals, but not all journals are indexed in PubMed. Unfortunately, CINAHL, the specialized database for nursing and allied health, is only available by subscription (see http://www.cinahl.com/)
3. Critically appraise the literature	In order to have confidence in the results of the literature, you first need to determine the quality of the data. Not all research is created equal! Therefore, when accessing an intervention trial, it is important to determine the following: ■ Were the clients randomly assigned to the study groups? ■ Was this assignment concealed? ■ Were there co-interventions? Were they equal for all groups? ■ Was follow-up complete and was it of sufficient duration? ■ Were there losses during the follow-up or withdrawals that would affect the results? ■ Were clients analyzed in the groups to which they were originally assigned? ■ Was the outcome assessor blinded? (Higgins & Green, 2005) For qualitative studies you should ask the following questions: ■ Is the research question clear and adequately substantiated? ■ Is the design appropriate for the research question? ■ Was the sampling appropriate for the research design and question? ■ Were data collected and managed systematically? ■ Were data analyzed appropriately? ■ Is the description of the results thorough? (DiCenso, Guyatt, & Ciliska, 2004) If you have found a systematic review, determine the following: ■ What study designs were synthesized? ■ Was the literature search described? ■ How was the validity of the studies assessed? ■ Were the results consistent across studies? ■ Were individual or aggregate data used in the analysis? (Oxman & Guyatt, 1991)

(Continued)

TABLE 3-2	FIVE STEPS IN EVIDENCE-BASED PRACTICE (CONTINUED)
	For clinical practice guidelines, you will want to consider the following questions: ■ Are the scope and purpose clearly outlined? ■ Were all stakeholder perspectives sought? ■ Were the guidelines developed following systematic methods that would minimize bias (as in those outlined for systematic reviews)? ■ Were the recommendations clearly presented and easy to follow? ■ Are the guidelines applicable in your circumstances? ■ Were the guidelines developed in an environment that was free from potential conflicts of interest? (AGREE Collaboration, 2003)
4. Decide whether and how to use the information	To decide whether the information you found is likely to help you with the question at hand, determine the size and precision of the treatment results; that is, ask whether the effects of the treatment were both statistically and clinically important. Decide whether your clients are similar to the clients in the study, whether the treatment is feasible in your setting, and whether all clinically important outcomes (e.g., harms and benefits) were considered. Finally, based on local practice, administrative constraints, and client preferences, ask whether the anticipated benefits are worth the harms and costs. If you are looking at qualitative research, decide what meaning and relevance the results have for your client care, whether the results will help you understand the context of your client care, and whether the study will enhance your knowledge about your client care (DiCenso, Guyatt, & Ciliska, 2004).
5. Evaluate the effects of your decision	Deciding how you will evaluate the effects of your decision should be as carefully thought-out as the other steps. Can you determine what would have happened if you had taken another route? Are the parameters by which you are evaluating your decision appropriate for the clinical question you asked in Step 1?

Source: Five steps in evidence-based practice (AGREE Collaboration, 2003; DiCenso, Guyatt, Ciliska, 2004; Higgins & Green, 2005; Oxman & Guyatt, 1991; Straus & Sackett, 1998).

systematic review; others assign the highest level to a well-conducted randomized controlled trial. This situation is very confusing for those who must use these sources of evidence to inform their practice. Understanding the differences is important (Glasziou, Vandenbroucke, & Chalmers, 2004; Schünemann, Best, Vist, & Oxman, 2003; Upshur, 2003).

An international group of epidemiologists and clinicians, calling themselves the Grading of Recommendations Assessment, Development and Evaluation (GRADE) Working Group, have been working on a "common sense approach" to grading the evidence and strength of recommendations. GRADE's 10 systematic and sequential steps guide a group from the initial establishment of the guideline development team and clinical priorities,

through the literature search, appraisal and synthesis, to determining the balance of benefits, harms, costs, and final recommendations and implementation.

As with other methods that grade evidence, the GRADE Working Groups consider the study design, quality, consistency, robustness of the results, and the applicability to the population at hand. The biggest advantage to this new approach is the stepped method of combining these elements. The quality of the evidence for each important outcome decreases by one level for limitations in study quality, important inconsistencies, lack of generalizability, imprecise or sparse data, or a high probability of reporting bias.[9] Readers wishing more information on the process are directed to the GRADE website, http://www.gradeworkinggroup.org/.

TABLE 3-3	RESEARCH TERMINOLOGY IN EVIDENCE-BASED PRACTICE
Absolute Risk Reduction (ARR)	The absolute arithmetic difference (i.e., the risk difference) in rates of harmful outcomes between experimental and control groups. Use of this term is restricted to a beneficial exposure or intervention.
Allocation concealment	Randomization is concealed when the person making the decision about enrolling a client is unaware of whether the next client enrolled will be entered in the intervention group or the control group (e.g., by using techniques such as central randomization or sequentially numbered opaque, sealed envelopes). When randomization is not concealed, clients with better prognoses may tend to be preferentially enrolled in the active treatment arm resulting in exaggeration of the apparent benefit of the intervention (or even falsely concluding that the intervention is efficacious).
Bias	A systematic error in the design, conduct, or interpretation of a study that may cause a systematic deviation from the underlying truth.
Case control study	A study designed to determine the association between an exposure and an outcome in which clients are sampled by outcome. Those with the outcome (i.e., the cases) are compared to those without the outcome (i.e., the controls) with respect to exposure to the suspected harmful agent.
Case reports	Descriptions of individual clients.
Case series	A study reporting on a consecutive collection of clients treated in a similar manner, without a control group. For example, a clinician might describe the characteristics of an outcome for 25 consecutive clients with diabetes who received education for prevention of foot ulcers.
Clinical practice guidelines	Systematically developed statements or recommendations to assist practitioner and client decisions about appropriate health care for specific clinical circumstances. Clinical practice guidelines present indications for performing a test, procedure, or intervention, or the proper management for specific clinical problems.
Cohort study	A study that identifies two groups (i.e., cohorts) of clients: one group received the exposure of interest and one group did not receive the exposure. The cohort study follows the two groups forward for the outcome of interest (also called a longitudinal study).
Co-intervention	An intervention other than the intervention under study that may be differentially applied to the intervention groups and the control groups and, thus, potentially introduces bias in the results of a study.
Comparative research	A research design that either compares two or more groups, compares a single group at two or more points in time, or compares a single group under different circumstances or experiences.
Confidence Interval	A range between two values within which it is probable that the true value lies for the population of clients from which the study clients were selected.
Confounder	A factor that distorts the true relationship of the study variable of interest by virtue of also being related to the outcome of interest. Confounders are often unequally distributed among the groups being compared. Randomized studies are less likely to have their results distorted by confounders than are observational studies.
Control group	Subjects in an experiment who do not receive the experimental treatment and whose performance provides a baseline against which the effects of the treatment can be measured.
Dependent variable	The outcome variable of interest; the variable that is hypothesized or thought to depend on or be caused by another variable, called the independent variable (also called the outcome).
Descriptive research	Research studies that have as their main objective the accurate portrayal of the characteristics of people, situations, or groups, and the frequency with which certain phenomena occur.

(Continued)

TABLE 3-3	RESEARCH TERMINOLOGY IN EVIDENCE-BASED PRACTICE (CONTINUED)
Dichotomous outcomes	"Yes" or "no" outcomes that either happen or do not happen, such as pregnancy, pressure ulcer, and death.
Dose-response gradient	The risk of an outcome increasing as the quantity or the duration of exposure to the putative harmful agent increases.
Effect size	The difference in outcomes between the intervention and control groups divided by some measure of variability, typically the standard deviation.
Generalizability	The degree to which the results of a study can be generalized to settings or samples other than those being studied.
Incidence	The number of new cases of a disease occurring during a specified period of time; expressed as a percentage of the number of people at risk during that time.
Independent variable	The variable that is believed to cause or influence the dependent variable; in experimental research, the independent variable is the variable that is manipulated.
Intention-to-treat analysis	The analyzing of study participant outcomes based on the group to which the participants were randomized, even if they dropped out of the study or for other reasons did not actually receive the planned intervention. This analysis preserves the power of randomization, thus maintaining the likelihood that important unknown factors that influence outcome are equally distributed across comparison groups.
Internal validity	The ability of a study to provide valid results, dependent on whether it was designed and conducted well enough that the study findings accurately represent the direction and magnitude of the underlying true effect.
Interrupted time series	A study design in which data are collected at several times both before and after the intervention. Data collected before the intervention allow the underlying trend and cyclical (e.g., seasonal) effects to be estimated, whereas data collected after the intervention allow the intervention effect to be estimated, while accounting for underlying secular trends. The time series–design monitors the occurrence of outcomes or end points over a number of cycles and determines whether the pattern changes coincident with the intervention.
Matched case-controlled study	A research technique that uses select sample characteristics to match experimental subjects with a control group (matched sample).
Meta-analysis	A statistical technique for quantitatively gathering the results of multiple studies that measure the same outcome and combining those results into a single pooled estimate or a summary estimate.
Nonrandomized controlled trial	An experiment in which assignment of clients to the intervention groups is at the convenience of the investigator or according to a preset plan that does not conform to the definition of being random.
Number Needed to Treat (NNT)	The number of clients who need to be treated over a specific period of time to achieve one additional good outcome. When discussing NNT, the intervention, its duration, and the good outcome should be specified. NNT is the inverse of the absolute risk reduction.
Observational studies	Studies in which a participant or clinician preference determines whether a participant is assigned to the intervention group or the control group.
Odds ratio	A ratio of the odds of an event in an exposed group to the odds of the same event in a group that is not exposed.
Outcome evaluation	An assessment of the impact of an intervention, which examines the changes that occurred as a result of the intervention and whether the intervention is having the intended effect. It answers the question, What is the impact of this intervention? It may also answer the question, Are the benefits of the intervention worth the costs?

(Continued)

TABLE 3-3	**RESEARCH TERMINOLOGY IN EVIDENCE-BASED PRACTICE (CONTINUED)**
Phenomenology	An approach to inquiry that emphasizes the complexity of human experience and the need to understand the experience holistically, as it is actually lived.
Power	The ability of a study to reject a null hypothesis when it is false (and should be rejected). Power is linked to the adequacy of the sample size: if a sample size is too small, the study will have insufficient power to detect differences between groups, if differences exist.
Prevalence	The proportion of persons in a population who are affected with a particular disease at a specified time. Prevalence rates obtained from high-quality studies can inform pretest probabilities.
Probability	The quantitative estimate of the likelihood of either a condition existing (e.g., in a diagnosis) or of subsequent events occurring (e.g., in an intervention study).
Prognostic study	A study that enrolls clients at a particular point in time and follows them forward to determine the frequency and timing of subsequent events.
Program evaluation	Research that investigates how well a program, practice, or policy is working.
Qualitative research	The investigation of phenomena in a non-quantitative, in-depth, and holistic fashion, through the collection of rich narrative materials. Examples of data collection include observation, interviews, and document analysis.
Quality improvement project	The selection of a particular diagnostic group, unit, or other measurement that needs scientific investigation to identify needed improvement.
Quantitative research	The investigation of phenomena that lend themselves to test well-specified hypotheses through precise measurement and the quantification of predetermined variables that yields numbers suitable for statistical analysis.
Quasi-experiment	A study in which subjects are systematically, rather than randomly, assigned to treatment conditions, although the researcher manipulates the independent variable and exercises certain controls to enhance the internal validity of the results.
Random allocation (or Randomization)	Allocation of individuals to groups by chance, usually with the aid of a table of random numbers. Not to be confused with systematic allocation (e.g., an allocation based on even and odd days of the month) or an allocation at the convenience or discretion of the investigator.
Randomized controlled trials	Experiments in which individuals are randomly allocated to receive or not receive an experimental preventive, therapeutic, or diagnostic procedure and then followed to determine the effect of the intervention.
Research utilization	The use of some aspect of a research or scientific investigation in an application unrelated to the original research.
Relative Risk Reduction (RRR)	The proportional reduction in rates of harmful outcomes between experimental and control participants. Used with a beneficial exposure or intervention.
Statistical significance	A description of results obtained in an analysis of study data that are unlikely to have occurred by chance, and the null hypothesis is rejected. When statistically significant, the probability of the observed results, given the null hypothesis, falls below a specified level of probability (most often $P < 0.05$).
Systematic review	A review of a clearly formulated question that uses systematic and explicit methods to identify, select, and critically appraise relevant research, and to collect and analyze data from the studies included in the review. Statistical methods (i.e., meta-analyses) may or may not be used to analyze and summarize the results of the included studies.

(Continued)

TABLE 3-3	RESEARCH TERMINOLOGY IN EVIDENCE-BASED PRACTICE (CONTINUED)
Time series design	A quasi-experimental design that involves the collection of information over an extended period of time, with multiple data collection points both before and after the introduction of a treatment.
Variable	A characteristic or attribute of a person or object that varies (i.e., takes on different values) within the population under study (e.g., body temperature, heart rate).

Source: Higgins, J. P. T., & Green, S. (Eds.). *Cochrane Handbook for Systematic Reviews of Interventions 4.2.5* [updated May 2005]. Retrieved from http://www.cochrane.org/resources/handbook/hbook.htm, August 19, 2006; Loiselle, C. G., Profetto-McGrath, J., Polit, D. F., Tatano Beck. C. (2004). *Canadian Essentials of Nursing Research.* Philadephia: Lippincott Williams & Wilkins.

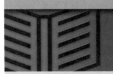

LITERATURE APPLICATION

Citation #1: Thomas, L., Cullum, N., McColl, E., Rousseau, N., Soutter, J., & Steen, N. (1999). Guidelines in professions allied to medicine. *Cochrane Database of Systematic Reviews, Issue 1.* Art. No.: CD000349. DOI: 10.1002/14651858.CD000349.

Discussion: The objective of this review was to identify and assess the effects of strategies to introduce clinical practice guidelines in nursing (including health visiting), midwifery, and other professions allied to medicine. The authors survey 18 studies that included 467 health professionals. They conclude that there is some evidence that guideline-driven care is effective in changing the process and outcome of care provided by professions allied to medicine. However, caution is needed in generalizing findings to other professions and settings.

Implications for practice: The issuing of clinical guidelines to nurses, midwives, dieticians, and other health care professionals allied to medicine may reduce variations in practice and improve client care. This review found that, despite limited research, some evidence suggests that guidelines can improve care and that professional roles can be substituted effectively.

Citation #2: Foxcroft, D. R., & Cole, N. (2000). Organisational infrastructures to promote evidence based nursing practice. *Cochrane Database of Systematic Reviews, Issue 3.* Art. No.: CD002212. DOI: 10.1002/14651858.CD002212.

Discussion: The objective of this review was to identify and summarize organizational infrastructure developments aimed at promoting evidence-based nursing practice. No studies were found to be sufficiently rigorous to be included in this systematic review. Seven case studies were identified but excluded from the review because of poor design and lack of controls. Several conceptual models on organizational processes to promote evidence-based practice and a number of organizational infrastructural interventions were described, but none was evaluated properly.

Implications for practice: There are no clear implications for practice. The next step in this field should be to conduct well-planned evaluations of well-planned interventions.

KNOWLEDGE TRANSFER AND EVIDENCE-BASED DECISIONS IN POLICY

During the 1990s, a number of federally funded organizations were created in Canada to enable evidence-based decision making and policy development. In 1994, the Canadian government set up the National Forum on Health, an advisory committee with a mandate to involve and inform Canadians and to advise the federal government on innovative ways to improve our health care system and the health of Canada's people. The Forum completed its task in 1997. Its recommendations incorporated the values of Canadians and the importance of evidence-based decision making into the long-term plans for the restructuring of Canada's health care

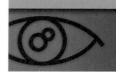

CRITICAL THINKING

You have just started work in a new palliative care hospital. You have been working in the community for many years and have enjoyed an environment where you were a respected member of the health care team, received encouragement and assistance to attend conferences, and had the opportunity to lead a couple of Nursing Best Practice Guideline initiatives in your agency. As you begin to take account of your new surroundings, you notice some aspects of care that you thought were revised years ago! You are conscious of being "the new kid on the block," but you finally summon the courage to ask your preceptor how evidence-based nursing is practised and supported on the floor. She looks at you suspiciously and says, "We've been giving excellent care around here for many years. Our clients are kept comfortable and their families appreciate what we do for them. We can't see any good reason to change."

What do you do now?

system. Today, Health Canada uses scientific expertise to inform its decisions on health standards, health policy, regulations, and health programs, and to provide evidence-based information to help Canadians make well-informed health care decisions.[10]

For many of the newly created organizations, part of their mandate included the obligation to create and disseminate research so that it could be readily used by decision-makers at all levels. This approach to dissemination is now commonly known as Knowledge Transfer and Exchange (KT&E), although there are a number of synonymous terms in use. The KT&E process is built on the concept that decision-makers are more likely to incorporate research results into their decisions if they have a vested interest in the process (i.e., if they have input into the important questions and other steps of the research). In 1997, the Canadian Health Services Research Foundation (CHSRF) was created to "support the evidence-informed management of Canada's healthcare system by facilitating knowledge transfer and exchange—bridging the gap between research and healthcare management and policy."[11] In 1999, the Canadian Population Health Initiative (CPHI) was created to promote the development of evidence-based healthy public policy with a population health focus. CPHI's 2001 report, *An Environmental Scan of Research Transfer Strategies*, which surveyed 17 organizations across Canada, is an excellent resource for anyone who wishes to gain an understanding of the KT&E process.[12]

The Canadian Institutes of Health Research (CIHR), the federal health research funding agency established in 2000, incorporated both the creation and translation of new research into its mandate.[13] The CIHR and the Canadian Agency for Drugs and Technologies in Health (CADTH) are primary funders of the Canadian Cochrane Centre and the Cochrane review groups, methods groups, and fields located in Canada.[14] The CHSRF and CIHR co-fund a number of nursing research chairs that have set up research programs to examine nursing practice, nursing resources, and effective strategies to transfer the knowledge into policy and practice.

An important player in this field is the Nursing Health Services Research Unit (NHSRU) at the University of Toronto and McMaster University. Its goals are to: (i) conduct research and other forms of inquiry, (ii) provide the information necessary for evidence-based policy and management decisions about the effectiveness, quality, equity, utilization, and efficiency of health care and health services in Ontario, with a particular focus on nursing services, and (iii) develop a joint mechanism for knowledge transfer between the Ontario Ministry of Health and Long-Term Care (MOHLTC) and the NHSRU to ensure the best and most recent evidence is

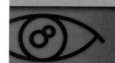

CRITICAL THINKING

You are a community health nurse visiting Mrs. McTavish to change the dressings on her stasis ulcers. She is upset when you get there and hasn't prepared things as she usually does for your visit. You have barely taken off your coat when she starts talking.

"My daughter went to her doctor recently because she was having really heavy periods again. I suffered from the same problems when I was her age. They weren't sure I could have any children. In those days, they kept trying to find out if I had any glandular problems and when I would have a really bad bleed, they would bring me into hospital for a D&C. She has been on contraceptives forever. I really worry about her. Don't they say that if you are on hormones for too long you increase your risks of cancer, heart disease, bone fractures, and things like that? Her doctor also said he might consider a hysterectomy. She's only 35. She's too young to go through menopause."

Where do you turn for your information?

What do you tell her?

On what evidence are you basing your care of her stasis ulcers?

used to guide evidence-based policy and management decision making.

The NHSRU has proven to be a valuable source of evidence for policy decisions on understanding and planning for health human resources, quality work environments for nurses, performance standards and practice, and the impact of organizational restructuring and downsizing, to name a few.[15,16] When asked, policymakers also voice concerns about incorporating evidence into their decisions. Risks, benefits, and costs are often vague and difficult for them to contextualize; they lack a framework by which to quickly assess the local applicability of the results; the information is often not available when they need it; they have many competing interests to consider when developing policy (e.g., research evidence); they are not trained as researchers and are often not in the position long enough to understand the full scope of the issues (Lavis, Davies, Gruen, Walshe, & Farquhar, 2006). The hope is that this situation will gradually change as a result of the efforts of the organizations described above.

According to the Canadian Institute for Health Information, health care spending in Canada was expected to reach $148 billion in 2006, an increase of $8 billion or 5.8 percent over 2005, or $4,411 per person.[17] It behooves all clinical health care providers to carefully consider the findings of both nursing and medical research and then deliver quality outcomes. Policymakers, clinicians, nursing leaders, and nursing managers must promote the use of evidence-based practice to develop best practices at all levels of care. Many health care organizations support research programs, the results of which are used locally and internationally. Not all organizations have the resources to conduct large research projects, but, at the very least, they should be engaged in evaluating current practices and programs to ensure they are meeting the best standards of care. Changes in practice can only be facilitated through the collaboration of all disciplines working together in an atmosphere that fosters evidence-based health care delivered to obtain quality outcomes.

KEY CONCEPTS

■ The focus on evidence-based practice is expected to remain a driving force in the health care arena in the foreseeable future.

■ Nursing can make significant contributions to the advancement of evidence-based care.

■ Nursing leaders and managers can promote a culture receptive to the practice of evidence-based care, and all nurses can support this culture.

■ Ultimately, evidence-based care is the gold standard in clinical care.

■ By accepting the challenge to provide evidence-based care, nursing can pursue its future, confident of its ability to contribute to an increasingly complex health care system.

KEY TERMS

best research evidence
evidence-based care
evidence-based medicine
evidence-based nursing practice

evidence-based practice
organization evidence
political evidence

REVIEW QUESTIONS

1. What is the major purpose of evidence-based practice?
   A. To increase variability of care
   B. To create a missing link in clinical care
   C. To determine which medical models can be applied by nursing
   D. To provide evidence-based care that is incorporated with clinical competency, client preferences, and local resources

2. Concerning evidence-based practice, which of the following is an accurate statement?
   A. Evidence-based practice takes the place of continuous quality improvement.
   B. Because we can already demonstrate effective and efficient care, evidence-based practice is redundant.
   C. Leaders and managers in nursing are not clinicians, generally speaking, and so do not have a role in evidence-based practice processes.
   D. Generally speaking, evidence-based practice is recognized by nursing, medicine, and health policymakers as state-of-the-art clinical practice

3. Which of the following organizations develops clinical practice guidelines?
   A. National Guideline Clearinghouse
   B. Public Health Agency of Canada
   C. Registered Nurses' Association of Ontario
   D. Guidelines Advisory Committee
   E. Canadian Medical Association

4. Which of the following is a research design that always involves testing of a clinical treatment with assignments of research subjects to either experimental or control conditions?
   A. Longitudinal study
   B. Randomized controlled trial

C. Meta-analysis
D. Time series design

REVIEW ACTIVITIES

1. Review Table 3-2, on pages 62–63. Are the steps for evidence-based practice clear to you? Consider a client that you recently cared for. What clinical questions do you have about that client's care? How would you try to answer them? Are any clinical pathways or standards in use to help you care for this client?

2. To understand some of the studies used in evidence-based care, it is necessary to understand some of the research terminology. Review the research terminology in Table 3-3, on pages 64–67. Think of a clinical question related to a client you cared for. What kind of research study would best answer your question? Check the library and see whether you can answer your question.

3. Go to the RNAO Best Nursing Practice Guidelines website. Consider a client you cared for your clinical experience. Which level of evidence supports the care delivery approaches to this client? How can you incorporate this guideline into your daily practice?

EXPLORING THE WEB

- Agency for Healthcare Research and Quality: *http://www.ahcpr.gov/*

- Appraisal Tools: *http://www.phru.nhs.uk/casp/casp.htm*

- Canadian Health Services Research Foundation: *http://www.chsrf.ca/home_e.php*

- Canadian Institute for Health Information: *www.cihi.ca*

- Canadian Institutes of Health Research: *http://www.cihr-irsc.gc.ca/*

- Canadian Medical Association infobase of clinical practice guidelines: *http://mdm.ca/cpgsnew/cpgs/index.asp*

- Canadian Population Health Initiative: *http://secure.cihi.ca/cihiweb/dispPage.jsp?cw_page=cphi_e*

- Centre for Evidence Based Nursing: *http://www.york.ac.uk/healthsciences/centres/evidence/cebn.htm*

- Centre for Reviews and Dissemination: *http://www.york.ac.uk/inst/crd/*

- Cochrane Collaboration: *http://www.cochrane.org/index.htm*

- CONSORT Statements: *http://www.consort-statement.org/*

- GRADE Working Group: *http://www.gradeworkinggroup.org/intro.htm*

- Guidelines Advisory Committee: *http://www.gacguidelines.ca/*

- Health Canada: *http://www.hc-sc.gc.ca/sr-sr/index_e.html*

- Institute for Work & Health: *http://www.iwh.on.ca*

- National Guideline Clearinghouse: *http://www.guideline.gov/*

- Newcastle-Ottawa Scale (Observational Studies): *http://www.ohri.ca/programs/clinical_epidemiology/oxford.htm*

- Nursing Best Practice Guidelines: *http://www.rnao.org/bestpractices/index.asp*

- Nursing Health Services Research Unit: *http://www.nhsru.com/*

- OHA Hospital Reports: *http://www.oha.com/oha/reprt5.nsf*

- Quality in Qualitative Evaluation: A Framework for Assessing: *http://www.pm.gov.uk/files/pdf/Quality_framework.pdf*

- QUOROM & MOOSE Statements: *http://www.consort-statement.org/Initiatives/complements.htm*

- Health Outcomes for Better Information and Care: *http://www.health.gov.on.ca/english/providers/project/nursing/nursing_mn.html*

REFERENCES

AGREE Collaboration. (2003). Development and validation of an international appraisal instrument for assessing the quality of clinical practice guidelines: The AGREE project. *Quality & Safety in Health Care, 12*(1), 18–23.

Canadian Health Services Research Foundation. (2004, March 11). *What counts? Interpreting evidence-based decision-making for management and policy: Report of the 6th CHSRF Annual Invitational Workshop*, pp. 1–14. Retrieved from http://www.chsrf.ca/knowledge_transfer/pdf/2004_workshop_report_e.pdf, June 26, 2007.

Canadian Nurses Association. (2002). *Position statement on evidence-based decision-making and nursing practice*. Retrieved from http://www.cna-nurses.ca/cna/, August 19, 2006.

Dicenso, A., Guyatt, G., & Ciliska, D. (2004). *Evidence-based nursing: A guide to clinical practice*. Philadelphia: Elsevier Publishing & AMA Press.

Estabrooks, C. A. (1998). Will evidence-based nursing practice make practice perfect? Canadian *Journal of Nursing Research, 30*(1), 15–36.

Estabrooks, C. A., Scott-Findlay, S., & Winther, C. (2004). A nursing and allied health sciences perspective on knowledge utilization. In L. Lemieux-Charles & F. Champagne (Eds.), *Using knowledge and evidence in health care* (pp. 242–280). Toronto: University of Toronto Press.

Evidence-Based Medicine Working Group. (1992). Evidence-based medicine: A new approach to teaching the practice of medicine. *JAMA, 268*(17), 2420–2425.

Glasziou, P., Vandenbroucke, J., & Chalmers, I. (2004). Assessing the quality of research. *British Medical Journal, 328*(7430), 39–41.

Higgins, J. P. T., & Green, S. (Eds.). *Cochrane Handbook for Systematic Reviews of Interventions 4.2.5* [updated May 2005]. Retrieved from http://www.cochrane.org/resources/handbook/hbook.htm, August 19, 2006.

Joint Provincial Nursing Committee. (2001). Progress report on the nursing task force strategy in Ontario: Good nursing, good health: A good investment. Toronto: Joint Provincial Nursing Committee.

Lavis, J. N., Davies, H. T. O., Gruen, R. L., Walshe, K., & Farquhar, C. (2006). Working within and beyond the Cochrane collaboration to make systematic reviews more useful to healthcare managers and policy makers. *Healthcare Policy, 1*(2), 21–33.

Naylor, C. D. (1995). Grey zones of clinical practice: Some limits to evidence-based medicine. *The Lancet, 345*(8953), 840–842.

Ontario Ministry of Health and Long-Term Care. (2002). *Health outcomes for better information and care project*. Retrieved from http://www.health.gov.on.ca/english/providers/project/nursing/overview/overview.html, August 19, 2006.

Oxman, A. D., & Guyatt, G. H. (1991). Validation of an index of the quality of review articles. *Journal of Clinical Epidemiology, 44*, 1271–1278.

Rafael, A. R. F. (2000). Evidence-based practice: The good, the bad, the ugly. *Registered Nurse,* September/October, 7–9.

Rappolt, S. (2002). Family physicians' selection of informal peer consultants: Implications for continuing education. *Journal of Continuing Education in the Health Profession, 22*(2), 113–120.

Sackett, D. L., Rosenberg, W. M. C., Gray, J. A. M., Haynes, R. B., & Richardson, W. S. (1996). Evidence-based medicine: What it is and what it isn't. *British Medical Journal, 312,* 71–72.

Schünemann, H. J., Best, D., Vist, G., & Oxman, A. D. (2003). Letters, numbers, symbols and words: How to communicate grades of evidence and recommendations. *CMAJ, 169*(7), 677–680.

Silagy, C., & Haines, A. (Eds.). (1998). *Evidence-based practice in primary care.* London: BMJ Books.

Stetler, C. B., Brunell, M., Giuliano, K., Morsi, D., Prince, L., & Newell-Stokes, V. (1998). Evidence-based practice and the role of nursing leadership. *Journal of Nursing Administration, 28*(7/8), 45–53.

Straus, S. E., & Sackett, D. L. (1998). Getting research findings into practice: Using research findings in clinical practice. *BMJ, 317*, 339–342.

Thomas, J., Harden, A., Oakley, A., Oliver, S., Sutcliffe, K., Rees, R. et al. (2004). Integrating qualitative research with trials in systematic reviews. *British Medical Journal, 328*(1010), 1012.

Udod, S. A., & Care W. D. (2004). Setting the climate for evidence-based nursing practice: What is the leader's role? *Canadian Journal of Nursing Leadership, 17*(4),64–75.

Upshur, R. E. (2003). Are all evidence-based practices alike? Problems in the ranking of evidence. *CMAJ, 169*(7), 672–673.

SUGGESTED READINGS

Angel, B. F., Duffey, M., & Belyea, M. (2000). An evidence-based project for evaluating strategies to improve knowledge acquisition and critical-thinking performance in nursing students. *Journal of Nursing Education, 39*, 219–228.

Bakken, S., & McArthur, J. (2001). Evidence-based nursing practice: A call to action for nursing informatics. *Journal of the American Medical Informatics Association, 8*, 289–290.

Beason, C. (2000). Creating an innovative organization. *Nursing Clinics of North America, 35*, 443–452.

Bonell, C. (1999). Evidence-based nursing: A stereotyped view of quantitative and experimental research could work against professional autonomy and authority. *Journal of Advanced Nursing, 30*(1), 18–23.

Bradham, D., Mangan, M., Warrick, A., Geiger-Brown, J., Reiner, J. I., & Saunders, H. J. (2000). Linking innovative nursing practice to health services research. *Nursing Clinics of North America, 35*, 557–568.

Ciliska, D. (2006a). Educating for evidence-based practice. *Journal of Professional Nursing, 21*(6), 345–350.

Ciliska, D. (2006b). Evidence-based nursing: how far have we come? What's next? *Evidence-Based Nursing, 9*, 38–40.

Cook, D., Mulrow, C., & Haynes, B. (1997). Systematic reviews: Synthesis of best evidence for clinical decisions. *Annals of Internal Medicine, 126*(5), 376–380.

Cullum, N. (2000). Users' guides to the nursing literature: An introduction. *Evidence-based Nursing, 3,* 71–72.

Dobbins, M., Davies, B., Danseco, E., Edwards, N., & Virani, T. (2005). Changing nursing practice: Evaluating the usefulness of a best practice guideline implementation toolkit. *The Canadian Journal on Nursing Leadership, 18*(1), 34–45.

Dobbins, M., & DeCorby, K. (2004). A knowledge transfer strategy for public health decision makers. *Worldviews on Evidence-Based Nursing, 2*, 100–108.

Goode, C. J. (2000). What constitutes the "evidence" in evidence-based practice? *Applied Nursing Research, 13*, 222–225.

GRADE Working Group. (2004). Grading quality of evidence and strength of recommendations. *BMJ, 328*, 1490–1497. Retrieved from http://bmj.bmjjournals.com/, August 19, 2006.

Greer, N., Mosser, G., Logan, G., & Halaas, G. W. (2000). A practical approach to evidence grading. *Joint Commission Journal on Quality Improvement, 26*, 700–712.

Grimshaw, J. (2004). So what has the Cochrane Colloboration ever done for us? A report card on the first 10 years. *CMAJ, 171*(7), 747–701.

Haynes, E. (2000). Research as a key to promoting and sustaining innovative practice. *Nursing Clinics of North America, 35*, 453–463.

Jadad, A. R., Cook, D. J., & Browman, G. P. (1997). A guide to interpreting discordant systematic reviews. *CMAJ, 156*(10), 1411–1416.

Jadad, A. R., Moore, R. A., Carroll, D., Jenkinson, C., Reynolds, J. M., Gavaghan, D. J. et al. (1996). Assessing the quality of reports of Randomized Clinical Trials: Is blinding necessary? *Controlled Clinical Trials, 17,* 1–12.

Kitson, A. (2000). Towards evidence-based quality improvement: Perspectives from nursing practice. *International Journal for Quality in Health Care, 12*, 459–464.

Kizer, K. (2000). Promoting innovative nursing practice during radical health system change. *Nursing Clinics of North America, 35*, 430–449.

Lemieux-Charles, L., & Champagne, F. (eds.). (2004). *Using knowledge and evidence in health care.* Toronto: University of Toronto Press.

McIntosh, H. M., Woolacott, N. F., & Bagnall, A. M. (2004). Assessing harmful effects in systematic reviews. *BMC Medical Research Methodology, 4,* 19.

Munro, B. H. (2005). *Statistical methods for health care research* (5th ed.). Philadelphia: Lippincott Williams & Wilkins.

Popay, J., Rogers, A., & Williams, G. (1998). Rationale and standards for the systematic review of qualitative literature in health services research. *Qualitative Health Research, 8*(3), 341–351.

Rosen, W., & Donald, A. (1995). Evidence based medicine: An approach to clinical problem solving. *British Medical Journal, 310,* 1122–1125.

Rosenfeld, P., Duthie, E., Bier, J., Bowar-Ferres, S., Fulmer, T., Iervolino, L. et al. (2000). Engaging staff nurses in evidence-based research to identify nursing practice problems and solutions. *Applied Nursing Research, 13*(4), 197–203.

Shaw, B. L., Taylor, W., & Roach, C. (2006). Focus on clinical best practices, patient safety and operational efficiency. *Healthcare Quarterly, 10*(special issue), 50–57.

Shorten, A., Wallace, M. C., & Crookes, P. A. (2001). Developing information literacy: A key to evidence-based nursing. *International Nursing Review, 48,* 86–92.

"STROBE statement: STrengthening the Reporting of OBservational studies in Epidemiology." Retrieved from http://www.strobe-statement.org/, February 16, 2006.

Urbshott, G. B., Kennedy, G., & Rutherford, G. (2001). The Cochrane HIV/AIDS review group and evidence-based practice in nursing. *Journal of the Association of Nurses in AIDS Care, 12*(6), 94–101.

van Tulder, M., Furlan, A., Bombarier, C., Bouter, L., & the Editorial Board of the Cochrane Collaboration Back Review Group. (2003). Updated methods guidelines for systematic reviews in the Cochrane Collaboration Back Review Group. *Spine, 28*(12), 1290–1299.

CHAPTER ENDNOTES

1. Agency for Healthcare Research and Quality, "Evidence-based Practice Centres, Overview, Centres." Retrieved from http://www.ahrq.gov/clinic/epc/, April 21, 2007.

2. Canadian Agency for Drugs and Technologies in Health, "About CADTH." Retrieved from http://www.cadth.ca/index.php/en/cadth, April 21, 2007.

3. Registered Nurses Association of Ontario, "Nursing Best Practice Guidelines." Retrieved from http://www.rnao.org/Page.asp?PageID=861&SiteNodeID=133, April 21, 2007.

4. Cochrane Collaboration, "What Is the Cochrane Collaboration?" Retrieved from http://www.cochrane.org/docs/descrip.htm, August 19, 2006.

5. Campbell Collaboration, "About the Campbell Collaboration." Retrieved from http://www.campbellcollaboration.org/About.asp, August 19, 2006.

6. Cochrane Collaboration, "What Is the Cochrane Collaboration?" Retrieved from http://www.cochrane.org/docs/descrip.htm, August 19, 2006.

7. Cochrane Library, "About Cochrane." Retrieved from http://www3.interscience.wiley.com/cgi-bin/mrwhome/106568753/AboutCochrane.html, March 23, 2007.

8. Ibid.

9. GRADE Working Group, "Grading the Quality of Evidence and the Strength of Recommendations." Retrieved from http://www.gradeworkinggroup.org/intro.htm, April 21, 2007.

10. Health Canada, Canada's Health Infostructure, "National Forum on Health." Retrieved from http://www.hc-sc.gc.ca/hcs-sss/ehealth-esante/infostructure/nfoh_nfss_e.html, April 21, 2007.

11. Canadian Health Services Research Foundation, "About CHSRF." Retrieved from http://www.chsrf.ca/home_e.php, April 21, 2007.

12. Canadian Population Health Initiative, "About CPHI." Retrieved from http://secure.cihi.ca/cihiweb/dispPage.jsp?cw_page=cphi_about_e, April 21, 2007.

13. Canadian Institutes of Health Research, "An Overview of CIHR, Mandate." Retrieved from http://www.cihr-irsc.gc.ca/e/30240.html#slide1_e, April 21, 2007.

14. Canadian Cochrane Centre, "Funding and Support." Retrieved from http://www.ccnc.cochrane.org/en/support.html, April 21, 2007.

15. Nursing Health Services Research Unit, "Welcome to the Nursing Health Services Research Unit." Retrieved from http://www.nhsru.com/, April 21, 2007.

16. Canadian Health Services Research Foundation. Retrieved from http://www.chsrf.ca/home_e.php, April 21, 2007.

17. Canadian Institute for Health Information, "Health Care Spending to Reach $142 Billion This Year." Retrieved from http://secure.cihi.ca/cihiweb/dispPage.jsp?cw_page=media_07dec2005_e, April 21, 2007.

CHAPTER 4

Nursing and Health Care Informatics

Leslie H. Nicoll, PhD, MBA, RN
Adapted by: Heather Crawford, BScN, MEd, CHE

From then on, when anything went wrong with a computer, we said it had bugs in it. (Admiral Grace Murray Hopper, on the removal of a two-inch-long moth from an experimental computer at Harvard University, September 9, 1945)

OBJECTIVES

Upon completion of this chapter, the reader should be able to:

1. List the components that define a nursing specialty and discuss how nursing informatics meets these requirements.

2. Discuss educational opportunities for nurses interested in pursuing a career in nursing informatics.

3. Describe highlights in the history of modern computing.

4. Discuss how ubiquitous computing and virtual reality have the potential to influence nursing education and practice.

5. Use established criteria to evaluate the content of health-related sites found on the Internet.

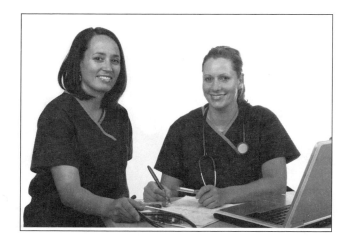

What is the most important card in your wallet? Your driver's licence? Your nursing registration? Your library card? In a few years, it might be your electronic health record. This record, a collection of all of your interactions with the health care system, would be available electronically to health care professionals anywhere in Canada. A swipe of the card in a barcode reader, and your complete health history would be available, no matter where you are or the nature of your complaint. At each encounter, the card would be updated, ensuring that every health care provider you come in contact with has the most complete and current health information available for your care.

Does this scenario sound like science fiction, or do you think it will be a reality within the coming years?

Like it or not, computers are here to stay. Computers have changed the way we communicate, obtain information, work, and, most recently, shop. As evidence, during 2001, 2.2 million Canadian households spent close to $2 billion on online shopping. As evidence, during 2005, almost 7 million Canadians spent just over $7.9 billion on online shopping. In 2003, Canadian households spent $3 billion shopping on the Internet. Canadian households placed almost 50 million orders over the Internet in 2005, up from 21 million orders in 2003. Eighty percent of Canadians expressed a concern about the use of credit cards on the Internet (Statistics Canada, 2006b). As of June 2007, more than 1 billion people worldwide had Internet access, up 214 percent from 2000 (Internet World Stats, 2007).

Consumers are also going online for health content. Among those who accessed the Internet from home, 63 percent of women and 53 percent of men searched for information about health or medical conditions (Statistics Canada, 2006a). Although most people online search for health information, industry experts predict other forms of "e-health"—connecting with providers or receiving case management online—will continue to experience rapid development (Bard, 2000).

Computers and the Internet are changing health care delivery, too. For example, in 2003, David Kaufman, a professor in the Faculty of Education at Simon Fraser University, in British Columbia, received funding to study how game and simulation technology can be used to educate people in the field of health. One of the researchers is working on a computer game for nine- to twelve-year-olds to teach them about contagious diseases, such as HIV/AIDS and West Nile virus. (Assessment of Technology in Context, Simon Fraser University, 2003). In another study, in the fall of 2005, Sunnybrook and Women's College Hospital was the first hospital in Ontario to evaluate a new software program, called New Age, which claims to improve client safety by instantly alerting clinicians of abnormal lab results. New Age is handheld software that will display Sunnybrook and Women's College Hospital's electronic client record data, including lab results, radiology reports, admission and discharge information, and client-specific transcription—all in an integrated fashion. The software allows physicians to monitor a client's condition in real-time and creates instant alerts (Bristow, 2005).

Nurses are not immune to the changes that computers are bringing to both everyday life and nursing practice. Computer technology can help nurses to achieve the goals of quality client care and positive client outcomes. Whether you are a student learning a clinical procedure using a computer-based instruction program or an administrator using a spreadsheet and database to plan a budget, computer technology is an essential part of professional nursing practice, both on the individual and institutional level.

Although nearly everyone is involved with computers to some degree today, some have chosen to specialize within the field of computer science, information, and technology. Within nursing, this specialty is known as nursing informatics. Nurses in informatics have taken on a wide variety of roles and are involved in a myriad of activities, ranging from the design and implementation of clinical information systems to research on the use of technology to improve client outcomes. Although this specialty is fairly new within the profession, informatics nurses are already having a major impact on the way care is planned and delivered in the current health care environment.

This chapter will introduce you to both dimensions of computing in professional nursing: the world of nursing informatics as well as the world of computing "for the rest of us." Although it may not be your career choice to become an informaticist, professional registered nurses of the 21st century will not be effective in their roles without a solid base of knowledge related to computers and technology and their impact on nursing practice, client care, and client outcomes.

WHAT IS NURSING INFORMATICS?

The term *informatics* was derived from the French word *informatique*. Gorn (1983) first defined the term as computer science plus information science. Informatics involves more than just computers—it includes all aspects of technology and science, from the theoretical to the applied. Another important part of the field of informatics concerns learning how to use new tools and maximizing the capabilities provided by computers and related information technologies (Ball, Hannah, & Douglas, 2000).

Nursing informatics refers to that component of informatics designed for and relevant to nurses. The first definition of nursing informatics was developed by Ball and Hannah in 1984 (Ball & Hannah, 1984). Various authors modified and embellished the definition during the ensuing decade (see Table 4-1). The definition proposed by the 1999 National Nursing Informatics Project (NNIP) discussion paper has been generally accepted in Canada. The sponsors for this project included the Canadian Association of Schools of Nursing (CASN), the Canadian Nurses Association (CNA), the Registered Nurses Association of British Columbia (RNABC), the Academy of Canadian Executive Nurses (ACEN), and the Nursing Informatics Special Interest Group of the Canadian Organization for Advancement of Computers

in Health (COACH). Note that this definition includes many components of nursing informatics: information management, knowledge from sciences other than nursing, and the importance of informatics within all areas of nursing practice. For nurses studying to become informatics specialists and for those developing curricula for education in nursing informatics, the definition also provides guidance (Gassert, 2000).

THE SPECIALTY OF NURSING INFORMATICS

Specialties in nursing cover a range of interests and clinical domains, such as critical care nursing, community health nursing, and nursing administration. Key attributes of a specialty were identified by Styles (1989) as follows:

- Differentiated practice
- A research program
- Representation of the specialty by at least one organized body
- A mechanism for credentialing nurses in the specialty
- Educational programs for preparing nurses to practise in the specialty

In 1992, the American Nurses Association (ANA) acknowledged that nursing informatics possessed these attributes and designated nursing informatics as an area

TABLE 4-1	EVOLUTION OF A DEFINITION: NURSING INFORMATICS

The discipline of applying computer science to nursing process
(Ball & Hannah, 1984)

A focus that uses information technology to perform functions with nursing
(Hannah, 1985)

The application of the principles of information science and theory to the study, scientific analysis, and management of nursing information for the purposes of establishing a body of nursing knowledge
(Grobe, 1988)

The combination of nursing science, information science, and computer science to manage and process nursing data, information, and knowledge to facilitate the delivery of health care
(Graves & Corcoran, 1989)

Nursing Informatics (NI) is the application of computer science and information science to nursing. NI promotes the generation, management and processing of relevant data in order to use information and develop knowledge that supports nursing in all practice domains.
(National Nursing Informatics Project (NNIP) discussion paper, 1999)

of specialty practice. The Canadian Nurses Association has 17 areas of specialty nursing certification; however, nursing informatics is not yet one of them.

In 2001, the Canadian Nursing Informatics Association (CNIA) was formed. The mission of the CNIA is to be the voice for nursing informatics in Canada. The Canadian Nurses Association granted emerging group status to the CNIA in recognition of the work undertaken by the group. In 2003, CNIA was granted affiliate status by the CNA. The CNIA is also affiliated with the Canadian Organization for Advancement of Computers in Health (COACH). Through this strategic alliance, the CNIA is the Canadian nursing nominee to the International Medical Informatics Association–Special Interest Group in Nursing Informatics. In 2002–03, the CNIA conducted a study, *Educating Tomorrow's Nurses: Where's Nursing Informatics?*[1] This project built on the 1999 National Nursing Informatics Project. It was influenced by the Canadian Nurses Association national Health Information: Nursing Components (HI-NC) policy initiative and Health Canada's Office of Health and the Information Highway (OHIH) work in conjunction with the Canadian Nurses Association (Vision 2020—ICT in Nursing) and with the University of Victoria Summit on health informatics competencies (Canadian Nursing Informatics Association, 2003).

EDUCATION IN INFORMATICS

Both formal and informal opportunities exist for education in nursing informatics. The first formal programs to offer specific degrees in nursing informatics were established within the past 15 years, and the number of programs has been increasing steadily. However, because educational options have been limited, many nurses practising in informatics have prepared for their role through on-the-job training or by receiving education outside of nursing. For example, a nurse may have a bachelor's degree of science in nursing (BSN) plus a second degree in computer science or information technology. Nurses have been successful in educating themselves using formal and informal resources. Nurses considering a career in informatics need to carefully consider the options that are available and plan their educational program accordingly.

FORMAL PROGRAMS   There are few formal programs in nursing informatics in Canada. However, an informatics graduate course is offered at the University of Toronto, and the University of Victoria has a School of Health Information Science. Some U.S. organizations offer weeklong or weekend educational events at Canadian venues, but these organizations are not bona fide educational institutions.

The Nursing Working Informatics Group of the American Medical Informatics Association (NWIG-AMIA) describes formal educational programs in nursing informatics as Category I, Category II, and Category III.

Category I programs are those graduate programs with a specialist nursing informatics focus. Six Category I programs are based at the following institutions of higher learning: Excelsior College (formerly Regents College), Albany, NY; New York University, New York, NY; St. Louis University, St. Louis, MO; University of Colorado Health Sciences Center, Denver, CO; University of Maryland, Baltimore, MD; and University of Utah, Salt Lake City, UT. Although each program is unique, they share some similarities. For example, students pursuing an education at the master's level will take approximately 42 semester credit hours of course work, which are divided among core courses (e.g., theory, research, policy, and advanced nursing), courses in nursing informatics (e.g., programming, database design, systems analysis and design, clinical decision making, informatics models, and practice activities), and support courses. Similarly, students at the University of Utah and the University of Maryland may pursue doctoral studies with substantive course work in nursing informatics. Again, courses are taken in nursing theory, research, statistics, and nursing informatics. As with any doctoral degree, a dissertation is required.

Category II programs are graduate and undergraduate programs and courses that allow a student to pursue a concentration (or a minor) in nursing informatics. In these programs, students take 6 to 12 credits of course work in informatics. Category II programs are available at Case Western Reserve University, Cleveland, OH; Duke School of Nursing, Durham, NC; Loyola University Chicago, Chicago, IL; Northeastern University, Boston, MA; Slippery Rock University, Slippery Rock, PA; University of Arizona, Tucson, AZ; University of Iowa, Iowa City, IA; University of Pennsylvania, Philadelphia, PA; and University of Phoenix (Phoenix Online), Phoenix, AZ.

Category III programs offer individual courses in nursing informatics at both the graduate and undergraduate level. The NWIG-AMIA has identified seven such programs (Georgia College and State University, Milledgeville, GA; Lewis College, Romeoville, IL; Oregon Health Sciences University, Portland, OR; Western Michigan University, Kalamazoo, MI; Wichita State University, Wichita, KS; University of North Carolina, Chapel Hill, NC; and University of Vermont, Burlington, VT). A few nursing informatics courses are offered in Canada: at Athabasca University in Alberta; at Kwantlen University College in British Columbia; and at Ryerson University and Mohawk College in Ontario. It is likely that this list is incomplete. Because nursing informatics has become such a popular area of study, and informatics courses and programs are being added to postsecondary curricula every year, if you are interested in formal study in informatics, check with schools and colleges of nursing in your locale to see what is available.

Although these are the only formal programs available at this time, many universities offer courses in computer science and information technology. Interested students are able to self-design programs that meet their individual learning needs. Programs at the University of Texas at Austin, University of California San Francisco, and the University of Wisconsin at Madison have been identified as having particularly strong concentrations of courses available in informatics (Gassert, 2000).

The Canadian Nursing Informatics Association's education bursary is directed at advancing the informatics education of a selected nurse recipient. The registered nurse or registered practical nurse must be a member in good standing in the Canadian Nurses Informatics Association, and be enrolled or accepted in an informatics certificate, diploma, or degree program.[2]

INFORMAL EDUCATION Many opportunities are available for nurses in Canada to be involved in informal education. In Ontario, the government has announced that the 14 Local Data Management Partnerships will link information technology and health care professionals from the 14 Local Health Integration Networks. Many hospitals now have formal positions in clinical informatics. Organizations have also implemented eHealth Councils. All of these initiatives present opportunities for nurses to learn through an informal route.

For many nurses, graduate education is not an option or personal choice, but they still desire to become more knowledgeable about informatics. For these nurses, many informal opportunities exist, including networking through professional organizations, keeping abreast of the literature by reading journals, and attending professional conferences.

Organizations vary in the scope of services offered to members and the types of educational programs offered. Nelson and Joos (1992) describe five types of organizations:

1. *Special interest groups* such as the Nova Scotia Nursing Informatics Special Interest Group, the Ontario Nursing Informatics Group, and the Saskatchewan Nursing Informatics Association. Non-nursing organizations that have special interest groups of interest to nurses include the Ontario Hospital Association, the Canadian Medical Association, the Canadian Society of Telehealth, and The Canadian Organization for the Advancement of Computers in Health (COACH).
2. *Information science and computer organizations*, such as the Canadian Information Processing Society (CIPS).
3. *Health computing organizations*, such as the Canadian Institute for Health Information (CIHI) and Smart Systems for Health Agency.
4. *User groups*, which consist of individuals working with a specific language, software, or vendor. One such group of interest to nurses is the Microsoft

Healthcare Users Group (MS-HUG), which focuses on applications of Microsoft products in health care environments.
5. *Local groups*, such as the nursing informatics special interest groups.

Nurses interested in learning more about informatics should become active in at least one related organization. As a member, a nurse has access to the meetings, publications, and educational offerings that the organization provides. Being on mailing lists and visiting organizations' websites also allows a nurse to keep abreast of different opportunities available through each organization.

Reading journals and newsletters is another way to become more knowledgeable about informatics. Offerings include trade magazines that are not related to health but are important sources of information, such as *PC Magazine* or the online magazine *Byte,* and specialized nursing journals, such as *CIN: Computers, Informatics, Nursing,* which offers continuing education contact hours in every issue. The American Medical Informatics Association (AMIA) publishes the *Journal of the American Medical Informatics Association,* a publication source for much of the research that has been conducted related to informatics. A nurse interested in informatics should become familiar with the journals that are available, subscribe to those that are most interesting, and read others in the library. Unfortunately, more information is published every month than anyone could possibly hope to keep abreast of—and that is where networking comes in! Colleagues can alert others to articles of interest that are in journals they might not regularly read.

Finally, conferences are excellent sources of education. At a conference, nurses are able to hear the latest information directly from experts in the field. Larger conferences usually have vendor exhibits that provide hands-on demonstrations for a variety of commercial products. Conferences vary in size, focus, location, and cost. For those interested in nursing informatics, nursing conferences are especially helpful. COACH: Canada's Health Informatics Association and the Canadian Institute for Health Information have an annual conference related to e-Health. Traditional themes have related to electronic health records, privacy, and telehealth. However, in 2007, new areas of focus included "e-health applications that are beginning to deliver on the expected benefits of improved client outcomes, improved client safety and improved cost effectiveness in the delivery of care."[3]

CERTIFICATION

Whether a nurse has pursued a formal or informal educational path in nursing informatics, many practising in the specialty choose to become certified. Certification in a specialty is a formal, systematic mechanism whereby nurses can voluntarily seek a credential that recognizes their quality and excellence in professional practice and continuing education (American Nurses Credentialing Center, 1993). For many nurses, becoming certified is both a professional milestone and a validation of their qualifications, knowledge, and skills in a defined area of nursing practice. The American Nurses Credentialing Center (ANCC) and the Canadian Nurses Association (CNA) offer certification examinations for a variety of specialties in nursing. The ANCC offers certification examinations in informatics. To be eligible for the nursing informatics examination, which was first offered in 1995, a nurse must meet the following requirements:

- Possess an active registered nursing licence in the United States or its territories
- Have earned a baccalaureate or higher nursing degree
- Have practised actively as a registered nurse for at least two years
- Have practised at least 2,000 hours in the field of nursing informatics within the past 5 years or completed at least 12 semester hours of academic credits in informatics in a graduate program in nursing and have practiced a minimum of 1,000 hours in informatics within the past 5 years
- Have earned 20 contact hours of continuing education credit applicable to the specialty area within the past 2 years (American Nurses Credentialing Center, 2001b)

The nurse who successfully passes the examination is certified as a generalist in informatics nursing. The ANCC is planning to offer an examination for a specialist in informatics nursing in the future. Once certified, the nurse must be recertified every five years. In the first year the examination was offered, 83 nurses became certified in informatics (Newbold, 1996). Currently, there are more than 400 nurses who are certified in the specialty (American Nurses Credentialing Center, 2001a).

CAREER OPPORTUNITIES

Career opportunities in the fields of computer science and information technology are growing at an exponential rate, and nursing is no exception. Nurses working in informatics can look forward to multiple job opportunities, with new roles continuously being developed as technology changes and matures. Changes in health care delivery have caused shifts in computer systems to case management, clinical systems, clinical data repositories, care mapping, and outcomes measures (Hersher, 2000).

Career opportunities for nurses in informatics exist in a number of different types of industries. Health care institutions, such as hospitals, are an obvious choice, but nurses also work for vendors of clinical information systems, insurance companies, and consulting firms.

CLINICAL INFORMATION

Clinical information systems are changing the way health care is delivered, whether in the hospital, the clinic, the provider's office, or the client's home. With capabilities ranging from advanced instrumentation to high-level decision support, a **clinical information system (CIS)** offers nurses and other clinicians information when, where, and how they need it. Increasingly, CIS applications function as the mechanisms for delivering client-centered care and for supporting the move toward the electronic health record (EHR).

What exactly is a CIS? Definitions vary, often from organization to organization. Semancik (1997) describes a CIS as a collection of software programs and associated hardware that supports the entry, retrieval, update, and analysis of client care information and associated clinical information related to client care. The CIS is primarily a computer system used to provide clinical information for the care of a client.

CLINICAL INFORMATION SYSTEMS

A CIS can be client-focused or departmental. In client-focused systems, automation supports client care processes. Typical applications found in a **client-focused clinical information system** include order entry, results reporting, clinical documentation, care planning, and clinical pathways. As data are entered into the system, data repositories are established that can be accessed to identify trends in client care. The **departmental clinical information system** evolved to meet the operational needs of a particular unit, such as the laboratory, radiology, the pharmacy, health records, or the finance or accounting department. Early systems often were standalone systems designed for an individual department. A major challenge facing CIS developers is to integrate these stand-alone systems to work with each other and with the newer client-focused systems.

ELECTRONIC HEALTH RECORD

A CIS is not the same as an **electronic health record (EHR)**. Ideally, the EHR will include all information about an individual's lifetime health status and health care. The EHR is a replacement for the paper health record as the primary source of information for health care, meeting all clinical, legal, and administrative requirements. However, the EHR is more than today's health record. Information technology permits much more data to be captured, processed, and integrated, which results in information that is broader than that found in a linear paper record.

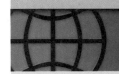

REAL WORLD INTERVIEW

M ount Sinai Hospital uses technology to provide its staff with the best possible environment to care for its clients. Sinai e-learning enables busy clinical staff to combine the best of computer-based learning with the best of instructor-based training. Through Sinai e-learning, it is simple for clinicians to get up to speed with new and upgraded applications, and test their knowledge in scenarios that accurately reflect real-world clinical situations—accelerating training, ensuring competency, and guaranteeing clinical staff can spend the maximum time caring for clients.

Dr. Lynn Nagle

Former Senior Vice-President, Technology and Knowledge Management, Mount Sinai Hospital

Source: Nagle, L. (2005). Dr. Lynn Nagle and the case for nursing informatics. *Canadian Journal of Nursing Leadership, 18* (1), 16–18. Reprinted with Permission.

The EHR is not a record in the traditional sense of the term. *Record* connotes a repository with limitations of size, content, and location. The term traditionally has suggested that the sole purpose for maintaining health data is to document events. Although documentation is an important purpose, the EHR permits health information to be used to support the generation and communication of knowledge.

The health care delivery system is dramatically changing, with a strong emphasis on improving outcomes of care and maintaining health. The EHR needs to be considered in a broader context and is not applicable only to clients, that is, individuals with the presence of an illness or disease. Rather, in the EHR, the focus is on the individuals' health, encompassing both wellness and illness.

As a result of this focus on the individual, the EHR is a virtual compilation of nonredundant health data across a person's lifetime, including facts, observations, interpretations, plans, actions, and outcomes. Health data include information on allergies, history of illness and injury, functional status, diagnostic studies, assessments, orders, consultation reports, and treatment records. Health data also include wellness information, such as immunization history, behavioural data, environmental information, demographics, health insurance, administrative data for care delivery processes, and legal data

(e.g., consents). The who, what, when, and where of data capture also are identified. The structure of the data includes text, numbers, sounds, images, and full-motion video. These structures are thoroughly integrated so that any given view of health data may incorporate one or more structural elements.

Within an EHR, an individual's health data are maintained and distributed over different systems in different locations, such as a hospital, clinic, physician's office, and pharmacy. Intelligent software agents with appropriate security measures are necessary to access data across these distributed systems. The nurse or other user who is retrieving these data must be able to assemble the data in such a way as to provide a chronology of health information about the individual.

The EHR is maintained in a system that captures, processes, communicates, secures, and presents the data about the client. This system may include the CIS. Other components of the EHR system include clinical rules, literature for client education, and expert opinions. When these elements work together in an integrated fashion, the EHR becomes much more than a client record—it becomes a knowledge tool. The system is able to integrate information from multiple sources and provides decision support; thus, the EHR serves as the primary source of information for client care.

A fully functional EHR is a complex system. Consider a single data element (i.e., a datum), such as a person's weight. The system must be able to record the weight; store it; process it; communicate it to others; and present it in a different format, such as a bar graph or chart. It may also be necessary to convert a weight from kilograms to pounds or vice versa. All of this processing must be done in a secure environment that protects the client's confidentiality and privacy. The complexity of these issues and the development of the necessary systems help to explain why few fully functional EHR systems are in place today.

DATA CAPTURE

Data capture refers to the collection and entry of data into a computer system. The origin of the data may be local or remote, with the data coming from client-monitoring devices; from telemedicine applications; directly from the individual recipient of health care; and even from others who have information about the recipient's health or environment, such as relatives, friends, and public health agencies. Data may be captured by multiple means, including key entry, pattern recognition (e.g., voice, handwriting, or biological characteristics), and medical device transmission.

All data entered into a computer are not necessarily structured for subsequent processing. Document-imaging systems, for example, provide for creation of electronically stored text but have limitations on the ability to process that text. Data capture includes the use of controlled vocabularies and code systems to ensure common meaning for terminology and the ability to process units of information. As noted earlier, great strides have been made in the development of standardized nursing languages. These languages provide structured data entry and text processing that result in common meaning and processing.

Data capture also encompasses authentication to identify the author of an entry and to ensure that the author has been granted permission to access the system and change the EHR.

STORAGE

Storage refers to the physical location of data. In EHR systems, health data are distributed across multiple systems at different sites. For this reason, there need to be common access protocols, retention schedules, and universal identification.

Access protocols permit only authorized users to obtain data for legitimate uses. The systems must have backup and recovery mechanisms in the event of failure. Retention schedules address the maintenance of the data in active and inactive forms and the permanence of the storage medium.

A person's identity can be determined by many types of data, in addition to common identifiers such as name and number. Universal identifiers or other methods are required for integrating health data of an individual distributed across multiple systems at different sites.

INFORMATION PROCESSING

Computer processing functions provide for effective retrieval and processing of data into useful information. These functions include decision support tools, such as alerts and alarms for drug interactions, allergies, and abnormal laboratory results. Reminders can be provided for appointments, critical path actions, medication administration, and other activities. The systems also may provide access to consensus- and evidence-driven diagnostic and treatment guidelines and protocols. The nurse could integrate a standard guideline, protocol, or critical path into a specific individual's EHR, modify it to meet unique circumstances, and use it as a basis for managing and documenting care. Outcome data communicated from various caregivers and health care recipients themselves also may be analyzed and used for continuous improvement of the guidelines and protocols.

INFORMATION COMMUNICATION

Information communication refers to the interoperability of systems and linkages for exchange of data across disparate systems. To integrate health data across multiple systems at different sites, identifier systems (e.g., unique numbers or other methodology) are essential for health care recipients, caregivers, providers, and sites. Local,

regional, and national health information infrastructures that tie all participants together using standard data communication protocols are key to the linkage function. Hundreds of types of transactions or messages must be defined and agreed to by the participating stakeholders. Vocabulary and code systems must permit the exchange and processing of data into meaningful information. EHR systems must provide access to point-of-care information databases and knowledge sources, such as pharmaceutical formularies, referral databases, and reference literature.

SECURITY

Computer-based health record systems provide better protection of confidential health information than paper-based systems because of their support controls that ensure that only authorized users with legitimate uses have access to health information. Security functions address the confidentiality of private health information and the integrity of the data. The design of security functions must ensure compliance with applicable legislation, regulations, and standards. Security systems must ensure that access to data is provided only to those who are authorized and have a legitimate purpose for using the data. Security functions also must provide a means to audit for inappropriate access.

Three important terms are used when discussing security: privacy, confidentiality, and security. It is important to understand the differences between these concepts.

- *Privacy* refers to the right of individuals to keep information about themselves from being disclosed to anyone. If a client had an abortion and chose not to tell a health care provider this fact, the client would be keeping that information private.

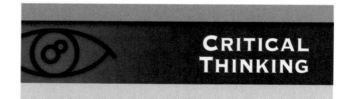

CRITICAL THINKING

In your clinical practice, you have likely interacted with a clinical information system to both enter and access data for the client you were caring for.

What security systems were in place to maintain the confidentiality of client data, for example, passwords, identification cards, and other features? Do you believe the security system was effective? Was it updated on a regular basis? Did the security system present any barriers to your obtaining necessary information for providing quality client care—for example, were the results of certain tests or past history restricted in any way?

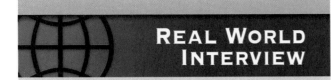

REAL WORLD INTERVIEW

Elizabeth Borycki, an RN and assistant professor at the University of Victoria's School of Health Information Science, has studied the impact of technology on client care and says EHRs can allow nurses to make well-informed, timely decisions about client care. Technology also makes it easier to access nursing research relevant to their clients. But Borycki cautions that some research suggests technology can lead to medical errors if it isn't designed in a clinician-friendly way. That's why she says it's essential for nurses to provide their expertise when new client documentation methods are being developed and introduced. "Nurses can identify aspects of technology that don't allow for its easy introduction to the clinical practice setting," she says. "They can identify functions, features, and components of technology that don't meet nursing's needs, and suggest elements that should be changed."

Source: Shaw, J. (2006). From paper to programming. *Registered Nurse Journal, 18* (2), 15. Reprinted with Permission.

■ *Confidentiality* refers to the act of limiting disclosure of private matters. After a client has disclosed private information to a health care provider, that provider has a responsibility to maintain the confidentiality of that information.

■ *Security* refers to the means of controlling access and protecting information from accidental or intentional disclosure to unauthorized people and from alteration, destruction, or loss. When private information is placed in a confidential EHR, the system must have controls in place to maintain the security of the system and not allow unauthorized people access to the data (CPRI Work Group on Confidentiality, Privacy & Security, 1995).

INFORMATION PRESENTATION

The wealth of information available through EHR systems must be managed to ensure that authorized caregivers (e.g., nurses) and others with legitimate uses have the information they need in their preferred presentation form. For example, a nurse may prefer to see data organized by source, caregiver, encounter, problem, or date. Data can be presented in detail or summary form. Tables, graphs, narrative, and other forms of information presentation must be accommodated. Some users may need to know only of the presence or absence of certain data, not the nature of

the data itself. For example, blood donation centres test blood for HIV, hepatitis, and other conditions. If a donor has a positive test result, the centre may not be given the specific information regarding the test but just general information that a test result was abnormal and that the client should be referred to an appropriate health care provider.

CANADA HEALTH INFOWAY

Canada Health Infoway, Inc., established in 2001, invests with public sector partners across Canada to implement and reuse health information systems that support a safer, more efficient health care system. The members of Infoway are the 14 Canadian provincial, territorial, and federal ministers of health. Infoway is currently working with its partners on projects in nine targeted areas: Registries, Diagnostic Imaging Systems, Drug Information Systems, Laboratory Information Systems, Telehealth, Public Health Surveillance, Interoperable EHR, Innovation and Adoption, and Infostructure.[4] Their goal is to have an interoperable EHR in place across 50 percent of Canada (by population) by the end of 2009.[5]

INTERFACE BETWEEN THE INFORMATICS NURSE AND THE CLINICAL INFORMATION SYSTEM

Information demands in health care systems are pushing the development of CISs and EHRs. The ongoing development of computer technology—smaller, faster machines with extensive storage capabilities and the ability for cross-platform communication—is making the goal of an integrated electronic system a realistic option, not just a long-term dream. As these systems evolve, informatics nurses will play an important role in their development, implementation, and evaluation.

Informatics nurses, because of their expertise, are in an ideal position to assist with the development, implementation, and evaluation of CISs. Their knowledge of policies, procedures, and clinical care is essential as workflow systems are redesigned within a CIS. It is not unusual for nurses within an institution to have more hands-on interaction with and knowledge of different departments than any other group of employees in an institution. Jenkins (2000) suggests that the process model of nursing (i.e., assessment, planning, implementation, and evaluation) works well during a CIS implementation; thus, nurses have a familiar framework from which to understand the complexity of a major system change.

TRENDS IN COMPUTING

As noted earlier, computers have moved from the realm of a "nice to know" luxury item to a "need to know" essential resource for professional practice. Nurses are knowledge workers who require accurate and up-to-date information for their professional work. The explosion in information—some estimate that all information is replaced every 9 to 12 months—requires nurses to be on the cutting edge of knowledge to practise ethically and safely. Trends in computing will also affect the work of professional nurses and not just through the development of CISs and EHRs. Research advances, new devices, monitoring equipment, sensors, and "smart body parts" will all change the way that health care is conceptualized, practised, and delivered.

Within this context, not every nurse will need to be an informatics specialist, but every nurse must be computer literate. Computer literacy is defined as the knowledge and understanding of computers combined with the ability to use them effectively (Joos, Whitman, Smith, & Nelson, 1996). Computer literacy may be interpreted as different levels of expertise for different people in various roles. At the most basic level, computer literacy involves knowing how to turn on a computer, start and stop simple application programs, and save and print information. For health care professionals, computer literacy requires an understanding of systems used in clinical practice, education, and research settings. In clinical practice, for example, electronic health records and clinical information systems are widely used. The computer-literate nurse is able to use these systems effectively and can address issues discussed earlier, such as confidentiality, security, and privacy. At the same time, the nurse must be able to effectively use applications typically found on personal computers (PCs), such as word-processing software, spreadsheets, presentation graphics, and statistical programs used for research. Finally, the computer-literate nurse must know how to access information from a variety of electronic sources and how to evaluate the appropriateness of the information at both the professional and client level. The remainder of this chapter is designed to help you gain a broader understanding of computer literacy and the computing environment of PCs and the online world, and includes a discussion of future trends.

DEVELOPMENT OF MODERN COMPUTING

Weiser and Brown (1996) have characterized the history and future of computing as having three phases. The first phase, known as the "mainframe era," is characterized by many people sharing one computer. Computers were found behind closed doors and run by experts with specialized knowledge and skills. Although we have mostly moved beyond the mainframe era, it still exists in CISs (hence, some of the problems discussed previously) and other situations with large mainframe systems, such as banking, weather forecasting, and academic institutions.

The archetypal computer of the mainframe era must be the ENIAC, developed at the University of Pennsylvania in 1945. The Electronic Numerical Integrator and Computer (ENIAC) was conceived by John Mauchly, an American physicist, and built at the Moore School of Engineering by Mauchly and J. Presper Eckert, an engineer. The ENIAC is regarded as the first successful digital computer. It weighed more than 60,000 pounds and contained more than 18,000 vacuum tubes. About 2,000 of the computer's vacuum tubes were replaced each month by a team of six technicians. Despite one vacuum tube blowing approximately every 15 minutes, the functioning of the ENIAC was still considered to be reliable! Many of the ENIAC's first tasks were for military purposes, such as calculating ballistic-firing tables and designing atomic weapons. Because the ENIAC was initially not a stored program machine, it had to be reprogrammed for each task.

Phase II in modern computing is the "PC era," which is characterized by one person to one computer. In this era, the personal computing relationship is personal and intimate. Similar to a car, the computer is seen as a special, relatively expensive item, which requires attention but provides a valuable service in one's life.

The first harbinger of the PC era was in 1948, with the development of the transistor at Bell Telephone Laboratories. The transistor, which could act as an electric switch, replaced the costly, energy-inefficient, and unreliable vacuum tubes in computers and other devices, including televisions. By the late 1960s, integrated circuits, tiny transistors, and other electrical components arranged on a single chip of silicon replaced individual transistors in computers. Integrated circuits became miniaturized, enabling more components to be designed into a single computer circuit. In the 1970s, refinements in integrated circuit technology led to the development of the modern microprocessor, integrated circuits that contained thousands of transistors. Weiser and Brown (1996) date the true start of the second phase as 1984, when the number of people using personal computers surpassed the number of people using shared computers.

Manufacturers used integrated circuit technology to build smaller and cheaper computers. The first PCs were sold by Instrumentation Telemetry Systems. The Altair 8800 appeared in 1975. Graphical user interfaces were first designed by the Xerox Corporation in a prototype computer, the Alto, developed in 1974. This prototype computer incorporated many of the features found on computers today, including a mouse, a graphical user interface, and a user-friendly operating system. However, the Xerox Corporation made a corporate decision to not pursue commercial development of the PC, the rationale being that the core business strategy of Xerox was copiers, not computers. One only has to look at how PCs have proliferated throughout the world to realize that this choice may not have been the smartest business decision ever made. In fact, this whole episode has become a bit of a computer history legend (Hiltzik, 2000; Smith & Alexander, 1988). Continuing development of sophisticated operating systems and miniaturization of components (modern microprocessors contain as many as 10 million transistors) have enabled computers to be developed that can run programs and manipulate data in ways that were unimaginable in the era of the ENIAC.

UBIQUITOUS COMPUTING

Phase III has been dubbed the era of **ubiquitous computing (UC),** characterized by many computers to each person. In 1996, Weiser and Brown (1996) estimated that the crossover with the PC era would occur between 2005 and 2020. Their prediction was not far off; many of their forecasts have already become reality. According to Weiser and Brown, in the ubiquitous computing phase, computers would be everywhere—in walls, chairs, clothing, light switches, cars, appliances, and so on. In the UC era, computers are so fundamental to our human experience that they will "disappear" and we will cease to be aware of them. The result will be "calm technology," in which computers do not cause stress and anxiety for the user but, rather, recede into the background of life.

For those who are skeptical that this era has either already come or will come to pass, consider two other ubiquitous technologies: writing and electricity (Weiser, 1991). In Egyptian times, writing was a secret art, known and performed only by specially trained scribes who lived on a level close to royalty. Clay tablets and, later, papyrus were precious commodities. Many people died without ever having seen a piece of paper in their lives! Now, paper and writing are everywhere. Within the course of an average day, most people use and discard hundreds of pieces of paper, never giving them a second thought. Electricity has a similar history. When electricity was first invented in the 19th century, entire factories were designed to accommodate the presence of light bulbs and bulky motors. The placement of workers, machines, and parts was designed around the need for electricity and motors. Today, electricity is everywhere. It is hidden in the walls and stored in tiny batteries. The average car has more than 22 motors and 25 solenoids.

We only have to look around a typical house to see how UC is becoming part of our lives. Microprocessors exist in every room: appliances in the kitchen, remote controls for the TV and stereo in the den, and clock radios and cordless phones in the bedroom. And the bathroom? Matsushita of Japan has developed a prototype toilet (dubbed the "smart toilet") that includes an online, real-time health-monitoring system. It measures the user's weight, fat content, and urine sugar level; plots the recorded data on a graph; and sends the data instantaneously to a health care provider for monitoring (Watts, 1999).

Another dimension of UC is the Internet. Each time you connect to the Internet, you are connecting with millions of information resources and hundreds of information delivery systems. A person truly does become one person to hundreds of computers. It is ironic that the interface to the UC world of the Internet is still through a PC. But this is changing. Wireless, infrared connections eliminate wires; handheld devices eliminate the bulky PC. We have become wireless and mobile—UC is a reality.

VIRTUAL REALITY

According to Weiser (1991), virtual reality (VR) is roughly the opposite of ubiquitous computing. Virtual reality puts people inside a computer-generated world, whereas UC puts the computer out in the world with people. Virtual reality, although still limited in its development, has enormous potential in health care applications.

Virtual reality, despite its recent popularization, is not new. Similar to the Internet, it had its beginnings within the U.S. Department of Defense with innovations developed during the 1960s. During the time of the Cold War, great fear focused on the possibility of a nuclear attack. Military leaders sought to develop systems that would remain intact in the face of great destruction. The Internet, a worldwide network of computers, was developed so that the electronic communication infrastructure could not be destroyed. Electronic mail (e-mail) was created to ensure rapid and secure communication in

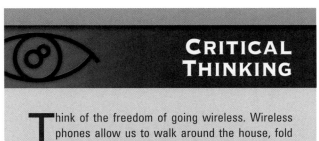

CRITICAL THINKING

Think of the freedom of going wireless. Wireless phones allow us to walk around the house, fold laundry, make the bed, straighten up a room, and yes, even go to the bathroom, all while talking on the phone. Remember being tethered by a phone cord?

Many businesses still do not provide their workers with wireless technology. Think of possible reasons why. Would wireless applications in health care settings improve the efficiency of care delivery systems? Why or why not?

the event the wire-based telephone system was destroyed. Virtual reality simulations were developed so that jet pilots' training would mimic a world turned upside down: flying through fire, mushroom clouds, and poisonous gases in planes that might lack air-to-ground control systems.

Current virtual reality systems have developed from these early applications. With VR, a person can see, move through, and react to computer-simulated items or environments. Using certain tools, such as a head-mounted computer display and a handheld input device, the user feels immersed in and can interact with this world. The virtual world can represent the current world or a world that is difficult or impossible to experience firsthand—for example, the world of molecules, the interior of the human body, or the surface of Pluto. By putting the sensors on the person (e.g., a head-mounted computer display and/or sensors in gloves, shoes, and glasses), the person can move and experience the world in a typical way—by walking, moving, and using the senses of touch, sight, smell, and hearing.

To date, VR applications have been more developed in medicine and other fields, but interest is growing for its applications in nursing. Within medicine, VR has allowed physicians to develop minimally invasive surgical techniques. Traditionally, surgery is performed by making incisions and directly interacting with the organs and tissues. Recent innovations in video technology allow direct viewing of internal body cavities through natural orifices or small incisions. The surgeon operates on a virtual image, manipulating instruments either directly or via virtual environments. In the latter case, a robot reproduces the movements of humans using virtual instruments. The precision of the operation may be augmented by data or the images can be superimposed on the virtual client (Satava, 1995).

Applications in medical education also exist. Virtual reality allows information visualization through the display of enormous amounts of information contained in large databases. Through 3-D visualization, students can understand important physiological principles or basic anatomy. Students can go inside a human body to visualize structures and see how they work. Changes in physiologic functioning can also be observed. For example, a student can visualize the vascular system of a client going into shock (Satava, 1993, 1995).

A popular use of VR in psychology has been in exposure therapy for clients with specific phobias. Hodges and colleagues (1995) used a VR reality simulation to treat clients with a fear of flying. Other researchers have found significant improvements in clients with agoraphobia using exposure therapy and VR (North, North, & Coble 1996).

At the University of Dayton Research Institute, Dayton, OH, researchers collaborated with the Miami Valley Transit Authority to assist disabled students to learn to ride the bus. Using a simulation of a public bus, students were able to learn how to get on, get off, and negotiate the interior, which gave them increased confidence and skills when faced with a real bus for the first time (Buckert-Donelson, 1995).

Applications in nursing are similar. For students learning clinical procedures, VR provides the opportunity to practise invasive and less commonly occurring procedures in the lab so they will have both the skill and confidence necessary when encountering a client requiring the procedure. Likewise, VR will enhance client education materials. Diabetic clients needing to understand the physiologic processes of the pancreas could visualize the organ to more fully understand their disease and treatment. Clients requiring painful or unusual procedures could experience a VR simulation as a means of preparation. By providing an alternate environment, VR also has the potential to mitigate or minimize the side effects of certain procedures, such as chemotherapy in clients with cancer.

THE INTERNET

The Internet will continue to change the way we communicate and obtain information. Many mistakenly believe that the Internet is a recent development. But, like VR, it has been around for almost four decades. The modern Internet started out in 1969, as a U.S. Defense Department network called ARPAnet. Scientists built ARPAnet with the intention of creating a network that would still be able to function efficiently if part of the network were damaged. Since then, the Internet has grown, changed, matured, and mutated, but the essential structure of interconnected domains randomly distributed throughout the world has remained the same. ARPAnet no longer exists, but many of the standards established for that first network still govern the communication and structure of the modern Internet.

In 1989, English computer scientist Timothy Berners-Lee introduced the World Wide Web (WWW). Berners-Lee initially designed the WWW to aid communication between physicists who were working in different parts of the world for the European Laboratory for Particle Physics, known in French as Conseil Européen pour la Recherche Nucléaire (CERN). As it grew, however, the WWW revolutionized the use of the Internet. During the early 1990s, increasingly large numbers of users who were not part of the scientific or academic communities began to use the Internet, in large part because of the ability of the WWW to easily handle multimedia documents. Other changes have also influenced the growth of the Internet, such as the U.S. government's High-Performance Computing Act of 1991; the decision to allow computers other than those used for research and military purposes to connect to the network; and the development of user-friendly software and tools that allowed less experienced computer users to obtain information quickly and easily.

USING THE INTERNET FOR CLINICAL PRACTICE

A major use of the Internet is to obtain information. In clinical practice, this dimension of the Internet is becoming essential to ensure that you have accurate and up-to-date information for your nursing work. To use information that exists on the Internet, skills must be developed for searching quickly and efficiently. A variety of strategies can be used for searching, including quick and dirty searching, links, and brute force. Keep in mind that you must be persistent: no single search strategy will work all the time, nor is any one search engine more effective than any other. Search engines are good starting points, but you can augment their effectiveness by adding a few other strategies to your Internet exploration tool kit.

THE P-F-A ASSESSMENT

One strategy to develop your search is to conduct a "purpose-focus-approach" (P-F-A) assessment. To determine your purpose, ask yourself why you are doing the search and why you need the information. Consider questions such as the following:

- Is it for personal interest?
- Do you want to obtain information to share with coworkers or a client?
- Are you verifying information given to you by someone else?
- Are you preparing a report or writing a paper for a class or project?

Based on your purpose, your focus may be as follows:

- Broad and general (e.g., basic information for yourself)
- Lay-oriented (e.g., to give information to a client) or professionally oriented (e.g., to locate information for colleagues)
- Narrow and technical, with a research orientation

Purpose combined with focus determines your approach. For example, information that is broad and general can be found using brute force methods or quick and dirty searching. Lay information can be quickly accessed at a few key sites, including MEDLINE*plus* and consumer health organizations. Similarly, professional associations and societies are a good starting point for professionally oriented information. Scientific and research information usually requires literature resources that can be found in databases such as MEDLINE or CINAHL (Cumulative Index to Nursing and Allied Health Literature).

QUICK AND DIRTY SEARCHING

Quick and dirty searching is a very simple but surprisingly effective search strategy. First, start with a search engine, such as Google (www.google.ca). Next, type in the term of interest. At this point, do not worry about being overly broad or general. You will retrieve an enormous number of found references (called hits), but you are interested only in the first 10 to 20. Look at the uniform resource locators (URLs), that is, the addresses of the sites that are returned by your search, and try to decipher what they mean. Pay attention to the domains: .com is commercial; .org refers to an organization; and .ca identifies a Canadian website. Quickly visit a few sites. Look for the information you need and useful links. If a site is not relevant, use the back button on your browser to return to your search results and go to the next site. When you find a site that appears to be useful, begin to explore the site. Many sites will connect you to other sites, using links, or hot buttons. If you click on a link, it will take you to a related site. Most sites have links you can follow to connect to other relevant sites. This process—quick search, quick review, clicking, and linking—can provide a starting point for finding useful information in a relatively short period of time.

BRUTE FORCE

Brute force searching is another alternative: type in an address in the URL box (the address box at the top of the browser window) and see what happens. The worst outcome is an annoying error message, but you may land on a site that is exactly what you want. To be effective, think of how URLs work: they usually start with www (for World Wide Web), then a word or phrase in the middle is followed by a domain. Perhaps you are trying to find a school of nursing at a certain university. What is the common name for the university? The very logical URL for the University of Victoria is www.uvic.ca. Organizations are also quite logical in their URLs: www.caccn.ca is the Canadian Association of Critical Care Nurses (CACCN); www.srna.org is the Saskatchewan Association of Registered Nurses (SRNA).

LINKS AND BOOKMARKS

As noted earlier, just about every website has links to other websites of related interest. Take advantage of these links, because the site developer has already done some work finding other useful resources. Combine quick and dirty searching or brute force with links to find the information you need. Each site you visit will have more links, and in this way, the resources keep building. Visiting a variety of sites will open up the vistas of information that are available. When you find a site of interest, bookmark it or add it to your list of favourites. A bookmark list, or list of favourites, is like a personal address book. Each time you find a site that is particularly useful, you can add it to your list of favourites, using the appropriate feature in your browser. Eventually, you will have a comprehensive list of sites that are relevant to your work and interests. Use this list to quickly return to websites in the future.

RESOURCES FOR PROFESSIONALS AND CONSUMERS

The preceding discussion has focused on strategies to use when you are faced with a "needle in a haystack" searching situation—just dive in and see what you find. The advantage of this method is that it is fast and easy. The disadvantages include sites of dubious quality that may be accessed, and the process, though fast, is not terribly efficient.

Another approach is to develop a short list of well-known, well-researched sites that can be used as starting points for further exploration. Such a list is useful to share with others so that they can begin their own exploration. These should be sites that you have determined are trustworthy and reliable, for example, organizations and associations with which we are all familiar, such as the Canadian Cancer Society (CCS). The CCS has client education and consumer information materials that can be obtained through www.cancer.ca. In addition to the traditional types of resources available from the CCS website, you can also e-mail the society to request more information, sign up for regular updates and news, read news items, and obtain updated statistical information. The website is truly a value-added version of the CCS. Practically any health organization you can think of has created a virtual storefront on the Internet. Professional associations, in nursing, medicine, and other disciplines, are also becoming comprehensive resource websites. Canadianrn.com (www.canadianrn.com) has a handy list of Canadian associations in nursing and related disciplines. Other resources include Canadian government agencies, such as the Canadian Institutes for Health Research (CIHR) (www.cihr-irsc.gc.ca) and Canada Health Infoway (www.infoway-inforoute.ca). Once again, all these agencies have been busy creating virtual institutes. A useful resource is Canadian Health Services Research Foundation (www.chsrf.ca/links/gov_e.php), which can point you to news, information, tools, and databases.

Although these resources are the web versions of known and useful organizations, some virtual resources exist only on the Internet. One such site that is particularly impressive is MEDLINE*plus* (http://medlineplus.gov), developed by the National Library of Medicine. A similar resource, specific to oncology, is OncoLink at the University of Pennsylvania (www.oncolink.org). OncoLink, created in 1994, was the first multimedia oncology information resource on the Internet. It continues to be true to its original mission to "help cancer patients, families, health care professionals and the general public get accurate cancer-related information at no charge" (Oncolink, 2001).

LITERATURE RESOURCES

Thinking back to P-F-A, if you are searching for scientific, technical, or research-oriented information, then you must search literature databases. The first place to turn to is the National Library of Medicine, which is the home of the **MEDLARS (Medical Literature Analysis and Retrieval System),** a computerized system of databases and databanks offered by the National Library of Medicine (NLM). A person may search the computer files either to produce a list of publications (bibliographic citations) or to retrieve factual information on a specific question. The most well-known of all the databases in the MEDLARS system is MEDLINE, NLM's premier bibliographic database covering the fields of medicine, nursing, dentistry, veterinary medicine, and the preclinical sciences. Journal articles are indexed for MEDLINE, and their citations are searchable using NLM's controlled vocabulary, called MeSH (Medical Subject Headings). MEDLINE contains all citations published in *Index Medicus* and corresponds in part to the International Nursing Index and the Index to Dental Literature. Citations include the English abstract when it is published with the article (approximately 76 percent of the current file). MEDLINE contains more than 11 million records from 7,300 health science journals. The file is updated weekly. An individual can search MEDLINE for free, using PubMed, a specially designed search engine (http://www.ncbi.nlm.nih.gov/sites/entrez). With this search engine, there are no fees to the user to access the MEDLINE database.

Two other literature resources to investigate are the U.S. National Guideline Clearinghouse (NGC) (www.ngc.gov) and the Canadian Agency for Drugs and Technologies in Health (CADTH) (http://www.cadth.ca/), which until April 2006 was known as the Canadian Coordinating Office for Health Technology Assessment (CCOHTA). Whereas MEDLINE includes citations to articles in professional journals, the NGC is a comprehensive database of evidence-based clinical practice guidelines and related documents produced by the Agency for Healthcare Research and Quality (AHRQ) in partnership with the American Medical Association (AMA) and the American Association of Health Plans (AAHP). The NGC mission is to provide physicians, nurses, and other health professionals and health care providers; health plans; integrated delivery systems; purchasers; and others an accessible mechanism for obtaining objective, detailed information on clinical practice guidelines and to further their dissemination, implementation, and use.

CADTH is a primary resource for unbiased health information on drugs, devices, health care systems, and best practices. It is funded by the Canadian federal, provincial, and territorial governments.

A variety of other literature resources are available on the Internet, some of which have fees attached. However, do not automatically assume that you must pay the fee. Your workplace or school may have licensing agreements in place with different vendors, and as an employee or student you may have access to the literature resources. Check with your library or information services department to see whether any of these arrangements apply.

The final element of searching for literature online is locating full-text articles. The databases discussed (e.g., MEDLINE and others) do not contain full–text articles— they provide only literature citations. However, most academic journals now have full-text articles online, available to university students through their library access. You can also visit the publisher's website to see whether access to the journal is available, or research the old-fashioned way, that is, by taking a trip to the library and photocopying articles. A final option is to access a service such as Ingenta (http://www.ingentaconnect.com/) to access its collection of scholarly research materials. This resource allows you to conduct a search. It identifies which articles can be sent to you, and what the fees will be (including article fees, service charges, and copyright fees).

EVALUATION OF INFORMATION FOUND ON THE INTERNET

When using Internet resources, one must always use critical thinking skills to evaluate the information that is found. The wide-open nature of the Internet means that just about anyone with a computer and online access can create a home page and post it for the world to see. Although there are many excellent health- and nursing-related sites, others do not measure up in terms of accuracy, content, or currency.

In recent years, criteria for website evaluation have proliferated. They range from the simple and cursory to the elaborate and expansive. I have found a simple mnemonic, "Are you PLEASED with the site?" to be very helpful (see Table 4-2).

The mnemonic makes the seven criteria very easy to remember, and I have found these criteria, in hundreds of hours of surfing and evaluating, to be extremely comprehensive (Nicoll, 2000, 2001). To determine whether you are PLEASED, consider the following:

- *P—Purpose.* What is the author's purpose in developing the site? Are the author's objectives clear? Many people will develop a website as a hobby or a way of sharing information they have gathered. The true purpose of the site should be immediately evident. At the same time, consider your purpose; that is, think back to your P-F-A assessment. Congruence should exist between the author's purpose and yours.
- *L—Links.* Evaluate the links at the site. Are they working? Links that do not take you anywhere are called dead links. Do they link to reliable sites? Critically evaluate the links at sites hosted by organizations, businesses, or institutions because these entities are usually presenting themselves as authorities on the subject at hand. Some pages, such as those created by individuals, are really nothing more than a collection of links. These can be useful as a starting point for a search, but it is still important to evaluate the links that are provided at the site.
- *E—Editorial (site content).* Is the information contained in the site accurate, comprehensive, and current? Is there a particular bias, or is the information presented in an objective way? Who is the consumer of the site: is it designed for health professionals, clients, consumers, or other audiences? Is the information presented in an appropriate format for the intended audience? Look at details, too. Are there misspellings and grammatical errors? "Under construction" banners that have been there forever? These types of errors can be very telling about the overall quality of the site.

TABLE 4-2	WEBSITE EVALUATION: ASK YOURSELF, "AM I PLEASED WITH THE SITE?"
P	Purpose
L	Links
E	Editorial (site content)
A	Author
S	Site navigation
E	Ethical disclosure
D	Date site last updated

■ *A—Author.* Who is the author of the site? Does that person or group of people have the appropriate credentials? Is the author clearly identified by name and is contact information provided? One suggestion is to double-check an author's credentials by doing a literature search in MEDLINE. When people advertise themselves as "the leading worldwide authority" on a topic, they should have a few publications to their credit to establish their reputations. It is surprising how many times this search brings up nothing.

Be wary of how a person's credentials are presented. Consider a site where Dr. X is touted as an expert. Upon further exploration, you may find that, in fact, Dr. X does have a PhD (or an MD or an EdD), but the discipline in which this degree was obtained has nothing to do with the subject matter of the site. Remember that there is no universal process of peer review on the Internet and people can present themselves in any way that they want. Be suspicious.

Keep in mind that the webmaster and the author may be two (or more) different people. The webmaster is the person who designed the site and is responsible for its upkeep. The author is the person responsible for the content and the expert in the subject matter provided. In your evaluation, make sure you determine the qualifications of these people.

■ *S—Site.* Is the site easy to navigate? Is it attractive? Does it download quickly or have too many graphics and other features that make it inefficient? A site that is pleasing to the eye will invite you to return. Sites that cause your computer to crash should be viewed with a skeptical eye.

■ *E—Ethical.* Is contact information available for the site developer and the author? Is full disclosure available on the author and the purpose of the site? Is this information easy to find or is it buried deep in the website? Many commercial services, particularly pharmaceutical companies, have excellent websites with very useful information. Some of them, however, exist only to sell their product, although this purpose may not be immediately evident.

■ *D—Date.* When was the site last updated? Is it current? Does the information need to be updated regularly? Generally, with health and nursing information, information needs to be updated both frequently and regularly. You should be concerned with sites that have not been updated within 12 to 18 months. The date the site was last updated should be prominently displayed. Keep in mind that different pages within the site may be updated at different times. Be sure to check the date on each of the pages that you visit.

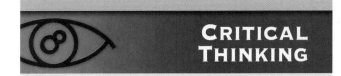

CRITICAL THINKING

PubMed has made the vast resources of the NLM available, for free, to anyone with a computer and Internet access. Some argue that scientific publications, such as the *New England Journal of Medicine*, are too technical and sophisticated for laypeople. Others contend that the resources of the NLM are maintained with taxpayer dollars and, therefore, should be available to all taxpayers.

Which point of view do you support? Why? As a health care professional, what resources for understanding and clarification would you suggest to your clients who are accessing abstracts and article citations from the professional health care literature?

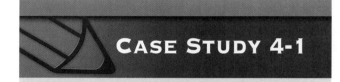

CASE STUDY 4-1

You are working in a women's health clinic with a number of nurse practitioners and family physicians. The clinic receives at least two to three telephone calls a day from women with a urinary tract infection (UTI). The question comes up, Do all these women need to be seen by a practitioner or can some of the cases be managed by telephone? You are asked to be on a committee to explore this issue and possibly come up with a protocol. Where do you begin? Is a protocol for telephone management of UTI realistic?

As you become more proficient at evaluating websites, you may have additional criteria to add to this list or criteria that are important to you for a specific purpose, but, in general, this simple group of seven criteria is surprisingly comprehensive. Test them for yourself. Do a quick search on a topic of interest, visit a number of sites, and determine just how PLEASED you are with what you find.

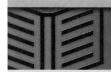

LITERATURE APPLICATION

Citation: Diaz, J. A., Griffith, R. A., Ng. J. J., Reinert, S. E., & Friedmann, P. D. (2002). Patients' use of the Internet for medical information. *Journal of General Internal Medicine, 17* (3), 180–185.

Discussion: Clients from a primary care internal medicine private practice in the United States were randomly selected and mailed a confidential survey. Of the 512 clients who returned the survey, 53.5 percent stated that they used the Internet for medical information. Those using the Internet for medical information were more educated (P <. 001) and had higher incomes (P < .001). Sixty percent felt that the information on the Internet was the "same as" or "better than" the information received from their doctors. Of those using the Internet for health information, 59 percent did not discuss this information with their doctor. Neither gender, nor education level, nor age less than 60 years was associated with clients sharing their Web searches with the physicians. However, clients who discussed this information with their doctors rated the quality of information higher than those who did not share this information with their physicians.

Implications for Practice: Primary care health care providers should recognize that clients are using the Internet as a source of medical and health information, and should be prepared to offer suggestions for Web-based health resources and to assist clients in evaluating the quality of medical information available on the Internet.

KEY CONCEPTS

- Computers are no longer a novelty but a fact of life, with exponential growth on a worldwide basis.

- Within nursing, the combination of computer science and information science with clinical expertise allows us to develop systems that have the ultimate goal of improving client outcomes.

- Nursing informatics is the application of computer science and information science to nursing. It promotes the generation, management, and processing of relevant data in order to use information and develop knowledge that supports nursing in all practice domains.

- Nurses can pursue formal education in nursing informatics at both the graduate and undergraduate levels. Informal education in informatics can be pursued through self-study, attendance at conferences, and reading the informatics literature.

- Certification in nursing informatics is voluntary and recognizes superior achievement and excellence in the specialty.

- The history of modern computing is described in three phases: phase I, the era of the mainframe computer; phase II, the era of the personal computer; and phase III, ubiquitous computing. The phase of ubiquitous computing,

characterized by many computers to one person, was predicted to occur between 2005 and 2020. Many believe that this phase has already begun.

- Virtual reality simulations have been used in education and client care. Minimally invasive surgery has been developed in large part through the technology of virtual reality.

- Effective searching for information on the Internet requires that you target your search. One technique is to conduct a P-F-A: a purpose-focus-approach assessment to determine what you are looking for and the best way to find it.

- PubMed is a search engine developed by the National Library of Medicine that allows you to search the databases of the MEDLARS system, including MEDLINE. It is free to anyone with Internet access.

- Information found on the Internet should be critically evaluated. Ask yourself, "Am I PLEASED with the site?"

  P—Purpose

  L—Links

  E—Editorial (site content)

  A—Author

  S—Site navigation

  E—Ethical disclosure

  D—Date site last updated

KEY TERMS

client-focused clinical
  information system
clinical information system (CIS)
computer literacy
data capture
departmental clinical
  information system
electronic health record
  (EHR)

information
  communications
MEDLARS (Medical
  Literature Analysis and
  Retrieval System)
storage
ubiquitous computing
  (UC)

REVIEW QUESTIONS

1. E-health includes which of the following activities?
   A. Obtaining health information online
   B. Shopping for health products online
   C. Online case management
   D. All of the above

2. Certification in nursing informatics is
   A. mandatory in certain states or for certain jobs.
   B. voluntary and recognizes superior achievement in the specialty.
   C. a component of Category II education in informatics.
   D. automatic after practising in the field for five years.

3. A person who is HIV-positive and chooses not to reveal this information to a nurse during an admission assessment is keeping this information
   A. anonymous.
   B. secure.
   C. confidential.
   D. private.

4. If a client came to you asking for a website to learn more about diabetes, which of the following would be appropriate for you to suggest?
   A. MEDLINE at the National Library of Medicine
   B. OncoLink
   C. MEDLINE*plus*
   D. All of the above

5. Decipher the following URL: www.uvic.ca. This is the URL for which of the following websites?
   A. University of Victoria
   B. Victoria Visitors and Convention Bureau
   C. Victoria State Government
   D. Victoria Nurses Association

6. You are interested in learning more about amyotrophic lateral sclerosis (ALS). You find a website where the author states that he is a worldwide leading researcher into causes for this disease. As part of your evaluation of the author's credentials, you
   A. take him at his word.
   B. e-mail him and ask for a list of references.

C. ask several colleagues whether they are familiar with his research.
D. conduct an author search on MEDLINE.

REVIEW ACTIVITIES

1. An immediate priority of Canada Health Infoway, Inc. is the development and implementation of effective electronic health record solutions in Canada. Is there a fully functional electronic health record system in place in your community today? If not, what are the barriers to implementation? Check the Canada Health Infoway, Inc. website at http://www.infoway-inforoute.ca/en/home/home.aspx.

2. A popular area of research in nursing informatics has been the attitudes of nurses toward computers and technology. Another topic that has been studied widely is ergonomics, that is, the relationship of a person's body to the computer equipment and negative health outcomes that may occur (e.g., repetitive motion injury is a common problem associated with computer use). As we move into the era of ubiquitous computing, do you think these research areas will continue to receive priority? Why or why not?

EXPLORING THE WEB

■ Pick a specialty area in nursing that interests you. Visit the Canadian Nurses Association (http://www.cna-nurses.ca) to determine whether the CNA certifies nurses in this specialty. If yes, what are the requirements? If no, is there another organization that credentials nurses in this specialty? Do a search to find another organization and its requirements for certification.

■ Find a current health news item, either in the newspaper or in a report on the television or radio. Search the Internet to find the original source of the news item. Was the way it was reported (e.g., newspaper, television, or radio) accurate? What information was included? What was omitted?

REFERENCES

American Nurses Credentialing Center. (1993). *Statement of philosophy.* Washington, DC: American Nurses Publishing.

Assessment of Technology in Context, Simon Fraser University. (2003). "ATIC in the Press." Retrieved from http://www.sfu.ca/~aticdl/Aticinthepressindex.htm, June 27, 2007.

Ball, M. J., & Hannah, K. J. (1984). *Using computers in nursing.* Reston, VA: Reston Publishers.

Ball, M. J., Hannah, K. J., & Douglas, J. (2000). Nursing and informatics. In M. Ball, K. Hannah, S. Newbold, & J. Douglas (Eds.),

Nursing informatics: Where caring and technology meet (3rd ed., pp. 6–14). New York: Springer-Verlag.

Bard, M. R. (2000). The future of e-health. *Cybercitizen Health, 1*(1), 1–13.

Bristow, L. (Nov/Dec. 2005). Sunnybrook tests new patient-safety alert system. *Canadian Healthcare Technology.* Retrieved from http://www.canhealth.com/current%20issue.html, November 6, 2005.

Buckert-Donelson, A. (1995). Heads up projects: Disabled learn to use public transportation. *VR World, 3*(3), 4–5.

Canadian Nursing Informatics Association. (2003). *Educating tomorrow's nurses: Where's Nursing Informatics?* Project G3-6B-DP1-0054, p. 8. Retrieved from http://www.cnia.ca/OHIHfinaltoc.htm, June 27, 2007.

CPRI Work Group on Confidentiality, Privacy & Security. (1995). *Guidelines for establishing information security policies at organizations using computer-based patient records.* Schaumburg, IL: Computer-based Patient Record Institute.

Diaz, J. A., Griffith, R. A., Ng, J. J., Reinert, S. E., & Friedmann, P. D. (2002). Patients' use of the Internet for medical information. *Journal of General Internal Medicine, 17*(3), 180–185.

Gassert, C. (2000). Academic preparation in nursing informatics. In M. J. Ball, K. J. Hannah, S. Newbold, & J. Douglas (Eds.), *Nursing informatics: Where caring and technology meet* (3rd ed., pp. 15–32). New York: Springer-Verlag.

Gorn, S. (1983). Informatics (computer and information science): Its ideology, methodology, and sociology. In F. Machlup & U. Mansfield (Eds.), *The study of information: Interdisciplinary messages* (pp. 121–140). New York: Wiley.

Graves, J. R., & Corcoran, S. (1989). The study of nursing informatics. *Image: The Journal of Nursing Scholarship, 21,* 227–231.

Grobe, S. J. (1988). Introduction. In H. E. Petersen & U. G. Jelger (Eds.), *Preparing nurses for using information systems: Recommended informatics competencies* (p. 4). New York: National League for Nursing.

Hannah, K. J. (1985). Current trends in nursing informatics: Implications for curriculum planning. In K. J. Hannah, E. J. Guillemin, & D. N. Conklin (Eds.), *Nursing uses of computer and information science* (pp. 181–187). Amsterdam: Elsevier.

Hersher, B. (2000). New roles for nurses in health care information systems. In M. J. Ball, K. J. Hannah, S. Newbold, & J. Douglas (Eds.), *Nursing informatics: Where caring and technology meet* (3rd ed., pp. 80–87). New York: Springer-Verlag.

Hiltzik, M. (2000). *Dealers of lightning: Xerox PARC and the dawn of the computer age.* New York: Harper Business.

Hodges, L., Rothbaum, B., Kooper, R., Opdyke, D., Meyer, T., North, M. et al. (1995). Virtual environments for treating the fear of heights. *IEEE Computer, 28*(7), 27–34.

Internet World Stats. (2007). "Internet Usage Statistics." Retrieved from http://www.internetworldstats.com/stats.htm, June 27, 2007.

Jenkins, S. (2000). Nurses' responsibilities in the implementation of information systems. In M. J. Ball, K. J. Hannah, S. Newbold, & J. Douglas (Eds.), *Nursing informatics: Where caring and technology meet* (pp. 207–223). New York: Springer-Verlag.

Joos, I., Whitman, N., Smith, M., & Nelson, R. (1996). *Computers in small bytes: The computer workbook* (2nd ed.). New York: National League for Nursing.

Lau, F. (2006). A collaborative approach to building capacity in health informatics. *Electronic Healthcare, 4*(4), 88–92.

Nagle, L. (2005). Dr. Lynn Nagle and the case for nursing informatics. *Canadian Journal of Nursing Leadership, 18*(1), 16–18.

National Nursing Informatics Project (NNIP) discussion paper. (1999). Project sponsored by CAUSN, CNA, Registered Nurses Association of British Columbia, Academy of Canadian Executive Nurses, and the Nursing Informatics Special Interest Group of COACH.

Nelson, R., & Joos, I. (1992). Strategies and resources for self-education in nursing informatics. In J. M. Arnold & G. A. Pearson (Eds.), *Computer applications in nursing education and practice* (pp. 9–19). New York: National League for Nursing.

Newbold, S. K. (1996). The informatics nurse and the certification process. *Computers in Nursing, 14*(2), 84–85, 88.

Nicoll, L. H. (2000). *Nurses' guide to the Internet* (3rd ed.). Philadelphia: Lippincott, Williams & Wilkins.

Nicoll, L. H. (2001). Quick and effective website evaluation. *Lippincott's Case Management, 6*(4), 220–221.

North, M. M., North, S. M., & Coble, J. R. (1996). Effectiveness of virtual environment desensitization in the treatment of agoraphobia. *Presence, Teleoperators, and Virtual Environments, 5*(3), 127–132.

OncoLink (2001). "About Oncolink." University of Pennsylvania Cancer Center. Retrieved from http://www.oncolink.org/about/index.cfm, June 29, 2007.

Sanli, M. (2005). Mount Sinai Hospital develops "Sinai e-Learning": Making it simpler for busy clinical staff to master healthcare applications. *Healthcare Quarterly, 8*(2), 82–84.

Satava, R. (1993). Virtual reality surgical simulator: The first steps. *Surgical Endoscopy, 7,* 203–205.

Satava, R. (1995). *Medicine 2001: The king is dead.* In R. M. Satava, K. Morgan, H. B. Sieburg, R. Mattheus, & J. P. Christensen (Eds.). *Interactive technology and the new paradigm for healthcare* (pp. 334–339). Washington, DC: IOS Press.

Semancik, M. (1997). *The history of clinical information systems: Legacy systems, computer-based patient record and point of care.* Seattle, WA: SpaceLabs Medical.

Shaw, J. (2006). From paper to programming. *Registered Nurse Journal, 18*(2), 14–17.

Smith, D., & Alexander, R. (1988). *Fumbling the future: How Xerox invented, then ignored, the first personal computer.* New York: Morrow.

Statistics Canada. (2006a). "Canadian Internet Use Survey." *The Daily,* August 15, 2006. Retrieved from http://www.statcan.ca/Daily/English/040708/d040708a.htm, June 27, 2007.

Statistics Canada (2006b). "E-commerce: Shopping on the Internet." *The Daily,* November 1, 2006. Retrieved from http://www.statcan.ca/Daily/English/061101/d061101a.htm, June 27, 2007.

Styles, M. M. (1989). *On specialization in nursing: Toward a new empowerment.* Kansas City, MO: American Nurses Foundation.

Ward, B. O. (1999). "Internet-positive patients" driving you crazy? Find out how to get online and cope. *Internet Medicine: A Critical Guide, 4*(7), 1, 6.

Watts, J. (1999). The healthy home of the future comes to Japan. *Lancet, 353*(9164), 1597–1600.

Weiser, M. (1991). The computer for the 21st century. *Scientific American, 265*(3), 94–102.

Weiser, M., & Brown, J. (1996, October 5). *The coming age of calm technology.* Retrieved from http://www.ubiq.com/hypertext/weiser/acmfuture2endnote.htm, July 19, 2002.

SUGGESTED READINGS

Biem, H. J., Klimaszewski, A., & Chen, F. (2004). Computer telephony in healthcare. *Electronic Healthcare, 3*(2), 80–86.

Canadian Health Network website. http://www.canadian-health-network.ca/servlet/ContentServer?cid=1038611684536& pagename=CHN-RCS/Page/HomePageTemplate&c=Page& lang=En, retrieved July 20, 2007.

Canadian Nurses Association. (2001) What is nursing informatics and why is it so important? *Nursing Now: Issues and Trends in Canadian Nursing, 11,* 1–4.

Canadian Nurses Association. (2002). Demystifying the electronic health Record. *Nursing Now: Issues and Trends in Canadian Nursing, 13,* 1–4.

Canadian Nurses Association. (2003). Measuring nurses' workload. *Nursing Now: Issues and Trends in Canadian Nursing, 15,* 1–4.

Health Canada. (2006). "eHealth Resources: Initiatives." Retrieved from http://www.hc-sc.gc.ca/ohih-bsi/res/init_e.html, June 29, 2007.

Hebda, T., Czar, P., & Mascara, C. (1998). *Handbook of informatics for nurses & health care professionals.* Menlo Park, CA: Addison-Wesley.

Lau, F. (2006). A collaborative approach to building capacity in health informatics. *Electronic Healthcare, 4*(4), 88–92.

Lau, F., Protti, D., & Coward, P. (2005). A review of information management practices for health ministries. *Healthcare Management Forum, 18*(2), 14–21.

National Institute of Nursing Research. (1993). *Nursing informatics: Enhancing patient care* (NIH Publication No. 93-2419). Bethesda, MD: National Institutes of Health.

Office of Health and the Information Highway (OHIH), Health Canada. (2006). "eHealth." Retrieved from http://www.hc-sc.gc.ca/hcs-sss/ehealth-esante/index_e.html. July 20, 2007.

Pastore, M. (2002). "Internet Part of the Family in Canada." Retrieved from http://www.clickz.com/stats/big_picture/geographics/article/php/964381, April 15, 2005.

Pederson, L., & Leonard, K. (2005). Measuring information technology investment among Canadian academic health sciences centres. *Electronic Healthcare, 3*(3), 94–101.

Protti, D. (2003). Issues, musings and trends IT & EHR Governance: Who should the leaders be? *Healthcare Management Forum, 16*(1), 40–42.

Protti, D. (2004). England's revolutionary change in approach to the electronic health record. *Healthcare Management Forum, 17*(1), 32–35.

Sandhu, J. S., Anderson, K., Keen, D., & Yassi, A. (2005). Implementing information technology to improve workplace health: A web-based information needs assessment of managers in Fraser Health, British Columbia. *Healthcare Management Forum, 18*(4), 6–10.

Shaw, C. (2004). Who needs health information management professionals?—Every Healthcare Entity Does! *Healthcare Quarterly, 7*(3), 107–108.

Shop.org. (2002). "Statistics: Holiday 2002, Transactions and Spending." Retrieved from http://www.shop.org/learn/stats_intshop_canada.asp, August 14, 2006.

Staggers, N., & Gassert, C. (2002). Results of a Delphi study to determine informatics competencies for nurses at four levels of practice. *Nursing Research, 51*(6), 383–390.

Strating, D., MacGregor, J., & Campbell, N. (2006). Bridging Information "islands": Designing an electronic health record that meets clinical needs. *Electronic Healthcare, 4*(4), 94–98.

Zytkowski, M. (2003). Nursing informatics: The key to unlocking contemporary nursing practice. *AACN Clinical Issues Advanced Practice in Acute Critical Care, 14*(3), 271–281.

CHAPTER ENDNOTES

1. Canadian Nursing Informatics Association. (2003). *Educating tomorrow's nurses: Where's nursing informatics?* Canadian Nursing Informatics Association, p. 8. Retrieved from http://www.cnia.ca/OHIHfinaltoc.htm, June 27, 2007.

2. Canadian Nursing Informatics Association, "CNIA Nursing Informatics Education Bursary." Retrieved from http://www.cnia.ca/education.htm, June 26, 2005.

3. e-Health 2007: Paths to Transformation website, "Welcome." Retrieved from http://www.e-healthconference.com/, June 28, 2007.

4. Canada Health Infoway, "Who We Are: Our Core Business." Retrieved from http://www.infoway-inforoute.ca/en/ WhoWeAre/Overview.aspx, April 1, 2007.

5. Ibid.

CHAPTER
5

Population-Based Health Care Practice

Patricia M. Lentsch Schoon, MPH, RN
Adapted by: Victoria E. Pennick, RN, MHSc

The selection of groups for care should be based on the questions: What difference might nursing care be expected to make in this situation? Is it more or less than would be expected in other groups?
(Ruth B. Freeman, 1957)

OBJECTIVES

Upon completion of this chapter, the reader should be able to:

1. Discuss the social mandate to provide population-based health care at the global, national, provincial, and local levels.

2. Describe how population-based nursing is practised within the community and the health care system.

3. Identify vulnerable and high-risk population groups for whom specific health promotion and disease prevention services are indicated.

4. Outline a multidisciplinary population-based planning and evaluation process that includes partnerships with the community and health care consumers.

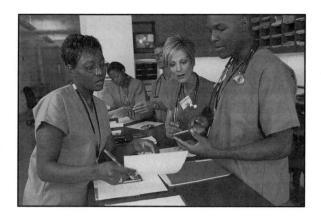

You are completing a clinical experience with the public health nurse in an elementary school located in a large metropolitan area. This school has 1,600 students from kindergarten to grade six. Forty percent of the families in the surrounding neighbourhood are in the low-income bracket; 46 percent immigrated to Canada within the past five years; 92 percent rent, rather than own their homes; virtually all of them live in high-rise apartments. Sixty-eight percent are Canadian citizens. Of those considered to be visible minorities: 42 percent are South Asian, 11 percent are Filipino, 4 percent are Black, 4 percent are Asian, and 3 percent are Middle Eastern. Twenty-two percent of the total population in the area is under the age of 14; 93 percent of the students speak English as a second language. The school nurse encourages you to think about some of the social problems these children might encounter that will affect their health and the nursing actions you might take to help them overcome those problems. (Toronto District School Board, 2006a, 2006b)

> *What health problems might you expect to identify in this group of schoolchildren?*
>
> *What social and environmental factors might contribute to these health problems?*
>
> *What nursing actions directed at groups of children, rather than individuals, could you take to help these children?*

Nurses have acted to improve the health of populations and communities since the time of Florence Nightingale. Nightingale's actions to improve the health care of soldiers on the battlefields of the Crimean War and of the poor and infirm in London were directed at vulnerable population groups. Nightingale's actions were based on the recognition that vulnerable population groups were not able to advocate effectively for themselves. She became their advocate. Nightingale was able to intervene to improve the health status of disenfranchised groups of people by influencing the health policies of the English government and changing the health care delivery systems in London and on the battlefield. That same spirit of advocacy and call to action is alive today among nurses throughout the world.

The primary thrust of this advocacy is on behalf of vulnerable groups in our society—those who, because of biological, social, and environmental factors, are not able to attain a level of health generally enjoyed by many of us. Nurses are united in partnership with other health care disciplines, the community, and health care consumers to achieve population-based global, national, provincial, and local health care goals. This chapter provides readers with an understanding of the theory and practice of population-based health care.

Population-based care requires active partnership of both providers and recipients of care. The phrase *health care consumer* includes recipients of care and those who make health care–related decisions at the individual or group level.

POPULATION HEALTH

Through the Alma-Ata Declaration, proclaimed in 1978, the international community, led by the World Health Organization (WHO), made a commitment to the principles of primary health care and global strategies that would see "health for all people of the world" (World Health Organization, 1978). In 1986, the WHO's First International Conference on Health Promotion was held in Ottawa. The Ottawa Charter, building on the principles of primary health care, was a blueprint for health promotion that has stood the test of time (World Health Organization, 1986). Building on previous meetings, participants at the Fourth International Conference on Health Promotion, held in 1997, in Jakarta, Indonesia, examined what was known about health promotion, re-examined the determinants of health, and invited the private sector to contribute resources needed to promote health in the 21st century (World Health Organization, 1997). In September 2005, the Declaration of Montevideo, co-sponsored by the Pan American Health Organization (PAHO) and the WHO stated that the principles outlined in the Declaration of Alma-Ata must be integrated into the health systems of a community rather than implemented as a separate program or objective (Pan American Health Organization, 2005).

Population health is the concept that a population—or a community—as a whole, has a particular state of health. This concept goes beyond the health of individuals and looks at the health of the entire population. The health of a population is strongly affected by social and environmental factors that are now widely known as **determinants of health.** Within our society, groups of vulnerable individuals are at increased risk of experiencing health disparities because of their lack of stable income, lack of education, reduced access to secure jobs, and inadequate housing.

In the Declaration of Alma-Ata, primary health care (PHC) was defined as "essential health care based on practical, scientifically sound and socially acceptable methods and technology, made universally accessible to individuals and families in the community through their full participation and at a cost that the community and country can afford to maintain at every stage of their development in the spirit of self-reliance and self determination" (World Health Organization, 1978). The Ottawa Charter defined **health promotion** as "the process of enabling people to increase control over and to improve their health."[1]

Individual **health risk factors** are variables that increase or decrease the probability of illness, disability or death. Risk factors may be either modifiable (i.e., they can be changed) or non-modifiable (i.e., they cannot be changed). Modifiable risk factors include smoking, lack of exercise, unsafe sexual practices, alcohol and drug use, and lack of health screening. Non-modifiable risk factors include age, sex, race, or other inherent physical characteristics. On the other hand, determinants of health are variables that include biological, psychosocial, environmental (physical and social), lifestyle, behavioural, and health system factors that may cause changes in the health status of individuals, families, and communities or populations. In the Jakarta Declaration, determinants or prerequisites for health were specifically identified as peace, shelter, education, social security, social relations, food, income, the empowerment of women, a stable eco-system, sustainable resource use, social justice, respect for human rights, and equity. Poverty was identified as the greatest threat to health.[2]

The Ottawa Charter set out five strategies for health promotion:

1. Build healthy public policy.
2. Create supportive environments.
3. Strengthen community action.
4. Develop personal skills.
5. Reorient health services.[3]

The Jakarta Declaration built upon the strategies from the Ottawa Charter and set the following five priorities:

1. Promote social responsibility for health.
2. Increase investments for health development.
3. Consolidate and expand partnerships for health.
4. Increase community capacity and empower the individual.
5. Secure an infrastructure for health promotion.[4]

Health status is the level of health of an individual, family, community, or population. It is a combination of individual and societal factors, and one's perception of how they all fit together. **Quality of life** is the level of satisfaction one has with the actual conditions of one's life, including satisfaction with socioeconomic status, education, occupation, home, family life, recreation, and the ability to enjoy life, freedom, and independence. Quality of life assessment reviews the perceived and actual ability to be autonomous and independent in making life choices; one's sense of happiness, satisfaction, and security; and the ongoing ability to strive to reach one's potential. **Health-related quality of life** refers to one's level of satisfaction with those aspects of life that are influenced either positively or negatively by one's health status and risk factors.

Functional health status is the ability to care for oneself and meet one's human needs. Functional abilities are the combined abilities to be independent in both activities of daily life and in the instrumental activities of daily living. **Activities of daily living** are activities related to toileting, bathing, grooming, dressing, feeding, mobility, and verbal and written personal communication. **Instrumental activities of daily living (IADLs)** are activities related to food preparation and shopping; cleaning; laundry; home maintenance; verbal, written, and electronic communications; financial management; and transportation, along with activities to meet social and support needs, manage health care needs, access community services and resources, and meet spiritual needs. Functional health status affects health-related quality of life.

The WHO's International Classification of Functioning, Disability and Health (ICIDH-2), adopted in 2001, recognizes the importance of defining health domains and health-related domains and their interrelationship to further our understanding of health status. Using the ICIDH-2 framework, health status is the result of the interaction between personal characteristics and environmental factors, the three main domains being impairment (i.e., body function and structure), activities (i.e., person-level functioning), and participation (i.e., societal functioning).[5]

Health and illness are on a continuum, with total health at one end and severe illness on the other. All of the aforementioned factors interact to determine an individual's position on the health–illness continuum.

Nurses working with our most vulnerable populations must develop strategies to target finite health care resources effectively. Despite the fact that we have universal health insurance in Canada, **vulnerable population groups** are often underserved. They often have a diminished health status and are at increased risk for morbidity and mortality because of multiple and complex medical and social problems. These people are vulnerable because of their poverty, lack of education, lack of opportunity, and their history of mental health and drug and alcohol abuse. Vulnerable population groups include Aboriginal people, elderly people, poor children, and people with disabilities (Shah, chapter 6). These groups often exist at the margins of mainstream society and have a reduced ability to participate in, or influence, decisions that affect their health care status.

Population-based health care initiatives to help and work with these groups exist at the global, national, provincial, and local level. Table 5-1 gives examples of population-based health care initiatives.

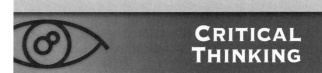

CRITICAL THINKING

Mrs. Jones is 85 years old. She has severe arthritis and deformities in her feet and has difficulty getting around. She lives in her own home in a large Canadian city, but knows she can call on her neighbour of many years to help her with shopping and errands. She has a home helper come in half a day a week to help with the light housekeeping. She is still able to do her own cooking. Her children, a grown son and daughter, live in a small neighbourhood north of the city and visit frequently. Each day, Mrs. Jones goes to the local YMCA, where she is greeted warmly by the other women, who are all much younger than she is. She participates in aquafit classes, walks on the indoor track, and relaxes in the whirlpool. Mrs. Jones admits that she experiences severe pain from her arthritis and that she would "just stiffen up" if she didn't get into the water every day. Mrs. Jones feels she is lucky to be able to live at home and participate in a daily exercise program. She would never consider herself disabled!

What determinants of health would you identify and what is their impact in Mrs. Jones's situation?

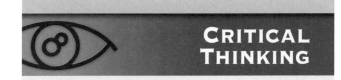

CRITICAL THINKING

You are caring for Joe, a 50-year-old quadriplegic man who lives at home with his aging parents. As visiting home health nurses, you and your colleagues visit every morning to help Joe with his morning care, which includes bowel and bladder care, bathing, dressing, and getting him into his wheelchair with his mechanical lift. Once he is up, he is able to propel his wheelchair around his home. His parents look after his meals, shopping, and errands; and his father helps him get back into bed in the evening. One morning, Joe is very upset. His mother fell down the stairs the previous evening and was hospitalized with a fractured shoulder. She was due to have it pinned later in the day. The hospital staff was not confident she would be able to return home.

What nursing advocacy initiatives might you undertake to ensure the provision of safe home care services for Joe and his father?

How might you justify the distribution of resources to assist Joe and his father to stay in their home?

As the primary care nurse caring for Joe's mother in hospital, what issues might you identify for this family? What strategies might you explore to solve them?

TABLE 5-1	POPULATION-BASED HEALTH CARE INITIATIVES
Global Groups	**Initiatives**
World Health Organization and the Pan American Health Organization (PAHO)	To help achieve the United Nations' Millennium Development Goals, members of PAHO and other WHO affiliate organizations agreed to advocate for the integration of primary health care (PHC) as an integral part of their health and social structure. Their strategies would be based on these elements: 1. Commitment to facilitate social inclusion and equity in health. 2. Recognition of the critical roles of both the individual and the community in the development of PHC-based systems.

(Continued)

TABLE 5-1	POPULATION-BASED HEALTH CARE INITIATIVES (CONTINUED)

	3. Orientation toward health promotion and comprehensive and integrated care.
	4. Development of intersectoral work.
	5. Orientation toward quality of care and client safety.
	6. Strengthening of human resources in health.
	7. Establishment of structural conditions that allow PHC renewal.
	8. Guarantee of financial sustainability.
	9. Research and development and appropriate technology.
	10. Network strengthening and partnerships of international cooperation in support of PHC. (Pan American Health Organization, 2005).
United Nations: Millennium Development Goals	The eight Millennium Development Goals (MDGs) form a blueprint agreed to by all the world's countries and all of the world's leading development institutions that these goals will be met by 2015. 1. Eradicate extreme poverty and hunger. 2. Achieve universal primary education. 3. Promote gender equality and empower women. 4. Reduce child mortality. 5. Improve maternal health. 6. Ensure environmental sustainability. 7. Develop a global partnership for development. (United Nations, 2005)
National Groups	**Initiatives**
Public Health Agency of Canada	The Public Health Agency of Canada (PHAC) was created in September 2004, with an overall goal of leading federal efforts to prevent and control disease and injuries and to promote health. Its priorities for 2005–06 are the following: 1. To develop and lead Canada's long-term strategic public health initiatives. 2. To develop, enhance, and implement integrated and disease-specific strategies. 3. To develop and enhance the capacity of the new Agency to meet its mandate. (Canada. Public Health Agency of Canada, 2006)
Great Britain	The Saving Lives: Our Healthier Nation initiative focuses on the prevention of 300,000 deaths in a 10-year period (Mitchell, 1999).
U.S. Department of Health and Human Services	The Healthy People 2010 initiative highlights health indicators related to the leading causes of death, including health behaviours; physical, social, and environmental factors; and health systems factors. (U.S. Department of Health and Human Services, 2000)

(Continued)

TABLE 5-1	POPULATION-BASED HEALTH CARE INITIATIVES (CONTINUED)
American Public Health Association	This association comments on the state of public health in the United States and recommends the development of a universal health care system to provide for Americans who are uninsured and disenfranchised. (American Public Health Association, 2001)
Provincial and Territorial Groups	**Initiatives**
Northwest Territories Health and Social Services	Aboriginal Head Start (AHS) is an early intervention program for First Nations, Inuit, and Métis children and their families. It is primarily a preschool program that prepares young Aboriginal children for school by meeting their spiritual, emotional, intellectual, and physical needs. This program is funded by Health Canada. (Northwest Territories. Health and Social Services, 2006).
Yukon	The Yukon Government, in partnership with the Canadian Cancer Society, completed a 27-month mass-media tobacco-reduction campaign with funding from Health Canada. Its intent was to encourage and support smokers who wanted to move toward the goal of becoming smoke-free. (Canadian College of Health Service Executives, 2004, p. 219)
Nunavut	Tobacco and mental health—particularly suicide—are identified as key population health priorities. (Canadian College of Health Service Executives, 2004, p. 218)
British Columbia Centre for Disease Control	Chee Mamuk is a program developed to provide culturally appropriate on-site community-based education and training on HIV/AIDS and sexually transmitted diseases to Aboriginal communities, organizations, and professionals within British Columbia. (British Columbia Centre for Disease Control, 2002)
Alberta Health and Wellness	The Smoke-Free Places Act took effect on January 1, 2006. It sets a minimum standard for all of Alberta and protects minors from exposure to second-hand smoke. (Alberta. Health and Wellness, 2006)
Saskatchewan Health	A number of Saskatchewan initiatives provide support services to individuals and families affected by Fetal Alcohol Spectrum Disorder (FASD). Saskatchewan Health is participating in an Interdepartmental Committee on Fetal Alcohol Spectrum Disorder (ICFASD), which consulted with the community to identify key issues and gaps in services, and published a summary report of the findings. (Canadian College of Health Service Executives, 2004, p. 211)
Manitoba Health	As of 2006, under the province's Environment Act, communities in southern Manitoba could be issued a Ministerial Order to undertake adult mosquito control to prevent or alleviate the threat of West Nile virus to human health. The Order could require that adult mosquito control be undertaken within a specific community and a zone of approximately a 3-kilometre radius around the community. In special circumstances, an Order could target a specific area within a municipality. Health Canada has concluded that the use of malathion for adult mosquito control in residential areas using an application at an ultra-low volume would not pose a health concern. However, people

(Continued)

TABLE 5-1	POPULATION-BASED HEALTH CARE INITIATIVES (CONTINUED)
	who wish to reduce their exposure to malathion can take precautions. (Manitoba. Manitoba Health, 2006)
Ontario Advisory Committee on HIV/AIDS (OACHA)	In June 2002, the Ontario Advisory Committee on HIV/AIDS (OACHA) presented a proposed strategy to the minister of health and long-term care entitled A Proposed HIV/AIDS Strategy for Ontario to 2008. OACHA's proposed strategy has three main goals: to prevent the spread of HIV; to improve the health and well-being of people living with HIV/AIDS; and to address social inequities that make people vulnerable to HIV. The proposed strategy has been disseminated to HIV stakeholders across the province, and work to carry out aspects of the strategy has begun. (Canadian College of Health Service Executives, 2004, p. 213)
Quebec Ministère de la Santé et des Services Sociaux	In 2004, the Quebec Government made public its 2004–2009 Government Action Plan on Domestic Violence, consisting of 72 commitments based on four key focuses of intervention: prevention, detection, adaptation to special realities, and socio-judicial intervention. Eight government ministries, including three secretariats and their respective assistance and protection networks, are accountable for the commitments made in the plan. The priority of this action plan is the safety and protection of victims and their families. (Quebec. Ministère de la Santé et des Services Sociaux, 2007)
New Brunswick Department of Health	With the support and direction of the Canadian Pandemic Influenza Plan, provinces and territories, including New Brunswick, continue to work on their pandemic planning processes. The plan covers surveillance, public health activities, essential health services, communications, and community emergency responses. (New Brunswick. Department of Health, 2006)
Nova Scotia	The Nova Scotia Department of Health has provided funding to Community Health Boards for local health promotion and prevention initiatives that are consistent with their community health plans. (Canadian College of Health Service Executives, 2004, p. 215)
Prince Edward Island (PEI)	In the fall of 2004, more than 7,000 PEI students aged 7 to 19 years received Adacel as part of a clinical trial. Adacel is a vaccine that provides protection against tetanus, diphtheria, and whooping cough. The results of the study were encouraging. It was found that Adacel can be safely given to students in a period as short as two years after their last dose of vaccine. PEI students now have the most complete coverage for whooping cough in North America. (Canadian College of Health Service Executives, 2004, p. 215)
Newfoundland and Labrador	A provincial Wellness Plan is under development with the advice and support of a Wellness Advisory Council comprising members from government departments, community, and professional organizations. Priority actions have been identified and include Healthy Children, Healthy Schools, which has a particular focus on healthy eating and physical activity for children and youth, as well as the development of Regional Wellness Coalitions and a Teen Wellness Team. (Canadian College of Health Service Executives, 2004, p. 216–217)

POPULATION-BASED NURSING PRACTICE

Population-based nursing practice has been an integral part of nursing since the profession began. Florence Nightingale's use of aggregated statistics as population-based indices and outcome measures demonstrates her population-focused practice. Canadian community health nurses have a long and important history. Over the years, they have understood the importance of social, economic, environmental, and political determinants of health. They considered social activism and collaboration with community organizations and governments to be fundamental aspects of public health nursing practice (Falk Rafael, Fox, Mildon, & O'Donnell, 1998). In 1905, Ottawa's Anti-Tuberculosis League hired Canada's first tuberculosis (TB) nurse—a public health role—to visit the homes of TB clients, and in 1907, the Toronto Health Department became the first municipal health department in Canada to hire a TB nurse, Christina Mitchell. In 1909, Ontario extended public health nursing by starting medical inspection programs under the Department of Education, to counteract high levels of school absenteeism due to widespread childhood disease. Working outside the strict structure of hospitals, public health nurses were the most independent nurses of this period. In 1920, the Ontario Red Cross Society funded a one-year university program for public health nurses at the University of Toronto, a program that would continue to be recognized as the preferred postgraduate training for Ontario public health nurses until the 1960s.[6]

Today, nurses in community health work in a broad spectrum of situations. Their populations include school children, homeless and at-risk youth, individuals with mental health problems, individuals with alcohol and drug abuse problems, individuals in the sex trade, Aboriginal people, and new Canadians, to mention a few. According to statistics from the Canadian Institute for Health Information (CIHI), 30,544 (13.2 percent) of a total 230,957 registered nurses were working in the community in 2003. In January 2004, Community Health Nursing became one of the 17 nursing specialties certified by the Canadian Nurses Association.[7]

NURSING IN NONTRADITIONAL SETTINGS

(CHCs) are nonprofit organizations that provide primary health and health promotion programs for individuals, families, and communities. A health centre is established by the community and governed by a community-elected board of directors; the health centre receives its base funding from the Local Health Integrated Networks in Ontario and may obtain program-specific funds from other sources. Community Health Centres work with others in the community on health promotion initiatives within schools, in housing developments, and in the workplace. Depending on the needs of the community, staff will include a mix of nurses, physicians, health promoters, social workers, nutritionists, and vocational counsellors,

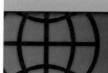

REAL WORLD EXAMPLE

In 1986, a group of homeless people in Toronto met to discuss health care issues they were facing. They felt discriminated against within the health care system, and given their circumstances, they were often unable to follow prescribed treatments. The group identified nurses as the people they would feel most comfortable approaching for health care.

Upon learning of the initial discussions, a group of volunteer nurses opened the first Street Health nursing station in September 1986, at a church in downtown Toronto. Other nursing clinics followed, located where homeless people congregated, in order to provide hands-on health care and assistance in accessing and navigating the existing health care system.

Street nurses provide services on the street, in alleys, along the lakeshore, in parks and ravines, and in homeless shelters and drop-in centres. Their clients' lives are characterized by extreme poverty, chronic unemployment, insecurity in housing, poor nutrition, high stress, and loneliness; they have more frequent and serious illnesses, and die younger, on average, than the general population. The nurses provide outreach nursing, mental health support and case management, HIV/AIDS prevention, support for those with Hepatitis C, and prevention strategies for those at risk for the disease on an individual basis, but are strong advocates for supportive public policy that will make a more lasting difference for the population as a whole.[8]

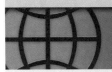

REAL WORLD EXAMPLE

A long-time street nurse and advocate for the homeless, Cathy Crowe, was granted the prestigious Atkinson Economic Justice award in January 2004. The award, which provides $100,000 per year, for up to three years, will allow her to strengthen her health care efforts on the street and continue her research and education work around public solutions to the homeless problem at the local and national level. Ms. Crowe worked as a street nurse for 15 years and was involved in numerous coalitions and public education work regarding the homeless. In 1998, she co-founded the Toronto Disaster Relief Committee, an organization that has dramatically increased the public's understanding of homelessness.[9]

These two real world examples demonstrate what nurses could do when they choose to advocate on behalf of their vulnerable clients. Policymakers can facilitate these initiatives by recognizing the true cost to society of non-action. Government departments are expected to manage their own budgets. There is little incentive to work across departments to assess how action in one area can affect outcomes in another. Nursing managers may find themselves in similar situations within their organizations. In the current atmosphere of accountability and the ultimate importance of the bottom line, all stakeholders—including the client, the service provider, and the payer—must come together to develop creative strategies. Regionalization of health and social services across Canada (the most recent example being the Local Integrated Health Networks in Ontario) has been cited by governments as initiatives to coordinate services to improve access and care. However, since in most cases the emphasis is on organizations that provide health care, with rare exceptions, organizations and initiatives that address determinants of health that fall outside the traditional health care system, will, by and large, be excluded.[10]

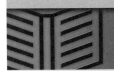

LITERATURE APPLICATION

Citation: Smith, D., & Davies, B. Participatory model: Creating a new dynamic in Aboriginal health. *Canadian Nurse, 102*(4), 36–39.

Discussion: This report outlines the challenges of using current research to inform nursing practice in Aboriginal communities, and highlights the utility of using a participatory model of research transfer to help overcome these challenges. An evidence-based prenatal workshop for community health nurses working in First Nations' communities in British Columbia was used as a venue to test the acceptability of the model and to increase the uptake of research to improve care.

Implications for practice: The nurses identified that "without participation, nothing would change" in the Aboriginal communities, that understanding the beliefs, lifestyle, and expectations of the individuals with whom they worked was "critical to success and capacity building."

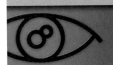

CRITICAL THINKING

Consider the previous literature application. Can this approach be used successfully when planning services for other vulnerable populations? Think of a vulnerable population with whom you work. What steps would you take to address one of their social determinants of health? As the nursing manager, what actions would you take to support your staff in this initiative?

to name a few; all staff are on salary. Traditionally, Community Health Centres were developed to help vulnerable groups within our communities overcome issues of access to service. As a result, Community Health Centres focus on providing primary care, linking with other community partners, advocating for determinants of health for their community, and empowering their clients to advocate on their own behalf.[11]

Aboriginal Health Centres are similar to CHCs but offer culturally appropriate primary care to Aboriginal families, individuals, and communities. Programs may include family medicine and nurse practitioner services, nutrition counselling, health education, disease prevention, mental health counselling, and traditional healing and others approaches, depending on the need of the community.[12]

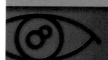

CRITICAL THINKING

The local food bank was scheduled to close in six months. The agency that had hosted it for the past decade was re-assessing its mandate and resources, and felt it could no longer provide this service. The community was devastated! With 40 percent of the local population identified as living in a low-income bracket, this closure was not good news. Sally, the local school nurse, and Carol, the outreach worker at the local Community Health Centre, hastily called a meeting of other community partners and clients. Over the next six months, the community was able to articulate their specific needs, identify why the food bank was important to them, and successfully convey their message to local politicians and the media. They successfully negotiated with another agency to host the service temporarily, until more permanent plans could be made—a commitment to which the community agencies and politicians agreed.

Do you think this was an effective effort? Why, or why not?

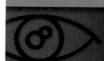

CRITICAL THINKING

Betty is a parish nurse who works in a low-income neighbourhood that is home to many new Canadians. Ten percent of the population is between the ages of 15 and 24. Most of the parents, although university-educated, have been able to find only menial jobs that pay poorly, necessitating long hours and often a second job. Many families are headed by a single parent. City-sponsored activities are available, but the registration process is frustrating for long-time city dwellers who are fluent in English and understand the system; It is virtually inaccessible to new Canadians who have poor command of English, little time, and no understanding of the system. The teens have limited access to age-appropriate health care and spend long hours left to their own devices—but are observed by the neighbourhood to make sure they act in culturally appropriate ways. Collaborative efforts between the parish nurse, public health, and the neighbouring community health centre resulted in the development of a youth health care clinic in one of the local secondary schools. Also in collaboration with other community agencies, Betty started "Saturday Night at the Movies" at a local community centre, giving the youth an opportunity to go to a chaperoned outing and still interact with their peers. When the local community health centre offered a number of small grants for community programs, the youth were successful recipients of a grant, when they applied for money to expand their recreational program.

What needs would you identify for this population?

What strategies from the Ottawa Charter have been employed in this example? What other strategies do you think should be considered?

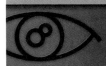

CRITICAL THINKING

While working at a health centre for homeless youth, the nurses identified the lack of parenting skills displayed by many of the teen parents. They knew from the literature and from their own experience that without good parenting, these children of children would never "spin out," and the cycle would be perpetuated. Through reviewing journals and conferring with colleagues who worked with the same population, they discovered a new teaching tool—a computer-programmed doll that cried and could not be consoled until the root cause was discovered and alleviated. The doll would only calm down if she was fed, her wet diapers changed, her tender loving care (TLC) needs were met, etc. The doll, used primarily in "family studies" classes in the secondary schools, as a tool to teach parenting skills to non-pregnant teens, cost $800. One of the other agencies had a doll donated, so the nurses were able to see her and glean information from the other agency's experience. The other agency staff raved about its utility. The nurses determined that they had to have one—but it was a little expensive for their meagre budget, and they couldn't justify buying the doll for a few of their clients, instead of medication and medical supplies that would benefit so many more. So, they decided to ask someone to donate it. They were sure the youth would be fascinated by it and would learn basic skills to deal with some of the challenges they would face in the months to come.

What health needs can you identify for this population?

What strategies, besides those outlined above, would you initiate to help meet these needs?

As the manager, what strategies and activities would you develop and implement to facilitate these initiatives?

PROGRAM PLANNING AND EVALUATION

The nursing process, which is integral to our care at the individual client level, is also used in population-based nursing practice to assess, diagnose, plan, implement, and evaluate programs developed to meet the needs of a community. Several models of program planning and evaluation are outlined in the literature, although all have similar components.

One model to consider when planning and evaluating programs to meet the needs of the community is the Precede-Proceed Model, developed by Lawrence Green and colleagues at the University of British Columbia. They outline nine steps to establish, evaluate, and maintain community programs. Steps one through five assess the health, social, and environmental issues; step six covers the implementation; while steps seven to nine address the evaluation (Green, 1999; Johnson, 2006;).

ASSESSMENT

Population assessment follows a structured model as a guide for data collection. Table 5.2 is a template for collecting population-level data on determinants of community health, as outlined in the Jakarta Declaration. In order to complete the full assessment, it is important to identify the issue, determine its importance to the community, back it up with epidemiological evidence if available, determine

the educational and organizational needs of the community if a program were to be implemented, and define the administrative and policy components of program implementation (Green & Kreuter, 1999).

PLANNING AND IMPLEMENTATION

During the planning and implementation stage, collaboration with all partners—including clients, care providers, and other community and government agencies—is imperative to the process. By determining buy-in and logistical factors and developing strategies to deal with them, you will help guarantee the success of your program. Defining measurable outcomes and a means of evaluation at this stage will facilitate the evaluation process.

EVALUATION

The programs should be measured in three ways: (infra)structure (e.g., manuals and finances); implementation processes (e.g., are people participating in the program?); and outcomes (e.g., did the program actually make a difference for the community?) (Green & Kreuter, 1999). Outcomes of population-based nursing practice focus on health status, functional abilities, and the quality of life of at-risk population groups. Justification is necessary, of both resources and budget. A cost-benefit analysis is appropriate, comparing improvements in health status, functional abilities, and quality of life of the targeted

TABLE 5-2	POPULATION-BASED NEEDS ASSESSMENT

Determinants of Health Information from observation and discussions with members of the community (i.e., primary data)	Is There Information to Assess These Determinants of Health? Information from health data sources (i.e., secondary data, such as census data and mortality data)	Assessment of Situation Review the data from the two sources of information. Do they agree or disagree? If they disagree, why?
Physical Environment: ■ Shelter ■ Stable Ecosystem ■ Peace ■ Sustainable Resource Social Environment: ■ Income ■ Education ■ Social Security ■ Social Relations Biological and Behavioural Determinants of Health Equity ■ Social Justice ■ Respect for Human Rights Genetic Endowment Access to Health Care Services		

Source: Johnson, I. (Ed.). (2006). *Determinants of Community Health, Year 1, Semester 2: Course Manual & Readings 2006–2007.* Toronto: University of Toronto.

at-risk population with expenditures of human and material resources. Ethical guidelines, as well as guidelines for culturally competent care, should be used to evaluate the efficacy of health provider interactions with vulnerable or marginalized population groups.

Data are collected that reflect the aggregated response of the total group for each specified outcome. Descriptive statistics, such as mean, range, and percentages may be used in the analysis of group data. These data may be collected at the program level, or may be forwarded to a provincial or national data collection program to allow between-program comparisons. Case studies illustrating how services provided to clients "made a difference" are also very effective.

Questions such as the following will help guide your data collection:

■ Did we find the high-risk, underserved, vulnerable population groups in the community/service area and provide timely and accessible services?
■ Did we offer service regardless of age, gender, race, ethnicity, health care status, or location?
■ Did our services meet the greatest unmet health needs of the community or the at-risk, vulnerable, underserved population groups?
■ Did their health status improve?
■ Were their health risks reduced?
■ Were they satisfied with the services they received?

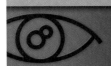

CRITICAL THINKING

Nursing diagnosis: Female students, aged 13 to 15, in Mid-town Middle School at risk for altered nutrition: less than body requirements related to nutritional habits, body image disturbance, sense of powerlessness, and lack of screening and outreach services as evidenced by:

- 10% of the female students are below the 5th percentile in weight but above the 25th percentile in height on standardized growth and development charts.
- 75% of the female students report that they routinely skip breakfast on three or more school days per week, and 50% routinely eat snacks from the vending machines for lunch.
- 90% of the female students agree with the statement, "I do not like my body the way it is."
- 80% of the female students agree with the statement, "It is very important to me and my friends to be thin."
- 20% of the female students report that their lives are out of control and one of the only things they have control over is their eating behaviours.

Goal: To reduce the risk for altered nutrition among 13- to 15-year-old female students at Mid-town Middle School.

Modifiable Risk Factors: Nutritional habits, body image disturbance, powerlessness, and lack of screening and outreach services

Protective Factors: Friendship and peer network, school nurse, social worker, counselling staff, school breakfast and lunch program, and primary care clinic open at school

Strengths, Assets, Resilience: Most of the girls are willing to talk to their parents about nutrition; students like their health and fitness class and the health and fitness instructor at school; school district has small amount of money to start an intervention program; most at-risk females visit the health office often and appear motivated to improve their health and fitness.

Outcomes	Interventions	Providers	Evaluation
1. By January 2008, 75% of the students will obtain lunch from the cafeteria rather than from the vending machines. (P)	■ Health teaching: nutrition ■ Collaboration: redesigning how and where students eat lunch ■ Policy development: change school policies about use of vending machines during lunch hour	■ School nurse ■ Health teachers ■ Administration ■ Food services ■ Student council ■ School nurse ■ School board	■ Student survey ■ Count numbers in cafeteria
2. By May 2008, 50% of students at risk will agree with the statement, "I like my body the way it is." (P)	■ Counselling: support group for at-risk students, peer counselling	■ Social workers ■ Psychologist ■ School nurse ■ Peer helpers ■ Peer helper instructor	■ Survey ■ Interview
3. By May 2008, 100% of the students at risk will agree with the statement, "I am more in charge of my life than I was six months ago." (P)	■ Counselling: support group for at-risk students, peer counselling	■ Social workers ■ Psychologist ■ School nurse ■ Peer helpers ■ Peer helper instructor	■ Survey ■ Interview

(Continued)

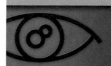

CRITICAL THINKING (CONTINUED)

Outcomes	Interventions	Providers	Evaluation
4. By January 2008, a screening and outreach program will be implemented to identify and refer students at risk for eating disorders. (S)	■ Outreach and referral: a school-wide program implemented for outreach and referral ■ Screening: the process for screening at-risk students will be developed and implemented ■ Provider education: workshop and information sheets will be provided to school staff ■ Social marketing: parents' association and school board will be targeted for information meetings	■ Administration ■ School staff ■ Peer counsellors ■ School nurse ■ Social workers ■ Psychologist ■ Health education teacher ■ Parents' association ■ School board	■ Provider survey ■ Log of students referred and analyzed ■ Evaluation at end of meeting of school board
5. By June 2008, 25% of students with weight below the 5th percentile and height above the 25th percentile on a standardized growth grid will weigh above the 5th percentile. (P)	■ Surveillance: a monitoring program for at-risk students will be developed and implemented	■ School nurse ■ Administration	■ Review of student progress records
			■ Exit survey
6. At the end of the session, 75% of participants in community health education will agree that adolescents with eating disorders are an important health priority in their community. (C)	■ Social marketing and health teaching: In June 2008, the community education department will hold a community meeting on eating disorders and adolescence.	■ Panel: health educator, school psychologist, social worker, school nurse, nutritionist, physician	

C: community-focused outcome; P: population-focused outcome related to individuals, families, small groups; S: system-focused outcome.

■ Did we manage to stay within our budget?
■ Did we use our resources in the most effective way?
■ Did we use our resources in a way that met the priority health needs of all of our high-risk client groups?
■ Did we target our services and use our resources to improve the health status of those who were the most underserved?
■ Did we have enough resources left over to meet the essential health needs of lower-risk population groups?

The evaluation process involves the multidisciplinary team, clients, and community partnerships. Regular evaluation of the program allows adjustments to be made, unmet needs of the at-risk groups to be identified, and further interventions developed if necessary. Community planning is an iterative process. Ongoing assessment of the structure, process, and outcomes is used to improve existing programs and develop new programs as the need arises.

The Critical Thinking feature shows an example of a school health program, developed following a nursing

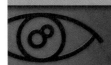

CRITICAL THINKING

In many developing countries, high rates of maternal and child morbidity and mortality are everyday realities. Access to health care may be many hours' walk away; supplies are often limited; and the health care providers may have been poorly trained. Nurses from the School of Nursing, University of Ottawa, recently embarked on a collaborative program with the Yunnan Provincial Public Health Bureau, in southern China, in an attempt to improve the health of these vulnerable members of society. Working collaboratively with their project partners in Yunnan, the Canadian team discovered that (i) isolation and mountainous terrain were major barriers to transportation and communication; (ii) health care personnel were poorly trained and poorly equipped to handle emergencies; and (iii) fees for health care providers were not adequate to reimburse them to leave their farms to deliver health care, and the fees for visits to either the midwife or the local hospital were prohibitive for the women themselves. Through their sharing of experiences in other poor settings, the Canadians were able to stimulate their Yunnan partners to think of ways to overcome some of these barriers. Their ideas were taken forth to the government, who agreed to pilot the strategies in a number of isolated communities. When the health of pregnant women and their children improved and mortality rates decreased, the government agreed to provide the programs throughout the province (Edwards & Roelofs, 2005).

Can you give other examples of international initiatives in which you or your colleagues have participated?

What are some of the access-to-care challenges faced by pregnant new Canadian women in your community? What initiatives in your community help these women to overcome these challenges? Were they successful? How was success measured?

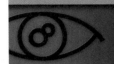

CRITICAL THINKING

Pregnant women in northern Aboriginal communities must be flown to southern centres (a 6- to 10-hour flight) to deliver their babies. This displacement takes them out of their familiar surroundings; away from their families and support systems; and places them in a foreign environment, surrounded by strangers who often speak in a language they don't understand. In the late 1980s, these women started to explore alternatives. Working with local nurses, midwives, doctors, local health centres, and the federal government, they were instrumental in establishing a local collaborative maternity program that ensured quality care for themselves and their babies, but kept them close to home.

Evaluation of the program showed that the women were receiving comprehensive perinatal care in their communities; perinatal and maternal mortality and morbidity rates became comparable to the rest of the province of Quebec; rates of premature births declined; numbers and costs of transfers to southern hospitals decreased; the program was considered successful because it had been developed collaboratively with the at-risk group it was meant to serve (Peterson & Mannion, 2005).

What access-to-care issues were identified by the community? What strategies were initiated to meet these needs? What other questions might you want to ask to determine whether this program was successful?

assessment, and its diagnosis of the teenage female population. Notice how the program addresses the issues at the levels of the community, the targeted population, and the system. The program also identifies measurable outcomes in order to evaluate the success of the program.

The goal for the World Health Organization (WHO) is the attainment by all peoples of the highest possible level of health. WHO defines health as a state of complete physical, mental, and social well-being and not merely the absence of disease or infirmity.[13] We know that personal, social, and political factors, commonly known as determinants of health, extend beyond the boundaries of traditional health care. As health care costs continue to rise, and governments around the world

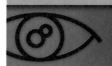

CRITICAL THINKING

Consider the implications of the following situation. Your community is experiencing a situation that is rapidly becoming known as a severe acute respiratory syndrome (SARS) epidemic. You are asked to forgo your home visits to your hospice clients for a few days so that you can help with contact follow-up. You have three hospice visits scheduled, one of them to a family with a child near death. Very little is known about SARS. Officials know it is passed by close contact with respiratory and oral secretions, but they are still unsure of the exact definition of "close contact," the incubation period, whether there can be third-party transfer, whether everyone who comes in contact is at the same risk of developing symptoms, and whether the symptoms will always be of the same severity. Your assistance, although voluntary, would be much appreciated by your colleagues who have been doing contact follow-up, without much relief, for three weeks now.

What decision would you make?

What alternative choices might you have in resolving this dilemma?

attempt to meet growing needs with finite budgets, society must recognize that, in order to attain good health, these factors are no less critical than high-quality health care. We must identify our vulnerable populations who are at highest risk for ill health; advocate for programs that will enable them to obtain food and income security, safe and sound housing, and strong support systems. We must enable them to find their own voice so they learn to advocate for themselves. We must not let our valuable human capital go untapped.

KEY CONCEPTS

- The focus of population-based health care is to reduce health disparities that exist among diverse population groups.

- The goal of population-based health care is for all members of a community to have equitable access to the resources they need to acquire and maintain the highest health status possible.

- Health promotion is the process of enabling people both to increase control over their health and to improve their health.

- Population-based nursing practice focuses on at-risk, vulnerable, and underserved population groups.

- Determinants, or prerequisites, for health include peace, shelter, education, social security, social relations, food, income, the empowerment of women, a stable ecosystem, sustainable resource use, social justice, respect for human rights, and equity.

- Population-based nursing practice starts with either a community health needs assessment that identifies health priorities and at-risk vulnerable population groups,

or the identification of the need by the vulnerable population groups themselves.

- Population-based health care involves multidisciplinary partnerships with the health care consumer and the community.

- To improve the health of the population as a whole, population-based intervention strategies need to be focused at the general population and integrated into the community health and social systems.

- Outcomes of population-based health care are measured at the population level. Three domains of population outcomes are health status, functional abilities, and quality of life.

- Nurses play key roles in the successful development and implementation of population-based health care services.

KEY TERMS

activities of daily living
Community Health Centres
determinants of health
functional health status

health promotion
health-related quality of life
health risk factors
health status

instrumental activities of
  daily living (IADLs)
population-based
  nursing practice

population health
vulnerable population
  groups

3. Survey your classmates using the health determinants assessment framework excerpt. Analyze your data and identify common health risk factors within the group.

REVIEW QUESTIONS

1. The goal of population health is
   A. access, cost, empowerment, equity.
   B. access, cost, equity, resilience.
   C. access, cost, equity, quality.
   D. for all members of a population to have equitable access to resources.

2. Population-based nursing interventions are directed at
   A. all individuals who need health services.
   B. people without health care insurance.
   C. the health needs of the total community.
   D. vulnerable groups within the community.

3. Major causes of health disparities include
   A. gender, race, ethnicity, and poverty.
   B. lack of sustainable health care systems.
   C. poverty, public policy, and national economic conditions.
   D. TB, diarrhea, malaria, and AIDS.

4. Priority population-based nursing interventions for at-risk families, with limited access to health care and many unmet health needs, should include
   A. advocacy, community organizing, social marketing, coalition building.
   B. disease and health event investigation, screening, referral, consultation.
   C. outreach, screening, referral and follow-up, health teaching, and counselling.
   D. screening, referral and follow-up, case management, surveillance.

REVIEW ACTIVITIES

1. Compare and contrast individual-focused nursing practice with population-based nursing practice. Compared to individual-focused nursing, what specific nursing knowledge and skills do you need to practice population-based nursing care?

2. If you were developing a framework for the empowerment of new Canadian women, what features would you include? How could you become a nursing advocate for the empowerment of new Canadian women at the local, national, and international levels?

EXPLORING THE WEB

- Canada Public Health Agency of Canada: *http://www.phac-aspc.gc.ca/about_apropos/index.html*

- Canadian Public Health Association: *http://www.cpha.ca/*

- Canadian Nurses Association: *http://www.cna-nurses.ca/cna/*

- Community Health Nurses' Initiatives Group: *http://www.chnig.org/*

- Community Health Nurses Association of Canada: *http://www.chnac.ca/*

- Health Canada: *http://www.hc-sc.gc.ca/*

- Local Health Integrated Networks: *http://www.health.gov.on.ca/transformation/lhin/lhin_mn.html*. Accessed 24March 2007.

- United Nations: *http://www.un.org*

- World Health Organization: *http://www.who.int/en/*

REFERENCES

Alberta. Health and Wellness. (2006). "Smoke-Free Places Act." Retrieved from http://www.health.gov.ab.ca/SmokeFree/smokefree.html, on July 30, 2006.

American Public Health Association. (2001). *The fourteen points for the campaign for universal health care—the nation's health.* Retrieved July 9, 2001, from http://www.apha.org/advocacy/priorities/issues/access/legislativereforming+thehealthcare.htm

British Columbia Centre for Disease Control. (2002). "Chee Mamuk." Retrieved from http://www.bccdc.org/content.php?item=96, on July 30, 2006.

Canada. Public Health Agency of Canada. "About the Agency." Retrieved from http://www.phac-aspc.gc.ca/about_apropos/index.html, July 30, 2006.

Canadian College of Health Service Executives. (2004). *Health systems update, 2004–2005* (12th ed.). Ottawa: Canadian College of Health Service Executives.

Edwards, N., & Roelofs, S. (2005). Participatory approaches in the co-design of a comprehensive referral system. *Canadian Nurse, 101*(8), 21–24.

Falk Rafael, A. R., Fox, J., Mildon, B., & O'Donnell, R. (1998). *Public health nursing: Position statement.* Toronto: The Community Health Nurses' Interest Group of the Registered Nurses Association of Ontario.

Freeman, R. B. (1957). *Public health nursing practice* (2nd ed.). Philadelphia: Saunders.

Green, L. W., & Kreuter, M. W. (1999). *Health promotion planning: An educational and ecological approach.* New York: McGraw-Hill.

Johnson, I. (Ed.). (2006). *Determinants of Community Health, Year 1, Semester 2: Course Manual & Readings 2006–2007.* Toronto: University of Toronto.

Manitoba. Manitoba Health. (2006). "West Nile Virus." Retrieved from http://www.gov.mb.ca/health/wnv/control.html, July 30, 2006.

Mitchell, P. (1999). UK government aims to prevent 300,000 deaths over ten years. *Lancet, 354,* 139.

New Brunswick. Department of Health. (2006). "Flu Prevention: It's in Your Hands." Retrieved from http://www.gnb.ca/0053/influenza/index-e.asp, July 30, 2006.

Northwest Territories. Health and Social Services Programs and Services. (2006). "Aboriginal Head Start." Retrieved from http://www.hlthss.gov.nt.ca/Features/Programs_and_Services/comm_wellness/ahs/default.asp, July 2, 2007.

Pan American Health Organization. (2005). *Regional declaration on the new orientations for primary health care (Declaration of Montevideo).* Washington, D.C., USA; September 2005. Retrieved from http://www.paho.org/english/ad/ths/os/PHC-orientation.htm, May 22, 2006.

Peterson, W. E., & Mannion, C. (2005). Multidisciplinary collaborative primary maternity care project: A national initiative to address the availability and quality of maternity services. *Canadian Nurse, 101*(9), 24–28.

Quebec. Ministère de la Santé et des Services Sociaux. (2007). "Domestic Violence." Retrieved from http://www.msss.gouv.qc.ca/en/sujets/prob_sociaux/domestic_violence.php, July 2, 2007.

Shah, C. P. (2003). *Public health and preventive medicine in Canada* (5th ed.). Toronto: Elsevier.

Smith, D., & Davies, B. (2006). Participatory model: Creating a new dynamic in Aboriginal health. *Canadian Nurse, 102*(4), 36–39.

Toronto District School Board. (2006a). "Thorncliffe Park Elementary School: Current School Profile." Retrieved from http://www.tdsb.on.ca/scripts/Schoolasp.asp?schno=1184, July 17, 2006.

Toronto District School Board. (2006b). "Thorncliffe Park Neighbourhood Profile." Retrieved from http://www.toronto.ca/demographics/cns_profiles/cns55.htm, July 17, 2006.

United Nations. (2005). "UN Millennium Development Goals." Retrieved from http://www.un.org/millenniumgoals/index.html, July 30, 2006.

U.S. Department of Health and Human Services. (2000). *Healthy people 2010: Understanding and improving health* (2nd ed.). Washington, DC: U.S. Government Printing Office.

World Health Organization. (1978). *Declaration of Alma-Ata: Report of the International Conference on Primary Health Care.* Alma-Ata, USSR, September 1978. Geneva: WHO. Retrieved from http://www.who.int/hpr/NPH/docs/declaration_almaata.pdf , August 2006.

World Health Organization. (1986). *Ottawa charter for health promotion.* Ottawa, Canada; November 1986. Retrieved from http://www.who.int/hpr/NPH/docs/ottawa_charter_hp.pdf, August 2006.

World Health Organization. (1997). *The Jakarta declaration on leading health promotion into the 21st century.* Jakarta, Indonesia; July 1997. Retrieved from http://www.who.int/hpr/NPH/docs/jakarta_declaration_en.pdf, August 2006.

SUGGESTED READINGS

Abbasi, K. (1999). Healthcare strategy—the role of the World Bank in international health. *British Medical Journal, 318,* 933–936.

Atkinson Charitable Foundation. (2004). "Street Nurse Cathy Crowe Receives Major Award for Work with the Homeless." Retrieved from http://www.atkinsonfoundation.ca/what_we_fund?PROGRAM_ID=24, on July 20, 2006.

Diem. E. (2004). *Community health nursing projects: Making a difference.* Philadelphia: Lippincott Williams & Wilkins.

Heymann, J., Hertzman, C., Barer, M. L., & Evans, R. G. (Eds). (2006). *Healthier societies: From analysis to action.* New York: Oxford University Press.

Hilfinger, D. K. (2001). Globalization, nursing, and health for all. *Journal of Nursing Scholarship, 33*(1), 9–11.

Kurland, J. (2000). Public health in the new millennium II: Social exclusion. *Public Health Reports, 115*(4), 298.

Leeseberg Stamler, L. (2004). *Community health nursing: A Canadian perspective.* Toronto: Pearson Education Canada.

Lindeman, C. A. (2000). The future of nursing education. *Journal of Nursing Education, 39*(1), 5–12.

Orchard, C. A., Smillie, C., & Meagher-Stewart, D. (2005). Community development and health in Canada. *Journal of Nursing Scholarship, 32*(2), 2005.

Registered Nurses Association of British Columbia. (1992). *Determinants of health: Empowering strategies for nursing practice.* Vancouver: Registered Nurses Association of British Columbia.

Robinson Vollman, A. (2003). *Canadian community as partner.* Philadelphia: Lippincott Williams & Wilkins.

Uys, L. R. (2001). Universal access to health care: If not now, when? *Reflections on Nursing Leadership, 27*(2), 21–23.

World Health Organization. (2000). *A massive effort for better health among the poor.* Retrieved from http://www.who.int/inf-new/conclu.htm, July 7, 2001.

Young, L. E., & Hayes, V. E. (2002). *Transforming health promotion practice: Concepts, issues, and applications.* Philadelphia: F. A. Davis Company.

CHAPTER ENDNOTES

1. *Ottawa Charter for Health Promotion.* Retrieved from http://www.who.int/hpr/NPH/docs/ottawa_charter_hp.pdf, August 2006.

2. *Jakarta Declaration on Leading Health Promotion into the 21st Century.* Retrieved from http://www.who.int/hpr/NPH/docs/jakarta_declaration_en.pdf, August 2006.

3. Ottawa Charter for Health Promotion, "Health Promotion Action Means." Retrieved from http://www.who.int/hpr/NPH/docs/ottawa_charter_hp.pdf, August 2006.

4. Jakarta Declaration on Leading Health Promotion into the 21st Century, "Priorities for Health Promotion in the

21st century." Retrieved from http://www.who.int/hpr/NPH/docs/jakarta_declaration_en.pdf, August 2006.

5. Tate, D. G., & Nieuwenhujsen, E. "The ICIDH–2: A New Classification of Disablement." Retrieved from http://www.psychosocial.com/policy/icidh.html, August 2006.

6. Ontario. Ministry of Health and Long-Term Care, "The History of Nursing in Ontario." Retrieved from http://www.health.gov.on.ca/english/public/program/hhr/nurses/history.html, August, 2006.

7. Canadian Nurses Association, "Obtaining CNA Certification." Retrieved from http://cna-aiic.ca/cna/nursing/certification/specialties/initials/default_e.aspx, August 2006.

8. Street Health, "About Us," Retrieved from http://www.streethealth.ca/home.htm, August 2006.

9. Atkinson Charitable Foundation, "Catherine (Betsy) Atkinson Murray's Remarks upon the Occasion of Cathy Crowe's Receipt of the Atkinson Economic Justice Award: Thursday, January 22, 2004." Retrieved from http://www.atkinsonfoundation.ca/pressroom/acfInTheNews/Betsys_Cathy_Crowe_Remarks..doc/view, August 2006.

10. Ministry of Health and Long-Term Care, "Local Health Integration Networks." Retrieved from http://www.health.gov.on.ca/transformation/lhin/lhin_mn.html, August 2006.

11. Ministry of Health and Long-Term Care, "Community Health Centres." Retrieved from http://www.health.gov.on.ca/english/public/contact/chc/chc_mn.html, August 2006.

12. Aboriginal Health Access Centres, "Programs and Services." Retrieved from http://www.ahwsontario.ca/programs/prog_top.html, September 2006.

13. World Health Organization, "About WHO." Retrieved from http://www.who.int/about/en/index.html, August 2006.

CHAPTER 6

Personal and Interdisciplinary Communication

Jacklyn L. Ruthman, PhD, RN

Adapted by: John P. Angkaw, RN, BScN, MEd(c) and Amy Curzon, RN

Effective communication among professionals is one way to establish and maintain the desired atmosphere of professional competence which ensures quality client care.
(Mary Ellen Grohar-Murray & Helen R. DiCroce, 2003)

OBJECTIVES

Upon completion of this chapter, the reader should be able to:

1. Detail current trends in society that affect communication.
2. Describe the communication process.
3. Identify the characteristics of verbal and nonverbal communication.
4. Increase effectiveness of communication by using basic communication skills.
5. Identify barriers to communication.
6. Describe typical nursing communication activities in the workplace.

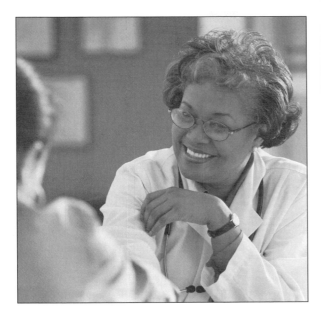

As a new graduate nurse working on a medical unit in your community hospital, you begin your shift by making rounds of your clients to perform initial assessments and obtain their vital signs. You enter the room of Mr. Davis, who has a long history of asthma and chronic obstructive pulmonary disease. He was admitted yesterday with aspiration pneumonia. While conducting a respiratory assessment, he tells you, "I don't think I'm going to survive this one. My body has gone through enough." His wife, who is at his bedside, replies, "What's wrong with you? Don't talk like that."

What are your thoughts about this situation?

What nonverbal cues might be used to help you interpret this message?

What communication skills will you use to respond appropriately?

Today's nurses use basic principles of communication to facilitate interactions with clients and their family members, peers, and practitioners in other disciplines. These principles allow nurses to adapt to trends that affect the profession of nursing and its practice. The dictionary defines communication as a process by which information is exchanged. Nurses follow a process of communication that is more universal than unique to nursing. They rely on communication skills to effectively promote client care and professionalism in a variety of settings for an increasingly diverse society. These skills enable nurses to engage in the complex, interactive process of communication that uses both verbal and nonverbal modes. Nurses are aware of the context in which communication occurs. Nurses must be aware of potential barriers to communication to be able to overcome those barriers. Awareness of the principles and skills of communication empowers nurses to manage a variety of communication demands in the workplace.

TRENDS IN SOCIETY THAT AFFECT COMMUNICATION

Good communication will grow in importance because of trends in our culture. Among the trends affecting nursing practice is the increasing diversity in society. Canada has been called the melting pot, and that has never been truer than now, when we see the influence of many different ethnic, racial, cultural, and socioeconomic backgrounds (Peach, 2005). Increased diversity causes once-dominant values and beliefs to be replaced or diluted with new values and beliefs. These differences become a source of possible misunderstanding that can be bridged by effective communication.

Another trend is our aging population. It is estimated that approximately 25 percent of the population will be 65 years of age or older by 2031. This figure would continue to grow to a figure between 35 to 50 percent by 2056 (Statistics Canada, 2006). Our aging society will challenge nurses to maintain effective communication to compensate for the diminished sensory abilities that typically accompany aging. Multiple sensory deficits can occur simultaneously so that clients may experience losses in a variety of combinations that include hearing, seeing, smelling, tasting, and touching. The potential diminished input challenges nurse and client alike to creatively compensate for these deficits.

At the same time that the population is aging, it is also shifting to an electronic mode, with computer technology playing an increasingly dominant role. As electronic communication assumes a greater role, nurses' ability to effectively communicate in writing will grow in importance. Reliance on written communication using electronic input shifts the source of input away from traditional visual, auditory, and kinesthetic modes to the written word. Therefore, tomorrow's nurses will require keen writing skills. These trends have influenced recommendations for current nursing competencies. Communication is so central to nursing that the majority of competencies required of nurse managers contain a communication component (Jeans & Rowat, 2005).

ELEMENTS OF THE COMMUNICATION PROCESS

Communication is the exchange of information or opinions. Communication is most often an interactive process that is a means to an end and is influenced by the context in which it occurs. Communication typically involves a

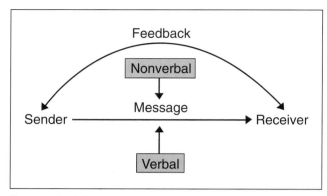

Figure 6-1 Basic Communication Model

sender, a message, a receiver, and feedback. Face-to-face communication allows the process to proceed almost immediately, that is, to be synchronous. Electronic media can be either synchronous or asynchronous. Figure 6-1 illustrates the communication process.

SENDER

A message originates with the sender. Laswell's classic model of communication (1948) describes the sender as the "who" in communication. When nurses initiate communication, they are the senders.

MESSAGE

The **message** originates with the sender. It consists of verbal and/or nonverbal stimuli that are taken in by the receiver. The message is the "what" in communication.

RECEIVER

The **receiver** takes in the message and analyzes it. When nurses listen to client-initiated conversations, they are the receivers. When the receiver reacts by returning a new message, the receiver and sender reverse roles.

FEEDBACK

The new message that is generated by the receiver in response to the original message from the sender is the **feedback.** Grohar-Murray and DiCroce (2003) state that feedback informs the sender that the receiver had understood the message transmitted. Feedback is effective when the two communicators are sensitive to each other's messages and they change behaviours based on the message exchanges.

CHANNELS OF COMMUNICATION

In almost every nursing interaction, there is **visual** (seeing), **auditory** (hearing), and **kinesthetic** (touching) input. According to Potter and Perry (2001), these sensory stimuli may be processed at different levels, with

the simplest level reporting what is actually seen, heard, or touched. The next level of sensory processing orders and structures information from the usual auditory or kinesthetic input and integrates the stimulus so that one reports observing, listening, or feeling. The highest level of processing interprets and integrates information from all the inputs leading to perception and - interpretation.

The processing occurs in each person who is communicating and may occur at different levels, depending on each person's cognitive abilities. For example, a toddler who is just beginning to communicate effectively using words delights in sharing labels such as "snow." This is the simplest level of communication. Upon touching the snow, the toddler might demonstrate an ability to integrate the experience with touching snow by exclaiming, "Snow cold." The mother delights in the child's sophistication and interprets the first encounter at the higher level of processing by responding to the child at the highest level and telling the child that's right and offering that snow is cold and white and beautiful and fun to play in.

THE VISUAL CHANNEL

All seeing people take in information from the surrounding environments through sight. The amount of detail available is limited primarily by how much one looks. For nurses, visual data offer a wealth of information that can lead to rapid interpretation. For example, a nurse who is caring for a fresh postoperative client looks at the dressing to validate that it is dry, intact, and free of discharge. The nurse interprets these negative findings as a stable situation.

THE AUDITORY CHANNEL

Hearing is another sensory channel that is focused on words that are spoken, as well as the volume, pitch, tone, rhythm, and speed with which they are delivered. Hearing involves identifying not only the words spoken but also how a message is delivered. Babies are typically born with the ability to hear, but they must learn to listen. Listening involves making sense out of what was said.

To listen effectively, the nurse must put together accurately what is said and how it is said. The nurse who is assessing the fresh postoperative client asks, "How would you rate your pain on a scale of 0 to 10, with 0 being no pain and 10 being the worst pain you can imagine?" The client replies, "Oh, I don't know, maybe a four." The nurse begins the feedback by inquiring of the client whether a pain rating of four is acceptable. The words the nurse speaks are also filled with cues based on the volume, rhythm, tone, pitch, and speed. The client tells the nurse that the pain is acceptable, but a nurse who is truly listening must also process cues based on the client's volume, rhythm, tone, pitch, and speed.

THE KINESTHETIC CHANNEL

All aspects of communication that relate to feelings are considered kinesthetic. At the most basic level, these feelings involve touch and physiological responses. Kinesthetic stimuli have cognitive and emotional components that are integrated to become feelings, or the quality of things as imparted through touch. For example, as the nurse repositions the client, the nurse may touch the client's skin and note that it is warm and dry. The nurse interprets these stimuli favourably. However, the nurse also notices that the client grimaces when moved. A client's body actions or body language communicate additional kinesthetic information. Body language is important because it may accompany, substitute, or modify input from other channels. Integrating information from all channels, the nurse perceives that the client may be in pain that is unacceptable. The nurse offers verbal feedback that matches that perception, thereby continuing the communication process using all channels until the exchange is complete.

MODES OF COMMUNICATION

The two traditional modes of communication, verbal and nonverbal, are exemplified in the nurse–client scenario in the Real World Interview. Because face-to-face encounters usually allow for verbal and nonverbal exchange, they have been regarded as the most effective modes of communication and hence have been preferred. When face-to-face encounters are not possible or practical, other approaches are used. Historically, the next most effective approach is the telephone, followed by voice messages, e-mail messages, and written documents. These electronic methods comprise the third mode of communication, which will grow in importance as nurses increasingly rely on technology, particularly computers, to communicate interpersonally. As was previously mentioned, using e-mail requires that nurses have keen writing skills.

VERBAL COMMUNICATION

Verbal communication relies on speaking words to convey a message. It also involves the use of the auditory channel previously discussed. The accuracy of the message is dependent on the sender's vocabulary and the receiver's ability to make sense of the words used to send the message. In addition, the verbal message is influenced by the sender's tone. According to Yogo, Hashi, Tsutsui, and Yamada (2000), when conveying a message, the tone is more influential than the content. Another factor that influences verbal communication is the pacing, or timing of a message. Verbal communication is a conscious process, so the sender has the ability to control what is said.

NONVERBAL COMMUNICATION

Nonverbal communication consists of aspects of communication that are outside what is spoken. The communicator's appearance, facial expressions, posture, gait, body movements, position, gestures, and touch all influence how the message is processed. And, although tone is more important than the words spoken, it has long been suggested that facial expression is even more important than either tone or the words used. Nonverbal communication tends to be unconscious and more difficult to control.

ELECTRONIC COMMUNICATION

As previously mentioned, communication is shifting to an electronic mode, with computer technology playing an increasingly dominant role. Clients are being monitored long distance and connecting to their health care providers using a variety of technologies, including telephone, voice mail, and e-mail. These methods, which may be asynchronous because caregiver and care receiver interact using technology rather than the traditional face-to-face or voice-to-voice encounter, require careful communication. For example, e-mail allows almost instantaneous communication around the world, but it also accommodates individual preferences with respect to the timing of the response. For example, a client can provide an update on a condition early in the day, and the caregivers can respond as their schedules permit. Using e-mail may save a client and caregiver from travel or loss of work; however, nurses acting in such a caregiver role need to have keen writing skills.

All the considerations that are important to effective writing are beyond the scope of this text; however, a few tips are worth sharing. The speed with which exchanges can now be made using computers has reduced the acceptable response time. Therefore, the first tip when communicating using computers is to respond in a timely manner. Next, keep in mind that accurate spelling, correct grammar, and organization of thought assume greater importance in the absence of verbal and nonverbal cues that are given in face-to-face encounters. Finally, always proofread your correspondences prior to sending them. Imagine yourself the recipient of the document. Look for complete sentences; a logical development of thought and reasoning; accuracy; and an appropriate use of grammar, such as punctuation and capitalization.

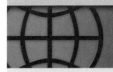

REAL WORLD INTERVIEW

The client is a 25-year-old male who came into the Emergency Department (ED) with the primary complaint of extreme shortness of breath. The differential diagnosis for his clinical presentation and laboratory data suggested possible acute respiratory distress syndrome (ARDS), pneumonia, or pulmonary edema. His condition was very poor, established by evidence of deteriorating arterial blood gas values despite aggressive oxygen therapies. His condition deteriorated so quickly that he required intubation and ultimately ventilator support.

The client was extremely ill and was admitted to the intensive care unit (ICU) for approximately two weeks. During his admission to the unit, he had periods of aggression and anxiousness related to the large breathing apparatus placed within his throat. In order to calm him, an order of sedation was administered on an as required basis. This sedation was essential according to the medical team in order to help normalize his arterial blood gases.

The client had written numerous notes to his family and the medical personnel requesting that the ventilator be removed. This request was not an act of suicide; rather, he denied he needed it and insisted he could breathe on his own.

While taking care of the client, I had the urge to remove the ventilator. I felt that the client at least deserved a trial without any assisted breathing devices. I had high hopes that removing the ventilator would either be successful in recovery, or an affirmation of his respiratory misfortunes.

The next day at rounds, I made mention of this idea to remove the ventilator at the client's request. Unfortunately my words fell on deaf ears. I wasn't about to give up, so I talked to the attending resident after rounds and still had no success.

I knew that a different approach was required. I spoke with the attending resident the following day since the blood gas values showed some improvement, and there was a chance for the team to accurately assess the client's mechanics of respiration. After a lengthy discussion, the attending resident finally decided to remove the ventilator.

In the end, the client did have poor mechanics of respiration. But, after some chest physiotherapy, the client was discharged four days later from the ICU.

Paul Jeffrey, RN, BScN (Hons), MN-ACNP(c), CEN

LEVEL OF COMMUNICATION

The level of communication depends on the audience for the message. Consequently, communication can be thought of as having three levels: public, intrapersonal, and interpersonal.

PUBLIC COMMUNICATION

The nurse educator presenting a workshop on signs and symptoms of menopause to a room full of middle-aged women engages in public communication. Her audience is a group of people with a common interest. As the presenter, she acts primarily as a sender of information. By design, feedback is typically limited in public speaking, though it does occur. Strategies abound to enhance public speaking skills, but it is beyond the scope of this text to discuss them.

INTRAPERSONAL COMMUNICATION

Intrapersonal communication can be thought of as self-talk. As the name suggests, this level of communication refers to how individuals communicate within themselves and can present as doubts or affirmations. New nurses may engage in intrapersonal communication while simultaneously doubting and affirming their ability to complete a procedure. For example, the first time newly registered RNs have to catheterize a client, they may simultaneously doubt their ability to insert a Foley catheter with one message, "I haven't done this for months," while affirming their ability to insert a Foley catheter with an "I can do this" message to themselves. They are engaging in intrapersonal communication. The so-called competing voices within them act as sender and receiver in this intrapersonal conversation, whose outcome will be influenced by the feedback that follows.

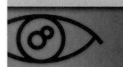

CRITICAL THINKING

Upon entering a client's room, you identify yourself as his nurse and greet the client. You then ask the client how he is feeling. He responds with a whisper and a grimace, "I've never felt better." You notice the client is slightly cyanotic. The client is supporting himself with his elbows so that he is sitting upright over the bedside table. You note he is using pursed lip breathing. Respirations are 36 per minute and shallow.

What kinds of problems occur when verbal and nonverbal communications are incongruent? How will you handle the incongruent verbal and nonverbal communications? Which message, the verbal or nonverbal, is more difficult to control?

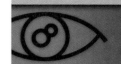

CRITICAL THINKING

A diabetic client who lives in the rural North is excited to have recently become connected to the World Wide Web with the acquisition of a computer and Internet services. His wife, who accompanies him to the office visit, wonders whether some of the monitoring that currently occurs during office visits might not be accomplished using e-mail. Winters are hard and travel is difficult, the client's circulation is poor, he fatigues easily, and using e-mail could save them the six-hour roundtrip to the primary care clinic. By using e-mail, they can maintain contact as needed without these drawbacks.

Do you agree with their idea? What are the advantages of this suggestion for the client? For the caregiver? What are the drawbacks of this suggestion for the client? For the caregiver? What safeguards can you think of to facilitate communicating using e-mail and to ensure quality care?

Simms, Price, and Ervin (2000) present communication with self, or intrapersonal communication, as the first important element in developing a sphere of communication. From self-awareness and understanding of oneself, a nurse can progress confidently to one-on-one interactions with others, and then into interactions with smaller and larger groups. See Figure 6-2 for some spheres of communication and their related skills.

INTERPERSONAL COMMUNICATION

Interpersonal communication involves communication between individuals, either person-to-person or in small

groups. Not surprisingly, nurses engage in this level regularly. Interpersonal communication allows for a very effective level of communication and incorporates all of the elements, channels, and modes previously discussed. The nurse, who observes a client grimace when he moves, interprets the nonverbal cue as indicating that the client is experiencing pain. Using verbal communication, she clarifies her perception by asking the client to describe and rate his pain. He describes it as tolerable and states he is expecting a visitor and he does not want to be drowsy. The communication goes back and forth until, ideally, both parties' understanding of the message match, achieving the goal of communication.

ORGANIZATIONAL COMMUNICATION

Avenues of communication are often defined by an organization's formal structure, which establishes who is in charge and identifies how different levels of personnel and various departments relate within the organization. When the chief executive officer of an organization announces that the company will adopt a new policy that all employees will follow, such an announcement is a downward communication. The message starts at the top and is usually disseminated by levels through the chain of communication.

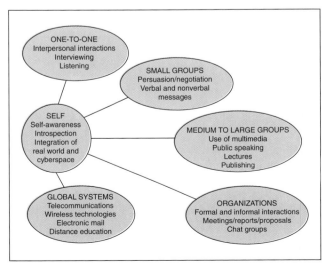

Figure 6-2 Spheres of Communication and Related Skills

Upward communication is the opposite of downward communication. The idea originates at some level below the top of the structure and moves upward. For example, when a nurse recommends a more efficient approach to organizing care to his nurse manager, who takes the recommendation to her superior, who uses the recommendation to develop a new policy, then upward communication has occurred. Lateral communication occurs among people with similar status. Two nurses who are discussing how to best change a client's dressing are engaged in lateral communication. Diagonal communication occurs when members of the team who may be on different levels of the organizational chart discuss a client care concern, such as discharge planning.

The organizational structure within nursing also determines who is responsible for representing nursing concerns in this type of interaction. For example, if the department practises within a primary nursing model, the primary nurse is responsible for representing nursing concerns. In team nursing, the team leader rather than the nurse delivering care is responsible.

A final avenue worth mentioning, which is not a formal avenue, is the grapevine. The **grapevine** is an informal avenue in which rumours circulate. It ignores the formal chain of command. The major benefit of the grapevine is the speed with which information is spread, but its major drawback is that it often lacks accuracy. For example, nurses who inform an oncoming shift about a rumour that layoffs or mandatory overtime is imminent, in the absence of any information from the hospital's administration, are participating in grapevine communication.

COMMUNICATION SKILLS

Because nurses are often placed in positions of leadership and are responsible for representing nursing's concerns to others, including the client, they must have the requisite skills to be effective communicators. No single correct method ensures effective communication. Rather, effective communication requires that both parties engaged in communicating use skills that enhance that particular interaction. Baker, Beglinger, King, Salyards, and Thompson (2000) believe that the most important considerations for facilitating communication are to be open and to be willing to give and receive feedback. Some of the most important skills that nurses rely on to facilitate communication are attending, responding, clarifying, and confronting skills. Additional skills are listed in Table 6-1.

ATTENDING

Attending involves active listening, the most important skill used by nurses to gain an understanding of the client's message. Active listening requires that the nurse pay close attention to what the client is saying. In addition, the nurse uses the sensory and visual channels, looking for congruence between what is said and how it is said. Attending involves the nurse's nonverbal cues. Facing the client and maintaining eye contact are two skills that facilitate attending. Sitting down and leaning forward sends a message that the nurse is willing to listen. Distracting behaviours, such as tapping, send a message

TABLE 6-1	ADDITIONAL COMMUNICATION SKILLS

Skill	Description
Supporting	Siding with another person or backing up another person: "I can see that you would feel that way."
Focusing	Centres on the main point: "So your main concern is . . ."
Asking open-ended questions	Allows for client-directed responses: "How did that make you feel?"
Providing information	Supplies knowledge that an individual did not previously have: "It's common for people with pneumonia to be tired."
Using silence	Allows for intrapersonal communication
Reassuring	Restores confidence or removes fear: "I can assure you that tomorrow . . ."
Expressing appreciation	Shows gratitude: "Thank you" or "You are so thoughtful."
Using humour	Provides relief and gains perspective; but may also cause harm so use humour carefully
Conveying acceptance	Makes known that one is capable or worthy: "It's okay to cry."
Asking related questions	Expands the listener's understanding: "How painful was it?"

that the nurse is not interested in the message; therefore, such behaviours should be avoided.

RESPONDING

Responding entails verbal and nonverbal acknowledgment of the sender's message. When a nurse nods affirmatively while listening, this nonverbal response says that the message has worth. A response can be as simple as an acknowledgment that the message was received, for example, "I hear you." Sometimes, however, responding involves more. Two verbal skills that elevate the level of responding are questioning and rephrasing. Questioning allows the nurse to clarify the message by asking related questions. Rephrasing involves restating what the nurse believes to be the important points. These techniques refine perceptions and enhance understanding.

CLARIFYING

Clarifying, by using such skills as restating, questioning, and rephrasing, helps the message become clear. As with most communication, clarifying can be accomplished using a variety of approaches. For example, if the nurse does not follow a client's account of his presenting complaint, the nurse can respond with "I lost you there." Perhaps the nurse tries to process information that is confusing or conflicting. The nurse can then restate what was heard, in an effort to clarify the information. Clarifying involves communicating as specifically as possible. Questioning and rephrasing, which were described previously, are used not only to respond but also to clarify.

CONFRONTING

Confronting describes working jointly with others to resolve a problem or conflict. Given that definition, confronting is an effective means of resolving conflict. It involves, first of all, identifying the conflict, which can arise from either perceived or real differences. A nurse might identify a conflict with a simple "we have a problem here." Next, the problem is clearly delineated so that those involved understand what it is and what it is not. Then, using knowledge and reason, attempts are made to resolve the problem. The goal is to achieve a win–win solution in which both parties' needs are met, which sounds easier than it sometimes is because emotions can get in the way and cloud reason. Cooling-off periods are sometimes needed between problem identification and conflict resolution. Acceptable motives for confronting are to resolve conflict, further growth, and improve relationships.

BARRIERS TO COMMUNICATION

Barriers are obstacles to effective communication. The nurse who can identify potential barriers to communication will be better equipped to avoid them or to compensate for them. Some of the most common barriers are gender, culture, anger, incongruent responses, and conflict.

GENDER

Gender interferes with communication when men and women lack the understanding that they sometimes process information differently. Gender differences and patterns do not preclude working together. Rather, both sides must realize the other's preference and make accommodations so that effective communication results.

Gender differences have been attributed, in part, to gender socialization in which males are provided with more opportunities to develop confidence and assertiveness than females. Fortunately, the feminist movement and increased sexual equality in Western society, in general, have lessened traditional sociological patterns of competitiveness and decisiveness in men and passivity and nurturing in women. However, remnants of the traditional model persist, particularly in health care settings. Nurses who lack assertiveness and confidence are encouraged to acquire the requisite skills to be assertive and confident to be an effective client advocate and also to communicate in a confident manner.

CULTURE

As was stated previously, our culture grows increasingly diverse. This diversity reduces the likelihood that clients and nurses will share a common cultural background. In turn, the number of safe assumptions about beliefs and practices decreases, and the probability for misunderstanding increases. For example, shortly after delivering a baby, women are often hungry and thirsty. Some cultures believe that women should eat hot foods and beverages to appropriately restore their energies, whereas other cultures believe cold foods and beverages are appropriate. A well-intentioned nurse who does not consult with the client about her preferences may arrange culturally inappropriate nourishment.

Broadly defined, culture encompasses different groups' beliefs and practices by gender, race, age, economic status, health, and disability. Poole, Davidhizar, and Giger (1995) suggest there are six cultural phenomena to consider when delegating to a culturally diverse staff: communication, space, social organization, time, environmental control, and biological variations. They emphasize that culture and communication are intrinsically intertwined (see the Literature Application).

Nurses are responsible for bridging gaps between themselves and their clients through first being accepting of differences. They can also overcome cultural differences by learning about other cultures. Finally, nurses bridge cultural differences by vigilantly using the skills previously described to facilitate communication.

ANGER

Anger is a universal, strong feeling of displeasure that is often precipitated by a situation that frustrates or prevents a person from attaining a goal or getting what is wanted from life. Anger is often a response to conflict and is influenced by one's beliefs. Ellis (1997) describes anger as an irrational response that arises from one of four irrational ideas: (1) the treatment one received was awful (awfulizing); (2) feeling that one can't stand having been treated so irresponsibly and unfairly (can't-stand-it-itis); (3) believing that one should not and must not behave as he did (shoulding and musting); and (4) because one acted in a terrible manner, he is a terrible person (undeservingness and damnation). Ellis maintains that beliefs remain rational as long as the evaluation of the action does not involve an evaluation of the person. Rational and appropriate responses are feelings of disappointment. Anger, on the other hand, can be unmanageable and self-defeating. According to Ellis, we all have the ability to choose our response to anger. Potter and Perry (2001) state that anger has the following nursing implications: (1) the nurse must not take the anger personally; (2) the nurse must meet the need that caused the angry response; and (3) when necessary, the nurse must encourage the client and the family to further express their feelings.

Anger can be dealt with in one of several ways. Three methods that may work from time to time but that may have serious and potentially destructive drawbacks are denying and repressing anger, which may lead to resentment; expressing anger, which may lead to defensiveness on the part of the respondent; and turning the other cheek, which may lead to continued mistreatment and lack of trust. Because anger stems from carrying things further and viewing the situation as awful, terrible, or horrible, Ellis (1997) advocates disputing irrational beliefs. Anger can stem from deep-seated feelings of unassertiveness. Assertion involves taking a stand, whereas aggression involves putting another person down. If unassertiveness is the source of anger, then a solution is to learn to act assertively.

INCONGRUENT RESPONSES

When words and actions in a communication do not match the inner experience of self or are inappropriate to the context, the response is incongruent. Some common incongruent responses are blaming, placating, being super reasonable, and using irrelevant information to make decisions. Blaming is finding fault or error and occurs when a response lacks respect for others' feelings. For example, a nurse who attributes a medication error to her overloaded assignment might blame the nurse who made the assignment, saying, "It's all her fault." This reaction can be avoided by standing up for one's rights while respecting the rights of others. Placating is soothing by concession, which occurs when one lacks self-respect. For example, a nurse who consents to a client assignment that she believes is unfair or unsafe just to

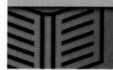

LITERATURE APPLICATION

Citation: Poole, V. L., Davidhizar, R. E., and Giger, J. N. (1995). Delegating to a transcultural team. *Nursing Management, 26*(8), 33–34.

Discussion: All cultural groups show evidence of six phenomena: communication, space, social organization, time, environmental control, and biological variations. However, the application and use of these phenomena vary within and among cultures. Nurses' cultural assessment is essential when delegating to a transcultural team. Suggestions for bridging variations are category specific. Regarding communication, the authors recommend assessing dialect, style, volume, the use of touch, context of speech, and kinesics. They identify that the two to three feet of socially acceptable space that some white American middle-class people find comfortable when talking is considered distant among other cultural groups, specifically African-Americans and the French. Although family may dominate as the primary social organization among many individuals and groups, others may hold an individualistic view. With respect to time, cultural groups may be focused on the past, present, or future. Environmental control is concerned with the locus of control, which can be internal or external. Finally, biological variations exist between racial and ethnic groups and can cause varying susceptibility to disease. All staff are encouraged to maintain an optimal level of wellness to maintain their ability to deal with client problems.

Implications for Practice: When delegating, all the previously mentioned phenomena must be considered for both individual and group interactions.

TABLE 6-2	ADDITIONAL BARRIERS TO COMMUNICATION

Barrier	Description
Offering false reassurance	Promising something that cannot be delivered
Being defensive	Acting as though one has been attacked
Stereotyping	Unfairly categorizing others based on their traits
Interrupting	Speaking before others have completed their message
Inattention	Not paying attention
Stress	A state of tension that gets in the way of reasoning
Unclear expectations	Ill-defined tasks or duties that make successful completion unlikely

keep the peace is placating. Placating can be overcome by paying attention to one's own needs and by negotiating what one believes to be a fair and safe assignment. Being super reasonable is to go beyond reason and lack respect for others' and one's own feelings. The nurse described previously, who, when approached by the house supervisor, agrees to whatever solution is offered, has become super reasonable when she says, "You're always right; I'll do whatever you need." This ineffective approach can be sidestepped by considering each other's feelings when arriving at a solution. Finally, using irrelevant information for decision making shows lack of respect for others' and one's own feelings. A nurse who challenges a colleague's abilities based solely on the colleague's out-of-work activities or political preference is using irrelevant information. Likewise, arguing against a colleague's ability to function as a charge nurse because of an incident that occurred a year prior during the nurse's orientation is often irrelevant. Respecting feelings and context can avert irrelevance.

CONFLICT

Conflict arises when ideas or beliefs are opposed. Not surprisingly, it occurs at different levels: interpersonal and organizational. As was previously stated, conflict resolution is one way to resolve conflict. To resolve conflict, the nature of the differences and the reasons for the differences must be considered. These differences arise for an array of reasons. Some of these reasons include variations in facts, goals, and methods to achieve goals, values, or standards (Grohar-Murray & DiCroce, 2003). Conflict resolution typically occurs using one of five distinct approaches: avoiding, accommodating, competing, compromising, and collaborating. Two conflict management strategies, avoiding and compromising, were used predominantly by all categories of nurses in this research study (Valentine, 2001).

Avoiding or retreating disregards the needs of self and others but sometimes offers the benefit of allowing tempers to cool. An example of avoidance is the nurse who walks away from a heated discussion with a peer, after a change-of-shift report. **Accommodating** satisfies the needs of others at the expense of self. The nurse who forfeits after-work plans to staff the unit by working overtime is accommodating. Accommodating can lead to disappointment or anger. **Competing** can lead to personal victory at the expense of others, which can lead to ill will. For example, two nurses who want the same weekend off may plead their cases to the nurse manager, each in hopes of getting her own way.

Compromising leads to a middle-ground solution in which each party makes a concession. The charge nurse who gives each of the nurses above a day off on the weekend they requested has resolved the conflict by compromising. Finally, **collaborating** resolves conflict so that both parties are satisfied. It involves seeking creative, integrative solutions, while also working through emotions. Collaborating is the best strategy for successful conflict resolution, but it is more difficult than it may appear. The charge nurse who clarifies the above nurses' requests for the same weekend off discovers one nurse wants the weekend off to attend her sister's wedding, whereas the other nurse wants to plan a getaway that can be moved to another weekend. Each nurse can be satisfied through collaboration.

Additional barriers to communication are seen in Table 6-2.

WORKPLACE COMMUNICATION

It is probably clear by now that how individuals communicate depends, in part, on where communication occurs and the relationship between the sender and the receiver.

Patterns of communication in the workplace are sensitive to organizational factors that define relationships. Nurses have diverse roles and relationships in the workplace that call for different communication patterns with superiors, coworkers, subordinates, physicians and other health care professionals, clients, families, and mentors.

SUPERIORS

Communicating with a superior can be intimidating, especially for a new nurse. Observing professional courtesies is an important first step. For instance, when a problem arises, begin by requesting an appointment to discuss the issue. This approach demonstrates respect and allows for the conversation to occur at an appropriate time and place. Dress professionally. Arrive for the appointment on time, and be prepared to state the concern clearly and accurately. Provide supporting evidence, and anticipate resistance to any requests. Separate your needs from your desires. State a willingness to cooperate in finding a solution and then match your behaviours to words. Persist in the pursuit of a solution.

COWORKERS

Nurses depend on their coworkers to collectively provide quality client care. Nowhere is this relationship more important than in the acute care setting, where nursing services are nonstop around the clock. Transfer of client care from nurse to nurse is one of the most important and frequent communications between coworkers. It depends on fluid communication in end-of-shift reports to achieve quality nursing care. However, time constraints demand that the change of shift report be accurate, informative, and succinct. How the nursing care is organized influences the person who receives the report. For example, nurses who practise using a team model will require that, at a minimum, the charge nurse or team leader receives the report.

The method of delivery of the report also varies from setting to setting and may include walking rounds, written communication, or tape recording. Regardless of the method used, information that is typically exchanged during a change of shift report, either in writing or orally, includes the client's age, gender, admitting problem, needs, other health care concerns, activity, diet, intake and output, IV therapy, treatments, tests, and family concerns. Significant physical findings and client responses to any of the items just listed are often elaborated. The organization of the information varies and may, for example, follow a head-to-toe model if assessment forms also use this organizing approach. The most important consideration for nurses as they organize their reports is to paint an accurate picture of the client's condition and needs.

SUBORDINATES

An excellent guide for directing communication with subordinates is the golden rule: Do unto others as you would have them do unto you. As a nurse who will be responsible for overseeing others' work, a valuable perspective to maintain is that all members of the team are important to successfully realize quality client care. Communication between nurses and subordinates will most likely involve delegating, which is covered in Chapter 13, and you are encouraged to review this material as it relates to subordinates. In addition to delegating, a few other communications skills are worth mentioning. Offering positive feedback, such as, "I appreciate the way you interacted with Mr. T. to get him to ambulate twice this shift," goes a long way toward team building, and it improves subordinates' sense of worth.

Nurses also have an opportunity to act as teachers to subordinates. Often in a hospital setting, nurses teach by example. Demonstrating the desired behaviour allows the subordinate to copy the behaviour. Allow time for return demonstrations to evaluate whether the subordinate has learned the intended skill. For example, as the nurse, you may demonstrate how to position a client with special needs, encouraging the subordinate to assist and ask questions. The next time repositioning is indicated, accompany the subordinate and observe that person's ability to successfully complete the task. Offer constructive feedback. Be patient. Remember your own learning curves when mastering new skills and behaviours, and allow those you supervise the opportunity to grow. Be open to the possibility that subordinates, particularly those with experience, may have a few pearls of wisdom to share with you as well. For example, this author is forever indebted to a nurse aide who shared how to really position clients comfortably. Likewise, a veteran registered practical nurse (RPN) who knew the politics of the institution mentored a batch of new graduates as they learned to be charge nurses on the evening shift.

PHYSICIANS AND OTHER HEALTH CARE PROFESSIONALS

One of the most intimidating experiences for new nurses is communicating with physicians. Despite gender and role challenges that have already been discussed, such communications need not be stressful events. The nurse's goal is to strive for collaboration, keeping the client goal central to the discussion. As was previously discussed, collaboration allows both parties to be satisfied. It involves seeking creative, integrative solutions while also working through emotions.

To communicate effectively with the physician, the nurse presents information in a straightforward manner, clearly delineating the problem, supported by pertinent evidence. This approach is especially important when reporting changes in client conditions. Nurses are responsible for knowing the classic symptoms of conditions, orally apprising the physician of changes, and recording all

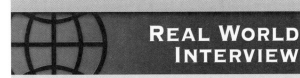

A night shift RN working in a busy emergency room was presented with a client who was hypertensive and complaining of a headache. When she did her initial triage assessment, including the client's vital signs, she found no abnormalities other than the slightly elevated blood pressure. The nurse was aware that in her place of work it was important to distinguish the truly urgent cases from those that could be sent to the waiting room. She further assessed the client's headache. She discovered that the client was not having any visual disturbances, such as photophobia, and his pupils were equal and reactive. She knew what to assess and look for and how to relate these findings to the physician in order to provide her client with the care necessary. By performing these assessments the nurse was prepared to discuss the basics, such as the client's chief complaint, his vital signs, his medications, and any changes from baseline. Know why you are worried about observed changes and communicate this to the physician.

Josh McDonald, MD

observations in the chart (Potter & Perry, 2001). Dr. Josh McDonald offers a recent real-life example from an occupational health care setting in the Real World Interview feature. It is important that the nurse remain calm and objective even if the physician does not cooperate.

Potter and Perry (2001) offer suggestions for handling telephone miscommunications. For example, if a physician sounds hurried over the phone, use clarification questions to avoid a misunderstanding. If a physician hangs up, document that the call was terminated and fill out an incident report. If the physician gives an inappropriate answer or gives no orders, for example, for a client complaint of pain, document the call, the information relayed, and the fact that no orders were given. In addition, document any other steps that were taken to resolve the problem, for example, notifying the charge nurse or nursing supervisor. If a physician cannot be reached, first follow the institution's procedure for treating the client and then document the actions taken.

CLIENTS AND THEIR FAMILIES

Communication with clients and their families is optimized by the many skills previously described in this chapter. A few additional skills have not yet been mentioned. The first is touch. Nurses routinely use touch as a way to communicate caring and concern. Occasionally, language barriers will limit communication to the nonverbal mode. For instance, a stroke client who cannot process words can still interpret a gentle hand on his shoulder.

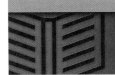

LITERATURE APPLICATION

Citation: Malone, G., and Morath, J. (2001). Pro-patient partnerships. *Nursing Management, 32,* 46–47.

Discussion: An effective nurse–physician partnership is a key factor influencing quality client care. When nurses and doctors work well with each other, their clients' death and readmission rates improve. Individual nurses can successfully collaborate with physicians by using assertive communication. Be open, honest, and direct. Promote lifelong learning in both nursing and medicine. Ask questions about your coworker's profession. Foster support for nurses and doctors. Reach out. Make and seek commitments with physician colleagues. Ask them to serve on several of your committees. Have them review your unit's operational systems. Realign your goals and work together. Form and strengthen a proactive, shared vision with your facility's physicians. Finally, stay focused. Remember, it is not about personality and power; it is about the clients.

As a nurse-physician team, you can establish a shared vision. Form joint practice committees and standardize care orders. Make collective decisions and maintain shoulder-to-shoulder dialogue.

Implications for Practice: In forging an environment of nurse–physician partnerships, consider adopting a 20-60-20 leadership outlook. Realize that 20 percent of employees resist change, complain, and criticize; 20 percent remain committed and cooperative; and 60 percent fall in between. Develop a strategy that models success with the receptive 20 percent and engages the middle majority.

Communication requires an openness and honesty with concurrent respect for clients and their families. In addition, clients' privacy needs to be honoured and protected by the nurse's actions and words. Information that clients share with nurses and other health care providers is to be held in confidence. Verbal exchanges regarding client conditions are private matters that should not occur in the hallway or just outside a client's room where they could be overheard by others. Nurses are obligated to not discuss client conditions with others, even family members, without the client's permission.

MENTOR AND PRODIGY

The final pattern of communication in the workplace that will be discussed is between mentor and prodigy. Mentoring is typically an informal process that occurs between an expert nurse and a novice nurse, but it may also be an assigned role. This one-on-one relationship

---

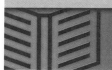

LITERATURE APPLICATION

Citation: DiBartola, L. (2001). Listening to patients and responding with care. *Joint Commission Journal on Quality Improvement, 27*(6), 315–323.

Discussion: Clinicians who want to improve their listening skills benefit from identifying the way in which clients are most comfortable interacting. A tool for assessing the client's preference is demonstrated. After the client's interaction style has been identified, the clinician uses this information to move closer to the way in which the client is most comfortable communicating. This article discusses a communication model for improving client communication. Figure 6-3 describes behavioural characteristics of the four communication modes.

The framework for this model is the continuum of two intersecting axes. The horizontal axis poles are inquisitive and assertive. The vertical axis poles are objective and subjective. People who are most comfortable communicating in an inquisitive way and tend to be objective are called investigators. Those who are most comfortable communicating in an inquisitive way but are subjective in nature are called unifiers. People who are most comfortable communicating in an assertive way and favour subjectivity are called energizers. Those who are most comfortable communicating in an assertive way and tend to be objective are called enterprisers. Behavioural markers can be used to identify someone's preferred communication mode (see Figure 6-4).

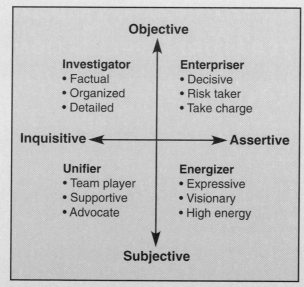

Figure 6-3 Behavioural Characteristics of the Four Communication Modes (From "Listening to Patients and Responding with Care," by L. DiBartola, 2001, *Joint Commission Journal on Quality Improvement, 27*(6), 319. Reprinted with Permission.)

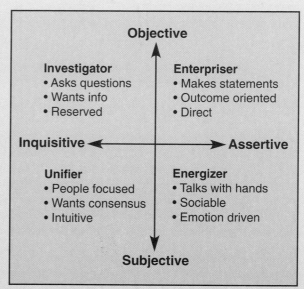

Figure 6-4 Behavioural Markers for the Four Communication Modes (From "Listening to Patients and Responding with Care," by L. DiBartola, 2001, *Joint Commission Journal on Quality Improvement, 27*(6), 322. Reprinted with Permission.)

(Continued)

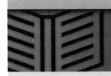

LITERATURE APPLICATION (CONTINUED)

Using your observation skills, determine where your client is on the inquisitive–assertive scale. Typical markers that would identify someone who is close to the inquisitive side are asking questions, attending carefully to detail, listening carefully to what the other person is saying, showing caution in making a decision without having adequate time to think about it, and preferring facts over intuition. On the other side of the scale, markers for someone who prefers to communicate in an assertive way are showing concern about wasting time, being quick to make a decision, being more interested in outcomes than in process, being willing to take risks, and making strong statements rather than asking questions.

In addition, you will want to make observations about the client's preference for objectivity or subjectivity. Whereas people with an objective preference are more interested in facts than intuition and in the project outcome than the process, people who are more subjective show more interest in the people who are working on the project than the project itself, are more willing to trust intuition than the facts, and show greater interest in being satisfied than in being right.

Nonverbal cues include the use of gestures or hands while talking for those on the assertive side, reserve and control for those on the inquisitive side, and high energy and expressiveness for those on the subjective side. To apply this model, think of an interaction that did not go well. Consider where both parties fit on the scale. The closer both parties are on the scale, the easier it will be for them to communicate.

Implications for Practice: After you understand the way in which both you and your client are most comfortable communicating, you can decide to communicate in a way that may be more comfortable for your client. You are not expected to change who you are; the goal of this approach is to know yourself, understand the client, and then move closer to the client. This approach will build trust and respect, and will result in the client feeling satisfied by the interaction.

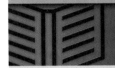

LITERATURE APPLICATION

Citation: Sobo, E. J., & Sadler, B. L. (2002). Improving organizational communication and cohesion in a health care setting. *Human Organization, 61*(3), 277–287.

Discussion: This article describes a project in one hospital, following reengineering. Employee morale had dropped, related to the reengineering exercise. As a result, it was decided to examine an opportunity to encourage employees to express their dissatisfaction, or any creative ideas that they might have, in the context of Employee Leadership Council meetings. An important consideration was that although this opportunity was created as a result of employee suggestion, the president and CEO of the hospital initiated the project.

Implications for Practice: The power of leading from strength cannot be overestimated. There is no one corporate culture, but cross-group exchange is required. Flexibility is important and, in fact, essential in any plan of change. An employee–leadership exchange forum, led by the CEO, can be a helpful strategy for enhancing employee leadership and employee–employer relations.

focuses on professional aspects and is mutually beneficial. The optimal novice is hardworking, willing to learn, and anxious to succeed (Shaffer, Tallarica, & Walsh, 2000). Communication entails using the skills previously described in this chapter to help the novice develop expert status and career direction by gleaning the mentor's wisdom. This wisdom is typically shared through listening, affirming, counselling, encouraging, and seeking input from the novice (Creasia & Parker, 1996).

Mentoring is facilitated by the novice and the mentor sharing the same work schedule. The novice is then exposed to the mentor, which allows for sharing and shadowing opportunities. The mentor can also anticipate added challenges with increasing responsibility that will likely

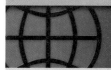

REAL WORLD INTERVIEW

A 16-year-old, first-time expectant mother presented to the labour and delivery department in labour, anticipating an uncomplicated delivery. The admitting nurse completed normal admissions information and, because of the client's age, assessed whether a social service consult was needed. The delivery commenced uneventfully, and a healthy baby girl was born. Since the mother indicated on admission that she wanted to breastfeed, the nurse assisted the mother to breastfeed during the immediate postpartum period prior to the baby being taken to the nursery.

In this clinical situation, because hospital stays are short, communication is critical for comprehensive and quality care to occur. Numerous health care providers are responsible for ensuring quality care in this setting. Nurses play a central role in coordinating communication between the client and her family; other nurses; the physician or nurse midwife; and other health care providers, such as the lactation consultant or the social worker. For example, a social worker could be contacted for challenging social situations identified during the admitting assessment, such as a report of physical abuse, incest, or active alcohol or substance use. The nurse also identifies potential teaching needs during the antepartum period, such as breastfeeding. These needs are communicated to the appropriate caregiver when responsibility for care is transferred between members of the health care team. The admitting nurse focuses on the client's immediate needs during labour. This client's age required specific attention to adolescent developmental needs. As with all clients, the nurse assesses readiness to learn. Whenever possible, she communicates using the client's preferred communication style, for example, video, reading material, or demonstration.

During labour, the nurse explained what to expect, encouraged the client and her support person through the stages of labour, and constantly reassured the client and her support person using verbal and nonverbal modes. She used multiple communication skills, that is, attending, responding, and clarifying. A team of health care workers was involved in this delivery. The nurse often functions as informer, recorder, and coach. She communicates labour progress to the physician or midwife and documents the progress while simultaneously supporting the client. Following delivery, communication with the client and her family continues. The nurse's responsibilities include ongoing assessment of the client's postpartum status and the initial assessment of the baby's status. The nurse is responsible for communicating to the nursery or postpartum nurse details of the pregnancy, the delivery, and the baby's initial status. The nurse may also prepare the mother for transfer to a postpartum combined care unit where other nurses will assume responsibility for care. Once again, communication regarding the multifaceted concerns of the new family unit is necessary in order to ensure quality care. Nurses' attention to accurate verbal reports and written records facilitates communication among the client, the client's family, coworkers, and physicians while maintaining confidentiality.

Kay Kember, RN

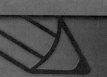

CASE STUDY 6–1

As a new graduate, you have finished your orientation and received notice that you have passed your CRNE (Canadian Registered Nurse Exam). The nursing care manager is relieved because two of the other regular nurses, one of whom is your preceptor, are pregnant and will soon be off on maternity leave. These absences will create a staffing crunch. Therefore, the nursing care manager is anxious to acclimate you to the role of team leader because you will soon be expected to assume those responsibilities.

How can your preceptor help you to take on this additional responsibility? What techniques will you use to enhance your communication with subordinates?

occur. Outlining these challenges with suggestions for how to manage them prepares the novice for the expanding responsibilities. Role-playing, in which the expert preceptor nurse describes a theoretical situation and allows the novice to practise a response to new and sometimes challenging situations, is another helpful strategy.

KEY CONCEPTS

- Nurses rely on basic principles of communication to facilitate interactions with clients and their family members, peers, and practitioners in other disciplines.

- Principles of communication allow nurses to adapt to trends that affect the profession of nursing and its practice, such as increasing diversity, an aging population, and computer technology.

- Nurses follow a process of communication that is more universal than unique to nursing. At the most basic level, this process involves a sender, a message, a receiver, and feedback. The input comes from visual, auditory, and kinesthetic stimuli, which are delivered using verbal and nonverbal modes. Nurses engage in three levels of communication: intrapersonal, interpersonal, and public.

- Nurses participate in upward, downward, lateral, and diagonal communications that are typically defined by their organization. Additionally, nurses may take part in informal exchanges using the grapevine.

- Nurses rely on communication skills, such as attending, responding, clarifying, and collaborating, to effectively promote client care and professionalism in a variety of settings.

- Barriers of gender, culture, conflict, and incongruent responses exist.

- Communication in the workplace involves many different relationships that shift the focus of effective communication. These relationships include communicating with superiors, coworkers, subordinates, physicians and other health care workers, and mentors.

KEY TERMS

accommodating	grapevine
attending	interpersonal communication
auditory	intrapersonal communication
avoiding	kinesthetic
clarifying	message
collaborating	nonverbal communication
competing	receiver
compromising	responding
confronting	verbal communication
feedback	visual

REVIEW QUESTIONS

1. Which of the following is a trend in society that affects communication?
   A. Decreasing interest in technology
   B. Increasing diversity among Canadians
   C. Increasing proportion of younger Canadians
   D. Decreasing need for writing skills

2. What element of the communication process returns input to the sender?
   A. Feedback
   B. Message
   C. Receiver
   D. Sender

3. Which of the following characteristics pertains to verbal communication?
   A. Eye contact
   B. Nodding
   C. Smiling
   D. Tone

4. Which of the following skills involves active listening and is an important skill used by nurses to gain an understanding of the client's message?
   A. Attending
   B. Clarifying
   C. Confronting
   D. Responding

5. Nurses must be concerned about barriers to communication
   A. because they enhance interactions.
   B. so that they can use them when communicating.
   C. so that they can compensate for them.
   D. Nurses do not need to be concerned.

REVIEW ACTIVITIES

1. Your nursing care manager has asked you to serve on a committee to explore how your unit might communicate more effectively. What current trends in our culture might affect the group's plan?

2. The charge nurse apologizes as she informs you that your assignment includes the "problem client" on the unit. What communication skills will you use to enhance communication with this client? How will you avoid barriers of communication with this client?

3. You found out that you passed your registration exams last month. When you report for your evening shift, you discover you are assigned to be the team leader. What considerations will be given as you communicate with subordinates?

EXPLORING THE WEB

■ What sites would you consider to improve your communication skills? It depends on what aspect of communication you want to improve. By using the *http://www.Yahoo.com* search engine and searching for the phrase *communication + skills,* more than 50 million sites were identified. Try it and look at the incredible online possibilities.

■ Keep up with what is happening in the field of nursing and technology. Visit *http://www.cnia.ca/.* What did you find?

■ Are you curious how effectively you communicate? Take an online communication test at *http://www.queendom.com/cgi-bin/tests/transfer.cgi.*

REFERENCES

Baker, C., Beglinger, J., King, S., Salyards, M., & Thompson, A. (2000). Transforming negative work cultures. *JONA, 30*(7/8), 357–363.

Creasia, J., & Parker, B. (1996). *Conceptual foundations of professional practice* (2nd ed.). St Louis, MO: Mosby.

DiBartola, L. (2001). Listening to patients and responding with care. *Joint Commission Journal on Quality Improvement, 27*(6), 315–323.

Ellis, A. (1997). *Anger: How to live with it and without it.* New York: Citadel Press, Kensington.

Grohar-Murray, E., & DiCroce, H. (2003). Leadership and management in nursing (3rd ed.). Upper Saddle River, NJ: Pearson Education Inc.

Jeans, M. E., & Rowat, K. M. (2005). *Leadership objective C: Competencies required of nurse managers.* Ottawa: Canadian Nurses Association.

Laswell, H. D. (1948). The structure and function of communication in society. In L. Bryson (Ed.), *The communication of ideas* (pp. 37–51). New York: Institute for Religious and Social Studies.

Malone, G., & Morath, J. (2001). Pro-patient partnerships. *Nursing Management, 32,* 46–47.

Peach, C. (2005). The mosaic versus the melting pot and the USA. *Scottish Geographical Journal, 121*(1), 3–27.

Poole, V. L., Davidhizar, R. E., & Giger, J. N. (1995). Delegating to a transcultural team. *Nursing Management, 26*(8), 33–34.

Potter, P., & Perry, A. (2001). *Canadian fundamentals of nursing* (2nd ed.). Toronto: Harcourt Canada Ltd.

Shaffer, B., Tallarica, B., & Walsh, J. (2000). Win-win mentoring. *Nursing Management, 31*(1), 32–34.

Simms, L. M., Price, S. A., & Ervin, N. E. (2000). *The professional practice of nursing administration* (3rd ed.). Clifton Park, NY: Delmar Learning.

Sobo, E. J., & Sadler, B. L. (2002). Improving organizational communication and cohesion in a health care setting. *Human Organization, 61*(3): 277–287.

Statistics Canada. (2006). *Population projections for Canada, provinces and territories, with detailed electronic tables.* Catalogue No. 91-520-SCB.

Valentine, P. E. B. (2001). A gender perspective on conflict management strategies of nurses. *Journal of Nursing Scholarship, 33*(1), 69–74.

Yogo, Y., Hashi, A. M., Tsutsui, S., & Yamada, N. (2000). Judgments of emotion by nurses and students given double-blind information on a patient's tone of voice and message content. *Perceptual and motor skills, 90,* 855–863.

SUGGESTED READINGS

Anderson, K. (1998). 16 tips for reaching agreement. *Nursing Management, 29*(10), 89.

Bellack, J. P., & O'Neil, E. H. (2000). Recreating nursing practice for a new century. *Nursing and Health Care Perspectives, 21*(1), 15–21.

Gray, J. (1992). *Men are from Mars, women are from Venus.* New York: HarperCollins.

Heller, B. R., Oris, M. T., & Durney-Crowley, J. (2000). The future of nursing education: 10 trends to watch. *Nursing and Health Care Perspectives, 21*(10), 9–13.

Kinney, M., & Hurst, J. (1979). *Group process in education.* Lexington, MA: Ginn Customs.

Malloch, K., Sluyter, D., & Moore, N. (2000). Relationship-centered care: Achieving true value in healthcare. *JONA, 30*(7/8), 379–385.

Moore, N. (2000). In Malloch, K., Sluyter, D., & Moore, N. (2000). Relationship-centered care: Achieving true value in healthcare (p. 384). *JONA, 30*(7/8), 379–385.

Yoder-Wise, P. S. (1999). *Leading and managing in nursing* (2nd ed.). St. Louis, MO: Mosby.

CHAPTER 7

Politics and Consumer Partnerships

Terry W. Miller, PhD, RN
Adapted by: Heather Crawford, BScN, MEd, CHE
Pat Frederickson, Former Executive Director/Registrar
College of Licensed Practical Nurses of Alberta
Rita McGregor, Former Director of Professional Practice—College
of Licensed Practical Nurses of Alberta

We also worked hard to engage Canadians in our consultations, because medicare ultimately belongs to them.... Strong leadership and the involvement of Canadians is key to preserving a system that is true to our values and is sustainable. (Commission on the Future of Health Care in Canada, 2002, p. xv.)

OBJECTIVES

Upon completion of this chapter, the reader should be able to:

1. Describe how politics defines health care services and affects nursing practice.
2. Recognize the need for nurses to be politically involved with the consumer movement in health care.
3. Describe the role of a nurse as a consumer advocate and political force.
4. Propose a political strategy for strengthening nurse–consumer relationships.
5. Articulate a service-oriented plan for providing nursing services to a selected consumer interest group.
6. Describe how demographic changes are affecting nurses and nursing services.

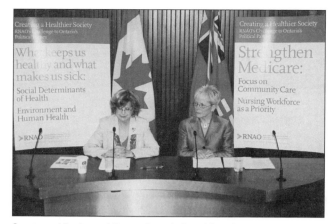

Courtesy of Registered Nurses Association of Ontario

The elderly man lying in a nursing home bed, pushing a call button and waiting for a nurse, is not thinking about anything other than the fact that he is not getting the service or care that he expected. He doesn't know whether the nursing shortage is affecting his care. He doesn't know the financial situation of the nursing home itself. He doesn't know the standards that the nursing home is expected to achieve.

Can we expect to improve the care of this elderly man given this scenario?

Does politics play a role in this elderly man's care?

Should nurses work with other consumer groups to improve care to elderly patients?

Politics is predominantly a process by which people use a variety of methods to achieve their goals. These methods inherently involve some level of competition, negotiation, and collaboration. Politics involves using power to influence, persuade, or change—it is the art of understanding relationships between groups in society and using that understanding to achieve particular outcomes (McIntyre & Thomlinson, 2003, p. 62). Nurses who can effectively compete, negotiate, and collaborate with others to acquire what they either want or need have developed strong political skills. They have the greatest ability to build strong bases of support for themselves, clients, and the nursing profession.

Politics exists because resources are limited and some people control more resources than others. **Resources** include people; money; facilities; technology; and rights to properties, services, and technologies. Individuals, groups, or organizations that have the ability to provide or control the distribution of desirable resources are politically empowered. The consumer movement in health care is a political movement about health care resources.

The purpose of this chapter is to support the need for nurses to be politically active for the good of both clients and the health care system. A major focus is how the consumer movement in health care creates new opportunities for nurses to advance nursing services by giving clients, including all people who receive health care, a stronger voice in their health care as consumers. Nurses are encouraged to develop a stronger political position by partnering with consumer groups instead of waiting for others to take the lead.

STAKEHOLDERS AND HEALTH CARE

Control of health care resources is spread among a number of vested interest groups called **stakeholders.** Everyone is a stakeholder in health care at some level, but some people are far more politically active about their stake in health care than others. See Table 7-1 for a list of some of Canada's most influential interest and lobbying groups. Many of these groups, as well as others, such as insurance companies, consumer groups, professional organizations, health care providers, and educational groups, exert political pressure on health policymakers—municipal, provincial, territorial, and federal legislative bodies—in an effort to make the health care system work to their advantage.

TABLE 7-1	**SOME OF CANADA'S INTEREST AND LOBBY GROUPS**
1. The Consumers' Association of Canada	6. C. D. Howe Institute
2. The National Citizens Coalition	7. Fraser Institute
3. The Health Action Lobby	8. Canada's Association for the Fifty-Plus
4. Canadian Health Coalition	9. Greenpeace Canada
5. Canadian Centre for Policy Alternatives	10. Aboriginal Youth Network

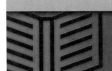

LITERATURE APPLICATION

Citation: Celebrating international nursing partnerships. (2006). *Canadian Nurse, 102*(6), 15–17.

Discussion: The purpose of this article was to demonstrate the commitment of the Canadian Nurses Association to work in cooperation with nurses around the world to promote global health and equity, and to advance the nursing profession for the benefit of all. Since 1976, the Canadian Nurses Association has worked with national nursing associations (NNAs) in Africa, the Americas, Asia, and Eastern Europe, as well as with funding organizations in Canada and overseas. These organizations have built alliances to increase the NNAs' ability to strengthen the nursing profession and improve the quality of health services and nursing delivered in partner countries. The article describes specific efforts to improve health care, strengthen nursing organizations, collaborate with other nursing leadership, and build gender equity. Finally, partnerships for today and the future are identified, including the Canada–Russia Initiative in Nursing, the Canada–South Africa Nurses HIV/AIDS Initiative, and the Strengthening Nurses and Nursing Associations Program.

Implications for Practice: Significant success has been made in the last 30 years to strengthen international nursing partnerships and improve health systems. Further work is required in the area of global health, and it is incumbent on all nurses and nursing associations to work collaboratively to build alliances that will strengthen health systems around the world.

Nurses should be interested in influencing governments because politicians pay attention to the health-related issues and concerns raised by their constituents and the organizations within their electoral boundaries. If the governments don't pay attention, they will not be re-elected. If nurses do not speak both individually and collectively, the voices of others will be heard by government, and the priorities and potential solutions posed by nurses will not be heard. Not all stakeholders in health care support the consumers' potentially dominant role in health care politics. Some contend that consumers do not necessarily know what is best for them. Instead, they support the idea that health care experts, such as physicians, are better able to direct health care policy. Others maintain that only those directly paying for the services should make policy decisions and that health care is not necessarily a right because services should be based on an individual's ability to pay.

The growing cost of health care has led to increasing political activism by nurses, other health care providers, as well as consumers. As noted in *Building on Values: The Future of Health Care in Canada*, known familiarly as the Romanow Report, "Canadians want and need a more accountable health care system (Commission on the Future of Health Care in Canada, 2002, p. xix). Nurses have come to understand how the control and distribution of resources in health care can dramatically affect their incomes, workloads, work environments, and clients. Nurses across the country have reported that the client load per nurse provider has increased significantly. However, without political influence, simply voicing these concerns does little to change health care at any level.

Nursing has a long history of uniting the various stakeholders and coordinating health care services around clients to ensure that clients obtain the health services they need; but, as pointed out by Ogren (2001), "many nurses have little knowledge about their history" (p. 7). Nurses who recognize they have a critical role in addressing the major issues in health care delivery at the bedside will ensure that nursing enters into discussions or partnerships with individuals and organizations that have control in the wider health care system. As partners, they will be able to compete, negotiate, and collaborate with other stakeholders at the system level to effect political change. These nurses are concerned with the price of health care at the system level and understand that resources are controlled and distributed through health policy decisions.

Many authors of nursing articles, some books, and a few research studies support nurses' involvement in public policy and health care politics (Fagin, 1998; Mason & Leavitt, 1999; Milstead, 1999; Williams, 1998). Several other authors promote greater inclusion of policy content and political process in nursing curricula (Brown, 1996; Gebbie, Wakefield, & Kerfoot, 2000; Jones, Jennings, Moritz, & Moss, 1997; Provost & Van Herk, 2006). Nurses' involvement in policy arenas, such as policymaking committees and institutional boards, includes advocating both for recipients of health care who are in need and have little or no voice and for those who need a stronger voice. Any professional nurse should understand and be able to articulate the relevance of politics to nursing practice. Making a difference in health care arenas is an outcome of involvement in policymaking. As

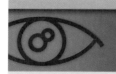

CRITICAL THINKING

Have you ever organized a local committee meeting, or a Nurses' Week event? Have you ever contacted your provincial member of Parliament or your local councillor regarding a provincial bill that affects health care or a safety issue in your neighbourhood? Have you ever been exhausted at the end of a busy day, after having managed complex client needs? Have you ever participated in an information picket? If you have engaged in any of these activities, then you have been involved in politics and the early stages of political action.

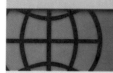

REAL WORLD INTERVIEW

Nurses generally associate being political with politics, and don't consider themselves in that realm. Being political has a much broader context; it means being an advocate for your beliefs. Every day nurses play an advocacy role, most often for client care, but that role can extend to advocating for change in the workplace or, in a much broader context, change in the health care system, or in professional or labour legislation.

Pat Frederickson
Former Executive Director/Registrar College of
Licensed Practical Nurses of Alberta

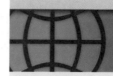

REAL WORLD INTERVIEW

"This morning I met with three very dedicated nurses from my riding.... [and] spoke about the vital role of nurses in the field of mental health services. Because of the stigma attached to mental illness, this is not always a very high profile area—some would say it's the silent health issue.... The nurses pointed out that four of five people in Ontario are affected at some level by mental illness. Our meeting this morning was a reminder of the far-reaching impact of the work done by Ontario's nurses in all aspects of health and wellness. Citizens of Durham riding are proud of the care and professionalism shown daily by nurses in our communities...."

John O'Toole,
MPP, Durham

Source: RNAO Registered Nurse Journal, May/June 2005, p. 27.
(Adapted from Hansard Issue L142A.) Reprinted with Permission.

Margaret Mead said, "never doubt that a small group of thoughtful committed citizens can change the world, indeed it's the only thing that ever has."

THE POLITICS AND ECONOMICS OF HUMAN SERVICES

Many nurses want to avoid the political nature of their work because they believe that human services should not be politically motivated. They also may ignore the business aspects of health care until they find themselves responsible for a budget. Yet all health care is inextricably linked to politics and economics and to the availability and services of providers. As a human service, health care has yielded remarkable returns in terms of improving overall quality of life as well as in extending life spans. As a business, health care has afforded millions of people, including nurses, with economic opportunities and lifelong careers.

Health care in Canada depends heavily on a continuous supply of resources from both public and private sectors. These resources include people, such as the providers of health care services, and the money to educate and pay these providers. Buildings, technology, administration, and equipment are just some of the other resources needed for the health care system to be serviceable. With health care requiring so many resources on such a large economic scale, thousands of people are directly involved in the allocation of those resources; hence, the politics of health care. Most of those people have good intentions, but they often disagree about how the resources can best be used to support health care.

Many consumers are aware that the ongoing redistribution of health care resources may not meet their health care needs, especially as they age and become more dependent upon related services. They are frightened by media reports of increasing national health care expenditures. Although most consumers do not directly pay for the majority of their health care, their individual portions of expenses incurred are rapidly increasing. Health policy is formulated, enacted, and enforced through political processes at the local, regional, provincial, territorial, and federal levels. For example, at the local or regional level, individual hospital boards or regional health authorities establish and implement policies regarding the availability of flu injections to high-risk populations in their area. At the provincial or territorial level, policies govern nurses within a province or territory by defining nursing practice, nursing education, and nursing registration. These policies are often governed by a provincial or territorial nurse practice act that designates a provincial or territorial nursing regulatory college or association as the authority for enforcing the policies. Federal policies are evident in the principles, rules, and regulations governing medicare, such as the Canada Health Act (1984). When bills affecting health care are being developed in provincial, territorial, and federal legislative bodies, nurses need to be aware of those actions and obtain copies of those bills, thus adding to their political knowledge base.

Ultimately, health care will be defined and controlled by those wielding the most political influence. If nurses fail to exert political pressure on the health policymakers, they will lose ground to others who are more politically active. It is unrealistic to believe that other stakeholders will take care of nursing while the competition for health care resources increases. Historically, some stakeholders in health care have never supported nursing as a profession or acknowledged professional roles for nurses. Nurses, like other health care providers, must compete, negotiate, and collaborate with others to ensure their future in health care.

CULTURAL DIMENSIONS OF PARTNERSHIPS AND CONSUMERISM

Prior to the 2001 Census, Canada had 1.8 million immigrants from around the world, with the majority coming from Asia. Most of these immigrants settled in the three largest metropolitan areas—Toronto, Montreal, and Vancouver. At that time, the total population of Canada was approximately 30 million (Canada. Statistics Canada, 2006). Even if immigrants are highly educated, they tend to have lower employment rates and lower salaries than individuals who were born in Canada. Leddy and Pepper (1998) recognized that "people's habits of promoting health, their ways of behaving when sick, their ways of recognizing and responding to illness, and their ways of defining health are strongly determined by their sociocultural background" (p. 35). Increasing racial and cultural diversity is indicated in the census data. Canada's Aboriginal population is much younger that the non-Aboriginal population. The average age of the Aboriginal population in 2001 was 24.7, which was 13 years younger than the average age of the non-Aboriginal population. About 71 percent of the country's entire Aboriginal population lived in urban areas (Canada. Statistics Canada, 2006, p. 285).

If nurses intend to form partnerships with consumer groups distinguished by cultural heritage, racial makeup, or ethnic background, they must understand and value diversity. Strong partnerships will frame nursing services in ways that respect cultural differences.

POLITICS AND DEMOGRAPHIC CHANGES

Certainly not all consumers agree about what health care should be, who should provide it, or how it should be paid for. The social, cultural, economic, psychological, and demographic characteristics of consumers largely determine their attitudes and inclination toward the health care system, its providers, and its services. Consumers also recognize some level of personal risk when changes are made in the system, especially involving access and wait times. If consumers, such as retired people, perceive that their out-of-pocket costs for health care

CASE STUDY 7–1

Jillian is a registered nurse who visits newborns and their moms in their home, as part of the Healthy Babies, Healthy Children program. She also belongs to the Childbirth Nurses Interest Group. The Canadian Pediatric Society, the American Academy of Pediatrics, and the United Kingdom's Foundation for the Study of Sudden Infant Death have released guidelines that encourage parents to sleep in the same room as their infant, but do not advocate parents and infants sleeping in the same bed. However, parents are still encouraged to breastfeed and cuddle their babies in bed. Jillian knows that many new moms have difficult initiating breastfeeding or require encouragement when the baby is fussy and doesn't latch on to the breast easily. Jillian has just heard that the local hospital's breastfeeding clinic is about to close related to lack of financial resources.

What would you do if you were Jillian?

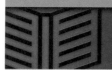

LITERATURE APPLICATION

Citation: Ferguson, S. L. (2001). An activist looks at nursing's role in health policy development. *Journal of Obstetric, Gynecologic, and Neonatal Nursing, 30*(5), 546–551.

Discussion: Nurses play a critical role in determining, developing, implementing, and evaluating health policies because of their knowledge of health care. A conceptual model (Longest, 1998) is useful to illustrate the public policymaking process. The model illustrated in this article depicts three phases: policy formulation, implementation, and modification.

Implications for Practice: Nurses will find the model illustrated in this article useful to influence public policy.

(e.g., for medication) either extends beyond their capacity to pay or will increase in the future, they are highly motivated to exert political pressure on their legislators to reverse the perceived trend.

The fastest growing consumer group for years to come is the elderly—people 65 years and older—due to lower fertility and higher life expectancy. The number of people aged 65 years and over has more than doubled in the past 35 years, reaching 4.1 million in 2003, which is close to 13 percent of the population (Canada. Statistics Canada, 2006, p. 280). During the same year, almost one in three Canadians was between the ages of 35 and 54, which corresponds to the baby-boomer generation. Within a few years, this group will reach retirement age. By 2011, those aged 65 and over will represent 15 percent of the total population (Canada. Statistics Canada, 2006, p. 280). The fastest growing group is aged 80 and over. From 1993 to 2003, the number of people aged 80 and over increased 43 percent to reach 932,000. The number of people aged 80 and over in 2011 is estimated to be 1.3 million (Canada. Statistics Canada, 2006, p. 280).

Without a doubt, this aging of the Canadian population is profoundly affecting health care at every level. The dramatic increase in the number of elderly people in the Western world means that about one-half of all people who have ever reached age 65 are alive today (Roszak, 1998).

Many seniors are joining consumer groups to have a greater political voice, influence health policy decisions, and ensure that they receive the health care services they will need for years to come. A growing number are bridging the gap of social isolation, prominent in the past, through the Internet as well as through involvement in consumer groups. They are establishing closer contact with the outside world and are managing to successfully strengthen their relationships with other stakeholders in health care.

The Canada's Association for the Fifty-Plus (CARP), with more than 400,000 members, constitutes a growing influential advocacy group for the 50-plus age group, and

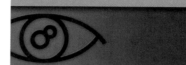

CRITICAL THINKING

How do you see the aging nursing workforce and the aging population affecting health care and your nursing practice? What are the political implications for health care providers with proportionally fewer people in the workforce and more people requiring health care services related to aging?

an ideal consumer partner for nursing in many ways. A large percentage of nurses are 45 years of age or older and within 5 years of qualifying for membership in the CARP. Few other consumer groups appear to have the potential that the CARP has for defining the health care system of the future.

NURSE AS POLITICAL ACTIVIST

Because of nurses' knowledge and expertise regarding the determinants of health, they are key informants when it comes to health and health care issues. Nurses have both a desire and a need to have meaningful involvement in decision making and informing decision-makers at various levels in health care organizations and in government when decisions affect nurses, their work life, and client care. Nurses have a valuable role in policy development, and increasingly, are finding the need to become more politically active. They have long felt that changes in the health care system were having a negative impact on their work life, their working conditions, and client care, especially during the 1990s, when cutbacks in health care led to the layoffs of nurses throughout the country. A serious negative impact affected the morale of nurses and ultimately client care: nurses were of the opinion that decisions had been made based on economics and that they were not being valued for their contribution to client care. That discontent lead to the formation of several studies, such as the Canadian Nursing Advisory Committee's (2002) *Our Health, Our Future: Creating Quality Workplaces for Canadian Nurses*, in 2002, followed, a few year later, by the National Nursing Sector Study (2005), *Building the Future: An Integrated Strategy for Nursing Human Resources in Canada*. Research conducted for these two projects provided detailed information on the work life, education, practice, and administration of nurses. This research provided valuable information so nurses could raise the awareness of issues affecting nurses and lobby for change.

Nurses have always enjoyed a high level of public trust, and they have leveraged this trust to their advantage. Over the past few years, the Canadian Nurses Association (CNA) has increasingly provided support for registered nurses to convey their messages to politicians, particularly during election campaigns. CNA encourages nurses to ask political candidates what they will do to improve the health of Canadians. This strategy is a very effective way of bringing the issues of nurses and health care to the attention of politicians and requiring politicians make a public statement on their position.

Practical nurses, psychiatric nurses, nurse educators, nursing students, and nursing administrators have national organizations on a much smaller scale, though they have been able to make their voices heard. Nurses have successfully lobbied for a nursing voice at the federal level, which resulted in Health Canada creating, in 1999, the Office of Nursing Policy, to strengthen the focus on nursing policy issues within Health Canada. This office advises Health Canada on various policy issues and programs, representing that perspective in various fora, contributing to health policy formulation and program development, and working closely with the nursing community in developing advice for the minister of health and long-term care and Health Canada."[1]

Nurses who are politically active have a definitive voice in their work environments for client welfare as well as for themselves. In addition to studying issues and voting, politically active nurses directly contact policymakers, such as the chairperson of the hospital board or legislators, through phone calls, letters, and e-mails. Politically active nurses join professional organizations and actively participate to ensure a more collective, unified voice supporting health care issues and policies that have value for consumers and nursing. Nurses who are most involved will be seen running for office, supporting political activities and candidates, assisting during campaigns, and helping to draft legislation.

As nurses develop politically, they come to understand the need for political strategy. The purpose of developing political strategies is to understand different ways to achieve one's goals, or the goals one is advocating for, while identifying the other stakeholders and their goals. Political strategy attempts to persuade the people supporting an issue, formulating a policy, or taking an action to take the position that supports those using the political strategy. To be feasible, a political strategy requires commitment by those using it, as well as their awareness of the other stakeholders. Effective political strategy implies considerable forethought and clarity of purpose in even the most ambiguous situations. Nurses who are most likely to wield political influence operate with strategy in mind before taking political action, voicing concerns, making demands, or even advocating for others. Unfortunately, some nurses may become involved in political issues or take overt political stands before adequately studying the political issue or the major stakeholders' positions regarding the issue.

Every nurse should be cognizant of the position of other involved groups regarding any relevant political health issue. Nurses need to listen to other policy perspectives and understand as many facets of the issue as possible when making health policy proposals. Proposals need to include a rationale to neutralize opposing views to ensure that unnecessary political fights can be avoided and that more collaboration will occur prior to any policy proposal being made to policymaking bodies, such as hospital boards or provincial legislatures. The more support obtained from the various stakeholders in any policy arena, the better chance of a workable policy being developed and implemented.

To be most politically effective, nurses must be able to clearly articulate at least four dimensions of nursing to any audience or stakeholder: what nursing is, what distinctive services nurses provide to consumers, how nursing benefits consumers, and what nursing services cost in relation to other health care services. Although anecdotal stories and emotional appeals may be effective with certain audiences, research-based evidence that supports the political position of the nursing profession exerts far more power.

POLITICS AND ADVOCACY

The nursing profession has embraced client advocacy for several decades, even though nurses risk compromising their employment positions when they advocate for clients. However, some concern has been voiced that the restructuring of health care is eroding the advocacy role of nurses (O'Connell, 2000). Part of that problem is that nurses doubt that they have the ability to advocate for their clients. They are not comfortable with the level of risk they associate with being a client advocate. The greatest nurses throughout the profession's history have been strong advocates for clients and have taken far greater risks than the potential loss of a particular job.

Interestingly, some clients have begun advocating for nurses, a role reversal. Those clients perceive nurses as overextended by the nature of their work environment and contend that something must be done to improve nurses' working conditions.

ADVOCACY AND CONSUMER ALLIANCES

Nurses must understand the political forces that define their relationships with consumers. Consumers expect the best people to be health care providers, but they are confused about the roles and responsibilities of professional nurses. Informed consumers understand how health policy directly affects them but are less likely to recognize how health policy affects nurses. Consumers may expect nurses to be their advocates only in the context of providing direct client care.

Working through their professional organizations, nurses can collaborate with consumer groups by creating alliances, which serve to promote the role of nurses as consumer advocates in health policy arenas and to strengthen the political position of both partners. These alliances create a stronger political voice than either group has alone. The partners gain power when interacting with any policymaking body because they represent (1) a larger **voting block**—a group that represents the same political position or perspective; (2) a broader funding base—a source of financial support; and (3) a stronger **political voice**—an increase in the number of voices supporting or opposing an issue—to any policymaking body. Increasingly, professional organizations in nursing recognize the value of partnering with consumers to build a better health care system. See Table 7-2 for steps in establishing an alliance with a consumer group.

TABLE 7-2	STEPS IN ESTABLISHING AN ALLIANCE WITH A CONSUMER GROUP
1. Listen	Become sensitized to the health care needs and political nature of the potential consumer ally.
2. Study	Seek both representative and opposing perspectives from consumer group meetings, focus groups, relevant literature, and interviews.
3. Assess	Determine the need, value, context, and boundaries for establishing the alliance.
4. Focus	Mutually identify the purpose and articulate the goals and specific, realistic objectives for the alliance.
5. Compromise	Work through nonessential and noncritical points and issues.
6. Negotiate	Agree on one's position and responsibilities in the alliance.
7. Plan	Develop a political strategy for achieving the goals and fulfilling the objectives.
8. Test	Test the political waters. Gather feedback on the plan from key people before taking action.
9. Model	Model the political work. Define the structure for working the political strategy with partners.
10. Direct the political action	Understand the bigger picture and concentrate on what can be changed.
11. Implement	Line up political support and take action.
12. Network	Be committed to the mutually recognized goal and consistently work to have an adequate base of support in terms of people, money, and time.
13. Build political credibility	Participate in local, provincial, and federal policy-making efforts that support the alliance and its political agenda.
14. Soothe and bargain	Downplay rivalry and address conflict in a timely, constructive manner.
15. Report, publicize, lobby	Report, publicize, and lobby the group's political cause, and draw public attention to the needs of the consumer group.
16. Reaffirm, redefine, or discontinue	Regularly evaluate work with consumer group.

CONSUMER DEMANDS

As recipients of health care, consumers demand to be treated as something more than passive recipients of health care. They are vocal in their requests that providers and organizations be more consumer-friendly and service-oriented, and they are seriously requesting a voice in how health care is delivered.

Nurses, working through professional organizations, such as the Canadian Nurses Association (CNA), have been strong supporters for clients' rights; however, other professional groups, such as the Canadian Medical Association (CMA) and the Canadian Healthcare Association (CHA), have received far more media recognition for their support of clients' rights, particularly regarding safety. This situation may be an indication that the CMA and CHA are better funded, wield more political power, and do a better job of presenting their positions on consumer issues to the media than the CNA.

Any political vision to make health care more consumer-friendly and service-oriented must address cost, access, choice, and quality. Perhaps the vision starts with a formula: the highest quality of care for all people at the least cost. Yet, defining—much less evaluating—quality is culturally bound and very complicated. A vision for high-quality, low-cost care will require multiple stakeholders collaborating to develop a workable philosophy, including a mechanism for checks and balances to minimize abuse and misuse and to encourage intelligent, ethical decisions by those wielding the most political power.

TURNING A CONSUMER-ORIENTED VISION INTO REALITY

Nurses have opportunities to be more than simply supporters of a consumer-oriented vision for health care; they can be co-creators. To make this vision real, nurses will need to be more educated and articulate about the value they add to the overall health care system. Encouraging other stakeholders and the policymakers to understand and promote the value of nursing to consumers will take considerable political work. This work will have to be more than anecdotal pleas, arguments in support of some consumer cause, or reactions to some particular health care issue or workplace injustice. Believing in a vision and working hard are not enough. Nurses must have a clear image of the vision; develop a sound philosophy; demonstrate intelligent, strategic thinking; and wield more political influence.

Although nurses may think they are the ones primarily affected by the changes in health care, a more powerful and, therefore, strategic position is to understand that everyone is affected, especially consumers. Rehtmeyer (2000) states that "nurses need to seize the opportunity to use the confusion in the health care arena as a source for trying or taking new directions" (p. 184). These new directions may include the strategies outlined in Table 7-3.

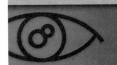

CRITICAL THINKING

Carling Provost and Kim Van Herk (2006) in their article, "Political Activism and Nursing," suggest that nursing students need to be more aware of how health policies affect both themselves as health professionals and society as a whole. According to Provost and Van Herk, nursing students need to become more involved in political organizations in order to have a positive impact on their level of political activity and need to be formally educated to be politically active. Their suggestions on how nurses can overcome barriers to being politically active include being aware of how policies are made and implemented within the Canadian system by building opportunities into nursing curricula so that students can observe the policymaking process; incorporating political activity hours into clinical placements; and exposing students to health policy education, such as writing a paper about a nurse who is a political leader.

What recommendations could you make to prepare students and nurses to be more politically aware and politically active in the health care system?

TABLE 7-3	**POLITICAL STRATEGIES FOR MOUNTING CONSUMER CAMPAIGNS**

1. Lobbying at provincial and federal levels for health care regulations and guidelines that serve a consumer group's interest
2. Consulting with representatives from a consumer group when health care regulations and guidelines are being debated or written
3. Monitoring the enforcement of health care regulations and exacting corrective or punitive action when noncompliance occurs
4. Encouraging providers to make changes in delivery of services voluntarily to meet changing consumer demands
5. Changing consumer perceptions and behaviours through the distribution of educational materials or other media

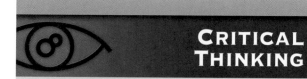

CRITICAL THINKING

Do you think that patients should be defined as clients or health care customers?

Would patients be less likely to sue health care providers if they were approached as clients or customers instead of patients?

THE CONSUMER DEMAND FOR ACCOUNTABILITY

When stakeholders are motivated and directed solely by their own perceived needs, competitive political strategies replace more collaborative approaches to addressing the consumer's health care needs. Accountability becomes a serious issue because the goal of pleasing stakeholders may supersede the goal of offering the highest quality services. People who will own the future of health care must address this growing problem of accountability. They will need to establish and sustain their credibility during a time when more people are distrustful of the health care system and legislators.

Most people comprehend that being accountable requires being held responsible for one's behaviour, decisions, and affiliations with others. Not withstanding, some nurses claim they are not culpable for their actions because they are merely doing what they must do as defined by their employer or some other larger entity.

These nurses fail to understand that professional accountability goes beyond responsibility in a particular employment situation. Accountability means that nurses will actively participate in risk identification and management, problem solving, and implementation of any changes that are required. It is not acceptable to identify that a risk exists, and then to sit back, and expect others to correct the situation. If there are risks for our clients, ultimately our care providers are also at risk. The Canadian Nurses Association and each of the provincial and territorial regulatory bodies have statements related to accountability.

Increasingly, consumers are demanding positive results and are holding those in the health care system accountable for better health care outcomes. Many organizations have ethics committees or statements related to ethics within their mission statements, but the existence of committees and statements will not satisfy the consumer who experiences negative outcomes. The strongest potential for litigation in health care comes from too few health care professionals accepting personal responsibility for ensuring that health care services are provided in a safe, competent manner at a system level as well as at a personal level. Health care professionals, including nurses, depend upon each other to ensure the quality, consistency, and overall effectiveness of health care within their work environments.

CREDIBILITY AND POLITICS

To have credibility, nurses must demonstrate professional competence and a degree of professional accountability

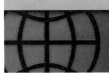

REAL WORLD INTERVIEW

Question: What role have civil servants played in your success?

Answer: During the formative years of the College of Licensed Practical Nurses of Alberta, we engaged the services of a consultant who had previously been a member of the Legislative Assembly (MLA). He provided us with some of the most valuable advice in developing government relationships. Although legislation and policy come from the elected officials, civil servants are the ones who have the ear of the ministers to provide them with advice and information. Therefore it is essential to have a collaborative working relationship in the key government departments. For us, they are primarily the departments of Health and Wellness and Advanced Education. We have worked with staff in the Health and Wellness department to develop legislation and make amendments over the years. Sometimes, recommendations for legislation come from the profession and sometimes they come from government. In our time with the College, we have gone through two complete writes of the regulations that govern our profession and the development of new umbrella legislation for all health professions. We have a very positive rapport with the staff in the department and always work through the process in a collaborative way. We would present our needs and suggestions for the legislation and our rationale, and work together to ensure a positive outcome for all, representing not only what is good for the profession, but also what is in the best interest of public safety.

Question: Where else have you been able to succeed with that kind of attitude?

Answer: We have used the same attitude with employers when working towards common goals, and working with other health care professions. Many barriers were removed in legislation, and the education greatly improved for LPNs [licensed practical nurses], with tremendous results in increased value and utilization of LPNs. There has been a return of the LPN to settings such as obstetrics and pediatrics, where they had previously been eliminated. We have also seen many new opportunities for LPNs in settings where they were not traditionally a part of the care team, such as public health and as team leaders in long-term care.

This positive and solution-oriented attitude has gained us the respect of other health disciplines, and allowed us to be agents of change, not only for the LPN but also for the betterment of all nurses and the health care system. We are now welcomed at all tables where decisions that affect nurses and health care are made, both provincially and nationally. Our motto is to work *with* the system, never against it.

Pat Frederickson
Former Executive Director/Registrar—College of Licensed Practical Nurses of Alberta

Rita McGregor
Former Director of Professional Practice—College of Licensed Practical Nurses of Alberta

that exceeds consumers' expectations. Nurses who are most able to successfully overcome these challenges assert their professional credibility in several ways. They are lifelong learners and demonstrate professional growth throughout their careers in nursing. They approach their career as a service to the public and to the nursing profession and as an honourable way to make a living. They take ownership of the situations in which they find themselves and work to resolve problems and overcome obstacles to providing the best care possible. Nurses strengthen their political position by taking ownership of their problems in serving consumers.

Nursing ownership, however, is not enough to guarantee the political credibility of nursing in the future because others see the political gains to be made from identifying themselves as consumer advocates.

A clear image of the vision you want to achieve and a sound philosophy for change are essential. Although it is always easy to bring problems forward, a far more effective approach is to clearly articulate the problem and present potential solutions. Consideration must be given to the options that are available and the most viable solutions. Seek out alliances with others who have the same vision and goals. Always maintain a consistent message and articulate it clearly, together with the benefits that can be expected. Persistence and patience are key when attempting to influence change, particularly through politics and political activity.

KEY CONCEPTS

- Individuals or groups take political action to achieve what they want or to prevent others from achieving a goal they do not agree with.

- Politics are inherent in any system in which resources are absolutely or relatively scarce and in which opposing interests compete for those resources.

- Nurses have a critical role in addressing the major system-level issues in health care delivery.

- Political, economic, and social changes in Canada are transforming the health care system.

- Nurses need to articulate what nursing is, the distinctive services nursing provides, how these services benefit consumers, and the cost of these services in relation to other health care services.

- If nursing is defined through politics to be less than critical or professional, nurses will be less empowered and paid less.

- The aging of the Canadian population constitutes a growing political force and affords nursing with an opportunity to become stronger in health policy arenas.

- To be politically effective, consumer alliances are critical for all stakeholders in health care.

- When a consumer group forms a political coalition with other groups, such as nurses, the political influence of both groups is strengthened.

KEY TERMS

political voice	stakeholders
politics	voting block
resources	

REVIEW QUESTIONS

1. Politics exists because
   A. it is required by law.
   B. resources cannot be limited by political process.
   C. some people control more resources than others.
   D. resources must be equally distributed among stakeholders.

2. The consumer movement in health care is
   A. a socialist movement about health care resources.
   B. growing because of the Internet and organizations such as the CARP.
   C. supported by all stakeholders in the health care system.
   D. losing its momentum.

3. The immigrant population in Canada
   A. includes 1.8 million racially and ethnically diverse people.
   B. will surpass the white majority in another 10 years.
   C. has resisted the consumer movement.
   D. is a well-organized, cohesive group of consumers.

REVIEW ACTIVITIES

1. Identify your local, provincial, and federal politicians. Write a letter or e-mail them to learn which health care legislation they support.

2. Research who is supporting current health care legislation. Are consumer protections being emphasized in any proposed legislation?

3. Identify a consumer group in which you are interested. Use the steps identified in Table 7-2 to establish an alliance with the group. What did you learn?

EXPLORING THE WEB

- Identify some websites for consumer groups. Canada's Association for the Fifty-Plus: *http://www.carp.ca/*
  The Health Action Lobby: *http://www.physiotherapy.ca/HEAL/english/index.htm*
  National Citizens Coalition: *http://morefreedom.org/*

- Note consumer tips at this site: *http://consumer.ic.gc.ca/epic/internet/inoca-bc.nsf/en/ca01485e.html*

- Note Health Canada's information on consumer participation and citizen engagement: *http://www.hc-sc.gc.ca/hcs-sss/qual/participation/index_e.html*

- Note this site for consumer reports: *http://www.consumer.ca/1652*

- Identify some sites for government bodies and health care agencies.

- Parliament of Canada: *http://www.parl.gc.ca/common/index.asp?Language=E*

- Health Canada: *http://www.hc-sc.gc.ca/*

REFERENCES

Brown, L. D. (1996). *Health policy in the United States: Issues and options*. New York: The Ford Foundation.

Canada. Statistics Canada. (2006). *Canada year book 2006*. Ottawa: Statistics Canada.

Canadian Nursing Advisory Committee. (2002). *Our health, our future: Creating quality workplaces for Canadian nurses: Final report of the Canadian Nursing Advisory Committee*. Ottawa: Advisory Committee on Health Human Resources.

Commission on the Future of Health Care in Canada. (2002). *Building on values: The future of health care in Canada*. Saskatoon:

Commission on the Future of Health Care in Canada. Commissioner: Roy J. Romano.

Fagin, C. (1998). Nursing research and the erosion of care. *Nursing Outlook, 46*(6), 259–261.

Ferguson, S. L. (2001). An activist looks at nursing's role in health policy development. *Journal of Obstetric, Gynoecologic, and Neonatal Nursing, 30*(5), 546–551.

Gebbie, K. M., Wakefield, M., & Kerfoot, K. (2000). Nursing and health policy. *Image: Journal of Nursing Scholarship, 32*(3), 307–314.

Jones, K., Jennings, B. M., Moritz, P., & Moss, T. M. (1997). Policy issues associated with analyzing outcomes of care. *Image: Journal of Nursing Scholarship, 29*(3), 251–276.

Kerfoot, K. (2000). On leadership—"Customerizing" in the new millennium. *MedSurg Nursing: The Journal of Adult Health, 9*(2), 97–99.

Leddy, S., & Pepper, J. M. (1998). *Conceptual bases of professional nursing* (4th ed.). Philadelphia: Lippincott.

Longest, B. (1998). *Health policymaking in the United States* (2nd ed.). Chicago: Health Administration Press.

Mason, D., & Leavitt, J. K. (1999). *Policy and politics in nursing and health care* (3rd ed.). Philadelphia: Saunders.

McIntyre, M., & Thomlinson, E. (2003). *Realities of Canadian nursing: Professional, practice, and power issues.* Philadelphia: Lippincott Williams &Wilkins.

Milstead, J. A. (1999). *Health policy & politics: A nurse's guide.* Gaithersburg, MD: Aspen.

Nursing Sector Study Corporation. (2005). *Building the future: An integrated strategy for nursing human resources in Canada.* Ottawa: Nursing Sector Study Corporation.

O'Connell, B. (2000). Research shows erosion to advocacy role. *Reflections on Nursing Leadership, 26*(2), 26–28.

Ogren, K. E. (2001). The risk of not understanding nursing history. In E. C. Hein (Ed.), *Nursing issues in the 21st century: Perspectives from the literature* (pp. 3–9). Philadelphia: Lippincott.

Provost, K. & Van Herk, K. (2006). Political activism and nursing. *Registered Nurse Journal, 18*(2), 22–23.

Registered Nurses Association of Ontario. (2005). Policy at work. *Registered Nurse Journal, 17*(3), 27.

Rehtmeyer, C. M. (2000). Seeing change as an opportunity. In F. L. Bower (Ed.), *Nurses taking the lead: Personal qualities of effective leadership* (pp. 173–198). Philadelphia: Saunders.

Roszak, T. (1998). *The longevity revolution and the true wealth of nations.* Boston: Houghton Mifflin.

Williams, R. P. (1998). Nursing leaders' perceptions of quality nursing: An analysis from academe. *Nursing Outlook, 46*(6), 262–267.

SUGGESTED READINGS

Abeln, S. H. (1994). Quality as a risk management tool. *Rehab Management, 7*(2), 105–106.

Alberta Association of Registered Nurses. (2004). *Turn up the heat! Political action and advocacy guide.* Edmonton: Alberta Association of Registered Nurses.

Anderson, E. T., & McFarlane, J. M. (2000). *Community as partner: Theory and practice in nursing.* Philadelphia: Lippincott, Williams & Wilkins.

Baird, K. (2000). *Customer service in health care: A grassroots approach to creating a culture of service excellence.* San Francisco: Jossey-Bass.

Buerhaus, P. I., Staiger, D. O., & Auerbach, D. I. (2000). Implications of an aging registered nurse workforce. *Journal of the American Medical Association, 283,* 2948–2954.

Canadian Nurses Association. (2005). "Position statement." *Accountability: Regulatory framework.* Ottawa: Canadian Nurses Association.

Canadian Nurses Association. (2006). Celebrating international nursing partnerships. *Canadian Nurse, 102*(6), 15–17.

Edwards, T. (2000). *Contradictions of consumption: Concepts, practices, and politics in consumer society.* Buckingham, UK: Open University Press.

Jennings, C. P. (Ed.). (2000 to present). *Policy, Politics and Nursing Practice.* (Quarterly journal available through Sage Publications, Thousand Oaks, CA).

Jones, K., Jennings, B., Moritz, P., & Moss, M. (1997). Policy issues associated with analyzing outcomes of care. *Image: Journal of Nursing Scholarship, 29,* 261–268.

Maney, A., & Bykerk, L. (1994). *Consumer politics: Protecting public interests on Capitol Hill.* Westport, CT: Greenwood Press.

Mason, D., & Leavitt, J. K. (1998). *Policy and politics in nursing and health care.* Philadelphia: Saunders.

Miller, T. W. (1996). Health policy, politics, and community health advocacy. In B. W. Spradley & J. A. Allender (Eds.), *Community health nursing: Concepts and practices* (pp. 635–657). Philadelphia: Lippincott.

O'Reilly, P. (2000). *Health care practitioners: An Ontario case study in policy making.* Toronto: University of Toronto Press.

Pope, T. (2000). The rising tide of consumerism: How will it affect long-term care decision making? *Long-Term Care Interface, 1*(1), pp. 36–40.

Shaw, J. (2005). RNs lead by example. *Registered Nurse Journal, 17*(6), 23.

Sherman, S. G., & Sherman, V. C. (1998). *Total customer satisfaction: A comprehensive approach for health care providers.* San Francisco: Jossey-Bass.

Smith, S., Heffler, S., & Freeland, M. (1999). The next decade of health spending: A new outlook. *Health Affairs, 18*(4), 86–95.

Spradley, B. W., & Allender, J. A. (1996). *Community health nursing: Concepts and practice.* Philadelphia: Lippincott.

Strasen, L. (1987). *Key business skills for nurse managers.* Philadelphia: Lippincott.

Wojner, A. W. (2001). *Outcomes management: Applications to clinical practice.* St. Louis, MO: Mosby.

World Health Organization. (1978). *Declaration of Alma Ata: Report of the International Conference on Primary Health Care.* Alma-Ata, USSR, September 1978. Geneva: WHO. Retrieved from http://www.who.int/hpr/NPH/docs/declaration_almaata.pdf, August 2006.

CHAPTER ENDNOTE

1. Health Canada, "About Health Canada, Office of Nursing Policy." Retrieved from http://www.hc-sc.gc.ca/ahc-asc/branch-dirgen/hpb-dgps/onp-bpsi/index_e.html, September 17, 2006.

UNIT III
Planning Care

CHAPTER 8

Nursing Leadership and Management

Linda Searle Leach, PhD, RN, CNAA
Adapted by: Eric Doucette, RN

Nursing requires strong, consistent and knowledgeable leaders who are visible, inspire others and support professional nursing practice. Leadership plays a pivotal role in the lives of nurses. It is an essential element for quality professional practice environments where nurses can provide quality nursing care. (Canadian Nurses Association, Position Statement on Nursing Leadership, June 2002)

OBJECTIVES

Upon completion of this chapter, the reader should be able to:

1. Define management.
2. Describe the management process.
3. Explain management theories.
4. Discuss motivation theories.
5. Define leadership and nursing leadership and explain their importance for organizations.
6. Differentiate between leadership and management.
7. Describe characteristics of effective leaders.
8. Identify factors that influence nursing leadership.
9. Identify leadership styles.
10. Explain Hersey and Blanchard's situational theory of leadership and its application in nursing leadership practice.
11. Identify Kouzes and Posner's five leadership practices.
12. Discuss transformational leadership theory.
13. Examine the link between nursing leadership and management.

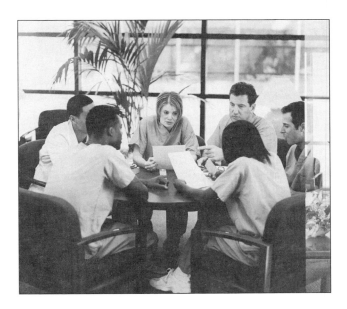

Gary, a 45-year-old father of three, was admitted to the cardiac observation unit earlier in the day. He had been diagnosed previously with heart disease and had experienced episodes of ventricular arrhythmias. That evening, while Gary was talking to his family on the phone, he suddenly stopped talking and went into ventricular tachycardia and cardiac arrest. Julie, his nurse, reacted immediately, by giving a precordial thump to his chest. Normal sinus rhythm appeared on the monitor before anyone else could respond to the code. Gary was then transferred to the coronary care unit (CCU).

Julie has been a registered nurse (RN) in the cardiac observation unit less than one year, and although she had participated in code arrests a few times, she had never witnessed one occur right before her eyes. Her knowledgeable action saved this client's life. The next morning, Julie was assigned to work a day shift in the CCU. Julie entered Gary's room, as the sun was just rising. As he awoke, she spent some quiet time with him. While he embraced the start of a new day, his thoughts must have been intense. What he chose to share was this acknowledgment: "You saved my life. Thank you." This precious moment was a celebration of both of their lives

> *Was Julie a leader in delivering client care? What leadership characteristics did this nurse demonstrate? Why is Julie considered a leader, even though she is not in an executive or a management position?*

Nursing professionals use their specialized knowledge, judgment, skills, and clinical experience to perform leadership roles. Many people think leaders are corporate executives, political representatives, military generals, or those who head organizations. However, effective nursing leadership is important in all nursing roles at all levels within an organization and across all domains of practice: direct practice, education, research, and administration. As stated in the Canadian Nurses Association (CNA) position statement on nursing leadership, "Nursing requires strong, consistent, and knowledgeable leaders who are visible, inspire others and support professional nursing practice" (Canadian Nurses Association, 2002). Leadership must become a shared responsibility. Nurses in all domains of practice and at all levels must maximize their leadership potential (Broughton, 2002). According to the CNA position statement, "To support excellence in professional practice, humanism must be restored to the work environment to help nurses feel safe, respected and valued" (Canadian Nurses Association, 2002).

Nurses have the potential to make a critical difference every day in the lives of their clients and their clients' families and in their practice environments. However, many nurses believe those critical differences are part of their ordinary work. Nurses are leaders, and by using their expert knowledge and leadership, they provide knowledgeable care that is extraordinary. Because rapid, dramatic change will continue in nursing and the health care industry, it is increasingly important for nurses to develop skill in leadership roles and management functions (Marquis & Huston, 2006). This chapter introduces the process of management and explains management theories and functions. Management will be defined, and current trends will be discussed. This chapter also discusses leadership and provides a framework to differentiate leadership and management. Leadership characteristics, styles of leadership, and leadership theories are described. In examining management and leadership, it will become evident that a symbiotic or synergistic relationship exists between the two concepts. The challenge for leaders and managers in today's complex practice settings is the integration of leadership and management skills to facilitate positive outcomes for clients, nurses, and the organization.

DEFINITION OF MANAGEMENT

Management can be defined as the systematic process of planning, organizing, leading, and controlling actions and resources to achieve organizational goals. Descriptive research about what managers do (Hales, 1986; McCall, Morrison, & Hanman, 1978; Mintzberg, 1973) has been a helpful way to expand our understanding of management. Managers often seem to work at a hectic pace and sustain that effort through long hours, frequently working without breaks. According to Yukl (1998), this practice reflects a preference by people in management positions, who become adept at continuously seeking information and are constantly engaged in interactions with others who need information, help, guidance, or approval. The typical manager is on the go.

Research by McCall, Morrison, and Hanman (1978) shows that the daily activities of managers are diverse and fast paced with regular interruptions. Priority activities are integrated among inconsequential tasks. In the scope of one morning, a manager may engage in serious and far-reaching decisions about downsizing personnel, respond to a client complaint, problem-solve a sick call, and participate in a celebration for an employee. Managerial work is driven by problems that emerge in random order, and that have a range of importance and urgency. These circumstances create an image of the manager as a firefighter, involved in immediate and operational concerns. A significant proportion of a manager's time is spent in interaction with others, and more of the work is concerned with handling information than in making decisions (McCall, Morrison, & Hanman, 1978).

In a landmark paper by Bruch and Ghoshal (2002), who studied busy managers in nearly a dozen large companies, they found that "fully 90% of managers squander their time in all sorts of ineffective activities. In other words a mere 10% of managers spend their time in a committed, purposeful and reflective manner" (p. 64). Effective managers need to balance both focus and energy. Focus is described by Bruch and Ghoshal as concentrated attention, or the ability to zero in on a goal and see the tasks through to completion. This description suggests that skilled managers have the wisdom to choose what to respond to and maintain active suppression to environmental distractions that can sidetrack the focused effort. Energy is described as the vivacity that is fuelled by intense personal commitment. Disequilibrium in focus and energy results in ineffective management.

THE MANAGEMENT PROCESS

In the early 1900s, the study of management, as a discipline, emerged with a focus on the science of management. In 1924, Mary Parker Follet wrote about management as an art of accomplishing things through people. Henri Fayol, a manager, wrote a book in 1916 called *General and Industrial Management*, in which he described the functions of planning, organizing, coordinating, and controlling as the **management process** (Fayol, 1916/1949). His work has become a classic in the way that we define the process of managing. Two other individuals, Gulick and Urwick, in some part as a result of their esteemed status as informal advisers to President Franklin D. Roosevelt, served to define the management process according to seven principles (Henry, 1992). Their principles form the acronym POSDCORB, which stands for planning, organizing, staffing, directing, coordinating (CO), reporting, and budgeting (Gulick & Urwick, 1937; Henry, 1992). Their work is also considered to be a classic description of management and remains a relevant description of how management is carried out today.

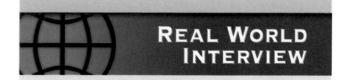

REAL WORLD INTERVIEW

As the CEO for the Brant Community Healthcare System, I have seen a number of dramatic changes occur within nursing leadership roles especially over the past decade. More informed health care consumers, contracting resources, increasing accountability in the public-funded health care system and finally, changes in legislation as well as professional regulation have contributed to the need to examine new organizational models and systems of care organization. The Chief Nursing Executive and the nursing leadership team have been invaluable to our organization, and success would not have been possible without their skilled application of management processes. Our nursing leaders have consistently provided knowledgeable and evidence-based guidance in planning, leading, organizing, and controlling change initiatives. Their perseverance and commitment contributed to our success as we navigated multiple changes, such as role reconfiguration, scope of practice expansion for Registered Practical Nurses, reengineered reporting structures, and merged physical plant facilities and client services. If you want to recruit and retain nurses, then strong nursing leadership is required as is a healthy working environment in which client-centred care can flourish and professional practice can continue to evolve.

Richard Woodcock
President and CEO, Brantford General Hospital, Brant Community Healthcare System

One of the most frequently referenced taxonomies of managerial roles is from an in-depth, month-long study of five chief executives by Henry Mintzberg. A taxonomy is a system that groups or classifies principles. Mintzberg's observations led to the identification of three categories of managerial roles: (1) information processing roles, (2) interpersonal roles, and (3) decision-making roles (Mintzberg, 1973). A role includes behaviours, expectations, and recurrent activities within a pattern that is part of the organization's structure (Katz & Kahn, 1978). The information processing roles identified by Mintzberg (1973) are those of monitor, disseminator, and spokesperson, and are used to manage people's information needs. The interpersonal roles consist of figurehead, leader, and liaison, and each of these roles is used to manage relationships with people. The decision roles are entrepreneur, disturbance handler, allocator of resources, and negotiator. Managers take on these roles when they make decisions.

More recently, Yukl (1998) and colleagues (Kim & Yukl, 1995; Yukl, Wall, & Lepsinger, 1990) described 13 managerial role functions for managing the work and for managing relationships. The role functions for managing the work are planning and organizing, problem solving, clarifying roles and objectives, informing, monitoring, consulting, and delegating. The role functions for managing relationships are networking, supporting, developing and mentoring, managing conflict and team building, motivating and inspiring, and recognizing and rewarding.

The amount of time a manager spends in particular roles varies by the manager's position in the organization, ranging from the lowest level manager, to the middle-level manager, to the highest or executive-level manager. However, in health care environments, this generalization needs to be tempered with an understanding of the impact on hospital restructuring, complexity of service delivery, client acuity, and the ever-growing span of control for the nurse manager. Again, nursing managers need to be cognizant of the required balance between focus and energy to maintain effectiveness.

Typically, a low-level managerial job is the first-line manager, and in health care organizations that position is the typical role of the nurse manager. Ideally, the nurse manager spends the majority of time in the clinical area, supervising, leading, and coaching staff as they deliver care, as well as maintaining active surveillance of the quality of care given. The reality of the situation is such that managers are often less accessible owing to the nature of their involvement on project teams, taskforces, and committees, and their competing priorities in balancing the costs and quality of health care. The next highest percentage of this manager's time is spent in planning, where other responsibilities, such as coordinating, evaluating, negotiating, and serving as a multispecialist and generalist, each require less than 10 percent of the nurse manager's time. In contrast, the middle-level manager, often called a director (e.g., the director of critical care nursing), spends less time supervising and more time in each of the other assignments, particularly planning, monitoring, and delegating. At the highest level of the organization, usually described as the executive level, planning and serving as a generalist are greatly expanded role functions, whereas monitoring is not the primary role function as it is for the other two levels. Nurses in executive-level roles in health care organizations usually have the title of chief nursing officer; in acute care hospitals, their title is often vice president and chief nursing officer.

MANAGEMENT THEORIES

The current theories of management practice have evolved from earlier theories. Management practices were actually a part of the governance in ancient Samaria and Egypt as far back as 3000 B.C. (Daft & Marcic, 2001). Most of our current understanding of management, however, is based on the classical perspective of management or the classical theories of management that were introduced in the 1800s, during the industrial age, as factories developed. The classical perspective includes three subfields of management: scientific management, bureaucratic theory, and administrative principles (Daft & Marcic, 2001; Wren, 1979).

SCIENTIFIC MANAGEMENT

While practising managers, such as Fayol, who was mentioned earlier, were describing the functions of managers, a man named Frederick Taylor was focusing his attention on the operations within an organization by exploring production at the workers' level. Taylor is acknowledged as the father of scientific management for his use of the scientific method and as the author of *Principles of Scientific Management* (1911). Productivity was the area of focus in scientific management. Taylor, an engineer, introduced precise procedures based on systematic investigation of specific situations. The underlying point of view is that the organization is a machine to be run efficiently to increase production.

Currently in Canada, the definition of nursing productivity/utilization is "workload over worked hours" (Canadian Institute for Health Information, 1999). Many nursing leaders recognize that this simple calculation does not account for the quality and outcomes of care delivered, nor for the impact of length of stay on total cost (O'Brien-Pallas et al., 2004). In a dynamic state, such as a care delivery setting, the individual and collective capacity of the nursing personnel (i.e., their scope, competence, experience, and their physician and psychosocial status) must be balanced against client needs and system characteristics (i.e., census, type of client mix, staff mix, occupancy, etc.). The maximum work capacity of any employee is 93 percent, because 7 percent is allocated in paid breaks during which no work is contractually expected (O'Brien-Pallas et al., 2004). O'Brien-Pallas and colleagues found that significant benefits, both fiscal and human, can be achieved by moderating productivity/utilization levels within a range of 85 percent, plus or minus 5 percent. This level suggests productivity targets may not be appropriate for specialty units, such as emergency departments or labour and delivery units, since their work flow demands can be variable.

Working independently of Taylor, Frank and Lillian Gilbreth also contributed significantly to the study of scientific management. They pioneered studies of time and motion that emphasized efficiency and culminated in "one best way" of carrying out work. Frank Gilbreth (1912) revolutionized surgical efficiency in the operating room, resulting in operations of shorter duration that substantially reduced risks from surgery for clients at that time.

BUREAUCRATIC THEORY

The beliefs of Max Weber, the German theorist recognized for the organizational theory of bureaucracy, were in stark contrast to the typical European organization that was based on a family-type structure in which employees were loyal to an individual, not to the organization and resources were used to benefit individuals rather than to advance the organization. Weber, however, believed efficiency was achieved through impersonal relations within a formal structure, competence should be the basis for hiring and promoting an employee, and decisions should be made in an orderly and rational way, based on rules and regulations. The **bureaucratic organization** was a hierarchy with clear superior-subordinate communication and relations, based on positional authority, in which orders from the top were transmitted down through the organization via a clear chain of command.

ADMINISTRATIVE PRINCIPLES

Administrative principles are general principles of management that are relevant to any organization. In addition to some of the principles described as comprising the management process (e.g., planning, organizing, directing, coordinating, and controlling), principles such as unity of command and direction were identified. Unity of command and direction refers to a worker receiving orders from only one supervisor, and related work being grouped under one manager. These are examples of general principles generated during the early 1900s, which were useful and relevant to all organizations (Fayol, 1916/1949).

LITERATURE APPLICATION

Citation: Laborde, A. S., & Lee, J. A. (2000). Skills needed for promotion in the nursing profession. *Journal of Nursing Administration, 30*(9), 432–439.

Discussion: This research was designed to identify skills (i.e., interpersonal versus technical) needed for job promotion within the nursing field. As a nurse changes positions from primarily clinical practice to a management role, interpersonal skills seem to be more important than technical skills to move up the organizational ladder. Although technical skills are necessary for those who supervise nurses, interpersonal skills become more important as tools to influence and lead others.

The hypotheses were as follows: more interpersonal skills would be important for promotion to upper-level management positions, whereas more technical skills would be important for promotion to lower-level management; a significant difference would exist between decision-makers' perceptions of the importance of the skills and the skills' objective importance to promotion decisions. A stratified random sample of 219 nurse administrators was obtained from a large hospital in the southeastern United States. Sixty scenarios with hypothetical candidates were used to approximate the promotion situations. Hypothetical candidates were described in terms of their interpersonal and technical skills, and the participants were asked to decide how likely they would be to recommend this candidate for a promotion by using a Likert-type 5-point scale in which 1 indicated "definitely not promote" and 5 indicated "definitely promote." No significant differences were found between the position and the number of interpersonal skills used. However, at the lower-level management position of clinical nurse 3 (CN3), a greater number of technical skills influenced promotion decisions than for the middle-management position.

Implications for Practice: The findings suggest that technical skills are more important for clinical nurse promotions than for nurse manager positions. The skills needed for success change as a nurse moves from clinical practice to a managerial position. Several strategies were proposed to increase managerial effectiveness. A dual career ladder would provide a mechanism for retaining technical skills and would provide the employee with a choice between developing technical skills and pursuing management. Succession planning may reduce the political influences and personal bias in the promotion process. Mentoring programs could provide valuable insights for new managers. Providing realistic job previews and complete job descriptions can clarify misunderstandings and reduce managerial burnout and turnover. Tourangeau et al. (2003) evaluated an intervention administered to a group of Canadian nurses designed to assist participants to value leadership and to develop knowledge, skills, and attitudes required for effective leadership. Tourangeau and colleagues found that it was possible to deliver leadership development interventions to both established leaders (i.e., formal leaders) and aspiring nurse leaders (i.e., informal leaders), which result in fairly rapid improvements in observed leadership practice. Additional research is needed to improve management development programs for nurses and to evaluate designs for how managers are selected.

Another key aspect of this perspective is attributed to Chester Barnard. Barnard (1938) is associated with the concept of the informal organization. The informal organization consists of naturally forming social groups that can become strong and powerful contributors to an organization. Barnard understood that these informal forces can be valuable in accomplishing the organization's goals and should be managed properly. He is also credited with the acceptance theory of authority, which identified people as having free will and being able to choose to comply with orders they are given (Daft & Marcic, 2001). This view of people as making a difference in organizations was a precursor to the human relations movement that emerged from experiments at a Chicago electric company, discussed in the next section. See Table 8-1 for an overview of management theories.

TABLE 8-1	MANAGEMENT THEORIES

Management Theory	Main Contributors	Key Aspects
Scientific management	Frederick Taylor (1856–1915) Frank Gilbreth (1868–1924) Lillian Gilbreth (1878–1972)	Machinelike focus Analysis of elements of an operation Training of the worker Use of proper tools and equipment Use of incentives Use of time and motion studies to make the work easier
Bureaucratic theory	Max Weber (1864–1920): German sociologist	Division of labour, hierarchy of authority, and chain of command Rationality, impersonal management Use of merit and skill as basis for promotion/reward Use of rules and regulations, focus on exacting work processes Career service, salaried managers
Administrative principles	Mary Parker Folle.t (1868–1933): Trained in philosophy/political science at Radcliffe	The science of management Principles of organization applicable in any setting
	Henri Fayol (1841–1925): French mining engineer, head of major mining company	Fayol's principles: unity of command, division of work, unity of direction, scalar chain, and management principles functions—planning, organizing, coordinating, and controlling
	Chester Barnard (1886–1961): Harvard economics, president of New Jersey Bell Telephone	Concerned with the optimal approach for administrators to achieve economic efficiency
	Luther Gulick and Lyndal Urwick (1937): *Papers on the Science of Administration*	Planning, organizing, supervising, directing, controlling, organizing, reviewing, and budgeting = POSDCORB
	James Mooney (1939): *Principles of Organization*	Four principles: coordination, hierarchical structure (scalar), functional (division of labour), staff/line principle
Human relations (replaced later by the term *organizational behaviour*)	Elton Mayo (1933) Fritz Roethlisberger (1939): Harvard University	Hawthorne studies led to the belief that human relations between workers and managers and among workers were the main determinants of efficiency. The Hawthorne effect refers to change in behaviour as a result of being watched.

HUMAN RELATIONS

The next focus in the development of management theory is the human relations movement. In contrast to the science of exact procedures, rules and regulations, and formal authority, which characterized scientific management, the theories from the human relations school of thought espoused the individual worker as the source of control, motivation, and productivity in organizations. During the 1930s, labour unions became stronger and were instrumental in advocating for the human needs of employees. During this time, experiments conducted at the Hawthorne plant of the Western Electric Company in Chicago led to a greater understanding of the influence of human relations in organizations.

Electricity had become the preferred power source over gas; the Hawthorne plant experiments were run to show people that more light was necessary for greater productivity. This approach was designed to increase the use of electricity. Researchers Mayo (1933) and Roethlisberger and Dickson (1939) measured the effects on production when the intensity of lighting was altered. They found that with more and brighter light, production increased as expected. However, production also increased each time they reduced the light, even when the light was extremely dim. Their research findings led to the conclusion that something else besides the light was motivating these workers.

The notion of social facilitation or the idea that people increase their work output in the presence of others was a result of the Hawthorne experiments. They also concluded that the effect of being watched and receiving special attention could alter a person's behaviour. The phenomenon of being observed or studied resulting in changes in behaviour is now called the **Hawthorne effect** (Hughes, Ginnet, & Curphy, 1999). Emerging from this study was the concept that people benefit and are more productive and satisfied when they participate in decisions about their work environment. This concept introduced the next phase in the evolution of management, called human relations management. In addition, social groupings, people's feelings, and their motivations became a focus of interest for future studies.

MOTIVATION THEORIES

The human relations perspective in management theory grew from the conclusion that worker output was greater when the worker was treated humanistically. This theory spawned a human resources point of view and a focus on the individual as a source of motivation. **Motivation** is not explicitly demonstrated by people but rather is interpreted from their behaviour. Motivation is the incentive that influences our choices and creates direction, intensity, and persistence in our behaviour (Hughes, Ginnett, & Curphy, 1999; Kanfer, 1990). Motivation is a process that occurs internally to influence and direct our behaviour in order to satisfy needs (Lussier, 1999). Motivation theories are not management theories per se; however, they are frequently included along with management theories.

There are two types of motivation theories: content motivation theories and process motivation theories (Lussier, 1999). The process motivation theories are expectancy theory and equity theory. The content motivation theories include Maslow's needs hierarchy and Herzberg's two-factor theory. Maslow's hierarchy of needs and Herzberg's two-factor theory are presented here along with Theory X, Theory Y, and Theory Z (see Table 8-2).

Motivation theories help explain why people act the way they do and how a manager can relate to individuals as human beings and workers. When you are interested in creating change, influencing others, and managing performance and outcomes, it is helpful to understand the motivation that is reflected in a person's behaviour. Motivation is a critical part of leadership because we need to understand each other in order to be good leaders and good followers. Covey (1990), in his national bestseller, *The Seven Habits of Highly Effective People*, defines habit number five as "Seek first to understand, then to be understood," which is a practice focused on the critical importance in empathetic communication, which is critical to effective leadership.

MASLOW'S HIERARCHY OF NEEDS

One of the most well-known theories of motivation is Maslow's hierarchy of needs. Maslow (1970) developed a hierarchy of needs that shows how an individual is motivated. Figure 8-1 applies Maslow's hierarchy of human needs to how organizations motivate employees. Motivation, according to Maslow, begins when a need is not met. For example, when a person has a physiological need, such as thirst, this unmet need has to be satisfied before a person is motivated to pursue higher-level needs. Certain needs have to be satisfied first, beginning with physiological needs, then safety and security needs, next belonging social needs, followed by esteem and ego needs before an individual is motivated by the needs at the next level. The need for self-actualization drives people to the pinnacle of performance and achievement.

HERZBERG'S TWO-FACTOR THEORY

Frederick Herzberg (1968) contributed to research on motivation and developed the two-factor theory of motivation. He analyzed the responses of accountants and engineers, and concluded that two sets of factors were associated with motivation. One set of motivation factors must be maintained to avoid job dissatisfaction: salary, job

TABLE 8-2	MOTIVATION THEORIES	

Motivation Theory	Main Contributors	Key Aspects
Selected content of motivation theories	Abraham Maslow (1908–1970)	Hierarchy of satisfaction of physiological, safety, belonging, ego, and self-actualization needs
Two-factor theory	Frederick Herzberg (1968)	Hygiene-maintenance factors = prevention of job dissatisfaction: provide adequate salary and supervision, safe and tolerable working conditions
		Motivators = job satisfaction: satisfying and meaningful work, development opportunities, responsibility, and recognition
Theory X	Douglas McGregor (1906–1964)	Theory X: leaders must direct and control as motivation results from reward and punishment
Theory Y		Theory Y: leaders remove obstacles as workers have self-control, self-discipline; their reward is their involvement in work
Theory Z	William Ouchi (1981)	Theory Z: Collective decision making, long-term employment, mentoring, holistic concerns, and use of quality circles to manage service and quality; a humanistic style of motivation based on Japanese organizations

security, working conditions, status, quality of supervision, and relationships with others. These factors have been labelled **maintenance or hygiene factors.** Factors such as achievement, recognition, responsibility, advancement, and the opportunity for development also contribute to job satisfaction. These factors are intrinsic and serve to satisfy or motivate people. Herzberg proposed that when these **motivation factors** are present, people are motivated and satisfied with their job. When these factors are absent from a work setting, people have a neutral attitude about their organization. In contrast, when the maintenance factors are absent, people are dissatisfied. Herzberg believed that by providing the maintenance factors, job dissatisfaction could be avoided, but that the presence of these factors will not motivate people.

New graduate nurses can use Herzberg's theory by evaluating the maintenance factors present in a health care organization when they apply for a job. The pay, working conditions, and the beginning relationship that has been established with the nurse manager are aspects of the job that the nurse should consider. If these maintenance factors are not adequate to begin with, then the nurse may become easily dissatisfied with the job. The higher-level needs that Herzberg describes as motivation factors should also be evaluated by the nurse before

joining an organization. Are opportunities available for the nurse to achieve professional growth, to take on new responsibilities, to advance, and to be recognized for one's contributions?

McGREGOR'S THEORY X AND THEORY Y

Continuing the emphasis on factors that stimulate job satisfaction and that motivate people to be involved and contribute productively at work, McGregor capitalized on his experience as a psychologist and university president to develop Theory X and Theory Y (McGregor, 1960). Theory X and Theory Y describe two different ways to motivate or influence others based on underlying attitudes about human nature. Each view reflects different attitudes about the nature of people. The **Theory X** view is that in bureaucratic organizations, employees prefer security, direction, and minimal responsibility. Coercion, threats, or punishment are necessary because people do not like the work that needs to be done. These employees are not able to offer creative solutions to help the organization advance. McGregor's beliefs about Theory X were related to the classical perspective of organizations that included scientific management, bureaucracy theory, and administrative principles.

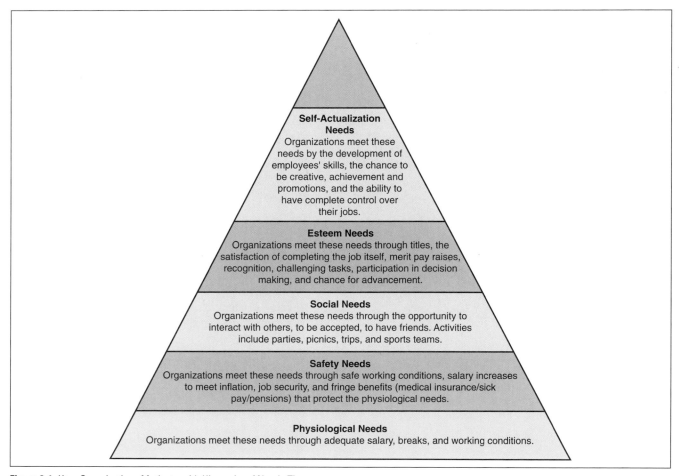

Figure 8-1 How Organizations Motivate with Hierarchy of Needs Theory.

Source: From Leadership: Theory, Application, Skill Building [p. 81], by R. N. Lussier and C. F. Achua, 2001, Cincinnati, OH: South-Western College.

The assumptions of **Theory Y** are that, in the context of the right conditions, people enjoy their work; can show self-control and discipline; are able to contribute creatively; and are motivated by ties to the group, the organization, and the work itself. In essence, this view espouses the belief that people are intrinsically motivated by their work. Theory Y was a guide for managers to take advantage of the potential of each person, which Mc-Gregor thought was being only partially utilized, and to provide support and encouragement to employees to do good work (McGregor, 1960).

OUCHI'S THEORY Z

Theory Z was developed by William Ouchi (1981) based on his years studying organizations in Japan. He identified that Japanese organizations had better productivity than organizations in the United States and that they were managed differently, through their use of quality circles, to pursue better productivity and quality. Theory Z focuses on a better way of motivating people through their involvement. Collective decision making is a hallmark of Theory Z, as is a focus on long-term employment that involves slower promotions and less direct supervision.

The organization and the worker are viewed more holistically. Through progressive development, the organization will be productive, and quality goals will be achieved. The organization invests in its employees and addresses both home and work issues, creating a path for career development. Democratic leaders, who are skilled in interpersonal relations, foster employee involvement (Ouchi, 1981).

THE CHANGING NATURE OF MANAGERIAL WORK

Current trends indicate that the number of managers in an organization, particularly at the middle level, is being reduced and that downsizing of staff has been a common phenomenon in most health care institutions across Canada. Hospitals are increasingly adopting structures with wider managerial spans of control (Pillai & Meindl, 1998; Spence Laschinger, Sabiston, Finegan, & Shamian, 2001), creating dramatic changes in the work environment and significantly affecting the relationship between nurses and managers. Blythe, Baumann, and Giovannetti (2001) found that as a result of an increased span of control, relations between managers and nurses became distant, and communications became less frequent and more formal. After reorganizations, those left in management positions are fewer in number and have taken on more responsibility over more areas, thereby increasing their respective spans of control.

As individual nurses become more involved in managing consumer relations and consumer care, managers will become managers of systems rather than managers of nurses per se. This shift will represent significant training and coaching as the role of the direct practice nurse evolves to integrate the managing of consumer relations and care. The nurse manager will be key as a change agent in managing the change process and sustaining the outcomes. As system managers, nurses will manage clinical systems, cost information systems, and data systems on consumer satisfaction and feedback.

Leadership responsibilities will be integrated among all organizational participants who function as **knowledge workers** and provide their professional expertise. This vision of true inter-professional practice will require all practitioners "to operate from a framework of trust, respect, authenticity, collaboration and common interest problem solving to effect positive outcomes for our mutual clients and our community of practitioners" (Doucette, 2006). Knowledge workers are those involved in serving others through their specialized knowledge. Among nurses, this specialized knowledge is the science of nursing, which is transacted via practice and art to serve clients and their families. Porter-O'Grady (2003) hypothesizes that knowledge has become the new currency, changing the traditional relationship between worker and employer, and between what people know and how they translate it into innovations and practices of work critical to the continuing viability of the organization. For now and for the immediate future, leadership responsibilities need to be dispersed among all nurses, who are knowledge workers by virtue of their professional nursing expertise.

DEFINITION OF LEADERSHIP

Leadership is commonly defined as a process of influence in which the leader influences others toward goal achievement (Yukl, 1998). Influence is an instrumental part of leadership and refers to a leader's ability to affect others, often by inspiring, enlivening, and engaging them to participate. The process of leadership involves the leader and the follower in interaction, which implies that leadership is a reciprocal relationship. Leadership can occur between the leader and another individual; between the leader and a group; or between a leader and an organization, a community, or a society. Defining leadership as a process helps us to understand more about leadership than the traditional view of a leader as a person in a position of authority, exerting command, control, and power over subordinates.

As professionals, nurses function as leaders when they influence others toward goal achievement. Nurses are leaders. There are many more leaders in organizations than those people who are in positions of authority. Each person has the potential to serve as a leader. In the nursing literature, definitions of the term *nursing leader* are highly varied. Definitions have reflected either a centring on the process or on the individual leader. Dunham and Klafehn (1990) defined a leader as an individual with decision-making capacity, shared values with nurses, a vision, and the ability to inspire others to work toward this vision. McCloskey and McCain (1987) and Huber et al. (2000) defined leadership as a process whereby the leader's role is to influence nurses to accomplish the goals of the organization. Fagin (1996) contended that nursing leaders are people who (a) have demonstrated skill in managing; (b) influence others in the advancement of the profession; (c) possess interpersonal skills within and outside the discipline; (d) have impressive publications; and (e) maintain an imposing reputation. Edwards (1994) saw nursing leadership as playing a central role in spearheading changes, predicting that "Two of the foremost tasks of a new nursing leadership will be to raise the consciousness of nurses through an ongoing critique of the present system and to offer philosophical and practical rationales for fundamental change based on nursing values and the central role that nursing plans in the health care process" (Edwards, 1994).

Leadership in nursing can take two forms; namely, formal and informal leadership. **Formal leadership,** describes a person in a position of authority or in a sanctioned, assigned role within an organization that connotes influence, such as a clinical nurse specialist (Northouse, 2001). Other formal leadership roles are nurse managers, acute care nurse practitioners, and professional practice leaders. An **informal leader** is an individual who demonstrates leadership outside the scope of a formal leadership role or as a member of a group rather than as the head or leader of the group. The informal leader is considered to have emerged as a leader when she is accepted by others and is perceived to have influence.

It is important to understand that not all leaders are managers but Manthey (1990) asserts that all managers need to be leaders. Another way to define leadership is through the differentiation of leadership and management (Zalenik, 1977). Bennis's work on differentiating the characteristics of managers versus leaders popularized the phrase "Managers are people who do things right and leaders are people who do the right thing" (Bennis & Nanus, 1985, p. 21).

Kotter (1990a) describes the differences between leadership and management in the following way: Leadership is about creating change, and management is about controlling complexity in an effort to bring order and consistency. According to Kotter, leading change involves establishing a direction, aligning people through empowerment, and motivating and inspiring them toward producing useful change and achieving the vision; whereas management is defined as planning and budgeting, organizing and staffing, problemsolving, and controlling complexity to produce predictability and order (Kotter, 1990b).

LEADERSHIP CHARACTERISTICS

According to Bennis and Nanus (1985), effective leaders share three fundamental qualities. The first quality is a guiding vision. A vision statement outlines what an organization wants to be and focuses on tomorrow (i.e., the preferred future); it is inspirational (i.e., it has reach) and provides a reference point to guide the nature of all decision making (Industry Canada, 2004). Nursing leaders focus on a professional and purposeful vision that provides direction toward the preferred future. The second quality is passion. Passion, as expressed by the leader, involves the ability to inspire and align people toward the

REAL WORLD INTERVIEW

At the Brant Community Healthcare System, Brantford, Ontario, we believe that nurses are critical to successful client-centered care, positive client outcomes, and effective inter-professional practice. As a result, we are committed to leadership development for nurses. With financial support from the Ministry of Health and Long-Term Care, we have designed and implemented an internship program for our new graduate nurses. This six-month preceptor program provides opportunities for general and specialized clinical knowledge transfer regarding the complexities of acute care and professional practice. A preceptor for each new graduate provides leadership, support, and guidance for being a professional and competent nurse. This new program is positioned for success as it is focused on socializing, educating, and developing competencies among our nursing graduates to help them to succeed and advance in our organization.

Mary K. Stewart
Vice President, Patient, CNO Services

promises of life. The third quality is integrity that is based on knowledge of self, honesty, and maturity, which is developed through experience and growth. McCall (1998) describes how self-awareness—knowing our strengths and weaknesses—can allow us to use feedback and learn from our mistakes. Daring and curiosity are also basic ingredients of leadership, which leaders draw on to take risks, learning from what works as much as from what doesn't work (Bennis & Nanus, 1985).

A requirement for all nursing leaders is Olympic thinking, which requires all nursing leaders to nurture an inspiriting vision of the preferred future, maintain a burning desire (i.e., a passion), and implement purposeful action towards vision achievement. To be a leader who lacks any one of these Olympic thinking elements is to be a leader who daydreams of the preferred future. Kraus (2006) asserts that research in sports psychology has shown that visualization can enhance success and performance (i.e., achievement of vision), and parallel research in positive psychology has confirmed that visualization can enhance success in everyday life, making it a valuable tool for those interested in motivation, self-help, and self-improvement. Kraus reports that visualization enhances confidence, boosts motivation, and engages the individual in a practice or discipline that keeps the leader focused on vision achievement.

Certain characteristics are commonly attributed to leaders. These traits are considered desirable and seem to contribute to the perception of being a leader. They include intelligence, self-confidence, determination, integrity, and sociability (Stodgill, 1948, 1974). Research among 46 hospitals designated as magnet hospitals for their success in attracting and retaining registered nurses emphasized the value of leaders who are visionary and enthusiastic, supportive and knowledgeable, have high standards and expectations, value education and professional development, demonstrate power and status in the organization, are visible and responsive, communicate openly, and are active in professional associations (Kramer & Schmalenberg, 1988; McClure, Poulin, Sovie, & Wandelt, 1983; Scott, Sochalski, & Aiken, 1999). Research findings from studies of nurses revealed that a caring nature, respectability, trustworthiness, and flexibility were the leader characteristics most valued. In one study, nurse leaders identified leadership characteristics as managing the dream, mastering change, designing organization structure, learning, and taking initiative (Murphy & DeBack, 1991). Research by Kirkpatrick and Locke (1991) concluded that leaders are different from non-leaders across six traits: drive, the desire to lead, honesty and integrity, self-confidence, cognitive ability, and knowledge of the business. Although no set of traits is definitive and reliable in determining who is a leader or who is effective as a leader, many people still rely on personality traits to describe and define leaders.

Another critically important leadership trait that is surfacing in the nursing literature is that of **emotional intelligence,** or EI. Salovey and Mayer (1990) describe EI as the ability both to recognize the meaning of emotions and their relationships and to reason and solve problems on the basis of emotions. Goleman (2006) further explored the concept of EI and hypothesized that EI can be learned and improves with age. Current studies consistently demonstrate that EI is the common trait or factor that distinguishes individuals as leaders, innovators, and effective managers.

The emotionally intelligent nurse will be obvious in the practice environment as the nurse who can identify, use, and regulate emotions to maximize critical thinking, resulting in sound decisions that support both positive outcomes and inter-professional collaboration in client care. As the complexities in practice and the delivery of care intensify, nursing leaders will need to guide with their heads and heart and to foster inter-professional practice, which is underpinned with teamwork, collaboration, high-quality client-centred care and positive outcomes for clients. This requirement of all nursing leaders amplifies the need for all nurses to maintain emotional awareness to develop and maintain emotional intelligence.

FACTORS THAT INFLUENCE THE QUALITY OF NURSING LEADERSHIP

Nursing history, education, use of self, organization structure and power, and organizational redesign are all factors that have contributed to the evolution of nursing leadership. Each will be examined briefly for its major contribution to the evolution of nursing leadership.

Nursing leadership has a strong and rich history with deep roots in both religious and military ground (Girvan, 1996). Meighan (1990) describes the influence that nursing's military roots played in the continuation of a command-and-control approach to achieve conformity in practice. The cost of this approach was the further distancing of nurses at the front line from decision making related to client care. Although the paradigm has shifted from controlling to empowering nurses to practise to their full scope, the change has not been a simple undertaking and has evolved in the face of hospital restructuring, new program reporting structures, and a mismatch between the demand and supply of nurses.

Nursing leaders must be lifelong learners with a thirst for knowledge and a desire to maintain and enhance leadership competencies. To effectively manage in chaotic and complex practice environments, leaders must be comfortable with and aware of the constant need for change, possess budget and financial skills, and remain committed to team building through effective management of personal growth (Gelinas and Manthey, 1997). The concept of future professional growth and

mentoring of nurse leaders has been the centrepiece in a number of continuing educational programs. Stordeur et al. (2000) investigated the idea that role modelling of transformational leadership behaviour would have a cascading effect on lower level managers. However, the study did not hold this hypothesis to be true, and Stordeur suggested that purposeful and coordinated effort was needed to provide leadership development and education to potential future nurse leaders. Dunham-Taylor (1995) found the idea that leadership competencies could be learned, and suggested that preceptorship, mentoring, and education are key strategies for the development of future nursing leaders.

The use of self is a strong factor that influences the quality of leadership. Upenicks (2003) argued that some specific leader attributes may be more effective than others in creating environments that lead to positive outcomes for nurses. In a study conducted with senior nurse executives, Upenicks concluded that a passion for nursing and the ability to articulate this passion to nurses and other members of the administration were coupled with leadership effectiveness and support of nursing. Nursing research has also demonstrated a strong link between the emotional intelligence (EI) of leaders and the success of an organization. The concept of EI was explored in the leadership characteristics discussed earlier in this chapter. The concept of self and the ability to transact self in an effective and authentic manner directly contributes to the quality of leadership.

Leaders must function in various practice environments where the characteristics of structure and power play a role in the quality of leadership. Variation of leadership styles is affected by the organizational structure and culture (i.e., the context) of the organization (Stordeur et al., 2000). Upenicks's study (2003) of nurse leaders from magnet and non-magnet hospitals confirmed that access to power, opportunity, information, and resources created an empowered environment with a climate that fosters leadership success and enhanced levels of job satisfaction among nurses. Upenicks also suggested that nurse leaders could have more power and credibility among peer executives if they learned how to think as professionals do in the business world.

Organizational redesign has been a major influence on the quality of nursing leadership. Nursing leaders have not only been changed by redesign but in the process of changing they have also had to lead the redesign of clinical care, delivery systems, and integrated care (Gelinas & Manthey, 1997). Leatt and Porter (2003) described the need for nursing leaders to have an ability to work effectively across disciplines given the increased emphasis on interdisciplinary team-based care, which is prevalent in health care organizational redesign. Tim Porter-O'Grady (2003) asserts that a new leadership role requires new skill sets. In our progress towards the preferred future, Porter-O'Grady espouses a need for leaders who are able to help others, see the need for change, challenge past practices, create a vision for the future, and construct new models for service delivery. Smith et al. (1994) describe the need for nurse leaders to have knowledge of nursing practice, but also to understand regulatory issues and business skills, and to have an understanding of risk, liability, strategic planning, and political acumen.

LEADERSHIP THEORIES

Many believe that the critical factor needed to maximize human resources is leadership (Bennis & Nanus, 1985). A more in-depth understanding of leadership can be gleaned from a review of leadership theories. The major leadership theories can be classified according to the following approaches: behavioural, contingency, and contemporary.

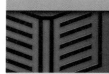

LITERATURE APPLICATION

Citation: Allen, D. W. (1998). How nurses become leaders: Perceptions and beliefs about leadership development. *Journal of Nursing Administration, 28*(9), 15–20.

Discussion: This article presents the factors that influence the development of leadership skills in nurses and the successful transition from a staff nurse role to a leadership role. Twelve registered nurses who had been in leadership positions for 9 to 29 years were interviewed. A core set of questions was used as a guide, followed by additional questions that helped to clarify misunderstanding of the answers provided. Five dominant factors were identified that greatly influenced the nurses' leadership development: (1) self-confidence; (2) innate leader qualities/tendencies; (3) progression of experiences and success; (4) influence of significant others; and (5) personal life factors. For most of the nurses, at least one individual fostered their sense of self-confidence through reinforcement and positive feedback. Education provided the participants with skills and knowledge that also contributed to their self-confidence. Innate leader qualities, going back as far as childhood, also contributed significantly to their leadership development. For example, most of the interviewed nurses, at some point in their life, were team captains or class officers. According to the author, a pattern of progressively successful experiences also emerged as a significant factor in leadership development. Education, especially when focused on leadership and management, provided the participants with new skills useful in their advancement. Mentors who recognized the strengths of the participants were able to improve their self-confidence and create opportunities for learning. Personal life factors, such as needing to work during the day shift or not being able to perform physically strenuous activities, led some of the participants to pursue nursing leadership and management. The factors that contributed to the development of these nurses were interconnected and promoted their gradual development as leaders.

Implications for Practice: Although many individual and environmental factors contribute to leadership development, each nurse can actively participate in designing and implementing a leadership development plan that facilitates forward progression of competence development and enhancement (i.e., from novice to expert). An important avenue of growth is acquiring a mentor, who can help to create a progression of experiences that develop leadership skills and judgment in working with other people and who can coach the importance of examining "the self" aspect of leadership quality. Coaching provides a powerful space between two individuals (i.e., the coach and the coachee), where an honest exploration of needs, motivations, desires, skills, and thought processes can be examined through the use of questioning techniques to facilitate critical thinking. Ultimately, coaching encourages commitment to action and the development of lasting personal growth and change. Pursuing education to learn new skills that involve leadership behaviours and management practices is another excellent way to develop into a nurse leader. Nursing associations, unions, specialty nursing groups, and the Canadian Nursing Students' Association are valuable training grounds for leadership. Nationally, the Canadian Nurses Association (CNA) has facilitated the exchange of knowledge through discussion papers, policy statements, think tanks, and its co-sponsorship of two national conferences: the Nursing Leadership Conference and the Health Care Middle Management Conference. The International Council of Nurses (ICN) also supports leadership development through projects such as its Leadership for Change program. These observations suggest the profound importance of leadership training and the need for a multi-level approach that begins with the individual nurse and moves to a global commitment as spearheaded by the ICN. Sharing a desire to change and improve nursing practice with others, through participation in professional nursing associations, is another important vehicle for development as a leader and a professional.

BEHAVIOURAL APPROACHES

Leadership studies from the 1930s by Kurt Lewin and colleagues at Iowa State University conveyed information about three leadership styles that are still widely recognized today: autocratic, democratic, and laissez-faire leadership (Lewin, 1939; Lewin & Lippitt, 1938; Lewin, Lippitt, & White, 1939). **Autocratic leadership** involves centralized decision making, with the leader making decisions and using power to command and control others. **Democratic leadership** is participatory, with authority delegated to others. To be influential, the democratic leader uses expert power and the power base afforded by having close, personal relationships. The third style, **laissez-faire leadership,** is passive and permissive, and the leader defers decision making. Lewin (1939) contrasted these styles and concluded that autocratic leaders were associated with high-performing groups but that close supervision was necessary and feelings of hostility were often present. Democratic leaders engendered positive feelings in their groups, and performance was strong, whether or not the leader was present. Low productivity and feelings of frustration were associated with laissez-faire leaders.

Behavioural leadership studies from the University of Michigan and from Ohio State University led to the identification of two basic leader behaviours: job-centred and employee-centred behaviours. Effective leadership was described as having a focus on the human needs of subordinates and was called **employee-centred leadership** (Moorhead & Griffin, 2001). **Job-centred leaders** were seen as less effective because of their focus on schedules, costs, and efficiency, resulting in a lack of attention to developing work groups and high-performance goals (Moorhead & Griffin, 2001).

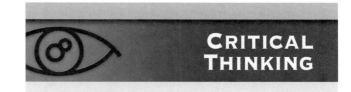

CRITICAL THINKING

Among the individuals commonly identified as leaders (Table 8-3), can you identify a set of traits that they all possess or traits that are associated with them? Are they perceived as leaders because they are characterized as having intelligence, self-confidence, determination, integrity, and charisma? What other traits do (did) they have?

The researchers at Ohio State focused their efforts on two dimensions of leader behaviour: initiating structure and consideration. **Initiating structure** involves an emphasis on the work to be done, a focus on the task and production. Leaders who focus on initiating structure are concerned with how work is organized and on the achievement of goals. This type of leader behaviour includes planning, directing others, and establishing the deadlines and details of how work is to be done. For example, a nurse demonstrating the leader behaviour of initiating structure could be a charge nurse who, at the beginning of a shift, sets up a client assignment.

The dimension of **consideration** involves activities that focus on the employee and emphasize relating to and getting along with people. This leader behaviour focuses on the well-being of others. The leader is involved in creating a relationship that fosters communication and trust as a basis for respecting other people and their

TABLE 8-3	**LEADERS AMONG US: PAST AND PRESENT**
Mother Teresa	Martin Luther King Jr.
Alexander Graham Bell	Sir John A. MacDonald
Chief Dan George	Mahatma Gandhi
Tiger Woods	Terry Fox
Roméo Dallaire	Florence Nightingale
Colin Powell	Pierre Elliott Trudeau
Pope John Paul II	Lester B. Pearson
Chris Hadfield	Joan of Arc
Frances Hesselbein	Julius Caesar
Margaret Thatcher	Alexander the Great
Henry Kissinger	Cleopatra
Nelson Mandela	The Queen

potential contribution. A nurse demonstrating consideration will take the time to talk with coworkers, be empathetic, and show an interest in others as people.

The leader behaviours of initiating structure and consideration define leadership style. The styles are as follows:

- Low initiating structure, low consideration
- High initiating structure, low consideration
- High initiating structure, high consideration
- Low initiating structure, high consideration

The Ohio State University studies associate the high initiating structure–high consideration leader behaviours with better performance and higher satisfaction outcomes than the other styles. This leadership style is considered effective, although it is not appropriate in every situation.

Another model based on these two dimensions is the managerial grid developed by Blake and Mouton (1985). Five styles identify the extent of structure, called concern for production, and the extent of consideration, called concern for people, demonstrated by the leader. The five leadership styles are the impoverished leader (1,1) for low production and low people concern; the authority compliance leader (9,1) for high production concern and low people concern; the country club leader (1,9) for high people concern but low production concern; the middle-of-the-road leader (5,5) for moderate concern in both dimensions; and the team leader (9,9) for high production and people concern. Figure 8-2 shows the leadership grid with the dimensions of people and production from low to high on a scale from 1 to 9. Team management (9,9) is usually a more effective leadership approach than an overemphasis on either concern for people or concern for production.

CONTINGENCY APPROACHES

Another approach to leadership is **contingency theory.** Contingency theory acknowledges that other factors in the environment influence outcomes as much as leadership style and that leader effectiveness is contingent upon,

or depends upon, something other than the leader's behaviour. The premise is that different leader behaviour patterns will be effective in different situations. Contingency approaches include Fielder's contingency theory, the situational theory of Hersey and Blanchard, path-goal theory, and the idea of substitutes for leadership.

Fielder's Contingency Theory. Fielder (1967) is credited with the development of the contingency model of leadership effectiveness. Fielder's theory of leadership effectiveness views the pattern of leader behaviour as dependent upon the interaction of the personality of the leader and the needs of the situation. The needs of the situation or how favourable the situation is toward the leader involves leader–member relationships, the degree of task structure, and the leader's position of power (Fielder, 1967). **Leader–member relations** are the feelings and attitudes of followers regarding acceptance, trust, and credibility of the leader. Good leader–member relations exist when followers respect, trust, and have confidence in the leader. Poor leader–member relations reflect distrust, a lack of confidence and respect, and dissatisfaction with the leader by the followers.

Task structure refers to the degree to which work is defined, with specific procedures, explicit directions, and measurable goals. High task structure involves routine, predictable, clearly defined work tasks. Low task structure involves work that is not routine, predictable, or clearly defined, such as creative, artistic, or qualitative research activities.

Position power is the degree of formal authority and influence associated with the leader. High position power is favourable for the leader, whereas low position power is unfavourable. When all of these dimensions—leader–member relations, task structure, and position power—are high, the situation is favourable to the leader. When these dimensions are low, the situation is not favourable to the leader. In both of these circumstances, Fielder showed that a task-directed leader concerned with task accomplishment was effective. When the range of favourableness is intermediate or moderate, a human relations leader who was concerned about people was most effective. These situations need interpersonal and relationship skills to foster group achievement. Fielder's contingency theory is an approach that matches the organizational situation to the most favourable leadership style for that situation.

HERSEY AND BLANCHARD'S SITUATIONAL THEORY

Situational leadership theory addresses follower characteristics in relation to effective leader behaviour. Whereas Blake and Mouton focus on leader style and Fielder examines the situation, Hersey and Blanchard consider follower readiness as a factor in determining leadership style. Rather than using the words *initiating structure* and *contingency,* they use *task behaviour* and *relationship behaviour.*

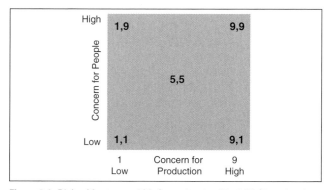

Figure 8-2 Blake, Mouton, and McCanse Leadership Grid. (From Leadership: Theory, Application, Skill Building [p. 75], by R. N. Lussier and C. F. Achua, 2001, Cincinnati, OH: South-Western College.)

High task behaviour and low relationship behaviour is called a telling leadership style. A high task, high relationship style is called a selling leadership style. A low task and high relationship style is called a participating leadership style. A low task and low relationship style is called a delegating leadership style.

Follower readiness, called job maturity, is assessed in order to select one of the four leadership styles for a situation. Consequently, nursing leaders must be able to assess the job maturity levels of individual nurses and match the leadership style of the nurse to the context of the situation. Regardless of an individual staff member's maturity level, some situations require the leader to adapt a telling style, as is the case with situations involving client safety or significant infractions of professional standards or practice regulations. According to Hersey and Blanchard's situational leadership theory (2000), groups with low maturity, whose members are unable or unwilling to participate or are unsure, need a leader to use a telling leadership style to provide direction and close supervision. This same style serves preceptors well, as they take on largely instructional roles with new graduates who have a limited basis of clinical experiences and are still working to master clinical competencies. The selling leadership style is a match for groups with low to moderate maturity who are unable but willing and confident and need clear direction and supportive feedback to get the task done. This type of leadership style may serve nurse leaders well in their efforts to launch new programs or revamp care delivery processes. The selling style serves the nurse leader well in promoting professional practice and practice development with nurses at the advanced beginner or competent levels, as described by Benner (1984). Participating is the leadership style recommended for groups with moderate to high maturity who are able but unwilling or are unsure and who need support and encouragement. The leader should use a delegating style with groups of followers with high maturity who are able and ready to participate and can engage in the task without direction or support. Nurses who have developed their practice, within their chosen domain, to the proficient and expert levels, therefore demonstrating both ability and willingness, may benefit from a delegational leadership style from their respective nurse managers.

An additional aspect of this model is the idea that the leader not only changes leadership style according to the followers' needs but also develops followers over time to increase their level of maturity (Lussier & Achua, 2001). Use of these four leadership styles helps a nurse manager to appropriately assign work to others and provide a trajectory for individual professional development.

PATH-GOAL THEORY   In this leadership approach, the leader works to motivate followers and influence goal accomplishment. The seminal author on path-goal theory is Robert House (1971). By using the appropriate style of leadership for the situation (i.e., directive, supportive, participative, or achievement-oriented), the leader makes the path toward the goal easier for the follower. The directive style of leadership provides structure through direction and authority, with the leader focusing on the task and getting the job done. The supportive style of leadership is relationship-oriented, with the leader providing encouragement, interest, and attention. Participative leadership means that the leader focuses on involving followers in the decision-making process. The achievement-oriented style provides high structure and direction as well as high support through consideration behaviour. The leadership style is matched to the situational characteristics of the followers, such as the desire for authority, the extent to which the control of goal achievement is internal or external, and the ability of the follower to be involved. The leadership style is also matched to the situational factors in the environment, including the routine nature or complexity of the task, the power associated with the leader's position, and the work group relationship. This alignment of leadership style with the needs of followers is motivating and is believed to enhance performance and satisfaction. The path-goal theory is based on expectancy theory, which holds that people are motivated when they believe they are able to carry out the work and when they think their contribution will lead to the expected outcome and that the rewards for their efforts are valued and meaningful (Northouse, 2001).

SUBSTITUTES FOR LEADERSHIP   **Substitutes for leadership** are variables that may influence followers to the same extent as the leader's behaviour. Kerr and Jermier (1978) investigated situational variables and identified some aspects as substitutes that eliminate the need for leader behaviour and other aspects as neutralizers that nullify the effects of the leader's behaviour.

Some of these variables include follower characteristics, such as the presence of structured routine tasks, the amount of feedback provided by the task, and the presence of intrinsic satisfaction in the work; other variables include organizational characteristics, such as the presence of a cohesive group, a formal organization, a rigid adherence to rules, and low position power. For example, an individual's experience can substitute for task-direction leader behaviour (Kerr & Jermier, 1978). Nurses and other professionals with a great deal of experience already have knowledge and judgment and do not need direction and supervision to perform their work. Thus, their experience serves as a leadership substitute. Another substitute for leader behaviour is intrinsic satisfaction that emerges from just doing the work. Intrinsic satisfaction occurs frequently among nurses when they provide care to clients and their families. Intrinsic satisfaction substitutes for the support and encouragement of relationship-oriented leader behaviour.

CONTEMPORARY APPROACHES

Contemporary approaches to leadership address the leadership functions necessary to develop learning organizations and lead the process of transforming change. These approaches include charismatic leadership and transformational leadership theory.

CHARISMATIC THEORY

A charismatic leader has an inspirational quality that promotes an emotional connection from followers. House (1977) developed a theory of charismatic leadership that described how charismatic leaders behave, their distinguishing characteristics, and situations in which such leaders would be effective. Charismatic leaders display self-confidence and strength in their convictions, and communicate high expectations and their confidence in others. They have been described as emerging during a crisis, communicating vision, and using personal power and unconventional strategies (Conger & Kanungo, 1987). One consequence of this type of leadership is a belief in the charismatic leader that is so strong it takes on an almost supernatural purpose, and the leader is worshipped as if superhuman. Worship can take both positive and negative forms. Examples of charismatic leaders who have been worshipped by some include Martin Luther King Jr., Sir Winston Churchill, and Jim Jones.

Charismatic leaders can have a positive and powerful effect on people and organizations. Lee Iacocca, former chief executive officer (CEO) of Chrysler Corporation, and the former CEO of Southwest Airlines, Herb Kelleher, are described as effective charismatic leaders. This type of leader can contribute significantly to an organization, even though all the leaders in an organization are not charismatic leaders and effective leaders do not exhibit all the qualities associated with charismatic leadership. Charisma seems to be a special and valuable quality that some people have and some people do not. Whether charismatic or not, leaders must be self-confident, energetic, knowledgeable, articulate, passionate, and honest. These are just a few of the character traits of charismatic leaders, and although not all effective leaders are charismatic, many have integrated various charismatic traits into their leadership style. This approach is critical to success, given today's complex and chaotic practice environments.

TRANSFORMATIONAL LEADERSHIP THEORY

Burns defined transformational leadership as a process in which "leaders and followers raise one another to higher levels of motivation and morality" (Burns, 1978, p. 21). Transformational leadership theory is based on the idea of empowering others to engage in pursuing a collective purpose by working together to achieve a vision of a preferred future. This kind of leadership can influence both the leader and the follower to a higher level of conduct and achievement that transforms them both (Burns, 1978). Burns maintained that there are two types of leaders: the traditional manager concerned with day-to-day operations, called the **transactional leader,** and the leader who is committed to a vision that empowers others, called the **transformational leader.**

Transformational leaders motivate others by behaving in accordance with values, providing a vision that reflects mutual values, and empowering others to contribute. Bennis and Nanus (1985) describe this new leader as a leader who "commits people to action, who converts followers into leaders, and who converts leaders into agents of change" (p. 3). According to research by Tichy and Devanna (1986), effective transformational leaders identify themselves as change agents; are courageous; believe in people; are value-driven; are lifelong

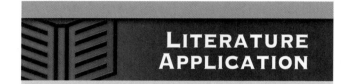

LITERATURE APPLICATION

Citation: Levi, P. (1999). Sustainability of healthcare environments. *Image: Journal of Nursing Scholarship, 31*(4), 395–398.

Discussion: Will nursing play a significant role in advancing the future of health care? Using indicators such as access to care, infant mortality, children's health, and statistics on children living in poverty, the author questions whether nursing, as a profession with more than 2.6 million members, will be instrumental in influencing policies to address these issues. The author identifies transitions occurring in the health care industry, including shifts from hospital dominance to care delivery in the community, from acute care to community-based and alternative care, from disease management to prevention, screening, and detection. These changes, along with advancing technologies from molecular and genetic research, are cornerstones in advancing our knowledge and changing health care practices.

Implications for Practice: The author calls for a strong culture of nursing in which nurses are socialized to succeed in a more complex environment. To have a significant role in the future of health care, nursing needs to encourage transformational leaders who create safe, effective, and ethical environments and nurses who involve themselves in forming and speaking out about health policy that continues to centre the client as the central reason for service delivery.

learners; have the ability to deal with complexity, ambiguity, and uncertainty; and are visionaries. Transformational leadership may be demonstrated by anyone in an organization regardless of a person's position (Burns, 1978). The interaction that occurs between individuals can be transformational and motivate both the leader and the follower to a higher level of performance (Bass, 1985).

Transformational leadership at the organizational level is about innovation and change. The transformational leader uses a vision based on shared values to align people and inspire growth and advancement. Both the inspiration and the empowerment aspects of transformational leadership lead to a commitment beyond self-interest, a commitment to a vision, and a commitment to action that creates change. Transformational leadership theory suggests that the relationship between the leader and the follower inspires and empowers an individual toward a commitment to the organization.

Nurse researchers have described nurse executives according to transformational leadership theory and have used this theory to measure leadership behaviour among nurse executives and nurse managers (Dunham & Klafehn, 1990; Dunham-Taylor, 1995, 2000; Leach, 2000; McDaniel & Wolf, 1992; McNeese-Smith, 1995; Trofino, 1995; Wolf, Boland, & Aukerman, 1994; Young, 1992). Additionally, transformational leadership theory has been the basis for nursing administration curricula and for investigation of relationships such as between a nurse's commitment to an organization and productivity in a hospital setting (Leach, 2000; McNeese-Smith, 1997; Searle, 1996). Cassidy and Koroll (1998) explored the ethical aspects of transformational leadership, and Barker (1990) comprehensively discussed nursing in terms of transformational leadership theory. Of the contemporary theories of leadership, transformational leadership has been a popular approach in nursing.

KOUZES AND POSNER'S FIVE LEADERSHIP PRACTICES

Kouzes and Posner's five leadership practices continue to gain popularity as a leadership model that underpins many leadership development training programs. Kouzes has found that people look for four characteristics in a leader. "First, people want a leader who is honest, trustworthy and has integrity. Second, people also want a leader who is forward looking, who has a vision of the future, foresight and thinks about the long term. Third, people want a leader who is competent, has expertise, knows what they are doing and last, is inspiring, dynamic, energetic, optimistic and positive about the future" (Kouzes & Posner, 2002). The five practices defined by Kouzes and Posner are 1) model the way; 2) inspire a shared vision; 3) challenge the process; 4) enable others

to act; and 5) encourage the heart. Modeling the way is about being authentic and true to your values and aligning actions with shared values. Inspiring a shared vision focuses the leader's attention to envision the future by imagining exciting and enabling possibilities and by enlisting others so that the vision is common to all and is appealing to the notion of shared aspirations. Challenging the process calls to the forefront the leader's sense of self, courage, risk-taking, and EI, as the leader searches for ways to change, grow, and improve. Recognizing the influence of structure and process (i.e., organizational context/structure), it is often difficult but necessary to challenge the established process, especially if that process is not in the best interests of professional practice and client-focused care. Enabling others to act is a transformational activity associated with quality leadership. Enabling others requires the manager to foster collaboration by promoting cooperative goals and building trust. In addition, the leader must strengthen individuals by sharing power and discretion (e.g., sharing decision making, delegation, critical thinking, and professional judgment). This requirement is pivotal to the success of interprofessional practice teams. Given the theories of motivation, Kouzes and Posner wrap up the five leadership practices with a commitment to encourage the heart. To create and sustain the effects of quality leadership, leaders must recognize the contributions of individuals by showing appreciation for individual excellence. Although many leaders ascribe to the current axiom, "there is no I in the word team," a fine balance exists between the need for individual and team recognition. Finally, encouraging the heart takes the form of celebrations of success and fostering a spirit of community. Collectively these five practices comprise what Kouzes and Posner call the "leadership challenge."

NURSING LEADERSHIP AND OUTCOMES

Snow (2001) commented that nursing has not kept pace with other industries in exploring the relationship between leadership and performance. The complexity of client care environments and the number of uncontrollable factors that exist may affect the ability of nursing researchers to design quality research initiatives that examine true cause-and-effect relationships between leadership and outcomes.

George et al. (2002) examined how the implementation of a shared leadership model influenced staff leadership behaviours and autonomy, and improved client outcomes. The intervention took the form of an educational series called the shared leadership concept program (SLCP), which consisted of four 8-hour-day mod-ules delivered over a period of two months. Three studies were completed between 1995 and 1999 by George et al. Each study used a different design, with the final study using a qualitative design with key information interviews. Interviews were conducted at three, six, and twelve months following the SLCP. Three key findings were reported: 1) an increase in nurse perception that leadership behaviour improved their ability to meet client needs and promoted faster recovery; 2) barriers to use of leadership skills in-cluded increased workloads, boring work, insufficient goal setting by managers, high turnover, and lack of responsi-bility; and 3) after completing the program, nurses were more assertive in addressing the barriers.

Perhaps one of the most important studies to date, which embodied both qualitative and quantitative approaches to examine the contextual factors influencing the delivery of nursing care, was described by Houser (2003). Analysis of themes from the interviews demon-strated the most common desirable leadership traits were excellent communication skills and an ability to articulate clear expectations and problem-solving skills. Most excit-ing about this study are the findings from the quantitative component that used the Leadership Practices Inventory (LPI) developed by Kouzes and Posner. Key findings sug-gest a positive relationship between strong leadership and staff expertise and stability. An inverse relationship was discovered between strong levels of expertise and negative client outcomes, such as hospital-acquired pneumonia and urinary tract infections, mortality, medication errors, and client falls. This study suggests strong committed leaders are required to develop professional leadership skills among staff and to guide professional development to impact positively on the expertise of staff.

Anderson, Issel, and McDaniel (2003) also made a significant contribution to the understanding of the rela-tionship between leadership and client outcomes. Their research in a long-term care environment focused on perceptions of open communication and participation in decision making. The client outcomes measured were resident behaviour, immobility complications, fractures, and restraint use. Correlations existed between larger facilities with experienced directors of nursing (DONs) who had good communication skills and a lower use of restraints. Experienced DONs with more experience and greater relationship-oriented leadership had a lower prevalence of complications associated with immobility. Finally, organizations with a relationship-oriented leader had a lower prevalence of fractures. Based on the work of these three nursing researchers, a relationship between nursing leadership and client outcomes has been demon-strated. However, further research is required to fully appreciate the extent of the relationship.

The emergence of the magnet hospital concept as originally described by Kramer and Schmalenberg (1988) has significantly facilitated nurse researchers to examine the relationship between leadership and nurse outcomes. Nurse outcomes include control over practice, autonomy, a culture of valuing nurses, and job satisfaction. The rela-tionship between leadership and nurse outcomes has been supported in current research work in both magnet and non-magnet hospitals (Aiken et al., 2001). A significant pos-itive relationship between head nurses exhibiting transfor-mational leadership style and job satisfaction was demon-strated in a descriptive study by Medley and Larochelle (1995). Spence Laschinger et al. (1999) implemented a de-scriptive study in a recently merged health care facility and explored the link between leader-empowering behaviours and staff nurse perceptions of workplace empowerment. Results suggested that staff believed their sense of work-place empowerment, job tensions, and judgment of their ability to get their work completed were related to the man-ager's use of empowering behaviours.

Kouzes and Posner's five leadership behaviours and their impact on job satisfaction, productivity and commit-ment were examined by Chiok Foong Loke (2001). Statistically significant differences were found between the managers' use of the five behaviours and employee out-comes of satisfaction, productivity, and organizational com-mitment. Kramer and Schmalenberg (2003) identified that clinical competence supports autonomous practice and that leadership is essential to facilitate personal growth op-portunities, which enhance maintenance of competence. McGillis Hall et al. (2001) demonstrated a statistically sig-nificant positive relationship between leadership and job satisfaction and a statistically negative influence on nurses' perception of job stress, role tension, and job pressure.

FUTURE DIRECTIONS

The organizations that nurses are a part of are constantly changing, and care delivery is increasing in its acuity and complexity. As a discipline, nursing is challenged to dis-cover innovative and effective ways to plan, implement, and evaluate care. The promise of transformational leadership, new knowledge management, and clinical care technolo-gies will help us to perform our work both effectively and efficiently, and will result in positive client outcomes.

Peter Drucker (1994) identifies the organization of the future as a knowledge organization composed of knowledge workers. Knowledge workers are those people who bring specialized, expert knowledge to an organiza-tion, and are valued for what they know. The knowledge organization will share, provide, and grow the information necessary to work efficiently and effectively. Drucker says that knowledge organizations, in which the knowledge worker is on the front lines with the expertise and the in-formation to act, will be the dominant organizational type (Drucker, 1994; Helgesen, 1995).

This description suggests that health care organizations are likely to be prime examples of knowledge-based organizations and will require a fundamental commitment to leadership development and knowledge management. In organizations such as these, the ideas of leadership being at the top and leadership being equated with the power of a position are obsolete notions. Workers with the expertise and information to act are the organization's leaders. They provide the service, interact with the customer, represent the organization, and accomplish its goals. Within such an organization, "leadership will be needed at all levels" (College of Nurses of Ontario, 1998), not just at the top and not just with certain positions in the organization. Every worker will play a role in fulfilling the purpose of the organization and, in so doing, will be both a leader and a follower. This future direction will challenge each nurse to assess, develop, and continually appraise and enhance his or her personal leadership competencies, style and effectiveness.

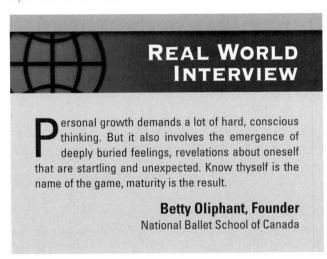

REAL WORLD INTERVIEW

Personal growth demands a lot of hard, conscious thinking. But it also involves the emergence of deeply buried feelings, revelations about oneself that are startling and unexpected. Know thyself is the name of the game, maturity is the result.

Betty Oliphant, Founder
National Ballet School of Canada

THE NEW LEADERSHIP

Margaret Wheatley, in *Leadership and the New Science* (1992), says, "There is a simpler way to lead organizations, one that requires less effort and produces less stress than the current practices" (p. 3). She presents a new view of leadership, one encompassing connectedness and self-organizing systems that follow a natural order of both chaos and uncertainty, which is different from the linear order in a hierarchy. The leader's function is to guide an organization using vision, to make choices based on mutual values, and to engage in the culture to provide meaning and coherence. This type of leadership fosters growth within each of us as individuals and as members of a group. The notion of connection within a self-organizing system optimizes autonomy at all levels because the relationships between the individual and the whole are strong (Wheatley, 1992).

For nursing, such systems might be the infrastructure that will foster interdisciplinary decision making and

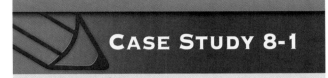

CASE STUDY 8-1

Sharon, a licensed practical nurse, was making rounds on her new client admitted to the continuing complex care unit. The client was a 95-year-old woman who had sustained a fall at home. Following three days of immobility on a hard surface, the client presented with a sacral pressure ulcer. On assessment of the client, Sharon noted the pressure ulcer was being managed with saline wet-to-dry dressings. On dressing change, Sharon found the ulcer was covered with necrotic tissue. Sharon immediately took a swab of the area, which returned positive for Methicillin-Resistant Staphylococcus Aureus (MRSA) and Streptococcus. She contacted the most responsible physician and presented a clear picture of the wound, and recommended debridement of the wound and consideration of topical negative pressure. A surgical consult was ordered by the physician, and surgical debridement was completed on day 4 following admission. Topical negative pressure was applied following consultation with the enterostomal therapist. On day 3, post-intervention granulation tissue was reported in the wound, and by day 11, the wound length and width had decreased by more than half and the depth decreased by 1.0 cm. The client was discharged to a long-term care facility with a completely closed wound.

What leadership characteristics did this licensed practical nurse demonstrate?

Why is leadership important at all levels throughout a health care organization?

How can a nurse develop this type of leadership skill?

strengthen the connection with nonprofessional workers. New possibilities may emerge that help nursing to move away from dependence on numbers of staff, numbers of patient care hours, cost and volume productivity measures, and the tools of both an industrial age and Newton's physics toward the new science focused on naturally occurring events, wholeness, and interaction.

GENERATIONAL LEADERSHIP ISSUES

Organizations have become more complex, and nursing's systems and ways of leadership must keep pace with the complexities and the advances of a highly technological, information-driven environment. Leadership will emerge from teams that self-organize and self-direct (Avolio,

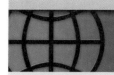

REAL WORLD INTERVIEW

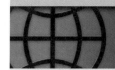

Clinical nurses have a role to play in guiding corporate decision making related to clinical practice. We teach students to be critical thinkers and agents for change, and encourage each nurse to use leadership skills, yet we fail to take advantage of these skills. Even today, when we think of leadership, we refer mostly to formal positions. Strict procedures, such as those in program management models that emphasize the bottom line, risk turning nursing leaders into generic executives. We need to evolve a model that replaces top-down hierarchies and linear reporting structures with teams of individual professionals who work in a fluid matrix. All nurses need to play a role in inter-professional teams to keep the nursing profession visible and active in decisions for client care. Rethinking approaches to leadership also means thinking about how to prepare nurses for their roles as future leaders. Each one of us should engage in this kind of creative thinking and not just leave it to schools of nursing, health care agencies, or nursing associations and unions. By sharing and debating our ideas and bringing them into the policy arena, we can also demonstrate a vital aspect of leadership.

Dr. Ginette L. Rodger
Vice President Professional Practice and Chief
Nursing Executive,
The Ottawa Hospital, Ottawa

REAL WORLD INTERVIEW

Leadership in nursing is probably one of the more personal forms of leadership. Nursing is one of the most intimate leadership relationships because of the vulnerability the client brings to the relationship. For clients who are dying or in terrible situations, the nurse provides two vital leadership characteristics: optimism and courage. For clients who have lost their courage, it is the nurse who shows courage and strength that supports the client and their family. Optimism and courage are the trademarks of great leaders. Nurses lead the client, their family, their nurse colleagues, and other health care providers. They have the courage to care in the face of fear and uncertainty, and in the face of disability or in death. Caring, hope, and support are a source of optimism that nurses provide. There are very few professions where you touch an individual's life so profoundly.

Jay Conger, PhD
Author, Learning to Lead

1999). Organizational teams will become diverse, both racially and ethnically, but also because different generations will participate in the workforce simultaneously.

The generation known as the baby boomers, born between 1946 and 1964, will work with different age-related groups, such as the baby-buster generation, also known as Generation X or Gen-Exers, born between 1965 and 1981 (Moats Kennedy, 1998). According to Moats Kennedy, the boomers and busters exhibit different values about work, motivation, lifestyle, and communication. For example, she points out that boomers tend to demonstrate loyalty to an employer, whereas busters regularly change organizations to advance their development. Additionally, busters have a more individual approach to work and tend to value a work–family balanced lifestyle more highly than boomers, who tend to work hard with a strong emphasis on money and acquiring possessions. Such different styles reveal differences in how learning occurs and the methods best suited for

busters, who are computer-skilled and comfortable with high-tech tools, versus boomers, who tend toward more personalized training methods.

Research among nurses has revealed that conflict and stress among these generations can occur regarding their feelings about work, job tenure, and work behaviours; for example, some boomers hold negative views about the degree of commitment and the self-centred focus exhibited by busters (Santos & Cox, 2000). Within a team-based approach to organizational work, leadership development must embrace an understanding of generational differences and support the idea of maximizing the strengths of boomers, busters, and the most recent group, generation nexters, born between 1980 and 2000.

NURSING LEADERSHIP AND MANAGEMENT: THE LINK

This chapter undertakes to set out a clear distinction between leadership and management and also provides an overview of the direct and proximate theories that underpin these concepts.

Over the past two decades, nursing has responded to changing technological and social forces affecting health care organizations. The response has required managers to develop new competencies related to the business of health care, including financial and marketing skills.

Providing care in a contracted resource situation has also required managers to possess excellent leadership skills, which are critical to effective team building in organizations. Successful team building is associated with successful recruitment, retaining a cohesive staff, and maintaining high-quality practice. Stout-Shaffer and Larrabee (1992) have identified the hallmarks of the new paradigm in health care organizations as semiautonomous work units, empowerment of all, trust, intuition and creativity, and planning with clients. The relationship between management and leadership is a rich source for debate among theorists in the literature. Tranbarger (1998) asserts that leadership is one of many functions of the manager's role; however, the contrary view is expressed by Gardner (1986), who contends that leadership requires more skills and, as a result, management is but one role of leadership. The notion that a manager guides, directs, and motivates, and that leaders empower others was described by Manthey (1990), who claims that every manager should be a leader. Bennis and Nanus (1985) are well known for their differentiation between managers and leaders, as in their assertion that "managers are people who do things right and leaders are people who do the right thing," which has become a mantra in leadership and management development courses. Marquis and Huston (1996) contend that strong management skills have been valued more than strong leadership skills in health care, which may be in keeping with the shift to more business management models, such as program management. Marquis postulates that leadership and management have a symbiotic or synergistic relationship. The synergistic notion suggests that the two concepts must be integrated so that the effective application of both skill sets results in dynamic management and inspirational leadership; both are required to steward professional development, job satisfaction, and navigate change. Gardner (1990) puts forward that individuals who have integrated both skill sets are distinguished from traditional managers.

Their distinguishing traits are 1) they think longer term; 2) they look outward to the larger organization; 3) they influence others beyond their own group; 4) they emphasize vision, values, and motivation; 5) they are politically astute; and 6) they think in terms of change and renewal.

The fundamental challenge within nursing is to determine the entry-to-practice leadership and management competencies and then to ensure basic undergraduate programs and continuing nursing education programs are focused on those competencies. At the end of the day, clients have a right to quality care delivered within safe and effective care environments. Nursing leaders and managers have an obligation to create, maintain, and enhance those care environments. In pursing effective leadership and management, and achievement of a voice in strategic organizational planning, individual nurses and the discipline, as a whole, must persevere and remain determined.

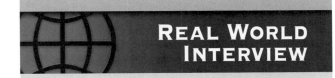

REAL WORLD INTERVIEW

Nothing in the world can take the place of persistence. Talent will not; nothing is more common than unsuccessful men with talent. Genius will not; unrewarded genius is almost a proverb. Education alone will not; the world is full of educated derelicts. Persistence and determination alone are omnipotent.

Calvin Coolidge, 30th president of the United States

KEY CONCEPTS

- Leadership is the fuel needed to sustain nursing through a constant evolution of care delivery systems.

- Nurses are leaders and make a difference to health care organizations through their contributions of expert knowledge and leadership. Leadership development is critical to developing knowledge workers.

- Leaders provide vision, inspire, and encourage. Change in health care organizations occurs because leaders value creativity and innovation.

- Management is a process used to achieve organizational goals. It involves the management functions of planning, leading, organizing, and controlling.

- Motivation is an internal process that contributes to our behaviour in an effort to satisfy our needs. Maslow's

hierarchy of needs reflects the belief that the needs that motivate us have an order, and lower-level needs have to be satisfied first or we will not be motivated to address higher-level needs. Herzberg's two-factor theory of motivation identifies maintenance factors, such as security and salary, which are needed to prevent job dissatisfaction; whereas motivators, such as development and opportunities to advance, contribute to job satisfaction.

- Leadership is a process of influence that involves the leader, the follower, and their interaction. Followers can be individual practitioners, professional groups or interprofessional practice communities, and members of society in general. Leadership can be formal and informal, occurring by being in a position of authority in an organization, such as the chief nursing officer, or outside the scope of a formal role, such as individual practitioners.

- Leadership and management are different. Management refers to the strategic actions employed to achieve organizational goals, whereas leadership is the effort to envision, inspire, and facilitate change. Current thinking suggests that individuals need to develop competencies in both leadership and management, and the resulting synergy facilitates the promotion of professional practice and safe client care at the individual practitioner and discipline level.

- Future directions for nurses in organizations will be influenced by technology and by the need for communities of practice and effective knowledge management structures and processes. Nursing leadership in the future will be needed at all levels within an organization, not just at the top or from managers. Every knowledge worker with specialized knowledge and expertise will be both a leader and a follower in knowledge organizations.

- Organizations are being viewed as self-organizing systems in which, initially, what looks like chaos and uncertainty is indeed part of a larger coherence and a natural order. Such a living system, when understood better by participants, will be a less stressful and more holistic environment in which to work.

- Work teams are becoming generationally diverse as more baby boomers are working alongside younger generations, called baby busters or Gen-Exers. Busters are less concerned with loyalty to an organization but value balance in their personal and work life. Boomers show commitment to their employer, work hard, and are motivated by financial rewards. These differences can be a source of stress among nurses.

KEY TERMS

administrative principles	leadership
autocratic leadership	maintenance or hygiene
bureaucratic organization	factors
consideration	management
contingency theory	management process
democratic leadership	motivation
emotional intelligence	motivation factors
employee-centred leadership	position power
formal leadership	substitutes for
Hawthorne effect	leadership
informal leader	task structure
initiating structure	Theory X
job-centred leaders	Theory Y
knowledge workers	Theory Z
laissez-faire leadership	transactional leader
leader–member relations	transformational leader

REVIEW QUESTIONS

1. Why is leadership development important for nurses if they are not in a management or formal leadership position?
   A. It is not really important for nurses.
   B. Leadership is important at all levels in an organization because nurses have expert knowledge and are interacting with and influencing the client.
   C. Nurse leaders leave their jobs sooner for other positions.
   D. Nurses who lead are less satisfied in their jobs.

2. Management, as a process that is used today by nurses or nurse managers in health care organizations, is best described as
   A. Scientific management.
   B. Decision making.
   C. Commanding and controlling others, using hierarchical authority.
   D. Planning, organizing, coordinating, and controlling.

3. Motivation is whatever influences our choices. What factors did Herzberg say would motivate workers and lead to job satisfaction?
   A. Being offered a substantial bonus when being hired.
   B. Realizing that no one ever gets fired from the organization and that job security is high.
   C. Having good relationships with colleagues and supervisors.
   D. Being offered opportunities for development and advancement.

4. Leadership is defined as
   A. Being in a leadership position with authority to exert control and power over subordinates.
   B. A process of interaction in which the leader influences others toward goal achievement.
   C. Managing complexity.
   D. Being self-confident and democratic.

5. According to Hersey and Blanchard and House, a participative leadership style is appropriate for employees who
   A. are not able to get the task done and are less mature.
   B. are able to contribute to decisions about getting the work done.
   C. are unable and unwilling to participate.
   D. need direction, structure, and authority.

6. According to Kouzes and Posner's model, leadership is founded upon five practices.
   True or False

7. The quality of leadership is linked to nurse and client outcomes.
   True or False

8. Which of the following is *not* an example of emotional intelligence (EI)?
   A. Appraising and expressing emotions in self and others.
   B. Integrating emotions into thought processes.
   C. Understanding emotions.
   D. Intelligence quotient.

9. Which of the following is *not* a characteristic of growing nurse leaders?
   A. Refraining from building strategic relationships.
   B. Seizing opportunities for change.
   C. Practising personal accountability.
   D. Advocating for safe, effective, and ethical client care.

10. The Canadian Nurses Association's position statement on leadership emphasizes that nurses in all domains and at all levels must maximize their leadership potential.

    True or False

REVIEW ACTIVITIES

1. Take the opportunity to learn about yourself by reflecting on the five predominant factors identified as being influential in a nurse's leadership development: self-confidence, innate leader qualities/tendencies, progression of experiences and success, influence of significant others, and personal life factors. Consider the factors that reinforce your confidence in yourself. What innate qualities or tendencies do you have that contribute to your development as a leader? Consider what professional experiences, mentors, and personal experiences or events can help you influence and change nursing practice.

2. Describe the type of leader you want to be as a nurse in a health care organization. Identify specific behaviours you plan to use as a leader. In what way are the theories of transformational leadership and the charismatic leadership useful to your development as a leader?

3. Rate each of these 12 job factors that contribute to job satisfaction by placing a number from 1 to 5 on the line before each factor.

Very important		Somewhat important		Not important
5	4	3	2	1

_____ 1. An interesting job I enjoy doing

_____ 2. A good manager who treats people fairly

_____ 3. Getting praise and other recognition and appreciation for the work I do

_____ 4. A satisfying personal life at the job

_____ 5. The opportunity for advancement

_____ 6. A prestigious or status job

_____ 7. Job responsibility that gives me freedom to do things my way

_____ 8. Good working conditions (safe environment, nice office, cafeteria)

_____ 9. The opportunity to learn new things

_____ 10. Sensible company rules, regulations, procedures, and policies

_____ 11. A job I can do well and succeed at

_____ 12. Job security and benefits

Write the number from 1 to 5 that you selected for each factor. Total each column for a score between 6 and 30 points. The closer to 30 your score is, the more important these factors (motivating or maintenance) are to you.

Motivating factors	Maintenance factors
1. _____	2. _____
3. _____	4. _____
5. _____	6. _____
7. _____	8. _____
9. _____	10. _____
11. _____	12. _____
Totals _____	_____

From *Leadership: Theory, Application, Skill Development* (pp. 15–16), by R. N. Lussier and C. F. Achua, 2001, Cincinnati, OH: South-Western College Publishing.

EXPLORING THE WEB

Search the Web, checking the following sites.

■ Emerging Leader: *http://www.emergingleader.com*

■ Leadership Directories: Who's who in leadership in Canada: *http://www.sources.com*

■ National Quality Institute Leadership Excellence Program: *http://www.nqi.ca*

■ Dorothy M. Wylie Nursing Leadership Institute: *http:/www. dwnli.ca*

■ Aboriginal Leadership Initiative in Canada: *http:/www.synergos.org/partnership/about/ aboriginalleadershipcanada.htm*

■ Registered Nurses' Association of Ontario: Best Practice Guidelines: *http://www.rnao.org/Page.asp?PageID= 861&SiteNodeID=133*

■ The Canadian Leadership Institute; *http:/www. cdnleadership.com*

REFERENCES

Aiken, L. H., Clarke, S. P., Sloane, D. M., Sochalski, J. A., Busse, R., Clarke, H., et al. (2001). Nurses' report on hospital care in five countries. *Health Affairs, 20*(3), 43–53.

Allen, D. W. (1998). How nurses become leaders: Perceptions and beliefs about leadership development. *Journal of Nursing Administration, 28*(9), 15–20.

Anderson, R. A., Issel, L. M., & McDaniel Jr., R. R. (2003). Nursing homes as complex adaptive systems: Relationship between management practice and resident outcomes. *Nursing Research, 52,* 12–21.

Avolio, B. (1999). *Full leadership development: Building the vital forces in organizations.* Thousand Oaks, CA: Sage.

Barker, A. (1990). *Transformational nursing leadership: A vision for the future.* Baltimore: Williams & Wilkins.

Barnard, C. (1938). *The functions of the executive.* Boston: Harvard University Press.

Bass, B. (1985). *Leadership and performance beyond expectations.* New York: Free Press.

Benner P. (1984). *From novice to expert: Excellence and power in clinical nursing practice.* Menlo Park, CA: Addison-Wesley.

Bennis, W., & Nanus, B. (1985). *Leaders: The strategies for taking charge.* New York: Harper & Row.

Blake, R. R., & Mouton, J. S. (1985). *The managerial grid III.* Houston, TX: Gulf.

Blythe, J., Baumann, A., & Giovannetti, P. (2001). Nurses' experiences of restructuring in three Ontario Hospitals. *Journal of Nursing Scholarship, 33,* 61–68.

Broughton, H. (2002). *Nursing leadership: Unleashing the power.* Ottawa: Canadian Nurses Association.

Bruch, H., & Ghoshal, S., (2002) Beware the busy manager. *Harvard Business Review, 80*(2), 63–69.

Burns, J. M. (1978). *Leadership.* New York: Harper & Row.

Canadian Institute for Health Information (2004). *MIS Guidelines for Canadian health care facilities.* Ottawa, Canada: Author.

Canadian Institute for Health Information. (1999). *MIS guidelines for Canadian healthcare facilities.* Ottawa, ON: Author.

Canadian Nurses Association (2002). *Position statement: Nursing leadership.* Ottawa: Canadian Nurses Association. Retrieved from http://www.cna-nurses.ca/CNA/documents/pdf/publications/PS59_Nursing_Leadership_June_2002_e.pdf, July 4, 2007.

Cassidy, V., & Koroll, C. (1998). Ethical aspects of transformational leadership. In E. Hein (Ed.), *Contemporary leadership behavior: Selected readings* (5th ed., pp. 79–82). Philadelphia: Lippincott.

Chiok Foong Loke, J. (2001). Leadership behaviours: Effects on job satisfaction, productivity and organizational commitment. *Journal of Nursing Management, 9,* 191–204.

College of Nurses of Ontario (1998). *Practice setting consultation program: An information guide.* Toronto: College of Nurses of Ontario.

Conger, J., & Kanungo, R. (1987). Toward a behavioral theory of charismatic leadership in organizational settings. *Academy of Management Review, 12,* 637–647.

Covey, S. R., (1990). *The seven habits of highly effective people* (lst ed.). New York: Simon & Schuster Inc.

Daft, R. L., & Marcic, D. (2001). *Understanding management* (3rd ed.). Philadelphia: Harcourt College.

Doucette, E., (2006). Role of the professional practice leader. *Brant Community Healthcare System What's Up Newsletter.* Brantford, Canada: Author.

Drucker, P. F. (1994). *The post-capitalist society.* New York: Harper & Row.

Dunham, J., & Klafehn, K. A. (1990). Transformational leadership and the nurse executive. *Journal of Nursing Administration, 20*(4), 28–34.

Dunham-Taylor, J. (1995). Identifying the best in nurse executive leadership: Part 2, interview results. *Journal of Nursing Administration, 25*(7/8), 24–31.

Dunham-Taylor, J. (2000). Nurse executive transformational leadership found in participative organizations. *Journal of Nursing Administration, 30*(5), 241–250.

Edwards, R. (1994). Image, practice and empowerment: A call to new leadership for the invisible profession. *Revolution, 4*(1), 18–20.

Fagin, C. M. (1996). Executive leadership: Improving nursing practice, education and research. *Journal of Nursing Administration, 26*(3), 30–37.

Fayol, H. (1916/1949). (C. Storrs, Trans.). *General and industrial management.* London: Pitman.

Fielder, F. (1967). *A theory of leadership effectiveness.* New York: McGraw-Hill.

Gardner, J. W. (1986). *The nature of leadership: Introductory considerations.* Washington DC: The Independent Sector.

Gardner J. W. (1990). *On leadership.* New York: The Free Press

Gelinas, L. S., & Manthey, M. (1997). The impact of organizational redesign on nurse executive leadership. *Journal of Nursing Administration, 27*(10), 35–42.

George, V., Burke, L. J., Rodgers, B., Duthie, N., Hoffman, M. L., Koceja, V., et al. (2002). Developing staff nurse shared leadership behaviour in professional nursing practice. *Nursing Administration Quarterly, 26*(3), 44–59.

Gilbreth, F. (1912). *Primer of scientific management.* New York: Van Nostrand.

Girvan, J. (1996). Leadership and nursing: Part 1: History and politics. *Nursing Management, 3*(1), 10–12.

Goleman, D. (2006). *Emotional intelligence: Why it can matter more than IQ.* New York: Bantam Books,

Gulick, L., & Urwick, L. (Eds.). (1937). *Papers on the science of administration.* New York: Institute of Public Administration.

Hales, C. P. (1986). What managers do: A critical review of the evidence. *Journal of Management Studies, 23,* 88–115.

Helgesen, S. (1995). *The web of inclusion: A new architecture for building organizations.* New York: Doubleday Currency.

Henry, N. (1992). *Public administration and public affairs* (5th ed.). Englewood Cliffs, NJ: Prentice Hall.

Hersey, P., & Blanchard, K. (2000). *Management of organizational behavior* (8th ed.). Englewood Cliffs, NJ: Prentice Hall.

Herzberg, F. (1968, January/February). One more time: How do you motivate employees? *Harvard Business Review,* 53–62.

House, R. H. (1971). A path-goal theory of leader effectiveness. *Administrative Science Quarterly, 16,* 321–338.

House, R. H. (1977). A 1976 theory of charismatic leadership. In J. Hunt & L. Larson (Eds.), *Leadership: The cutting edge* (pp. 21–26). Carbondale, IL: Southern Illinois University Press.

Houser, J. (2003). A model for evaluating the context of nursing care delivery. *Journal of Nursing Administration, 33*(1), 39–47.

Huber, D. L., Maas, M., McCloskey, J., Scherb, C. A., Goode, C. J., & Watson, C. (2000). Evaluating nursing administration instruments. *Journal of Nursing Administration, 30*(5), 251–272.

Hughes, R. L., Ginnett, R. C., & Curphy, G. J. (1999). *Leadership: Enhancing the lessons of experience* (3rd ed.). San Francisco: Irwin McGraw-Hill.

Industry Canada. (2004). *Steps to competitiveness: Explanation step one—Defining vision and mission.* Ottawa: Industry Canada. Retrieved from http://strategis.ic.gc.ca/epic/site/stco-levc.nsf/en/qw00046e.html, August 18, 2007.

Kanfer, R. (1990). Motivation theory in industrial and organizational psychology. In M. D. Dunnette & L. M. Hough (Eds.), *Handbook of industrial and organizational psychology: Vol. 1* (pp. 53–68). Palo Alto, CA: Consulting Psychologists Press.

Katz, D., & Kahn, R. L. (1978). *The social psychology of organizations* (2nd ed.). New York: John Wiley.

Kerr, S., & Jermier, J. (1978). Substitutes for leadership: Their meaning and measurement. *Organizational Behavior and Human Performance, 22,* 374–403.

Kim, H., & Yukl, G. (1995). Relationships of self-reported and subordinate-reported leadership behaviors to managerial effectiveness and advancement. *Leadership Quarterly, 6,* 361–377.

Kirkpatrick, S. A., & Locke, E. A. (1991). Leadership: Do traits matter? *The Executive, 5,* 48–60.

Kotter, J. (1990a). *A force for change: How leadership differs from management.* Glencoe, IL: Free Press.

Kotter, J. (1990b). What leaders really do. *Harvard Business Review, 68,* 104.

Kouzes, J. M., & Posner, B. Z. (2002). *The leadership challenge* (3rd ed.). San Francisco: Jossey-Bass Inc.

Kramer, M., & Schmalenberg, C. (1988). Magnet hospitals: Part II institutions of excellence. *Journal of Nursing Administration, 18*(2), 11–19.

Kramer, M., & Schmalenberg, C. (2003). Securing "good" nurse/physician relationships. *Nursing Management, 34*(7), 34–38.

Kraus, S. (2006). Success lessons from the Winter Olympics: Visualization. Retrieved from http://ezinearticles.com/?Success-Lessons-from-the-Winter-Olympics:-Visualization&id=148344, March 10, 2007.

Laborde, A. S., & Lee, J. A. (2000). Skills needed for promotion in the nursing profession. *Journal of Nursing Administration, 30*(9), 432–439.

Leach, L. S. (2000). *Nurse executive leadership and the relationship to organizational commitment among nurses.* Unpublished doctoral dissertation, University of Southern California, Los Angeles.

Leatt, P., & Porter, J. (2003). Where are the healthcare leaders? The need for investment in leadership development. *Healthcare Papers, 4*(1), 14–31.

Levi, P. (1999), Sustainability of healthcare environments. *Image: Journal of Nursing Scholarship, 31*(4), 395–398.

Lewin, K. (1939). Field theory and experiment in social psychology: Concepts and methods. *Journal of Sociology, 44,* 868–896.

Lewin, K., & Lippitt, R. (1938). An experimental approach to the study of autocracy and democracy: A preliminary note. *Sociometry, 1,* 292–300.

Lewin, K., Lippitt, R., & White, R. (1939). Patterns of aggressive behavior in experimentally created social climates. *Journal of Social Psychology, 10,* 271–299.

Lussier, R. N. (1999). *Human relations in organizations: Applications and skill building* (4th ed.). San Francisco: Irwin McGraw-Hill.

Lussier, R. N., & Achua, C. F. (2001). *Leadership: Theory, application, skill development.* Cincinnati, OH: South-Western College.

Manthey, M. (1990). The nurse manager as leader. *Nursing Management, 21*(6).

Marquis, B. L., & Huston, C. J. (1996). *Leadership roles and management functions in nursing* (2nd ed.). Philadelphia: J.B. Lippincott.

Maslow, A. (1970). *Motivation and personality* (2nd ed.). New York: Harper & Row.

Mayo, E. (1933). *The human problems of an industrial civilization.* New York: Macmillan.

McCall, M. W., Jr. (1998). *High flyers: Developing the next generation of leaders.* Boston: Harvard Business School Press.

McCall, M. W., Jr., Morrison, A. M., & Hanman, R. L. (1978). *Studies of managerial work: Results and methods* (Tech. Rep.). Greensboro, NC: Center for Creative Leadership.

McCloskey, J. C., & McCain, B. E. (1987). Satisfaction, commitment and professionalism of newly employed nurses. *Image, 19*(1), 20–24, 178.

McClure, M., Poulin, M., Sovie, M., & Wandelt, M. (1983). *Magnet hospitals: Attraction and retention of professional nurses.* Kansas City, MO: American Nurses Association.

McDaniel, C., & Wolf, G. (1992). Transformational leadership in nursing service. *Journal of Nursing Administration, 12*(4), 204–207.

McGillis Hall, L., Doran, D., Baker, G. R., Pink, G. H., Sidani, S., O'Brien-Pallas, L., et al. (2001). *A study of the impact of nursing staff mix models and organizational change strategies on patient, system and nurse outcomes.* Toronto: Faculty of Nursing, University of Toronto and Canadian Health Research Foundation.

McGregor, D. (1960). *The human side of enterprise.* New York: McGraw-Hill.

McNeese-Smith, D. (1995). Job satisfaction, productivity, and organizational commitment: The result of leadership. *Journal of Nursing Administration, 25*(9), 17–26.

McNeese-Smith, D. (1997). The influences of manager behavior on nurses' job satisfaction, productivity, and commitment. *Journal of Nursing Administration, 27*(9), 47–55.

Medley, F. & Larochelle, D. R. (1995). Transformational leadership and job satisfaction. *Nursing Management, 26*(9), 64JJ-64NN.

Meighan, M. (1990) The most important characteristics of nursing leaders. *Nursing Administration Quarterly, 15*(1), 63–69.

Mintzberg, H. (1973). *The nature of managerial work.* New York: Harper & Row.

Moats Kennedy, M. (1998). Boomers versus busters: Addressing the generation gap in healthcare management. *Healthcare Executive, 13*(6), 6–10.

Mooney, J. (1939). *Principles of organization.* New York: Harper.

Moorhead, G., & Griffin, R. W. (2001). *Organizational behavior: Managing people in organizations* (6th ed.). Boston: Houghton Mifflin.

Murphy, M., & DeBack, V. (1991). Today's nursing leaders: Creating the vision. *Nursing Administration Quarterly, 16*(1), 71–80.

Northouse, P. (2001). *Leadership: Theory and practice* (2nd ed.). Thousand Oaks, CA: Sage.

O'Brien-Pallas, L., Thomson, D., McGillis Hall, L., Pink, G., Kerr, M., Wang, S. et al. (2004). *Evidence-based standards for measuring nurse staffing and performance.* Toronto: Faculty of Nursing, University of Toronto and Canadian Health Services Research Foundation.

Ouchi, W. (1981). *Theory Z: How American business can meet the Japanese challenge.* Reading, MA: Addison-Wesley.

Pillai, R., & Meindl, J. (1998). Context and charisma: A "meso" level examination of the relationship of organic structure, collectivism, and crisis to charismatic leadership. *Journal of Management, 24,* 643–671.

Porter-O'Grady, T. (2003). A different age for leadership, Part 2. *Journal of Nursing Administration, 33*(3), 173–178.

Roethlisberger, J. F., & Dickson, W. J. (1939). *Management and the worker.* Cambridge, MA: Harvard University Press.

Salovey, P., & Mayer, J. (1990). Emotional intelligence. *Imagination, Cognition and Personality, 9,* 185–211.

Santos, S. R., & Cox, K. (2000). Workplace adjustment and intergenerational differences between matures, boomers, and Xers. *Nursing Economic$, 18*(1), 7–13.

Scott, J. G., Sochalski, J., & Aiken, L. (1999). Review of magnet hospital research: Findings and implications for professional nursing practice. *Journal of Nursing Administration, 29*(1), 9–19.

Searle, L. (1996). 21st century leadership for nurse administrators. *Aspen's Advisor for Nurse Executives, 11*(4), 1, 4–6.

Smith, P. M., Parsons, R. J., Murray, B. P., Dwore, R. B., Vorderer, L. H., & Wallock Okerlund, V. (1994). The nurse executive, an emerging role. *Journal of Nursing Administration, 24*(11), 56–62.

Snow, J. L. (2001). Looking beyond nursing for clues to effective leadership. *Journal of Nursing Administration, 31*(9), 440–443.

Spence Laschinger, H., Sabiston, J. A., Finegan, J, & Shamian, J. (2001). Voices from the trenches: Nurses' experiences of hospital restructuring in Ontario. *Canadian Journal of Nursing Leadership. 14*(10), 6–13.

Spence Laschinger, H., Wong, C., McMahon, L., & Kaufmann, C. (1999). Leader behavior impact on staff empowerment, job tension and work effectiveness. *Journal of Nursing Administration, 29*(5), 28–39.

Stodgill, R. M. (1948). Personal factors associated with leadership: A survey of the literature. *Journal of Psychology, 25,* 35–71.

Stodgill, R. M. (1974). *Handbook of leadership: A survey of theory and research.* New York: Free Press.

Stordeur, S., Vandenberghe, C., & D'hoore, W. (2000). Leadership styles across hierarchical levels in nursing departments. *Nursing Research, 49,* 37–43.

Stout-Shaffer, S., & Larrabee, J. (1992). Everyone can be a visionary leader. *Nursing Management, 23*(12), 54–58.

Taylor, F. (1911). *Principles of scientific management.* New York: Harper & Row.

Tichy, N., & Devanna, D. (1986). *Transformational leadership.* New York: Wiley.

Tourangeau, A., Lemonde, M., Luba, M., Dakers, D., & Alksnis, C. (2003). Evaluation of a leadership development intervention. *Canadian Journal of Nursing Leadership, 16*(3), 91–104.

Tranbarger, R., (1998). The nurse executive in a community hospital. In M. Johnson (Ed.), *Series on nursing administration* (Vol. 1). Menlo Park, CA: Addison Wesley.

Trofino, J. (1995). Transformational leadership in health care. *Nursing Management, 26*(8), 42–47.

Upenicks, V. (2003). Nurse leader's perceptions of what comprises successful leadership in today's acute care environment. *Nursing Administration Quarterly, 27,* 140–152.

Wheatley, M. J. (1992). *Leadership and the new science: Learning about organization from an orderly universe.* San Francisco: Berrett-Koehler.

Wolf, G., Boland, S., & Aukerman, M. (1994). A transformational model for the practice of professional nursing. Part 1. *Journal of Nursing Administration, 24*(4), 51–57.

Wren, D. (1979). *Evolution of management thought.* New York: Wiley.

Young, S. (1992). Educational experiences of transformational nurse leaders. *Nursing Administration Quarterly, 17*(1), 25–33.

Yukl, G. (1998). *Leadership in organizations* (4th ed.). Upper Saddle River, NJ: Prentice Hall.

Yukl, G., Wall, S., & Lepsinger, R. (1990). Preliminary report on validation of the managerial practices survey. In K. E. Clarke & M. B. Clark (Eds.), *Measures of leadership* (pp. 223–238). West Orange, NJ: Leadership Library of America.

Zalenik, K. A. (1977). Managers and leaders: Are they different? *Harvard Business Review, 55*(5), 67–80.

SUGGESTED READINGS

Avolio, B. J., Zhu, W., Koh, W., & Bhatia, P. (2004) Transformational leadership and organizational commitment: Mediating role of psychological empowerment and moderating role of structural distance. *Journal of Organizational Behaviour, 25*(8), 951–968.

Bass, B. (1998). *Transformational leadership: Industrial, military, and educational impact.* Mahwah, NJ: Erlbaum.

Bauman, A., O'Brien-Pallas, L., Armstrong-Stassen, M., Blythe, J., Bourbonnais, R., Cameron, S., et al. (2001). *Commitment and care: The benefits of a healthy workplace for nurses, their patients and the system.* Ottawa, ON: Canadian Health Research Foundation and The Change Foundation.

Bower, F. L. (2000). *Nurses taking the lead: Personal qualities of effective leadership.* Philadelphia: Saunders.

Buerhaus, P. I. (2000). Implications of an aging registered nurse workforce. *Journal of the American Medical Association, 283,* 2948–2954.

Cadman, C., & Brewer, J. (2001). Emotional intelligence: A vital prerequisite for recruitment in nursing. *Journal of Nursing Management, 9*(6), 321–324.

Canadian Nursing Advisory Committee. (2002). *Our health, our future: Creating quality workplaces for Canadian nurses: Final report of the Canadian Nursing Advisory Committee.* Ottawa: Advisory Committee on Health Human Resources.

Collins, D., & Holton, E. (2004). The Effectiveness of managerial leadership development programs: A meta-analysis of studies from 1982 to 2001. *Human Resources Development Quarterly, 15*(2), 217–248.

Cronin, S. N., & Bechere, D. (1999). Recognition of staff nurse job performance and achievements: Staff and manager perceptions. *Journal of Nursing Administration, 29*(1), 26–31.

Evans, M. G. (1996). R. J. House's "A path-goal theory of leader effectiveness." *Leadership Quarterly, 7*(3), 305–309.

Ferguson-Paré, M., Mitchell, G., Perkin, K., & Stevenson, L. (2002). Academy of Canadian Executive Nurses (ACEN) background paper on leadership. *Canadian Journal of Nursing Leadership, 15*(3), 4–8.

Goleman, D. (1998). *Working with emotional intelligence.* New York: Bantam Books.

Gordon, S. (1997). *Life support: Three nurses on the front lines.* New York: Little, Brown.

Herbert, R., & Edgar, L. (2004). Emotional intelligence: A primal dimension of nursing leadership? *Canadian Journal of Nursing Leadership, 17*(4), 56–63.

Hesselbein, F., Goldsmith, M., & Beckhard, R. (Eds.). (1996). *The leader of the future: New visions, strategies, and practices for a new era.* San Francisco: Jossey-Bass.

Jeans, M., & Rowat, K. (2005). *Competencies required of nurse managers: Identifying the skills, personal attributes and knowledge required of nurse managers, and the enablers and barriers for nurse managers to acquire and sustain these competencies. The pulse of renewal: A focus on nursing human resources.* May, 2005. Special report. Toronto: Canadian Journal of Nursing Leadership.

Kanges, S., Kee, C. C., & McKee-Waddle, R. (1999). Organizational factors, nurses' job satisfaction and patient satisfaction with nursing care. *Journal of Nursing Administration, 29*(1), 32–42.

Kohles, M. K., Baker, W. G., Jr., & Donoho, B. (1995). *Transformational leadership: Reviewing fundamental values and achieving new relationships in health care.* Chicago: American Hospital.

Kramer, M. (1990). The magnet hospitals: Excellence revisited. *Journal of Nursing Administration, 20*(9), 35–44.

Kramer, M., & Schmalenberg, C. (1990). Fundamental lessons in leadership. In E. Simendinger, T. Moore & M. Kramer (Eds.), *The successful nurse executive: A guide for every nurse manager* (pp. 42–56). Ann Arbor, MI: Health Administration Press.

Laschinger, H., Finegan, J., & Shamian, J. (2001). The impact of workplace empowerment, organizational trust on staff nurses' work satisfaction and organizational commitment. *Health Care Management Review, 26*(3), 7–23.

Lemire Rodger, G. (2005). Leadership challenges and directions. In J. M. Hibberd & D. L. Smith (Eds.), *Nursing leadership and management in Canada* (3rd ed.). Toronto: Elsevier Canada.

Luthans, S. F., Hodgetts, R., & Rosenkratz, S. (1988). *Real managers.* Cambridge, MA: Ballinger.

O'Neil, E., & Coffman, J. (Eds.). (1998). *Strategies for the future of nursing: Changing roles, responsibilities, and employment patterns of registered nurses.* San Francisco: Jossey-Bass.

Parse, R. (1997). Leadership: The essentials. *Nursing Science Quarterly, 10*(3), 109.

Porter-O'Grady, T., & Wilson, C. K. (1995). *The leadership revolution in health care: Altering systems, changing behaviors.* Gaithersburg, MD: Aspen.

Rosenbach, W. E., & Taylor, R. L. (1998). *Contemporary issues in leadership* (4th ed.). Boulder, CO: Westview Press.

Senge, P. M. (1990) The fifth discipline. *The art and practice of the learning organization.* London: Random House

Storr, L. (2004). Leading with integrity: a qualitative research study. *Journal of Health Organization & Management, 18*, 415–434.

Urwick, L. (1944). *The elements of administration.* New York: Harper & Row.Villeneuve, M., & MacDonald, J. (2006). *Toward 2020: Visions for nursing.* Ottawa: Canadian Nurses Association.

CHAPTER
9

Strategic Planning and Organizing Client Care

Amy Androwich O'Malley, RN, MSN
Ida M. Androwich, PhD, RNC, FAAN
Adapted by: Heather Crawford, BScN, MEd, CHE

Our moral responsibility is not to stop the future, but to shape it…to channel our destiny in humane directions to ease the trauma of transition.

(Alvin Toffler)

OBJECTIVES

Upon completion of this chapter, the reader should be able to:

1. Describe the importance of an organization's mission and philosophy and their impact on the structure and behaviour of an organization.

2. Define the purpose of strategic planning and identify the steps in the strategic planning process.

3. Articulate the importance of aligning the organization's strategic vision both with the organization's own mission, philosophy, and values and with the goals and values of the communities served by the organization.

4. Have a basic understanding of common organizational structures and a framework for examining their purposes, their advantages, and their disadvantages.

Leadership in the health care organizations of the 21st century demands competent nurses with different skill sets from the past. Functioning in a leadership role in today's highly complex health care environment requires an understanding of how systems function and how to improve health care delivery. Yet, health care providers, including professional nurses, have been slow to integrate this information into their clinical practice. Planning for continuous improvement of quality, service, and cost-effectiveness is a critical competency of successful 21st century health care organizations and nurses.

The recent (2000) Canadian Adverse Events Study estimated that preventable adverse events cause between 9,000 and 24,000 deaths each year in Canada (Baker et al., 2004). In the United States, the National Advisory Council on Nurse Education and Practice and the Council on Graduate Medical Education concluded that client safety is dependent on the implementation of an interdisciplinary system that addresses the realities of practice and client care and that education and service must stress interdisciplinary approaches (National advisory councils in nursing and medicine collaborate, 2000). Other studies stress that the way a nurse's work is organized is a major determinant of client welfare (Havens & Aiken, 1999). Consequently, nurses in leadership positions must be educationally prepared to develop and implement sound models for the effective delivery of client care. Although many health care organizations collect large sets of data and are beginning to use scientific methods to improve the services they render, these activities are typically fragmented, isolated from day-to-day nursing management, and lacking alignment with any organizational strategy. The Canadian Nurses Association (CNA) concurs with the Canadian Adverse Events Study that errors occur as a result of system failure rather than human failure (Baker & Norton, 2001). This chapter will discuss the strategic planning process and the importance of aligning the organization's strategic vision with the mission, philosophy, and values of the organization and the communities served by the organization.

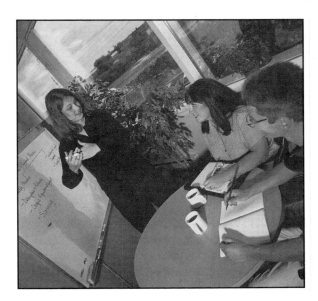

You are a staff nurse in a hospital that has just celebrated its 50th anniversary. Your organization is about to merge with a facility that is only five years old. You have been asked to participate on a committee to develop a mission statement for the new merged facility.

What are your thoughts about the invitation to participate?

What information do you need in order to do your job well?

What resources do you need?

Is this situation unusual? How can it be meaningful for you?

There are increasing opportunities for nurses to become involved in strategic and tactical planning for the delivery of health care services in their organizations and communities. Yet, to be effective in leadership roles, nurses need a basic understanding of the way in which organizations are structured, how organizational systems function, and how to engage in the strategic planning process. In the past, many health care organizations were structured in a highly formal, top-down, militaristic manner. These bureaucratic organizations worked well in a relatively stable environment when communication channels could be hierarchical; however, these organizations are not useful in a dynamic health care system in which information is rapidly changing. Increasingly, managers are recognizing the importance of obtaining subordinate input from all levels of the organization in order to give strategic plans meaning, and to increase the likelihood of implementation (Marquis & Huston, 2006). In addition, workers in today's health care systems are considered knowledge workers—professionals hired for their knowledge, skills, and expertise. They need a system that supports their ability to practise to the full extent of their professional accountability (Kanter, 1997).

ORGANIZATIONAL PURPOSE, MISSION, PHILOSOPHY, VALUES

Every organization has a purpose and a guiding philosophy. Most often, the purpose and philosophy are explicitly stated and detailed in a formal mission statement. Typically, this mission statement reflects the organization's values and indicates the behaviour and strategic actions that can be expected from that organization. Most health care organizations have mission statements that speak to providing high quality or excellence in client care. Some mission statements focus exclusively on providing care, whereas others assume a broader view and consider the education of health care professionals and the promotion of research as contributing to a broader mission. The mission of other organizations may be community-based, and these organizations consequently will focus on providing community outreach and population-based services to a specific community or population within a community.

MISSION STATEMENT

The **mission statement** is a formal expression of the purpose or reason for existence of the organization. It is the organization's declaration of its primary driving force or its vision of the manner in which it believes care should be delivered. (For examples of actual mission statements, refer to Exploring the Web, p. 186.)

PHILOSOPHY

The **philosophy of an organization** is typically embedded in the mission statement. It is, in essence, a value statement of the principles and beliefs that direct the organization's behaviour. A careful reading of the mission statement will usually provide a good understanding of the institutional philosophy or value system. Mission statements with phrases such as *with respect for the dignity of each elderly resident, a brighter future for all children,* or *vigorous rehabilitation to maximize each individual's utmost potential* provide clues to the type of service that one can expect from that organization. In the best of worlds, the behaviours of the organization are consistent with its stated mission, philosophy, and values.

VISION

The **vision** of an organization provides a clear picture of what the future will look like for that organization. It usually defines the key results achieved and the goals that are still to be accomplished, and describes the key behaviours that the organization needs to demonstrate to be successful. The boundaries of the organization will be clearly described.

VALUES

Values describe the boundaries the organization will have while pursuing its vision. Both core values (i.e., those values that will not be compromised) and aspirational values (i.e., those values that are wished for) will be described.

In order to be meaningful, values must be described in clear behavioural terms and must be measurable. Sometimes an organization's values are formally stated and explicit, as in a mission statement. At other times, the values are implicit and become part of the organizational culture. It is always important to assess an organization's values, as depicted in its mission statement, prior to considering employment; when important individual and organizational values collide, the result will likely be a constant source of frustration for both the employee and employer.

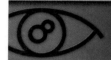

CRITICAL THINKING

Examine these two mission statements and then respond to the questions that follow.

Hospital A: "Our mission is to improve the health and well being of our community and provide quality health care, through co-operation with our partners—the community, providers, educators, and researchers. We will create a supportive team environment for clients, employees, and clinical staff. We will create and maintain an integrated, accessible, and affordable health system, with excellence as our constant goal."

Hospital B: "We are a Catholic health care community that respects the sacredness of all aspects of life. Inspired by the healing ministry of Jesus Christ, our staff, physicians, and volunteers are dedicated to service and to the support of one another. In this environment of service, support, and respect, we meet the physical, emotional, social, and spiritual needs of those served through compassionate care, teaching, and research."

Which of these institutions do you think would be more likely to organize a client lecture series on living with diabetes? Value the contributions of nursing? Provide experimental therapy for cancer? Be open to scheduling routine client care visits for preadmission orientation?

STRATEGIC PLANNING

As Lewis Carroll observed in *Alice's Adventures in Wonderland*, "If you don't know where you are going, any road will do." A health care organization needs to have a good idea of where it fits into its environment and the types of programs and services that are needed and demanded by its clients or stakeholders. This approach applies at both a broad organizational level and at a unit level. A nurse manager in an ambulatory medicine clinic needs to have an understanding of which programs and services are valued by the client population the clinic serves and how the unit's ongoing activities fit with the overall strategy of the larger organization. Staff also need to consider clients' needs when developing new services.

STRATEGIC PLANNING DEFINITION

The scenario described in the interview with Dr. Carruthers (see the Real World Interview) is an example of factors that affect strategic planning. A **strategic plan** can be defined as the sum total or outcome of the processes by which an organization engages in environmental analysis, goal formulation, and strategy development with the purpose of organizational growth and renewal. Robbins et al. (2002) define strategic planning as "plans that apply to the entire organization, that establish the organization's overall objectives, and that seek to position the organization in terms of its environment" (p. 55). Strategic planning is ongoing and is especially needed whenever the organization is experiencing problems or internal or external review problems.

THE PURPOSE OF STRATEGIC PLANNING

The purpose of strategic planning is twofold. First, it means that everyone shares the same idea or vision for where the organization is headed; and second, a good plan can help to ensure that the needed resources are available to carry out the initiatives that have been identified as important to the unit or agency. In addition, a clear plan allows the manager to select among seemingly equal alternatives based on the alternatives' potential to move the organization toward the desired end goal. Senge (2006) states that people with a strong sense of personal direction can join together to create a powerful synergy toward what "we truly want" (p. 197). **Reengineering** is the fundamental rethinking and redesign of the process under review to bring about radical and dramatic improvements and increases in value. Often called business process reengineering, it implies an approach that will allow dramatic changes and yield dramatic improvements in the manner in which the business

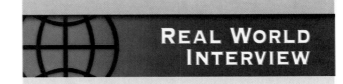

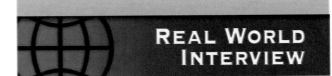

processes are carried out. Strategic planning is a major component of business process reengineering.

STEPS IN THE STRATEGIC PLANNING PROCESS

In any strategic planning process, steps need to be followed in a particular order. This process is similar to the nursing process, in which one assesses and plans before implementing an intervention. Similarly, when developing an organizational, unit, or program plan, it is important to progress in a systematic manner. The first step consists of an environmental assessment.

ENVIRONMENTAL ASSESSMENT

An environmental or a situational assessment requires a broad view of the organization's current environment. For example, when a school of nursing conducted an environmental analysis of the type of undergraduate nursing education that would be needed for the 21st-century professional nurse, it began planning a curriculum revision that would incorporate an increasing emphasis on community-focused care. In addition, this analysis of the environment led faculty to understand that new models for clinical education would be needed to promote improved and expanded linkages between education and practice. This analysis is in line with Donaldson and Fralic's (2000) belief that the health care

system is evolving, which makes uniting the academic and clinical practice settings more critical than ever.

SWOT ANALYSIS

A **SWOT analysis** is a tool that is frequently used to conduct environmental assessments. SWOT stands for strengths, weaknesses, opportunities, and threats. A SWOT analysis identifies strengths and weaknesses in the internal environment and opportunities and threats in the external environment. The SWOT analysis is useful both for initial brainstorming and for a more formal planning document. Figure 9-1 is an example of a SWOT analysis that could be conducted by a university health care centre (Jones & Beck, 1996). Following careful consideration of the SWOT analysis, the organization then re-evaluates its mission and vision to ensure they are congruent with the analysis.

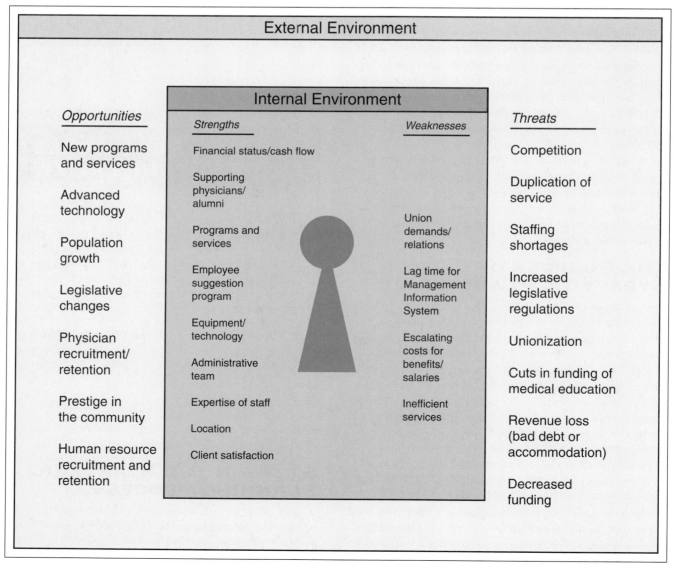

Figure 9-1 Key to Success in Strategic Planning: SWOT Analysis.

COMMUNITY AND STAKEHOLDER ASSESSMENT

A frequently overlooked but highly important area for analysis is the stakeholder assessment. A **stakeholder** is any person, group, or organization with a vested interest in the program or project under review. A **stakeholder assessment** is a systematic consideration of all potential stakeholders to ensure that the needs of each of these stakeholders are incorporated in the planning phase.

For a program to be successful, the involvement of those who will be affected is essential, whether the stakeholders are in the community or are the unit staff who will be affected by a proposed strategic plan. When stakeholders are not involved in the project planning, they do not gain a sense of ownership and may accept a program or strategic goals with only limited enthusiasm, or not at all.

OTHER METHODS OF ASSESSMENT

A number of methods can be used to support involvement in the strategic planning process. Thoughtful planning is required to determine which method to use when another method is appropriate.

SURVEYS AND QUESTIONNAIRES   Frequently, surveys or questionnaires are used when there is both a large number of stakeholders and a general idea of the options available. For example, staff might be polled to determine whether they would attend continuing education and which days and times would be most desirable.

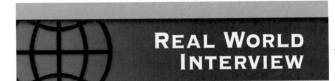

REAL WORLD INTERVIEW

As an administrator, it is imperative that I consider the needs of the staff when planning for the Nursing Practice Council. Although I have a vision of the roles and responsibilities of this Council, it is important that the staff share this vision, or create one of their own that is congruent with the mission of the organization. Staff represented on the Nursing Practice Council include those providing direct client care, nurse educators and clinical nurse specialists, nursing managers, and directors of nursing. In order to provide this opportunity to the staff, we had a two-day facilitated retreat off-site to formulate, and subsequently articulate, the mission, vision, and values of the Nursing Division within the Health Sciences Centre, and to articulate goals and objectives for the next two years.

Dorothy Johnson, PhD, MSN
Chief Nursing Officer, Health Sciences Centre

FOCUS GROUPS AND INTERVIEWS   Focus groups are small groups of individuals selected because of a common characteristic, such as a recent diagnosis of diabetes. People are invited to meet as a group and respond to questions about a topic in which they have an interest or an expertise. An example of a focus group would be a group of clients who have recently had experiences with childbirth. They might be asked to come together to discuss their obstetric experiences at the institution in the hope that the discussion will lead to insights or information that could be used for improving care in the future. Focus groups are usually more time-consuming and expensive to conduct than questionnaires or surveys. They work best when the topic is broad and the options are not clear.

ADVISORY PANEL   Large projects often benefit from an advisory panel, selected from various constituencies affected by a proposed program. The advisory panel does not have formal authority over a program, but it is instrumental in reviewing the planned program and making recommendations and suggestions. Because the advisory panel is deliberately selected to reflect representation from various stakeholders and areas of expertise, the panel is expected to be able to identify potential concerns and provide sound guidance for the program.

REVIEW OF LITERATURE RELATED TO IDENTIFIED PROGRAMS   A review of the literature should be completed prior to strategic planning or beginning any new project or program. This review will allow the project team to identify similar programs, their structures and organization, potential problems and pitfalls, and successes. In the case scenario described in the Johnson interview, prior to designing the program, it was helpful to have an understanding of the methods and strategies already identified in the literature as being effective in working with children and educators. Reviewing the literature is an ongoing process. As programs are tentatively identified, the literature is searched for best practices and best evidence of how to conduct a program, and then the program ideas are refined.

RELATIONSHIP OF STRATEGIC PLANNING TO THE ORGANIZATION'S MISSION

All strategic planning and goals and objectives must be examined with an eye to the purpose or mission of the organization. Organizations can get into trouble when they move too far from their core mission. Consequently, each new project needs to be evaluated in light of its congruence with the main mission that has been identified. It is fine for an organization to move to another project, but only if the new project is in line with the mission.

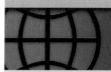

REAL WORLD INTERVIEW

Activities in a High/Scope Teacher Education Centre (High/Scope) include the advanced-level professional development of preschool and elementary teachers and administrators; research on the effectiveness of educational programs; and the development of curricula for infant, toddler, preschool, and elementary programs. These are but a few of the activities related to High/Scope. In 2005, Canada's first combined High/Scope training facility and child care centre opened at the Sheridan Institute of Technology & Advanced Learning (Sheridan) at the Davis campus in Brampton, Ontario. This was a result of a visionary partnership between the Regional Municipality of Peel and Sheridan College. The facility is designed to accommodate both a High/Scope curriculum environment for children and a High/Scope teacher education centre for adult learners. Sheridan provides a variety of specialized High/Scope educational workshops and advanced certifications, which support Early Childhood Educators in developing the skills necessary to provide high-quality programs and thereby influence the care and education the children receive. In cooperation with Sheridan, the municipally operated Learn. Play. Care. Child Care Centre offers a nurturing environment for the children, with High/Scope teacher-certified Early Childhood Educator (ECE) staff. This Centre offers a full range of services for children aged from 18 months to kindergarten. The Region of Peel Children's Services operates the child care centre, and the attached training room is operated by Sheridan. The program for the children can be observed by students in a realistic High/Scope environment. The High/Scope Educational Research Foundation authorizes Sheridan to deliver High/Scope training in Canada. This child care and training facility is the first joint venture of this type between a municipal government and a community college.

Brenda Stagg
Associate Dean, Sheridan College Institute of Technology
and Advanced Learning

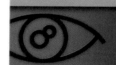

CRITICAL THINKING

You have just read about the High/Scope teacher education centre. Use the description of that centre to answer the following questions:

If this concept were expanded to include health care, what would be the first step to consider?

What opportunities do you envision?

Would these services add value? Who would you contact? What stakeholders would need to be included?

Do opportunities exist for nursing education?

Do you think that community involvement would be important to the success of this program? Why?

What do you think would be the response of the community? What kinds of strategies would you use for building community support?

How would you define success?

Otherwise, the new programs risk draining energy from the main focus of the mission.

PLANNING GOALS AND OBJECTIVES

After all strategic goals and objectives have been identified, they need to be prioritized according to strategic importance, resources required, and time and effort involved. A time line should be set to allow a thoughtful evaluation of each goal and objective and the degree to which each can be implemented in the specified time frame and with the available resources. To avoid misunderstandings and unmet expectations, this time line and its goals and objectives should be communicated to all stakeholders.

DEVELOPING A MARKETING PLAN

When the strategic planning process involves new programming for external audiences, and even if only an internal redesign or restructuring is involved, the strategic plan and the goals and objectives will need to be communicated to all involved constituencies. Such communication will be needed, for example, when an institution is planning to implement a new information system to ensure that it meets provincial government expectations for reporting data. Designing, implementing, training, and evaluating this new system will require substantive changes in both work flow and in the way that employees carry out their day-to-day work. If adequate thought has not been given to communication across the organization about the project, the chance of success is less and the risk of poor cooperation is greater. See Table 9-1 for a summary of the steps involved in strategic planning. See Table 9-2 for an illustration of aligning the balanced scorecard with typical strategic directions.

TABLE 9-1	SUMMARY OF STEPS IN STRATEGIC PLANNING

1. Perform an environmental assessment.
2. Conduct a stakeholder analysis.
3. Review the literature for evidence and best practices.
4. Determine congruence with the organizational mission.
5. Identify planning goals and objectives.
6. Estimate resources required for the plan.
7. Prioritize according to available resources.
8. Identify time lines and responsibilities.
9. Develop a communication plan.
10. Write and communicate the business or strategic plan.
11. Evaluate.

TABLE 9-2	ALIGNING THE BALANCED SCORECARD WITH TYPICAL STRATEGIC DIRECTIONS

Balanced Scorecard	Typical Strategic Directions
Clinical Utilization and Outcomes	Quality Patient Care/Improvement
Financial Performance and Condition	Organizational Effectiveness
Patient Satisfaction	Patient and Family Focused Care
System Integration and Change	Partnerships, Collaboration and Integration

Source: Brun, L. (2003). The dos and don'ts of strategic planning. *Healthcare Management Forum, 16*(4), 37–38. Reprinted with Permission.

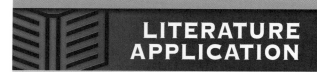

LITERATURE APPLICATION

Citation: LaPorta, J. A., King, G., Cathers, T., Havens, L., Young, L., & Aylward, S. (2003). A test of a centre's vision. *Healthcare Management Forum, 16*(1), 34–36.

Discussion: The Thames Valley Children's Centre (the Centre) conducted a "vision test" that would inform the community whether or not the Centre's vision was being achieved. This project was conceived as a result of the Centre's strategic planning and re-visioning exercise. The test focused on what the clients themselves viewed as key life outcomes, which related to employment, independent living, attendance at school, and participation in the community, to name a few.

Young people who were graduates of the Centre, were at least 16 years of age, were no longer clients of the Centre, and lived within 50 kilometres of the city of London were contacted. The survey was explained, and their level of interest in participating in the study was determined. As a result of the feedback received, the Centre determined it was meeting its vision for a significant portion of individuals.

Implications for Practice: The survey findings revealed that "it is a myth to think that people requiring rehabilitation services are less happy and less satisfied with their lives." When caring for a population undergoing rehabilitation, services need to target lifelong goals, such as productivity and self-determination, in addition to short-term goals related to function, such as mobility. One of the most important goals is to assist people to attain satisfaction in their lives.

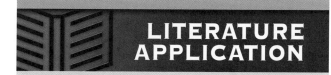

LITERATURE APPLICATION

Citation: Iron, K. (2006). ICES report: Health data in Ontario: Taking stock and moving ahead. *Healthcare Quarterly, 9*(3), 24–26.

Discussion: Policymakers, planners, administrators, and the public are able to see how well the health care system is performing by evaluating the information provided to them in balanced scorecards. Many system characteristics and data sources must be utilized in order to present a complete picture. Ontario has been a leader in reporting in many clinical areas, such as surgical procedures, cardiac care, and the use of drugs in the elderly. However, other key areas, such as chronic disease management and preventive care, cannot be fully evaluated because the relevant data are either of poor quality or are unavailable. This article describes how health information could be improved in Ontario, and the types of data that are required. One of the primary recommendations is to create a centralized and dedicated health information agency in order to have a real-time health service and clinical information system, vital for improving the health of Ontarians.

Implications for Practice: The importance of accurate collection, interpretation, and dissemination of data cannot be overemphasized. Although great strides have been made, the ability to measure how the health system works is necessary to understand and improve client outcomes and system efficiency.

ORGANIZATIONAL STRUCTURE

Organizations are structured or organized to facilitate the execution of their mission, strategic plans, reporting lines, and communication within the organization. This need for structure applies to both entire organizations as well as individual nursing units. Organizational structures can be described in a number of ways by identifying their selected characteristics, which tend to exist on a continuum. For example, under the category of type or level of authority in an organizational structure, a highly bureaucratic, highly authoritarian structure is at one end of the continuum, and a highly democratic, participative structure is at the other end. The highly authoritarian model is well suited for the purposes of the military, where it is seen most often. When decisions need to be made quickly, with clarity and not with challenges or discussion, as in a battle situation, a highly authoritarian organizational structure works well.

An example at the other end of the continuum would be a multidisciplinary group of professionals meeting to determine the care management of a client or client population. This group might be a hospice team task force made up of nurses, social workers, physicians, home care personal support workers, bereavement specialists, and chaplains, all meeting to discuss the care planning for a dying client. In this situation, team members of each discipline need to be able to freely contribute according to their particular area of knowledge and expertise. This type of organizational structure can function successfully only in a participative, democratic manner.

TYPES OF ORGANIZATIONAL STRUCTURES

Although a poor structure makes a high performance impossible, the best structure in the world will not ensure good performance (Drucker, 1973).

Most often, the existing organizational structures are communicated by means of an organizational chart. Figure 9-2 is an example of an organizational chart for a large acute care general hospital system. This organization has a tall bureaucratic structure with many layers in the hierarchy, or chain of command, and a centralized formal authority in the board of trustees. It represents a formal, top-down reporting structure.

MATRIX STRUCTURE

Because of the greater complexity of today's health care system, more organizations are using matrix structures. Figure 9-3 shows a matrix design (Shortell & Kaluzny, 2000).

FLAT VERSUS TALL STRUCTURE

Organizations are considered flat when there are few layers in the reporting structure. A tall organization would have many layers in the chain of command. An example of a flat organizational structure is a school of nursing that has no departments and many faculty members reporting to one dean of nursing.

DECENTRALIZED VERSUS CENTRALIZED STRUCTURE

The terms *centralized* and *decentralized* refer to the degree to which an organization has spread its lines of authority, power, and communication. A tall, bureaucratic design like that in Figure 9-2 would be considered highly centralized. A matrix design like that in Figure 9-3 would be on the decentralized end of the continuum. As can be seen in Figure 9-3, the nursing manager can interface with the Alzheimer's disease program manager without going through a central, hierarchical core, as would happen in a bureaucratic structure like that in Figure 9-2.

Other characteristics or attributes can be used to assess organizations. Many typologies exist that may be used for this purpose. For example, Shortell and Kaluzny (2000) suggest using external environment, mission/ goals, work groups/work design, organizational design, inter-organizational relationships, change/innovation, and strategic issues. Refer to Table 9-3 for an example of how these attributes can be assessed in four different health service organizations (Shortell & Kaluzny, 2000).

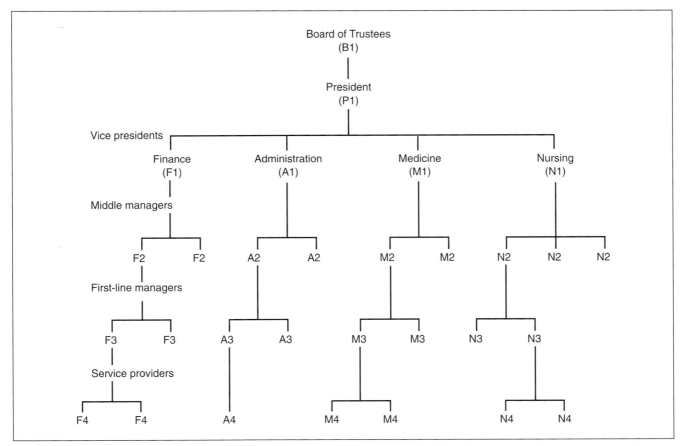

Figure 9-2 Organizational Chart, Formal Authority Structure: Acute Care General Hospital.

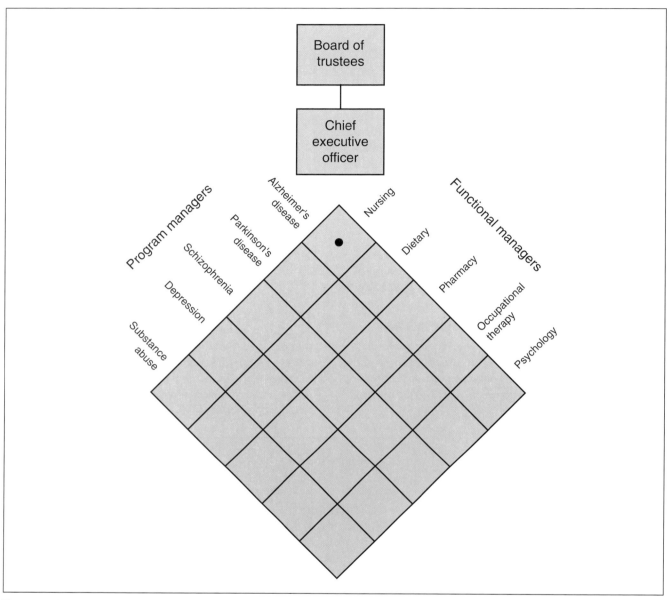

Figure 9-3 Matrix Design: A Psychiatric Center. An individual worker in this example is part of the Alzheimer program as well as a member of the nursing department.

DIVISION OF LABOUR

The way the labour force is divided or organized has an effect on how the mission is accomplished. The functional organizational chart in Figure 9-4 graphically depicts how the formal authority in this organization is structured (Shortell & Kaluzny, 2000). At the highest level, the board of trustees delegates authority to the chief executive officer, who delegates to the vice presidents and so on. At the vice presidential level, there are five department directors for each branch. The department directors each report to their respective vice

president. The nurse managers report to their department director of nursing. The charge nurse reports to the nurse manager of her unit. The treatment nurse and the medication nurse report to the charge nurse. In this functional design, the division of labour is efficient and specialized. A danger with a functional division of labour is that individuals may be so focused on their own specific area that they have little perspective on the overall picture. For example, a treatment nurse may focus on treatments and have little information about the total client.

TABLE 9-3	TYPOLOGY OF FOUR HEALTH SERVICES ORGANIZATIONS			
Attribute	**Regional Health Authorities**	**Home Health Care Agencies**	**Hospitals**	**Pharmaceutical Companies**
External environment	Complex High change Highly integrated	Relatively simple Moderate change Increasingly competitive	Complex High change	Moderate complexity Moderate change Highly competitive
Mission/goals	Acute and primary care emphasis; keep people well	Quality of life Maintaining functional status	Acute care emphasis; curing illness	Research and development (R&D) emphasis; new product development
Work group/work design	Program and cross-program teams; high need for coordination Coordination of care across continuum	Simple design; primarily one-on-one client contact	Departmental and cross-departmental teams; high need for coordination	Separation of functions possible; R&D versus sales; relatively low need for coordination
Organization design	Functional, divisional, and matrix, integrating primary care physicians, specialists, and all professions	Functional	Divisional and matrix	Divisional and strategic business units
Inter-organizational relationships	Vertically and horizontally integrated health system	Expand client base and gain economies of scale	Key to becoming part of vertically integrated health systems	Important for global expansion
Change/innovation	Respond to and create new client-focused and organization-focused care management approaches	Respond to demographic and social changes	Respond to the new paradigm; implement new roles within vertically integrated systems	Respond to new product development demands
Strategic issues	Fit into an expanded and changing health care delivery system	Demonstrate continuing value and, therefore, reimbursement for services	Fit into an expanded and changing delivery system	Decrease time to develop new drugs

In the matrix structure shown in Figure 9-3, the structure was less important; and the workforce roles and reporting relationships were based on the project or task to be accomplished, rather than on a rigid hierarchy. An example of a matrix structure is the planning involved in the preparation for a Canadian Council on Health Facilities Accreditation review. The organization teams could be composed of various individuals at varying levels of responsibility and from programs across the organization, but they could interact with staff at all levels and

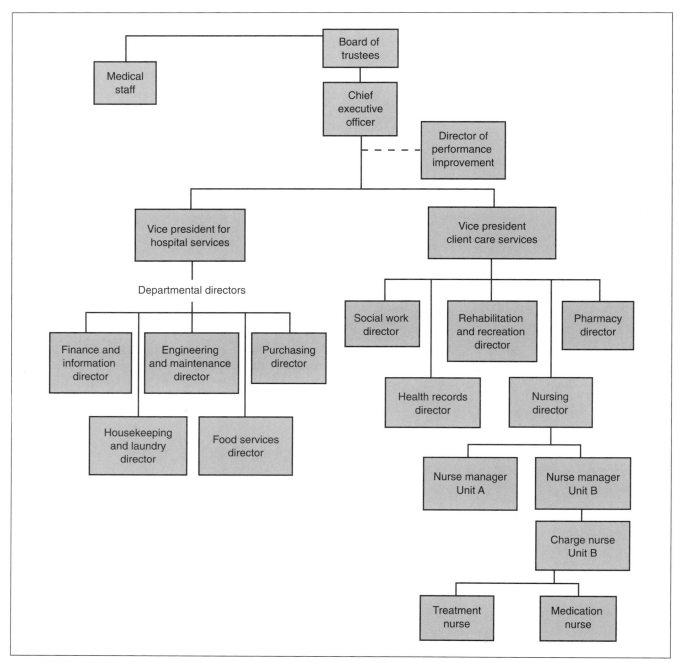

Figure 9-4 A Functional Design: Nursing Home

report as a task force for the purposes of the accreditation survey.

ROLES AND RESPONSIBILITIES

Note that exact roles and responsibilities within each level and division are not defined on the organizational charts beyond specifying the given division, for example, nursing. Scope of responsibilities, specific duties, and specific job requirements are found in documents such as individual job or position descriptions.

REPORTING RELATIONSHIPS

An organizational chart, such as the one that appears in Figure 9-4, shows the formal reporting relationships, which are shown with a solid line. Sometimes dotted lines are used in an organizational chart to depict dual or secondary reporting relationships. An example of such a relationship might be the role of the director of quality improvement, who reports directly to the chief executive officer but also has position accountabilities to the board of trustees. The formal reporting relationships may or may

CASE STUDY 9-1

A client presented to the Emergency Department with complaints of nausea, vomiting, and diarrhea over three hours. The triage nurse determined that the client was of low-risk, and referred him to the "fast track," an area that was completely staffed by licensed practical nurses. When a licensed practical nurse assumed the care of the client, she noticed that his vomitus was becoming blood-tinged, and she contacted the physician. The client's condition progressively worsened, and he was eventually admitted to the Intensive Care Unit.

What could have been done differently?

Was anyone at fault? Who?

Why is good communication especially important when there is a functional division of labour?

What types of problems could you expect if staff members focused on their own tasks and failed to communicate with each other about the client's emotional, psychosocial, educational, and discharge needs?

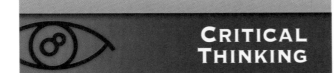

CRITICAL THINKING

A number of studies have demonstrated that primary nursing leads to improved client and nurse satisfaction.

Why do you think this might be? Can you think of any disadvantages to a primary nursing care model for organizing care?

not reflect the actual communications that occur within the institution.

DIVISION OF LABOUR BY GEOGRAPHIC AREA

Care delivery can be efficiently divided according to geography or location. Such a division of labour might consist of the hospital and ambulatory care; or at smaller unit levels, the North Team and the West Team. Frequently, care provided by home health agencies is divided by geographic district for travel efficiencies. At the health care system level, geographical division could mean that each major area, such as the hospital and the supporting ambulatory clinics (located two blocks away), would have separate supporting services, such as two pharmacies, one in the ambulatory clinic and one in the hospital. Both ambulatory clinic and inpatient areas could, and often do,

have separate health records departments. An obvious concern in such arrangements is lack of coordination and duplication of services.

DIVISION OF LABOUR BY PROGRAM Sometimes, care delivery is organized around programs. A division of labour by program is a type of functional division of work, but is based on a client's diagnosis or the specialty care required by a client. For example, care delivery might be divided into a cardiology program, a woman's health program, and an oncology program. Division of labour by program can lead to improved quality of care and decreased confusion for the client because the information and protocols used in the outpatient area would be consistent with the information and protocols used in the hospital and across the entire health care system. Figure 9-5 demonstrates a program design (Shortell & Kaluzny, 2000).

PRIMARY NURSING Primary nursing care describes a model of care in which one nurse is primarily responsible for all aspects of client care for a given client or clients. The client is assigned a primary nurse upon admission, and, when possible, that nurse will be the client's primary caregiver throughout the hospitalization. In this model, an associate nurse is usually assigned to assume care responsibilities when the primary nurse is not available.

Many factors affect strategic planning, such as highlighted by the SWOT analysis discussed in this chapter (page 174). Nurses need to prepare to address these many factors.

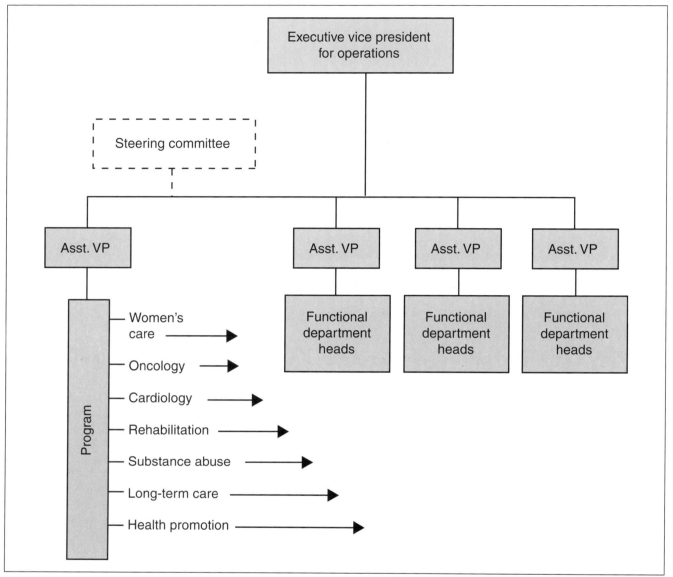

Figure 9-5 Program Design.

Y̶ou have been asked to take a leadership role in identifying potential concurrent disorder programs that could be implemented in the community-based mental health centre where you work as a community health nurse. You normally report to the mental health manager, but for this project you are designated as the coordinator of concurrent disorder programs. As you begin your assessment of potential programs, you will need to interact with a number of functional departments across the organization, such as dietary, pharmacy, occupational therapy, and psychology. In addition, you will have to examine the other mental health programs to ensure you are not duplicating services.

Given this situation, what would be some advantages of working in an institution that had a matrix design such as that depicted in Figure 9-3? What might be disadvantages?

KEY CONCEPTS

- Nurses have increasing opportunities to become involved in strategic planning for the delivery of health care services in their organizations and communities. To participate effectively, however, nurses need a basic understanding of the way in which organizations are structured, how organizational systems function, and how to engage in the strategic planning process.

- Every organization has a purpose and a guiding philosophy, which are typically explicitly stated and detailed in a formal mission statement.

- The mission statement reflects the organization's values and provides the reader with an indication of the behaviour and strategic actions that can be expected from that organization.

- A health care organization needs to have a good idea of where it fits into its environment and the types of programs and services that are needed and demanded by its customers or stakeholders.

- The pivotal value of strategic planning is that it requires an organization to focus on its raison d'être and its mission and to test how its operations are leading to accomplishment of that mission.

- The purpose of strategic planning is twofold. First, it means that everyone shares the same idea or vision of where the organization is headed; second, a good plan can help to ensure that the needed resources are available to carry out the initiatives that have been identified as important to the unit or agency.

- A stakeholder assessment is a systematic consideration of all potential stakeholders to ensure that the needs of each of these stakeholders are incorporated in the planning phase. For a program to be successful, the involvement of those who will be affected is essential.

- Organizations are structured or organized in a manner that is designed to facilitate the execution of their mission and their strategic plans.

- Organizational structures can be described in a number of ways by identifying selected characteristics.

KEY TERMS

focus groups
mission statement
philosophy of an organization
reengineering
stakeholder

stakeholder assessment
strategic plan
SWOT analysis
values
vision

REVIEW QUESTIONS

1. A document that describes the institution's purpose and philosophy is
   A. the organizational chain of command.
   B. the organizational chart.
   C. the mission statement.
   D. the strategic plan.

2. Which of the following is the outcome of the processes by which an organization engages in environmental analysis, goal formulation, and strategy development with the purpose of organizational growth and renewal?
   A. Stakeholder assessment
   B. SWOT analysis
   C. Strategic planning
   D. Mission development

3. The most formal and hierarchical organizational structure would be expected to have an organizational chart with
   A. a matrix design.
   B. many layers of command.
   C. a program design.
   D. a number of dotted lines representing reporting relationships.

4. SWOT means
   A. strengths, weaknesses, opportunities, threats.
   B. strengths, worries, outcomes, threats.
   C. strengths, weaknesses, opportunities, treatment.
   D. structures, worries, outcomes, threats.

REVIEW ACTIVITIES

1. Having a strategic plan in place can help an organization to make a decision between two alternatives. For example, an institution whose strategic plan calls for positioning itself as the leading cancer care provider in the area would be well served to advertise for nurses on the Canadian Association of Nurses in Oncology website (http://www.cano-acio.ca/) or in the *Canadian Journal of Oncology*, rather than in a local newspaper, even if the costs of advertising on the website or in the journal were higher. Identify another situation in which a strategic plan could guide an organization in its choices among alternative actions.

2. Write a beginning mission statement and strategic plan for your professional nursing career. Do you plan to care for vulnerable populations in the community, become an expert in critical care nursing, or seek advanced education to become a midwife? Once you have identified your mission, outline a strategic plan with objectives to attain your nursing goals. For example, you might want to conduct a SWOT analysis, looking at the external environment; your internal environment (i.e., your skills, talents, and preferences); and the strengths, weaknesses,

opportunities, and threats that exist in each. After you have completed this exercise, you will have a better idea of which opportunities to pursue. For example, if you know that you want to work in pediatrics, you might ask for a subscription to a pediatric journal for your birthday. Additionally, you may be able to select or have input into the selection of your final clinical rotation in school, or you may be more likely to search out meetings, conferences, or educational sessions in your area of interest.

3. You are asked to help establish the community advisory panel for your institution's proposed hospice program. How would you choose people to include on the community advisory panel? What groups of professionals and consumers would you want to see represented on a hospice community advisory panel? Identify at least 10 candidates and the stakeholder groups that they might represent. Remember to include both professionals and consumer/community representatives. Before inviting people to join the advisory panel, it would be helpful to assess their support for hospice concepts and their level of interest in becoming involved. How might you go about doing this?

4. Examine the organizational structure of an organization or institution with which you are familiar. How would you characterize it using the types of structures that were discussed in this chapter? Look at organizational communication, reporting structure, and division of labour. Is the organization a hierarchy or a matrix? Does the structure of the institution or organization assist it in meeting its goals? Why or why not?

EXPLORING THE WEB

- Upon completion of your nursing degree, you are planning to interview for a position at an area hospital. In preparation for your interview, you want to understand the hospital's mission and other information, all of which is readily available on the web. For example, if you were planning to apply at Capital Health Edmonton (*http://www.capitalhealth.ca/default.htm*), you would go to *http://www.capitalhealth.ca/Careers/default.htm*. The exact address of the mission statement of the health system is available at *http://www.capitalhealth.ca/AboutUs/MissionVisionValues/default.htm*.

- Another example is The Hospital for Sick Children in Toronto at *http://www.sickkids.ca/* (the exact web address of the mission statement is *http://www.sickkids.ca/abouthsc/section.asp?s=Who+We+Are&sID=11873&ss=Vision%2C+Mission+%26+Values&ssID=231*).

- Look at these web pages, paying particular attention to the descriptions they provide of the organizations' missions. What impressions do you form about these organizations and their missions? Does the stated mission seem to fit with the general feel that you get from the website? Could you easily find information about positions available? About the institution? Try this exercise with your local hospital or medical centre.

REFERENCES

Baker, G. R., & Norton, P. (2001). Making patients safer! Reducing error in Canadian healthcare. *Healthcare Papers, 2*(1), 10–31.

Baker, G. R., & Norton, P. (2004). Next steps for patient safety in Canadian healthcare. *Healthcare Papers, 5*(3), 75–80.

Baker, G. R., Norton, P. G., Flintoft, V., Blais, R., Brown, A., Cox, J., et al. (2004). The Canadian Adverse Events Study: The incidence of adverse events among hospital patients in Canada. *Canadian Medical Association Journal, 170*(11), 1678–1686.

Brun, L. (2003). The dos and don'ts of strategic planning. *Healthcare Management Forum, 16*(4), 37–38.

Chezem, J., Friesen, C., Montgomery, P., Fortman, T., & Clark, H. (1998). Lactation duration: Influences of human milk replacements and formula samples on women planning postpartum employment. *Journal of Gynecological and Neonatal Nursing, 27*(6), 646–651.

Donaldson, S., & Fralic, M. (2000). Forging today's practice-academic link: A new era for nursing leadership. *Nursing Administration Quarterly, 25*(1), 95–101.

Drucker, P. (1973). *Management tasks, responsibilities, and practices.* New York: Harper & Row.

Havens, D. S., & Aiken, L. H. (1999). Shaping systems to promote desired outcomes: The magnet hospital model. *Journal of Nursing Administration, 29*(2), 14–20.

Iron, K. (2006). ICES report: Health data in Ontario: Taking stock and moving ahead. *Healthcare Quarterly, 9*(3), 24–26.

Jones, R., & Beck, S. (1996). *Decision making in nursing.* Clifton Park, NY: Delmar Learning.

Kanter, R. M. (1997). *On the frontiers of management.* Boston: Harvard Business School Press.

LaPorta, J. A., King, G., Cathers, T., Havens, L., Young, C., & Aylward, S. (2003). A test of a centre's vision. *Healthcare Management Forum, 16*(1), 34–36.

Marquis, B. L., & Huston, C. J. (2006). *Leadership roles and management functions in nursing theory and application* (5th ed.). Philadelphia: Lippincott, Williams, & Wilkins.

National advisory councils in nursing and medicine collaborate to develop new approaches for enhancing patient safety. (2000). *Health Workforce Newslink, 7*(1), 5.

Robbins, S. P., DeCenzo, D. A., & Stuart-Kotze, R. (2002). Fundamentals of management: *Essential concepts and applications* (3rd Canadian ed.). Toronto: Prentice-Hall.

Senge, P. M. (2006). *The fifth discipline: The art & practice of the learning organization.* New York: Doubleday.

Shortell, S., & Kaluzny, A. (2000). *Health care management: Organization design and behavior,* (4th ed.). Clifton Park, NY: Delmar Learning.

SUGGESTED READINGS

Aikman, P., Andress, I., Goodfellow, C., LaBelle, N., & Porter-O'Grady, T. (1998). System integration: A necessity. *Journal of Nursing Administration, 28*(2), 28–34.

Bates, D., & Gawande, A. (2000). Error in medicine: What have we learned? *Annals of Internal Medicine, 132,* 763–767.

Bennis, W. (1999, Summer): The end of leadership: Exemplary leadership is impossible without full inclusion, initiatives, and cooperation of followers. *Organizational Dynamics,* 71–80.

Biem, H. J., Cotton, D., McNeil, S., Boechler, A., & Gudmundson, D. (2003). Day medicine: An urgent internal medicine clinic and medical procedures suite. *Healthcare Management Forum, 16*(1), 17–23.

Bodenheimer, T. (1999). The movement for improved quality in health care. *New England Journal of Medicine, 340,* 488–492.

Buerhaus, P., & Staiger, D. (1997). Future of the nurse labor market according to health executives in high managed-care areas of the United States. *Image: Journal of Nursing Scholarship, 29*(4), 313–318.

Buerhaus, P., Staiger, D., & Auerbach, D. (2000). Why are shortages of hospital RNs concentrated in specialty care units? *Nursing Economic$, 18*(3), 111–116.

Chassin, M. R. (1996). Quality of health care part 3: Improving the quality of care. *New England Journal of Medicine, 335*(14), 1060–1063.

Chassin, M. R., Galvin, R. W., & the National Roundtable on Health Care Quality. (1998). The urgent need to improve health care quality. *Journal of the American Medical Association, 280,* 1000–1005.

Chezem, J., Montgomery, P., & Fortman, T. (1997). Maternal feelings after cessation of breastfeeding: Influence of factors related to employment and duration. *Journal of Perinatal and Neonatal Nursing, 11*(2), 61–70.

Cormak, M., Brady, J., & Porter-O'Grady, T. (1997). Professional practice: A framework for transition to a new culture. *Journal of Nursing Administration, 27*(12), 32–41.

Drucker, P. (1973). *Management tasks, responsibilities, and practices.* New York: Harper & Row.

Duckett, L., Henly, S., Avery, M., Potter, S., Hills-Bonczyk, S., Hulden, R., et al. (1998). A theory of planned behavior-based structural model for breast-feeding. *Nursing Research, 47*(6), 325–336.

Fraser, B., & Hollett, R. G. (2003). Use of a program logic model to guide the development of a strategic plan for Wellington County Hospitals Network. *Healthcare Management Forum, 16*(3), 12–17.

Institute of Medicine. (1999). *To err is human.* Washington, DC: National Academy Press.

Jones, K. R., DeBaca, V., & Yarbrough, M. (1997). Organizational culture assessment before and after implementing patient-focused care. *Nursing Economic$, 15*(2), 73–80.

Kaplan, R. S., & Norton, D. P. (1996) *Translating strategy into action: The balanced scorecard.* Boston: Harvard Business School Press.

Korabek, B., Slauenwhite, C., Rosenau, P., & Ross, L. (2004). Innovations in seniors care: Home care/physician partnership. *Canadian Journal of Nursing Leadership, 17*(3), 65–78.

Kouzes, J. M., & Posner, B. Z. (2002) *The leadership challenge* (3rd ed.). San Francisco: Jossey-Bass, A Wiley Company.

Kreitzer, M. J., Wright, D., Hamlin, C., Towey, S., Marko, M., & Disch, J. (1997). Creating a healthy work environment in the midst of organizational change and transition. *Journal of Nursing Administration, 27*(6), 35–41.

Leape, L., Woods, D., Hatlie, M., Kizer, K., Schroeder, S., & Lundberg, G. (1998). Promoting patient safety by preventing medical error. *Journal of the American Medical Association, 280*(16), 1444–1447.

Levi, P. (1999). Sustainability of healthcare environments. *Image: Journal of Nursing Scholarship, 31*(4), 395–398.

Mills, A., & Blaesing, S. (2000). A lesson from the last nursing shortage: The influence of work values on career satisfaction with nursing. *Journal of Nursing Administration, 30*(6), 309–315.

Nicklin, W., & Stipich, N. (2005). Enhancing skills for evidence-based healthcare leadership: The Executive Training for Research Application (EXTRA) program. *The Canadian Journal of Nursing Leadership, 18*(3), 35–44.

Olson, L. L. (1998). Hospital nurses' perceptions of the ethical climate of their work setting. *Image: Journal of Nursing Scholarship, 30*(4), 345–349.

Prescott, P. (2000). The enigmatic nursing workforce. *Journal of Nursing Administration, 30*(2), 59–65.

Rambur, B. (1999). Fostering evidence-based practice in nursing education. *Journal of Professional Nursing, 15*(5), 270–274.

Regenstein, M. (2000). *Medical errors and patient safety: Issue for public hospitals.* Washington, DC: National Public Health and Hospital Institute.

CHAPTER 10

Effective Team Building

Karin Polifko-Harris, PhD, RN, CNAA
Adapted by: Heather Crawford, BScN, MEd, CHE

Exemplary leaders enable others to act. They foster collaboration and build trust. This sense of teamwork goes far beyond a few direct reports or close confidantes. They engage all those who must make the project work. . . . (Jim Kouzes & Barry Posner, 2002, p. 18)

OBJECTIVES

Upon completion of this chapter, the reader should be able to:

1. Identify the differences between groups, teams, and committees.
2. Discuss the stages of group development.
3. Review key concepts of effective teams.
4. Discuss ways in which a nurse manager can create an environment conducive to team building.

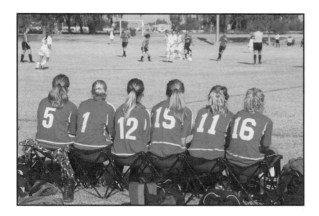

As a new nurse, you are making the day's assignments for a 34-bed medical-surgical unit. Working with you today will be another two registered nurses, two licensed practical nurses, and one unregulated care provider. You graduated only months ago but were recently promoted to the role of charge nurse. Today, one of the licensed practical nurses and the unregulated care provider are challenging your client care assignments, saying you do not have enough experience to make a fair assignment, and they are trying to get the two registered nurses to side with them. The two registered nurses often work together, as do the two licensed practical nurses. You know you made the best assignment given the staff available, yet you are wondering whether there is a better solution.

What are your thoughts on how to proceed?

What would be the best way to address their concerns?

How could you more actively involve them in the client assignment responsibility?

Essential leadership and management skills in nursing always include some element of effective teamwork. Working together in a successful team requires more than good luck or chance. As the health care delivery system continues to increase in complexity, issues such as changing reimbursement schedules, more seriously ill hospitalized clients, and a move from acute health care to non-acute health care delivery challenge nurse managers to alter how they provide nursing care to clients. A critical trend in human resource development is team training. Whereas Canadian business culture emphasizes the role of the individual in achieving success, the nursing profession has begun refocusing on teamwork and team building as a method for meeting the needs of a changing health care delivery model. Nurses generally do not work in isolation but provide care that is interdependent, providing a level of expertise to help the client achieve optimal wellness. This chapter discusses the key factors that contribute to a successful nursing team, including team building. It also discusses characteristics and skills of an effective team leader.

DEFINING TEAMS AND COMMITTEES

Katzenbach and Smith (1993) define a **team** as "a small number of people with complementary skills who are committed to a common purpose, performance goals, and approach for which they hold themselves accountable (p. 45)." Senge, Roberts, Ross, Smith, and Kleiner (1994) further elaborate that a team is a group that has a purpose and needs each member's contributions to succeed. On some teams, all members may have similar backgrounds and abilities, such as a nursing policy and procedure team. Other teams may comprise members who have a variety of skills and talents, to provide different perspectives and ideas on how to solve problems.

An **interdisciplinary team** is composed of members with a variety of clinical expertise. An advantage of an interdisciplinary team is the different strengths and viewpoints the team members contribute. Everyone on the interdisciplinary team (i.e., nurses, physicians, social workers, dieticians, case managers) is trained in his or her specialty and looks at care delivery with a different focus. Sometimes having so many viewpoints can be difficult, though; especially if a single decision is needed and everyone has a different opinion. The best way to work with an interdisciplinary team is to allow everyone to be heard, and to entertain various problem-solving methods and potential solutions. It is the role of the team leader to ensure that all members have the opportunity to participate to accomplish the work of the team.

To get the work of an organization completed, multiple committees may develop to assist in communication. A **committee** is a work group with a specific task or goal to accomplish. An ad hoc committee is generally temporary and formed for a specific purpose, for a specific time frame, or to accomplish a certain short-term goal. An example of an ad hoc committee may be the bed utilization committee that meets only until flu season is over. Unlike ad hoc committees, standing committees may be an integral component of the organizational structure; for example, a Quality Improvement Committee that meets on a monthly basis. Standing committees may be mandated through organizational bylaws, such as medical staff meetings. Other committees may exist because a formal process is needed for decision making, as in the Critical Care Committee. Regardless of the purpose of the committee, after the work has been completed, the group should be disbanded. Individuals are far too busy to continue to attend committee meetings after the mandate of the committee has been fulfilled.

A committee may also be advisory, such as a committee that meets to discuss concerns of the professional nursing staff (e.g., a Professional Practice Council) and then reports back to the Chief Nurse Executive (CNE).

STAGES OF TEAM PROCESS

All teams progress through predictable phases of development, much like people do, as they evolve from an immature stage to (one hopes!) a mature stage. It is critical to note that not all teams reach maturity for a variety of reasons: perhaps there is ineffective leadership, problematic members, unclear goals and directives, or lack of focus or energy. Similar to individuals on the continuum of maturity, some teams may become fully functional and mature quickly, bypassing a stage or two along the way. High-functioning teams, whose members are familiar with one another, are usually able to make decisions quickly and accurately; it may take longer for other teams, whose members need to get to know and trust one another before the actual work can take place.

Tuckman and Jensen (1977) identified five stages that a group normally progresses through as it reaches maturity. These stages are known as **group development** and consist of forming, storming, norming, performing, and adjourning (see Table 10-1). Lacoursiere (1980) identified these same developmental stages as orientation, dissatisfaction, production, and termination.

The first stage is one of **forming,** in which several critical phases begin: the expectation phase, the interaction phase, and the boundary formation phase. The expectation phase starts when the first meeting begins. Everyone is curious what the group is all about—how will it meet their needs, what they will need to do to fit in, and what they can gain from group membership. During the interaction phase, opinions begin to be formed as the group takes shape, and expectations and boundaries are more clearly defined. The group is establishing its identity, with the help of the group leader who provides the team with information on the purpose of the group and the vision and boundaries of what the group is expected to accomplish.

The second stage of group development is the **storming** phase. As everyone begins to feel more comfortable in the group setting, certain feelings and statements

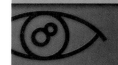

CRITICAL THINKING

You are the nurse who is working with Mr. Ward, a 76-year-old male who was admitted for congestive heart failure and chronic kidney disease. Mr. Ward is well known to the staff at Memorial Hospital for his multiple admissions. During this admission, his blood pressure was unusually high and he appeared sluggish. His wife is visiting her relatives out of town, and he is by himself. When you attend the daily client care conference, you note most of the interdisciplinary team is present: the community nurse case manager, the social worker, the nurse caring for him, the hospital chaplain, the dietician, the pharmacist, and his primary care physician.

What key issues are concerning you? What perspective does each of the team members bring to the discussion on the care of Mr. Ward? How would you proceed to develop or alter Mr. Ward's plan of care? Are there any other team members who may be able to assist you with Mr. Ward's care?

may result in members finding a position within the group to which they can contribute. The storming phase is generally difficult because of conflict that may, at times, be quite apparent. Differences among group members—including even the group leader, perhaps—become obvious, with people often taking sides on certain concerns or issues. Although this phase is tension filled and confrontational, a group often needs to journey through the storming phase to encourage resolution of the emerging problems and to actively solve the issues at hand.

Stage three is the **norming** phase, which follows the conflict and confrontation of the storming stage. Although the problems are not yet solved, and decisions may not

TABLE 10-1	STAGES OF GROUP PROCESS (DRAWING ON TUCKMAN & JENSEN, 1977, AND LACOURSIERE, 1980)			
Forming	**Storming**	**Norming**	**Performing**	**Adjourning**
■ Expectations	■ Tension	■ Positioning	■ Actual work	■ Closure
■ Interactions	■ Conflict	■ Goal setting	■ Relationships	■ Evaluation
■ Boundary formation	■ Confrontation	■ Cohesiveness	■ Group maturity	■ Outcomes review

have been made, members have a general understanding of the issues are and who will be progressing toward solving them. Positions within the group are now established, with members having a sense both of belonging and of setting goals to meet the expectations outlined in the forming stage. Conflict has converted into cohesiveness.

Performing is the fourth stage in the maturity of a group and is probably the most enjoyable phase. Interdependence is the foremost activity—members know what their role is and what they are supposed to do, and obvious progress is made toward the plan to achieve the overall group goal. The group is considered mature at this stage, and the individual members are now ready to focus on the actual work that will meet the group's objectives. Another strength of the performing stage is the emphasis placed on maintaining effective relationships with group members, as the individual members function as a whole (Tappen, 2001).

The final stage of group processing is **adjourning.** The group has met its objectives, and the primary focus is closure activities and the termination of team relationships. Closure is the process by which the team members review the team's progress. Were the goals and objectives of the team met? Would anything have been done differently if the team were to start over? During the final stage, the group should evaluate whether the stated purpose was accomplished. What were the outcomes of both the group process and the individuals' participation? Groups are often disbanded without this closing review, leaving some members feeling empty and without a feeling of accomplishment.

GROUP ROLES

As in any gathering, when people come together in a group, everyone takes on a different role. Some may want the role to be self-serving, as with the person who wants to be the centre of attention and insists on being the dominant force in any decision. Others play a role that is clearly supportive: they are there to contribute in any way they can to the betterment of the whole but do not need or want any limelight thrown their way. People may take on numerous other roles, though some roles are not always clearly defined.

FUNCTIONAL VERSUS DYSFUNCTIONAL MEMBERS

In any team, there are likely to be both participants who are functional and those who are somewhat dysfunctional in their behaviours. Sometimes the behaviours are unconsciously acted out—perhaps in the form of a defence mechanism, such as denial. At other times, a group member is quite clear and focused about the role being played, such as the antagonizer. In any case, the astute group leader needs to be aware of everyone's roles to facilitate the optimal group process possible.

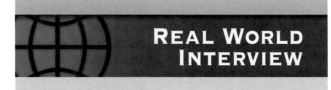

So what role would a functional group member perform? Several roles are critical to the successful meeting of a group's goal (Bradford, 1978). When a project first begins, a group member is needed to fill the role of initiator—the person who gets the ball rolling and defines the group's problem. A role complementary to the initiator is that of coordinator—the person who is aware of the project flow and who keeps it moving in the right direction. Likewise, the team needs a mobilizer, whose job is to keep things energized and who provides the spark needed to keep team members interested in the project. Other functional roles include the questioner, who asks the questions that are on everyone's mind; the antagonist, who looks at the situation in an opposite manner to everyone else; and the recorder, who chronicles the details of the group meeting and process. It is not necessary to have all the roles filled at all times in functional groups.

What are the dysfunctional roles that hinder the progress of a group? Unfortunately, numerous personality types can be difficult, especially during the group's formative stages. Criticizers find fault with everything and everybody, yet seldom contribute positively when asked. Everything is a strong "No!" and if it is not done their way, they believe it will not be done correctly. Passive members will rarely take a stand on anything. Their passivity and inability to make a decision is often frustrating. They will not say a word for fear of rebuttal.

Detailers get so caught up with the facts that it is hard for them to see the big picture or to keep heading toward the goal. Likewise, controllers monopolize the group discussion—no one else can be heard. The only opinion that matters is theirs. They need constant refocusing by

TABLE 10-2	STRATEGIES FOR COPING WITH DIFFICULT PERSONALITIES

Personality Type	Coping Strategies
Criticizer	Do not argue—it will only add fuel to the fire! Ask for input and practise active listening by reflecting on what you hear. Give criticizers a project to which they can directly contribute.
Passive one	Engage in communication, ask direct questions, ask for direct responses.
Detailer	Allow the detailer to give details at certain points in the meeting. Begin with the objective for the session, repeat information when necessary, and summarize.
Controller	Keep focused on the task at hand; note any inconsistencies in the controller's conversation.
Pleaser	Let pleasers know that their comments are safe from attack and that their opinions are valued.

the leader to keep them on track. Finally, pleasers want to do just that—please. They will not make a comment or decision that may be unfavourable to anyone else. Refer to Table 10-2 for suggestions on how to cope with difficult personalities.

KEY CONCEPTS OF EFFECTIVE GROUPS

A familiar saying is that "the whole is greater than the sum of the parts." An effective group is one in which all members are equally important, everyone's voice and opinions are heard, and progress is made toward the stated goal on a steady basis. How does one encourage the energy that comes from placing people of different backgrounds and specialties together to mutually solve problems and make decisions? What are the necessary skills to work with interdisciplinary team members in an increasingly complex health care delivery system?

GREAT TEAM GUIDELINES

An assumption is often made that any group of people who come together will inevitably become a team. This assumption is not necessarily true. Some groups will just remain workgroups, whereas most teams will initially function as effective working groups. A group is a collection of individuals who are in an interdependent relationship with one another. A team, on the other hand, goes beyond that; as shown in Table 10-3, team members share the ownership of the team's function and direction to increase their confidence and commitment (Mears, 1994).

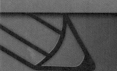

CASE STUDY 10-1

Your nurse executive has assigned you as the new team leader of the task force on client falls. This task force has been meeting for almost a year without making much progress. At your first meeting, you note that there are several challenging personalities in the group and wonder whether they will ever be able to work together effectively.

Jamie is a new graduate nurse and volunteers for everything so that he will be liked. Angela is the detailer, often asking everyone to repeat what they said so that she can get more information on the topic. Samantha is the passive one and just looks annoyed at having to be there. You noticed she was doing some of her client charting during the meeting. Annabelle attempts to keep the team on track, but with her soft-spoken voice, she is not well heard. Finally, no matter what anyone says, Beth is critical and comes up with a reason why something will not work.

Where do you begin?

How would you deal with the five group members?

What is your primary focus at the beginning of your time as team leader and why?

TABLE 10-3	TEAM VERSUS GROUP

Team	Group
Decisions made by concensus with all inputs heard and valued	Groups tend to have majority and minority opinions
Disagreements are carefully examined and resolution is sought	Criticism tends to be destructive and disagreements are not effectively dealt with
Objectives are well understood and accepted by the team	Group members do not necessarily accept common objectives
Free expression of ideas occurs and others listen to what is said	Personal feelings are hidden
Self-examination of how the group is functioning frequently occurs	Discussions are avoided regarding how the group is functioning
Roles are understood by all members	Individuals tend to protect their role and their niche in the group
Shared leadership occurs on an as-needed basis	Leadership is appointed

Source: Mears, P. (1994) *Healthcare teams: Building continuous quality improvement.* Orlando, FL: St. Lucie Press Inc. Reprinted with Permission by the author.

Great teams don't just happen; before anyone even meets, behind-the-scenes planning, preparation, and forward thinking have already taken place. Theories of effective teams have been discussed in the literature for several decades by Lewin (1951), McGregor (1960), Argyris (1964), Burns (1978), Bennis (1989), and Senge (2006). What are the guidelines for encouraging great teams? A great team accomplishes what it sets out to do, with everyone on the team participating to achieve the desired outcomes. See Figure 10-1 for great team guidelines.

First and foremost, the team must have a clearly stated purpose: what are the goals, what are the objectives, and how long and how often will the team meet? What is the vision of the team? What does the leader see the team accomplishing? An effective team keeps the larger organization's mission in mind as it progresses; otherwise, its goals will be inconsistent with those of the parent organization. Second is an assessment of the team's composition: what are the team members' personal strengths and weaknesses? How do the team members see themselves—all as individuals? Do they see themselves as part of a cohesive team? Are any additional members needed? What are the roles of each team member?

Third is the communication link. Are effective communication patterns in place? Is there a need to improve communication, either in written or verbal format? Does the team work well with e-mail and voice mail, or does it need the traditional paper trail to stay connected? Is communication open, with minimal hidden agendas by the members? Can the truth be told in order to reach a difficult decision, in a compassionate and sympathetic manner?

Active participation by all team members is a critical fourth item. Does everyone have a designated responsibility? Do people listen to one another, or is everyone trying to be heard at the same time? What are the relationships of the team members? Is there mutual trust and respect for members and their decisions, however unpopular? Are there turf issues that must be resolved before proceeding? *Turf*, according to Husting (1996), is the primary reason that early team-building efforts may not work. Therefore, it is important for the team leader to work on resolving turf-related problems first. The climate of the team should be relaxed but supportive, especially during brainstorming of new ideas or discussion of problems and problem solving.

Is there a clear plan as to how to proceed? This fifth element leads to an action plan that everyone agrees with early on and that is revisited at designated times. Feedback by team members and others affected by the team's decisions is necessary to keep focus. The sixth guideline is actually ongoing, in that assessment and evaluation are continuous throughout the team's history. Outcomes have to be consistent and related to the expectations of the organization. Creativity is also encouraged at the team level; perhaps a member has an idea for solving a problem, a solution that no one has ever tried. In a supportive environment, pros and cons of all reasonable ideas should be freely discussed. A team needs to periodically assess its progress.

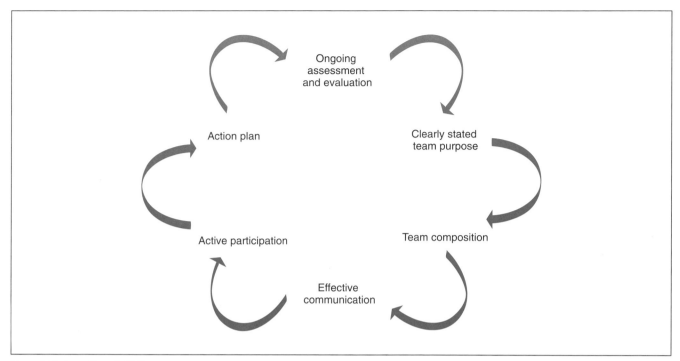

Figure 10-1 Great Team Guidelines

CREATING AN ENVIRONMENT CONDUCIVE TO TEAM BUILDING

Before any members can be effective in a team, whether the team is a committee or is part of the staff on a nursing unit, a team leader needs to ensure that the environment is conducive to team building. The attitudes, organizational culture, policies, and procedures all help to determine how successful the team will be in accomplishing its directives. Developing an environment that is supportive and exciting to work in is an ongoing process rather than a one-shot event.

Many hospitals employ authoritarian styles of management and leadership rather than true participatory or democratic styles. If the team members work in an authoritarian environment, they may be hesitant or uncomfortable in making decisions for themselves and may prefer the leader to make clear the parameters for decision making. Creativity and creative solutions to problems may be a challenge in this environment, but creativity is critical for progress to occur. Organizational hierarchy needs to be carefully looked at. Is it a formal or informal hierarchy? Who has the power to make decisions or to derail solutions? Having a top-heavy organizational structure and power base may discourage a team from being effective—too many people need to be informed of all the steps, decisions, and solutions of the team, and some may actually thwart progress from occurring.

Resources must be made available to the team to carry out its work. Is there a meeting space that is conducive to conversation and available on a regular basis? Is

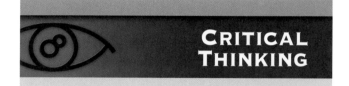

CRITICAL THINKING

The chief nurse executive has asked your nurse manager to initiate a new committee to review client safety issues in the hospital. She has asked you to join the committee. Although you are a nurse on a stroke rehabilitation unit, you know that challenging client safety issues are everywhere in the hospital. So far, no one else has volunteered to be on the committee, even though the nurse manager posted the request for members several weeks ago.

Who are you interested in having on the committee? Are they all registered nurses? Why or why not? How will you encourage people to join the committee? How will the nurse manager initiate the group process? Discuss several types of staff that you have worked with who were either functional or dysfunctional in a group and why.

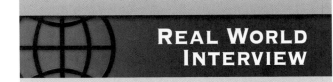

REAL WORLD INTERVIEW

When you start working with a team, it is really important to understand everyone's perspective—what their experiences are, where they work, what is important to them. You need to be observant and pay attention to both verbal and nonverbal communication. You need to be able to read between the lines.

John Fielding, RN
Risk Manager

necessary secretarial support available to set up the meetings and to record and distribute the minutes? Is there adequate staffing to allow team members the time to meet? Are the communication systems reliable?

Are the administrators supportive of the team's efforts? For example, if there is a problem in having key members attend meetings, whether it is lack of commitment or other conflicting duties, will the administrator support efforts to change this situation? Often, a staff nurse is assigned to a team that is focused on solving an institutional problem, such as restraint usage, but another nurse may not have been assigned to take care of the staff nurse's clients during the committee meetings.

Team members also need to see that progress is being made and that it is made on a consistent basis. Does the environment reward team members' contributions? Is team membership an expectation? Can the team's work be linked to the continuous improvement process so that members can see how they are making a difference in the client's care, the client's families, or community they serve; system enhancement; or overall improvement of the quality of the organization? Continuous improvement is a process in which the status quo is never accepted and in which the care delivered is always being reviewed for better ways to improve satisfaction, decrease errors, or smooth the care delivery processes. Likewise, it is imperative to notify administration if the team's progress is not coming along as expected. It is better to share the unfavourable news as early as it is discovered, unless there is a good chance the direction may be changed with time or additional changes. Involving others early in the process may deflect more serious issues later on, because other people may be able to offer additional resources or information that team members may not have access to.

Table 10-4 offers a team evaluation checklist to evaluate whether your team environment is healthy and receptive. Any areas checked *no* may be opportunities for further improvement.

TEAMWORK ON A CLIENT CARE UNIT

The role of the nurse is multifaceted. Depending on the scenario, a nurse may work directly or indirectly with a wide variety of staff on the health care team. A registered nurse (RN) is directly responsible for the care of the

TABLE 10-4	TEAM EVALUATION CHECKLIST		
Question		**Yes**	**No**
1. Is the environment/climate conducive to successful team building?			
2. Do the team members have mutual respect and trust of one another? Are the team members honest with one another?			
3. Does everyone actively participate in the decision making and problem solving of the team?			
4. Are the purpose, goal, and objectives of the team obvious to all participants?			
5. Are creativity and mutual support of new ideas encouraged by all team members?			
6. Is the team productive and does it see actual progress toward goal attainment?			
7. Does the team begin and end its meetings on time?			
8. Does the team leader provide vision and energy to the team?			

client, but that care encompasses ensuring that the physician orders and nursing orders are carried out and that documentation is completed accurately and appropriately for the shift. The RN ensures all ordered treatments and procedures have been completed; discharge planning is coordinated with the social worker, the community case manager, and the pharmacist; the client's family understands how to dress the client's wound; and finally, the client understands the discharge instructions. The role of the RN team leader incorporates the entire spectrum of care provided to the family by a wide variety of people. The effective nurse possesses excellent communication skills, both written and verbal; communicates in a manner sensitive to others' cultural and value differences; is aware of others' abilities; and shows genuine interest in the team members. An open and objective communication style is needed, and communication should be carried out in an unbiased, constructive manner.

EFFECTIVE TEAM MEETINGS

To run an effective team meeting, the team leader needs to plan and coordinate the work of the team. The leader needs to have a clear understanding of the purpose and goals of the team, facilitating members' full participation. People are more apt to accomplish objectives when the vision is clearly stated and mapped. The leader should embrace and understand the change process and be able to teach staff members, and inspire followers toward participative management according to how they work and communicate in groups (Marquis & Huston, 2006). Another critical function of the leader is to prepare the team members ahead of time, perhaps meeting

REAL WORLD INTERVIEW

One thing that I always try to keep in mind is that one can never overcommunicate. I try to communicate both up and down the ladder with different modalities, such as direct e-mail, communiques, open forums, newsletters, and voice mail messages to groups. The message always needs to be delivered in a positive way. People are more likely to eagerly anticipate further updates if your message is delivered positively, succinctly, and is of importance to them.

Leanne Danford, MScN
Director of Nursing

with them individually to fully engage them in the team. This time spent between the nurse leader and the team member is critical.

When the team meeting is in session, the leader will often be (1) the time keeper, ensuring that the meeting begins and ends when stated; (2) the coordinator, making sure that necessary items and information are available to the team; (3) the peacemaker, tempering opposite viewpoints that are discussed in meeting sessions; (4) the delegator, assigning tasks as needed, such as appointing someone to research a particular perspective of the problem being investigated, or ensuring that the minutes are available; (6) the feedback loop, providing information on the status of goals; and (7) the role model, inspiring others on the team to continue their focus on the goals of the team, especially when performance does not show progress.

An effective team does not attain results on its own. In addition to providing a supportive environment that nurtures success for its members, an effective team has a leader with vision. This leader has a clear idea of the team's strategic plan and will help others see the plan clearly, and to understand its place in the institution. The leader readily inspires trust and respects all members of the team, regardless of their status in the organization. Ross, Wenzel, and Mitlyng (2002) offer the following suggestions for building a successful team through effective leadership:

- Identification with a mission—Value the contributions of all team members: all members are critical to the success of the team regardless of their position on the team. Recognize that the mission of the organization is more important than personal ambition.
- Confidence and trust—Team members cross traditional organizational lines because there is a high level of interpersonal confidence and trust. Encourage interaction among group members: know when verbal and nonverbal behaviour is appropriate and inappropriate, and keep the flow of communication going. Turf issues are minimized.
- Promote debate—Discourage "we versus they" thinking: build teamwork that encourages inter-team participation and relationships. Team members are able to disagree with each other and debate issues from varying viewpoints. After a decision is made, the entire team supports one another and the decision, and moves the issues forward.
- Identify with team success—Acknowledge and celebrate team accomplishments: publicly and frequently acknowledge positive contributions by team members, and keep the team members abreast of the positive changes they are actively involved in making. Team members share the limelight and share credit for success with their colleagues.

■ It is imperative that effectiveness as a team member is evaluated, regardless of your role. Are you carrying your weight, or are you expecting others to carry out your directives?

DEVELOPING DECISION-MAKING AND PROBLEM-SOLVING SKILLS

Huber (2000) discusses a range of decision-making approaches that assist in accomplishing the stated goals and objectives during a nursing team's existence. Knowing when to have the entire team participate in the decision-making process or when to have only the leader make the decision varies depending on the situation and the desired outcome. The *autocratic* decision process is used by the leader in situations in which (1) the task or outcome is relatively simple (e.g., finding space to meet); (2) most team members would agree with the decision and provide consensus; and (3) a decision has to be made promptly.

In the *consultative* decision process, the leader will ask the opinions of the entire team, but the final decision lies with the leader. A fully developed team may use the *joint* decision process, in which there is mutual decision making by both team members and the leader, with everyone having an equal vote. This process encourages everyone

to fully accept the team's conclusion. The joint decision process is also the most creative because all have the opportunity to provide input and differing perspectives into the decision. On the opposite end from the autocratic decision process is the *delegated* decision process, in which the leader is not involved with the final verdict. Instead, the team is truly self-governed and accountable for its decisions. An example of a delegated decision process is the setting up of a unit orientation program for new graduate nurses. After the leader provides the necessary parameters, the team develops its own orientation program and merely reports its decision to the nurse executive.

What are some common problems teams have when charged with decision making and problem solving? A primary issue is that of actually coming to a decision. An autocratic decision is made by one person, regardless of input from others. A joint decision is made together by everyone, with some members winning (i.e., those whose idea was chosen) and some losing (i.e., those whose idea was not chosen). Another common style of decision making is that of consensus: in decisions by consensus, everyone must agree with the final outcome, or else everyone must agree to work together until an acceptable decision is made.

Teams must also grapple with the issue of low productivity, or minimal results. People sometimes cannot focus

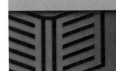

LITERATURE APPLICATION

Citation: Oandasan, I., Baker, G. R., Barker, K., Bosco, C., D'Amour, D., Jones, L. et al. (2006). *Teamwork in healthcare: Promoting effective teamwork in healthcare in Canada: Policy synthesis and recommendations.* Ottawa: Canadian Health Services Research Foundation.

Discussion: Teamwork and collaboration in health care are priority issues for Canadians and their decision-makers, with many reports calling for improved collaboration as a key strategy in health care renewal. Effective teamwork can improve the quality of client care, enhance client safety, and reduce workload issues for health professionals. This report was commissioned to answer three questions: What are the characteristics of an effective team and how do you measure its effectiveness? What interventions have been successful in implementing and sustaining teamwork in health care and what can we learn from other countries? and To what extent has teamwork been implemented in Canadian health care settings, and what are the barriers to implementation? The report was completed by an inter-professional research team who conducted interviews, and completed an in-depth review of "team" literature. They identified the challenges of building and maintaining effective teamwork, which included, but was not limited to lack of common definition of teams and teamwork; organizational factors that affect teamwork; and the implication of current policy and legislation on teams. The change required to support teamwork is collaboration. Leadership and commitment at all levels of the health care system are required.

Implications for Practice: Leadership and commitment are required from all levels of the health care system in order to foster effective teamwork and collaboration. Turf battles have to be eliminated. A common definition for health care teams, teamwork, and team effectiveness is required. Further work is required by all domains—leadership, education, practice, and research to influence the creation of effective teams and collaborative efforts.

in the right direction; if a team meets infrequently, an entire year can pass without the team accomplishing anything of significance. In contrast, some teams believe that group members do not have any other commitments except to work on their team's goals and objectives. These high-powered teams expect team members to devote a fair amount of non-meeting time to writing, researching, and producing results for the next team meeting, regardless of other organizational obligations.

SUCCESSFUL TEAM MEMBERSHIP

Within any group, some members are productive, results-oriented team players, and other members are perfectly content to let others do the work. Some members may be destructive, exhibiting such behaviour as being the aggressor, the disapprover, or the blocker of others' suggestions; being a recognition seeker; being a self-confessor of personal, non-group–oriented feelings or comments; being a playboy or playgirl; being a group dominator or help seeker; or using the group to meet personal needs or plead special interests (Northouse & Northouse, 1992).

If a team is to succeed, the right blend of personalities, experience, and temperaments is critical to work successfully toward a common goal. For example, if a new graduate nurse is placed on a critical committee responsible for developing a new sick call policy, senior staff nurses should also be included for their experience. If an entire team is composed of aggressive, visionary members who are not detail-oriented, many fine points may be missed. However, if a team is predominantly composed of people who get caught up with specific issues, the team members may miss the overall goal, because they are bogged down in details.

For a team to have positive outcomes, an astute team leader will keep in mind that some personality types complement others. One tool that some organizations use to assist them in devising effective work teams and team building is the Myers-Briggs Type Indicator, a psychological instrument that identifies different personality types. Successful teams are those that use the right blend of personalities to achieve their goals.

KEY CONCEPTS

- Teams, groups, and committees are essential to the effective functioning of any health care organization.

- Teams may be formed for a variety of reasons, including the need for professional affiliation, the need for socialization, and the need for psychological fulfillment.

- Teams, groups, and committees consist of people who come together for a common purpose and who need each other's contributions to achieve the overall goal.

- Each group goes through defined stages of increasing maturity.

- Group members can perform functional or dysfunctional roles, which may ultimately enhance or hinder the group's progress toward goal attainment.

- Great teams have clearly stated purposes, effective communication, an action plan, and continuously evaluate their progress.

- The team leader has certain designated responsibilities and tasks to ensure team productivity.

- An environment conducive to team building should be in place for maximum success.

- The team has various decision-making and problem-solving abilities and methods.

KEY TERMS

adjourning
committee
forming
group development
groups

interdisciplinary team
norming
performing
storming
team

REVIEW QUESTIONS

1. In forming a group, the leader should keep in mind that
   A. the group should decide the goals and objectives.
   B. the group is responsible for developing its vision.
   C. the group should be constructed of similar personality types.
   D. the group should encourage active participation by all members.

2. Which is the normal sequencing of group development?
   A. Forming, norming, storming, performing, adjourning
   B. Norming, forming, storming, performing, adjourning
   C. Forming, storming, norming, performing, adjourning
   D. Forming, storming, conforming, norming, adjourning

3. Which of the following group roles is considered functional?
   A. Initiator
   B. Detailer
   C. Pleaser
   D. Controller

4. One of the primary duties of effective team leaders to their team is to
   A. ensure that all the details are taken care of all the time.
   B. enable the team to envision their goals and objectives.
   C. take effective minutes of the meetings.
   D. allow everyone a chance to participate, even if the meeting goes longer than expected.

5. In maintaining an environment conducive to team building, it is important to
   A. have leaders with an autocratic management style.
   B. encourage creativity within the organization.
   C. reward employees who consistently revise the team's objectives.
   D. hold an evaluation session at the completion of the team's duration.

REVIEW ACTIVITIES

1. You are the manager of a 38-bed medical surgical unit. In light of recognition of scope of practice, you have hired three licensed practical nurses to fill positions in which only registered nurses worked before.

   ■ How would you plan for the LPNs to become part of the team?

   ■ What are some important considerations for you, your established staff, and the new employees?

   ■ What are some things you can do to assist them in becoming members of your team?

2. Because of the increase in client complaints about the quality of care, you have been asked to develop a team to address these client care issues.

   ■ What are your expectations of the five stages of group development?

   ■ How will you encourage the group members to progress though each stage?

3. On the unit on which you work as a registered nurse, the team is interdisciplinary in nature: you directly work with licensed practical nurses, unregulated care providers, a unit clerk, one housekeeper, one respiratory therapist, one community nurse case manager, and one clinical nurse specialist.

   ■ What are some of the advantages of working with interdisciplinary teams?

   ■ What are some of the challenges of working with interdisciplinary teams?

   ■ How does one best communicate with an interdisciplinary team?

EXPLORING THE WEB

■ Where would you find additional information on effective team building on the Internet?
http://www.management-training-consultants.com/effective-teams.htm

■ What type of leadership style do you have in a team situation?
http://www.nwlink.com/~donclark/leader/leadstl.html and *http://www.mindtools.com/pages/article/newLDR_84.htm*

REFERENCES

Argyris, C. (1964). *Integrating the individual and the organization.* New York: Wiley.

Bennis, W. (1989). *Why leaders can't lead.* San Francisco: Jossey-Bass.

Bradford, L. P. (1978). *Group development.* La Jolla, CA: University Associates.

Burns, J. M. (1978). *Leadership.* New York: Harper & Row.

Huber, D. (2000). *Leadership and nursing care management* (2nd ed.). Philadelphia: W. B. Saunders.

Husting, P. M. (1996). Leading teams and improving performance [Electronic version]. *Nursing Management, 27*(9), 35.

Katzenbach, J. R., & Smith, D. K. (1993). *The wisdom of teams: Creating the high-performance organization.* New York: Harper Business.

Kouzes, J. M., & Posner, B. Z. (2002). *The leadership challenge* (3rd ed.). San Francisco: Jossey-Bass/A Wiley Company.

Lacoursiere, R. B. (1980). *The life cycle of groups: Group development stage theory.* New York: Human Sciences Press.

Lewin, K. (1951). *Field theory in social sciences.* New York: Harper & Row.

Marquis, B. L., & Huston, C. J. (2006). *Leadership roles and management functions in nursing theory and application* (5th ed.). Philadelphia: Lippincott, Williams, & Wilkins.

McGregor, D. (1960). *The human side of enterprise.* New York: McGraw-Hill.

Mears, P. (1994) *Healthcare teams: Building continuous quality improvement.* Orlando, FL: St. Lucie Press Inc.

Northouse, P. G., & Northouse, L. L. (1992). *Health communication: Strategies for health professionals* (2nd ed.). Norwalk, CT: Appleton & Lange.

Oandasan, I., Baker, G. R., Barker, K., Bosco, C., D'Amour, D., Jones, L. et al. (2006). *Teamwork in healthcare: Promoting effective teamwork in healthcare in Canada: Policy Synthesis and Recommendations.* Ottawa: Canadian Health Services Research Foundation.

Ross, A., Wenzel, F. J., & Mitlyng, J. W. (2002). *Leadership for the future: Core competencies in healthcare.* Chicago: Health Administration Press.

Senge, P. M. (2006). *The fifth discipline: The art & practice of the learning organization.* New York: Doubleday/Currency.

Senge, P. M., Roberts, C., Ross, R. B., Smith, B. J., & Kleiner, A. (1994). *The fifth discipline fieldbook: Strategies and tools for building a learning organization.* New York: Doubleday/Currency.

Tappen, R. M. (2001). *Nursing leadership and management: Concepts and practice* (4th ed.). Philadelphia: F. A. Davis.

Tuckman, B. W., & Jensen, M. A. C. (1977). Stages of small group development revisited. *Group and Organizational Studies, 2*(4), 419.

SUGGESTED READINGS

Abrahamsen, C. (2003). Patient safety: Take the informatics challenge. *Nursing Management, 34*(4), 48–52.

Bellack, J., & O'Neil, E. (1999). Recreating nursing practice for a new century: Recommendations and implications of the Pew Health Professions Commission's final report. *Nursing & Health Care Perspectives, 21*(1), 14–21.

Bennis, W. (1989). *On becoming a leader.* Reading, MA: Addison-Wesley.

Brown, B. (1998). 10 trends for the new year: Nurse managers predict the skills, technology and mind-set you'll need to prosper in 1999. *Nursing Management, 29*(2), 33–36.

Carley, M. S. (1996). Teambuilding: Lessons from the theater [Electronic version]. *Training & Development, 50*(8), 41.

Dimock, H. G. (1985). *How to observe your group* (2nd ed.). Guelph: University of Guelph.

Dimock, H. G. (1987). *Groups: Leadership and group development* (rev. ed.). San Diego: University Associates.

Farrell, M. P., Schmitt, M. H., & Heinemann, G. D. (2001). Informal roles and the stages of interdisciplinary team development. *Journal of Interprofessional Care, 15*(3), 281–295.

Grohar-Murray, M. E., & DiCroce, H. R. (1997). *Leadership and management in nursing.* Stamford, CT: Appleton & Lange.

Harwood, A. (1997). Spot the saboteurs. *Nursing Times, 93*(25), 72–75.

Henderson, E. (2003). Communication and managerial effectiveness. *Nursing Management—UK, 9*(9), 30–35.

Jain, V. K., & Lall, R. (1996). Nurses' personality types based on the Myers-Briggs Type Indicator. *Psychology Reporter, 78*(3 pt. I), 938.

Keirsey, D., & Bates, M. (1978). *Please understand me: Character and temperament types.* Del Mar, CA: Prometheus Nemesis Books.

Kennedy, M. M. (2001). What do you owe your team? Survival tips for people who dread teamwork. *Physician Executive, 27*(4), 58–60.

Leeseberg Stamler, L., & Yiu, L. (2005). *Community health nursing: A Canadian perspective.* Toronto: Pearson/Prentice-Hall.

Lengacher, C. A., Mabe, P. R., VanCott, M. L., Heinemann, D., & Kent, K. (1995). Team-building process in launching a practice model. *Nursing Connections, 8*(2), 51–59.

Leppa, C. J. (1996). Nurse relationships and work groups disruption. *Journal of Nursing Administration, 26*(10), 23–27.

Millward, L. J., & Jeffries, N. The team survey: A tool for health care team development. *Journal of Advanced Nursing, 35*(2): 276–287.

Monty, V. (1994). Effective team building and personality types [On-line]. *Special Libraries, 85*(1), 1.

Morand, D.A. (2001). The emotional intelligence of managers: Assessing the construct validity of a nonverbal measure of people skills. *Journal of Business and Psychology, 16*(1), 21–33.

Myers, I. B. (1995). *Introduction to type.* Palo Alto, CA: Consulting Psychologists Press.

Opt, S. K., & Loffredo, D. A. (2000). Rethinking communication apprehension: A Myers-Briggs perspective. *Journal of Psychology, 134*(5), 556–570.

Prager, H. (1999). Cooking up effective team building. *Training & Development, 53*(12), 14.

Shope, T. C., Frohna, J. G., & Frohna, A. Z. (2000). Using the Myers-Briggs Type Indicator (MBTI) in the teaching of leadership skills. *Medical Education, 34*(11), 956.

Sovie, M. (1992). Care and service teams: A new imperative. *Nursing Economic$, 10*(2), 94–100.

Stein, S., & Book, H. (2000). *The EQ edge: Emotional intelligence and your success.* Toronto: Stoddart Publishing Co. Limited.

Wilson, R. D., Mateo, M. A., & Brumm, S. K. (1999). Revitalizing a departmental committee. *Journal of Nursing Administration, 29*(3), 45–48.

Woolf, R. (2001). How to talk so people will listen. *Journal of Nursing Administration, 31*(9), 401–402.

CHAPTER 11

Budget Concepts for Client Care

Corinne Haviley, RN, MS
Adapted by: Heather Crawford, BScN, MEd, CHE

There is nothing more difficult to take in hand, more perilous to conduct, or more uncertain in its success than to take the lead in the introduction of a new order of things. (Jean-Jacques Rousseau, 1712–1778)

OBJECTIVES

Upon completion of this chapter, the reader should be able to:

1. Describe the budget preparation process for health care organizations.
2. Define commonly used budgets for planning and management.
3. Describe key elements that influence budget preparation.
4. Identify services and products that generate revenue.
5. Identify expenses associated with the delivery of service.

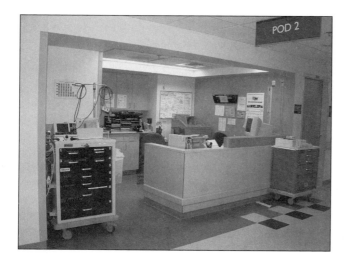

You are assigned to a new unit for your clinical experience. You wonder what types of services are provided to clients on this unit. You talk with your instructor and, if appropriate, the nursing manager of the unit to review the unit's budget. You review the unit's scope of service and budget.

What kinds of clients are cared for on this unit?

What kinds of services are provided to clients on this unit?

How does the unit's budget help ensure provision of care for clients on this unit? A key factor that influences client care is the cost involved in the delivery of service. Resources—people, equipment, and time—are required to support the services delivered by nurses. These resources cost money. The economic success of a health care organization depends on those who are involved with service delivery. The decline in health care funding, as well as escalating costs and increasing demands, have required hospitals to improve operational efficiency and to make economically sound decisions. The challenge in health care is to ensure that the quality of care and the calibre of the staff are not compromised in this ever-changing, cost-controlled environment.

Nurses need to understand how to manage the cost of client care as it relates to their own clinical practice. Nurses are accountable for the distribution and consumption of resources, whether those resources are time, supplies, drugs, or staff. It is essential that appropriate decisions be made regarding cost-effective practices. Cost containment affects the financial viability of a nursing department or unit. Hence, nurses need to be informed and partner with the management team to control expenses in relation to client care. A good management practice includes staff input when analyzing budget variances and generating ideas for saving money on medical-surgical supplies.

The purpose of this chapter is to provide an overview of the operating budget process, including budget development, implementation, performance, and evaluation.

Common financial language and tools are discussed so nurses can understand the process involved in cost-effective care.

Types of Budgets

Hospitals use several types of budgets to help with future planning and management, including operating, capital, and construction budgets.

Operating Budget

An **operating budget** accounts for the income and expenses associated with day-to-day activity within a department or organization. Revenue generation is based upon clients being in the correct accommodation and the expenses associated with equipment, supplies, staffing, and other indirect costs. Revenue may be reduced by the number of days that a client stays in the wrong accommodation. For example, if a patient has semi-private insurance, and is in a standard ward room, the organization loses the revenue from the insurance company for the accommodation.

Capital Budget

A **capital budget** accounts for the purchase of major new or replacement equipment. Equipment is purchased when new technology becomes available or when older equipment becomes too expensive to maintain because of age-related problems, such as inefficiencies resulting from the speed of the equipment or downtime (i.e., the amount of time equipment is out of service for repairs). Sometimes the expense or scarcity of replacement parts makes it prohibitive to maintain equipment. Finally, equipment may become antiquated because of its inability to either deliver service consistently, meet industry or regulatory standards, or provide high-quality outcomes.

Because a significant expense is associated with equipment acquisition, organizations want to make the best and most economical and informed decisions. Staff members from a variety of areas, including materials management, clinical specialties, the legal department, biomedical engineering, information technology, finance, and management can contribute important input when planning for equipment purchases. Equipment features, benefits, and limitations have to be understood as they relate to the needs and goals of a department or institution. Substantial analysis is required because multiple vendors, or companies, often sell similar or varying products with different terms, conditions, and warranty and maintenance agreements that can have short- and long-term effects.

Organizations differ regarding the dollar amount that is considered a capital purchase (Sullivan & Decker, 1997).

Capital purchases are based upon the equipment cost and the life expectancy (i.e., the shelf life) or how long the equipment is expected to perform over time. Generally, capital purchases cost more than $1,000 and last five years or longer. For example, in one organization, a stent costing $2,000 is a supply item used during a surgical procedure. This supply is considered an operational expense because its life expectancy is two years, whereas a computed tomography (CT) scanner costing more than $1,000 with a life expectancy of seven years is considered a capital expense.

CONSTRUCTION BUDGET

A **construction budget** is developed when renovation or new structures are planned. The construction costs generally include labour, materials, building permits, inspections, equipment, and contingency dollars. Expenses may be shifted to another department that absorbs the services on a temporary basis.

BUDGET OVERVIEW

An operating budget is a financial tool that outlines anticipated revenue and expenses over a specified period. A process called **accounting,** an activity that managers engage in to record and report financial transactions and data, assists with budget documentation. The budget translates operating plans into financial and statistical terms so that the budget can be calculated. Budgets serve as standards to plan, monitor, and evaluate the performance of a health care system. Details regarding a budget are specific to the area governed. Budgets account for the income generated as compared to the expenses needed to deliver the service. Budgets make the connection between operating plans and allocation of resources, which is especially important because health care organizations measure multiple key indicators of overall performance. For example, along with financial performance, organizations routinely evaluate quality client outcomes and customer and staff satisfaction. All these indicators are intertwined and hold value in terms of client care. Collectively, they reflect organizational success.

A **balanced scorecard** is a documentation tool providing a snapshot of pertinent information and activity at a particular point in time. A balanced scorecard identifies any of four perspectives about an organization: finances, customer satisfaction and services, internal operating efficiency, and learning and growth (Norton & Kaplan, 2001). Figure 11-1 shows the Neonatal Intensive Care Unit patient care team's balanced scorecard at the Winnipeg Health Sciences Children's Hospital, Winnipeg Regional Health Authority. This scorecard displays the indicators of neonatal transport team response times, pain assessment, parent satisfaction, radiology results communicated to parents, central line infection rates, access to appropriate ventilators, continuity of nursing care, and staff satisfaction. Figure 11-2 is a balanced scorecard showing a

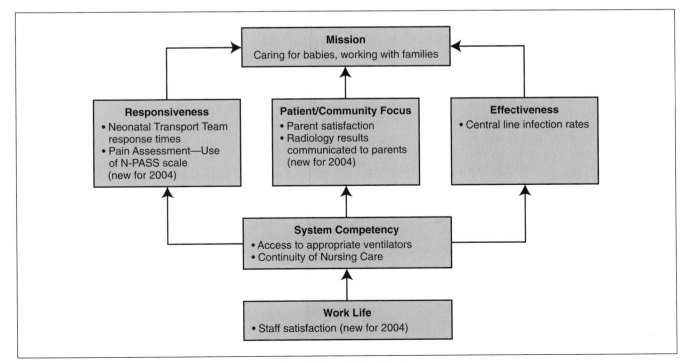

Figure 11-1 NICU (Neonatal Intensive Care Unit) Patient Care Team's Balanced Scoreboard.

Source: Sawatzky-Dickson, D. (2004). A balance with the NICU quality team. Child Health Quality Team. *Quality for Kids Newsletter, 3*(2): 2. Reprinted with Permission of the Winnipeg Regional Health Authority.

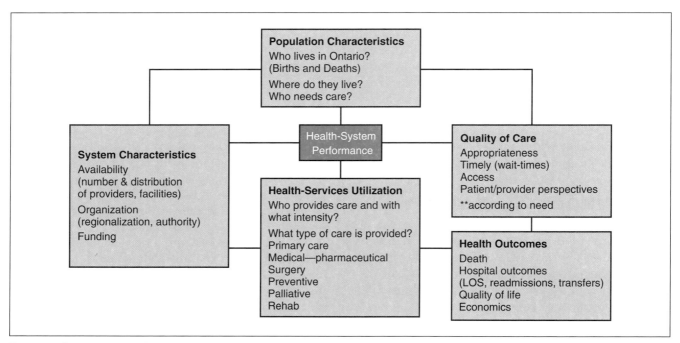

Figure 11-2 Characteristics for Examining Health-system Performance: A Balanced Scorecard Approach.

Source: Iron, K. (2006). ICES report: Health data in Ontario: Taking stock and moving ahead. *Healthcare Quarterly, 9*(3), 24–26. Reprinted with Permission.

variety of indicators that illustrate the connectivity between performance and quality outcomes.

Similar to controlling personal funds, such as managing one's chequing or savings account, budgeting helps to define services by projecting how much cash will be generated (i.e., revenue) and how much services will cost to operate (i.e., expenses). Budgeting requires forward thinking so that problems and obstacles can be anticipated and planned for. Budgets also serve as a benchmark to measure whether the planning expectations are being met. Typically, budgets are monitored monthly, so that if deficiencies arise, financial improvement plans can be instituted early. Corrective action is often initiated to prevent long-term effects in a particular area, such as waste or loss of supply items. The budget functions as a tool to foster collaboration because individuals within a department must work together to achieve its goals.

BUDGET PREPARATION

Formulating a budget involves a systematic approach that begins with preparation (Grohar-Murray & DiCroce, 1997). Budgets are generally developed for a 12-month period. The yearly cycle is based on a fiscal year as determined by the province or territory (e.g., April 1 through March 31) Shorter- or longer-term budgets may also be developed depending upon the organizational planning process.

Prior to the beginning of the budget year, most organizations devote approximately six months to preparing and developing the operating budget. To prepare a budget, organizations gather fundamental information about a variety of elements that influence the organization, including demographic information, volume and cost increases or decreases, regulatory influences, and strategic plans. Additionally, it is helpful to review the department's scope of service, goals, and history.

DEMOGRAPHIC INFORMATION

Pulling together demographic information relative to the population that the organization serves is most helpful because it identifies unique demographic characteristics that influence client behaviour, such as age, race, sex, and income. For example, an obstetrics practice would expect to attract women of childbearing age rather than an older male population. Therefore, understanding the demographics and market share (i.e., the percentage of the population living in the area that uses the organization's services) helps paint a clear picture regarding the client population.

REGULATORY INFLUENCES

The Canadian Council on Health Services Accreditation (CCHSA) accredits health facilities to ensure that organizations meet specific standards. In addition, the CCHSA can make recommendations that will affect the capital or operating budget of the facility. Regulatory requirements

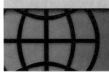

REAL WORLD INTERVIEW

Staff nurses need to understand their own department's client volume, the nature of their case load, the effects of client acuity, and how it may change. As client acuity changes, so does client care delivery. We may be able to anticipate the services that will be needed based upon client acuity and how those services will affect the client's stay. Communicating this information to management is most helpful. Remember that the budget process is fluid and not stagnant. Situations change and can alter the budget over time. A budget is not made in stone; it is only a guideline. Nurses can have an impact upon cost by understanding, through cost accounting, which supplies are being used with different types of admissions or procedures. Once calculated, this data can be shared with physicians. The use of standardized products can be compared when analyzing procedures or admissions by physicians and nurses. This process should assist in understanding both practice patterns and costs related to client care. Physicians and nurses control major costs.

Nurses need to be stewards in recognizing expenses. For example, nurses are key to the client's length of stay and when and how resources are allocated during a client's stay. Nurses need to act on issues before they become critical. Wastage is a good area to focus on because it adds to the cost of a client's stay. If a nurse wastes four gloves, the cost may be only $10 to cover the cost of the gloves. But think further about additional costs, such as packaging, shipping, stocking, charging the unit, and tracking, which may inflate the cost to $30. If this expense occurs during all 3 shifts times 30 beds, then the dollar amount adds up considerably. This cost in turn cuts into the ability of the unit to balance its budget.

Barb Seeley, BScN
Surgical Unit Manager

---

may change regarding who may deliver a specific service and in what type of setting; for example, a procedure may have to be performed in the hospital rather than in a physician's office if it is to be reimbursed by the insurance company; similarly, reimbursement may depend on whether a nurse practitioner or a physician is consulted.

Consumers' willingness to pay out of pocket when not covered by insurance affects revenue as well. For example, the cost of circumcision is no longer covered by health insurance, and if someone requires a cast, the cost of a plaster of Paris cast is covered, but a fibreglass cast is not.

STRATEGIC PLANS

Generally, hospitals have strategic plans that map out the direction for the organization over several years. Strategic plans guide the staff at all levels so that the entire organization can have a shared mission and vision with clearly defined steps to meet the goals.

Each department develops unit-specific plans to help the organization follow its overall strategic plan. For example, a goal may be to become the centre of excellence for gastroenterology endoscopy laboratories for the surrounding region. To meet the goal, one department may focus on client satisfaction and room turnaround time to increase volume and decrease client wait times for procedure appointments. This goal is part of the organization's overall plan.

SCOPE OF SERVICE AND GOALS

During the budget preparation phase, individual departments or sections should be thoroughly examined. Hospital systems are frequently divided into sections, departments, or units to compartmentalize them for organizational purposes. These subsections or units, commonly called **cost centres,** are used to track financial data.

Each department or cost centre defines its own scope of service (Figure 11-3 and Figure 11-4 provide examples of scopes of service). The scope of service is helpful because it provides information related to the types of service and the sites at which services are offered, including the usual treatments and procedures, hours of operation, and the types of client/customer groups.

Departmental goals may include the introduction of new technology or treatments, client education, and creation of a special client care environment. Staff members are generally questioned to determine whether they have any proposed quality initiatives that should be included in the plans for the upcoming year. Generally, new treatments, client education materials, and documentation tools require different types or amounts of supplies. Technically trained staff members are often needed to implement new services. Both the staff and supplies can

The gastrointestinal endoscopy suite may be defined as a specialized department that performs major procedures that are both diagnostic and therapeutic in nature, such as upper GI endoscopies, colonoscopies, flexible sigmoidoscopies, and endoscopic retrograde cholangiopancreatography (ERCP). Conscious sedation is typically delivered to clients to provide comfort during the procedures. The endoscopy suite is open Monday through Friday from 0700–1700 hours, and provides after-hours service for emergent cases. Pre-procedure, intra-procedure, and post-procedure care, including full recovery, is provided on site. Services are provided to critical in-house clients at the bedside via the staff assigned to travel to inpatient units. The department employs nurses, technicians, and receptionists, who work with gastroenterologists and surgeons to provide care. The unit is equipped with 10 procedure rooms, 25 recovery bays, and a gastrointestinal scope cleaning facility on site.

Figure 11-3 Endoscopy Suite Scope of Service.

A medical nursing unit provides primarily inpatient care to clients with acute or chronic medical problems, such as congestive heart failure, diabetes, pulmonary disease, cancer, and so on. The unit, equipped with 30 private and semi-private beds, a lounge, and conference/consultation rooms, is operational 24 hours per day, 7 days per week. Client education and support groups are held routinely in the library located directly on the unit. Team nursing is employed as the model of care. Nurses, licensed practical nurses, unregulated care providers, and unit clerks are employed, with a social worker and diabetes educator providing additional client support. Clients admitted to the unit for longer than 48 hours are discussed during daily multidisciplinary rounds. The rounds include community nurse case managers; psychosocial counsellors; and nutrition, nursing, and medical staff. Staff discuss client problems to facilitate future care, including discharge planning.

Figure 11-4 Medical Nursing Unit Scope of Care.

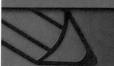

CASE STUDY 11–1

The manager from an inpatient unit asks for staff input into identifying ways to decrease the use of medical supplies and paper items. These items have been identified as exceeding the budget by 10 percent to 20 percent during the past three months. This is the first time that the staff members have been involved in helping with cost containment. Clinical nurses and assistants have been invited to participate.

When approaching an analysis of medical supply use, what might be the first step in the process? If you were to divide the staff into work groups, which members should be chosen to analyze the use of clerical supplies? How would you proceed if you were trying to determine the supply costs associated with starting an IV with continuous infusion?

have varying costs during the early induction phase through full implementation. Creating a new environment or "evidence-based best practice" experience may require additional funding that must be identified early in the planning stages. The manager is responsible for identifying the expenses associated with client care up-front so that they are budgeted.

HISTORY

Organizations typically use history or past performance as a baseline of experience and data to better understand activity in a department or unit. These data are used to assist in interpreting associated expenses with staff productivity and unit performance. Most often, adjustments are made to planned budgets because of the ever-changing cost of products and supplies. Bulk contracts are negotiated so

that predetermined reduced rates can be realized when organizations purchase large quantities of supplies. For example, if a hospital purchases a large quantity of one product, the vendor may reduce the price as an incentive. Additionally, knowledge about historical volume (e.g., procedures, admissions, or client visits and average length of stay) provides a perspective as to how a department has grown or declined over time. This information may help with anticipating future demand and capacity. The story behind a unit and how the department developed is equally important because the financial numbers are tracked over time. Often the culture and complexity of a unit unfold by interviewing staff who were involved in the unit during the past, including physicians, nurses, technologists, assistants, housekeeping, and nutritionists. This information may provide further insight into why and how decisions were made in the past. Hence, multiple phases of data gathering are imperative to build a budget.

Budget Development

After background data have been gathered, the development of the budget can follow, including the projection of revenue and expenses.

Revenue

Revenue is income generated through a variety of means, including billable client services, investments, and donations to the organization. Specific unit-based revenue is generated through billing for services such as special accommodation. The specific number and types of services and procedures have to be projected for the budget. Each type of service may have varying volume associated with it. For example, projecting the volume and type of procedure to be conducted in a gastrointestinal laboratory is based upon feedback from referring physicians and technical staff, in addition to conclusions from historical data.

Similarly, the same types of projections occur for in-patient units, including the number of clients anticipated to be admitted, along with the average length of stay (e.g., three to five days) and the projected occupancy rate. The type and amount of services and patient days can be measured. The number of patient days or the services delivered are tracked from a productivity and efficiency perspective.

It is important to note that the reimbursement rates of third-party payers affect revenue and can change from year to year. For example, the rate for semi-private accommodation may increase from $100 to $125 per day. Uniform rates are often used. Insurance companies dictate or negotiate rates with health care organizations on an annual basis, depending on whether they notice particular trends occurring, such as a hospital that offers only semi-private or private accommodation.

Expenses

Expenses are determined by identifying the costs associated with the delivery of service. Expenditures are resources used by an organization to deliver services and may include supplies, labour, equipment, utilities, and miscellaneous items.

Understanding what it takes to deliver client care services helps to ensure that appropriate budgets are in place to pay for the services. Expenses are commonly separated into line items, representing specific categories that contribute to the cost of the procedure or activity, such as paper supplies, medical supplies, drugs, and so on. This arrangement helps identify a service's significant expenses. For example, a colonoscopy may have a high medical supply cost, whereas chemotherapy administration may be associated with a high drug cost.

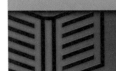

LITERATURE APPLICATION

Citation: Elser, R., & Nipp, D. (2001). Worker designed culture change. *Nursing Economic$, 19*(4), 161–163, 175.

Discussion: To effect operational efficiency and to improve employee performance, these authors propose specific actions to change the nursing culture. Work groups called resource utilization teams were organized to evaluate the unit values and the emotional components that affect relationships. Staff received educational support regarding communication and relationships so that differences and conflicts could be resolved. The staff was surveyed to determine their perceptions of their work environment based upon the cumulative responses. The team formulated a plan to staff the unit using the knowledge that they had gained and the budgetary dollars that had been allocated. The team further identified role responsibilities and tasks that should be assigned to change the unit operations.

The strength of this article is in the creative proposal to capitalize on the knowledge and insight of staff to influence unit productivity. Every department or unit has its own unique characteristics and culture that influence the ability to produce and deliver quality care. Engaging staff in problem solving and role development is key to successful financial and operational management.

Implications for Practice: Expenses and productivity can be analyzed creatively by using the workforce to improve operations and care. Imagine the potential if a work group were continually analyzing quality data points over time. The power of these work groups lies in their diverse members, who can see the department from different perspectives. When the work group is empowered, constructive measures can be identified to address problems that challenge departmental productivity, client flow, and expenses.

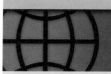

REAL WORLD INTERVIEW

It is not just my job to be responsible for the budget. I encourage my staff to know the costs of supplies, and to understand the rationale behind transferring clients to the correct accommodation. In addition, I teach them about patient days, and hours per patient day, so that they understand how the budget is formulated. I don't think the staff realizes how something simple can negatively affect our bottom line. For example, the nurses will stockpile such items as face cloths or incontinence pads in the client's bedside table. Admittedly, this practice saves some time for the nurse, but if the client is discharged prior to these items being utilized, the linen is returned to the company for relaundering, and the incontinence pads are discarded. Both will cost our unit precious dollars. I have asked the staff for suggestions on how to save money and supplies, and they have had some very creative solutions. In addition, they are more aware of wasteful activity, and our collective endeavour has helped reduce our supply usage.

Maureen Shaughnessy, MSN
Unit Manager—Cardiology

SUPPLIES

As new procedures are introduced, or when a manager wants to ascertain the actual supply expenses associated with a procedure or activity, zero-based budgeting may be instituted. Zero-based budgeting is a process used to drill down into expenses by detailing every supply item and the quantity of items typically used. A list of supplies is developed, including large and small items, along with the itemized expense. Supplies are often packaged in bulk and sold in quantity. Hence, the expense of the items has to be calculated and backed out of the bulk figure to accurately depict the expense.

Figure 11-5 illustrates the zero-based budgeting that may be necessary to understand all of the expenses associated with delivering a procedure. This example can be expanded further to calculate the total expense associated with the anticipated number of procedures. This calculation can be achieved by multiplying the number of anticipated procedures by the total expense per procedure, which leads to authentic projections.

HUMAN RESOURCES

Human resources are significant expenses associated with medical and nursing care. Health care services are very labour intensive. Salaries and benefits account for an estimated 80 percent of operating costs. Hence, it is very important to calculate the amount of time that all staff members—professional, technical, and support staff—are involved with the service. For example, the time that it takes to schedule an appointment, register a client, and escort a client to a procedure room or unit needs to be calculated into the overall cost of care for the client.

In the ambulatory area, staff time is calculated relative to the delivery of a specific procedure, including preparation for the procedure, intra-procedure care, and

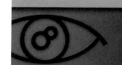

CRITICAL THINKING

Staff handling client care activities on a day-to-day basis are in an optimal position to identify the best practices that affect efficiency and cost-effectiveness. Managers can consult with staff and then organize processes to assist with unit-based improvement. Think back on the steps taken by a nurse during the first hour of a shift. Reflect on communication and how information is received. Examine the amount of time spent in client care versus other activities. Create a journal of activity from different time increments during a shift. Discuss your observations with your coworkers and manager. What problems in flow of activity and gaps in communication or efficiency did you find? How can you drill down further into understanding how the unit operates and ways to increase productivity? How could you improve your team's functioning?

post-procedure care. Pre-procedure preparation entails gathering of supplies, assembling equipment, and preparing the environment. Preparing the client may involve taking a history, completing a physical, administering medication or taking specimens, placing tubes or establishing an intravenous line, and positioning the client. Intra-procedure care is the actual care delivered after the procedure has been initiated. Post-procedure care may require educating and discharging a client, or extensive recovery activity requiring several hours of direct nursing

General Supplies	Quantity	Price	Drugs	Quantity	Price
4 Chux	4	$ 3.00	Fentanyl	1	$ 0.25
Tri Pour Container	1	$ 0.20	Versed	1	$ 2.10
Sterile Water 1,000 ml	1	$ 0.40		Total	$ 2.35
Normal Saline Vial	2	$ 0.10			
Cannister/Lid	2	$ 3.25			
Tubing	2	$ 0.50			
02 Cannula	1	$ 0.05	Printed Forms	Quantity	Price
Suction Catheter	1	$ 0.02			
Disposable Gowns	2	$ 3.80	Hospital Consent	1	$ 0.10
Gloves	6	$ 0.35	Procedure Consent	1	$ 0.75
4X4's	10	$ 0.25	Nursing Form	1	$ 0.75
Surgilube	2oz.	$ 0.15	Vital Sign Sheet	1	$ 0.05
Photos	2	$ 4.30	Doctors Orders	1	$ 0.15
Syringe 10cc	2	$ 0.15	History/Physical	1	$ 0.10
Syringe 60cc	1	$ 0.35	Discharge Instruction	1	$ 0.20
Emesis Basin	1	$ 0.10	Education Sheet	1	$ 0.80
Denture Cup	1	$ 0.15	Charge Voucher	1	$ 0.10
Recording Paper	1	$ 0.05	Procedure Education	1	$ 0.10
Alcohol Pads	2	$ 0.05		Total	$ 3.10
Slippers	1	$ 0.75			
Mask	2	$ 0.25			
Goggles/Face Shield	1	$ 1.20	Clerical Supplies	Quantity	Price
Cetacaine Spray	1	$ 0.10			
Bite Block	1	$ 2.00	Patient File	1	$ 0.80
Patient Bag	1	$ 0.20	Labels	2	$ 0.05
Cleaning Brush	1	$ 2.20	Xerox Paper	6	$ 0.05
	Totals	$23.92	Pen	1	$ 0.05
			Pencil	1	$ 0.05
			Marker	1	$ 0.05
IV Start	Quantity	Price	Highlighters	1	$ 0.05
				Total	$ 1.10
Tourniquet	1	$ 0.15			
Alcohol Wipes	2	$ 0.05			
Angiocath	1	$ 0.05			
IV Solution	1	$ 0.60			
IV Primary Set	1	$ 4.00			
Tegaderm	1	$ 0.15			
Tape	6 inches	$ 0.05	Grand Total		
Band-Aid	1	$ 0.05			
4X4	4	$ 0.10			
	Totals	$ 5.20			

Figure 11-5 Zero-Based Budgeting for GI Lab. (Adapted with permission of Northwestern Memorial Hospital, Chicago, IL.)

care and removal of equipment and supply items. Refer to Table 11-1 for a sample time analysis related to labour.

STAFFING The number of staff and the types of staff are often accounted for in a staffing model. This model outlines the number of staff required based upon the primary statistic, such as procedures or clients. An outpatient model may focus on the number of procedure rooms that require staff. One nurse may be required to staff a gastrointestinal laboratory procedure room, and one shared technician may staff two procedure rooms.

Models can help in analyzing productivity, as illustrated in the following:

- Scenario 1: One nurse is assigned to a procedure room during a 4-hour period, during which 8 clients are treated.

- Scenario 2: One nurse and a technical assistant are assigned to a procedure room for 4 hours, and 16 clients are treated.

The second scenario depicts greater productivity because the number of procedures delivered doubled by using two staff, recognizing that the assistant staff member will cost the organization less in terms of salary expense. Because labour is one of health care's greatest operational costs, enhancing productivity will likely produce savings.

For an inpatient unit, nurses may be assigned to a fixed number of clients during all three shifts. The ratios vary depending upon the shift and client acuity. The nurse-to-client ratio on a medical nursing unit may be one nurse to five (1:5) clients during the day and evening shift, whereas it may be 1:10 during the night shift. The

TABLE 11-1	TIME ANALYSIS PER PROCEDURE		
Pre-procedure Care	**Time (minutes)**	**Intra-procedure Care**	**Time (minutes)**
Appointment schedule	5	Positioning	5
Registration	10	Initiation of conscious sedation	10
Escort to change room	5	Procedure	10
Subtotal	20	Subtotal	25
Direct Client Preparation		**Post-procedure Care**	
History	5	Recovery	120
Client education and consent	10	Education	10
IV initiation	10	Changing and discharging	10
Subtotal	25	Subtotal	140

Grand total = 210 minutes per procedure

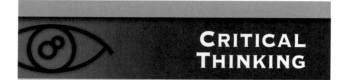

CRITICAL THINKING

"**S**taying in the loop" is key to becoming energized and feeling engaged as a part of the client care team and as a vital part of the organization (Nelson, 1997). When you walk onto a unit, ask a staff member what key quality initiatives the unit is working on to reflect continuous quality improvement. Ask what the unit's goals are and how staff participates in decisions so that the goals may be achieved. Think about how these initiatives may increase productivity, or staff or client satisfaction or decrease expenses. Ask the staff what impact their efforts are having. How is the staff involved in helping the organization to meet its goals?

nurse-to-client ratio may be 1:1 for all shifts on a critical care unit. Chapter 12 deals with effective staffing in more depth.

BUDGET APPROVAL AND MONITORING

Once developed, budgets are submitted to administration for review and final approval. The approval process may take several weeks because the unit budgets are combined to determine the overall budget for the health care organization. Senior management, representing finance and operations, often makes the final decisions regarding acceptance of a budget.

The unit or department manager is responsible for controlling the budget. Budget monitoring is generally carried out on a monthly basis to ensure that revenue is generated consistent with projected productivity and standards. Organizations often recognize a flexible budget, which allows for adjustments if the volume or census increases or decreases. If the volume increases, expenses will likely increase. If the volume decreases and expenses increase, then the manager needs to determine what actions are necessary to control or reduce costs. Many organizations require managers to complete a budget variance report, which identifies when categories are out of line and corrective action is needed. Figure 11-6 illustrates a variance report. The entire health care team is responsible for ensuring that expenses are kept within the budgeted amount and that the volume or census is maintained. The manner in which these controls are accomplished depends on the organization. Some institutions request that balanced scorecards be developed reflecting departmental activity at a glance. Variance reports or scorecards may be posted so that all staff members have an opportunity to review the budget and participate in any improvement needed.

Staff can meet to discuss implementation or reinforcement of strategies that can positively affect the budget (Elser & Nipp, 2001; Yoder-Wise, 1998). The following are some examples of such strategies:

■ Analyze time efficiency of staff involved in client care.
■ Plan for supplies needed for every client encounter and consciously eliminate unnecessary items.

	Budget	Actual	% Variance	Comments/Action
Revenue				
Inpatient				
Outpatient				
Other				
	List all line items over or under budget			
Expenses				
Salary				
Full-time equivalent employees (FTEs)				
Medical supplies				
Clerical supplies				
Purchased service				
Maintenance				
Miscellaneous				

Figure 11-6 Variance Report per Cost Centre.

- Learn how a department is reimbursed for services delivered, identifying covered and excluded expenses.
- Discuss quality and cost differences in supplies with other staff and management.
- Evaluate staff and equipment downtime.
- Analyze the causes of schedule delays, cancelled cases, and extended procedure times.
- Explore new products with vendor representatives and network with colleagues who have tried both new and modified products.
- Reduce the length of client stays by troubleshooting early.
- Assist staff in organizational planning.
- Enhance productivity through rigorous continuous quality improvement.
- Post overtime and high/low productivity analysis.

- Explore how time and motion studies may increase efficiencies by identifying gaps or duplication in effort.
- Ensure that staff have the right tools and that the tools are ready when needed.
- Analyze client supplies and review costs per client encounter (e.g., chemotherapy administration, dialysis, insertion of indwelling or peripheral catheter).
- Track various steps in client care that are time consuming or problematic for a unit (e.g., communication from front desk to recovery room, staff response to client call lights, number of staff responding to an emergency code).
- Acquire a working knowledge of how a department/unit monitors financial and quality indicators, and participate in the development of action plans to increase client satisfaction or to create the "best client experience."

KEY CONCEPTS

- Nurses play an integral role in the development, implementation, and evaluation of a unit or department budget.

- If nurses are not conscious of revenue and expenses, then deviation from financial performance will occur.

- Overall, organizational performance is dependent upon the insight and skills of staff members regarding client care quality and financial outcomes.

- Hospitals use several types of budgets to help with future planning and management, including operating, capital, and construction budgets.

- In the budget preparation phase, data are gathered related to a variety of elements that influence an organization, including demographic information, regulatory influences, and strategic initiatives. Additionally, it is helpful to understand the department's scope of service, goals, and history.

- During the budget preparation phase, individual departments or sections should be thoroughly examined. Hospital systems are frequently divided into sections, departments, or units to compartmentalize them for organizational purposes. These subsections or units, commonly called cost centres, are used to track financial data.

- Organizations typically use history or past performance as a baseline of experience and data to better understand activity in a department or unit.

- After background data have been gathered, the development of the budget can follow, including the projection of revenue and expenses.

- Expenses are determined by identifying the cost associated with the delivery of service. Expenditures are resources used by an organization to deliver services and may include labour, supplies, equipment, utilities, and miscellaneous items.

- After budgets are developed, they are submitted to administration for review and final approval. The approval process may take several weeks because the unit budgets are combined to determine the overall budget for the health care organization.

KEY TERMS

accounting
balanced scorecard
capital budget
construction budget
cost centres
operating budget
revenue

REVIEW QUESTIONS

1. An operating budget accounts for
   A. the purchase of minor and major equipment.
   B. construction and renovation.
   C. income and expenses associated with daily activity within an organization.
   D. applications for new technology.

2. Revenue can be generated through
   A. client accommodation.
   B. donations to service organizations.
   C. use of generic drugs.
   D. messenger and escort activities.

3. Cost centres are used to
   A. develop historical and demographic information.
   B. track expense line items.
   C. plan for strategic growth and movement.
   D. track financial data within a department or unit.

4. The purpose of monitoring a budget is to
   A. keep expenses above budget.
   B. maintain revenue above the previous year's budget.
   C. ensure revenue is generated monthly.
   D. generate revenue and control expenses within a projected framework.

5. Productivity can be measured by
   A. the number of beds in a hospital.
   B. the cost for services rendered.
   C. past performance and history regarding revenue.
   D. the volume of services delivered.

REVIEW ACTIVITIES

1. Look around your clinical agency. Do you see any balanced scorecards? What do they reveal about your agency?

2. Using the zero-based budgeting figure in this chapter, construct an analysis of one of the clinical procedures in your agency.

EXPLORING THE WEB

- Go to the site for the Canadian Council on Health Services Accreditation. What information did you find there? http://www.cchsa.ca/

- Review the site for the Academy of Canadian Executive Nurses. Was the information helpful? http://www.acen.ca/

- Review these sites for helpful information. What did you find there?
  Canadian College of Health Service Executives: http://www.cchse.org/

  Health Canada: http://www.hc-sc.gc.ca/

REFERENCES

Elser, R., & Nipp, D. (2001). Worker designed culture change. *Nursing Economic$, 19*(4), 161–163, 175.

Grohar-Murray, M. E., & DiCroce, H. R. (1997). *Leadership and management in nursing*. Stamford, CT: Appleton & Lange.

Iron, K. (2006). ICES report: Health data in Ontario: Taking stock and moving ahead. *Healthcare Quarterly, 9*(3), 24–26.

Nelson, B. (1997). *1001 ways to energize employees.* New York: Workman Publishing, pp. 30, 66, 151.

Norton, D., & Kaplan, R. (2001). *The strategy-focused organization: How balanced scorecard companies thrive in the new business environment.* Boston: Harvard Business School Press.

Sullivan, E. J., & Decker, P. (Eds.). (1997). *Effective leadership and management in nursing: Key skills in nursing management.* Menlo Park, CA: Addison Wesley, pp. 90–104.

Yoder-Wise, P. (1998). *Leading and managing in nursing,* (2nd ed.). St. Louis, MO: Mosby, pp. 226–243.

SUGGESTED READINGS

Barnum, B., & Kerfoot, K. (1995). Nursing division budgeting. In Barnum, B. & Kerfoot K. (Eds.), *The nurse as executive* (4th ed., pp. 188–198). Gaithersburg, MD: Aspen.

Camp, R. C. (1989). *Benchmarking: The search for industry best practices that lead to superior performance.* Milwaukee, WI: ASQC Quality Press.

Carruth, A., Carruth, P., & Noto, E. (2000). Nurse managers flex their budgetary might. *Nursing Management, 31*(2), 16–17.

DiJerome, L., Dunham-Taylor, J., Ash, K., & Brown., R. (1999). Evaluating cost center productivity. *Nursing Economic$, 117*(6), 334–340.

Dixon, N. M., (2000). *Common knowledge: How companies thrive by sharing what they know.* Boston: Harvard Business School Press.

Garvin, D. (2000). *Learning in action: A guide to putting the learning organization to work.* Boston: Harvard Business School Press.

Iowa Intervention Project. (2001). Determining cost of nursing instrumentations: A beginning. *Nursing Economic$, 19*(4), 146–160.

Jones, K. R. (1999). The capital budgeting process. *Seminars for Nurse Managers, 7*(2), 55–56.

Keeling, B. (2000). How to establish a position and hours budget. *Nursing Management, 31*(3), 26–27.

CHAPTER 12

Effective Staffing

Anne L. Bernat, RN, BSN, MSN, CNAA
Adapted by: Heather Crawford, BScN, MEd, CHE

High quality nursing care should be the goal of every nurse, educator and manager. High quality to me means care that is individualized to a particular client, administered humanely and competently, comprehensively and with continuity. Primary nursing is one means of accomplishing that quality of care. (Marie Manthey, 1980)

OBJECTIVES

Upon completion of this chapter, the reader should be able to:

1. Discuss utilization of workload measurement systems data by the staff nurse and the nurse manager.

2. Develop a staffing pattern for a critical care unit with 22 clients.

3. Evaluate staffing effectiveness on an inpatient unit using two client outcomes.

4. Compare and contrast models of care delivery.

5. Discuss the role of a case manager versus a unit staff nurse.

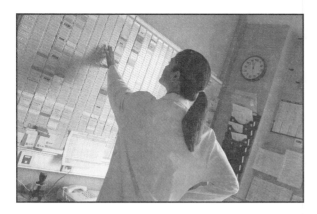

DETERMINATION OF STAFFING NEEDS

Nurse staffing has varied widely since the inception of nursing as a profession. Nursing staffing has ranged from one nurse to many soldiers, as in Florence Nightingale's time, to today, when you may see one nurse to one client in a critical care area. In today's rapidly changing health care environment, many variables must be considered in determining nurse staffing requirements. The effectiveness of the staffing pattern is only as good as the planning that goes into its preparation. The following key budget concepts and issues need to be reviewed and assessed when building or assessing a staffing pattern.

CORE CONCEPTS

A familiarity with the key terms—full-time equivalents (FTEs), worked hours, benefit hours, paid hours, direct and indirect care, and nursing hours per patient day (NHPPD)—is necessary to understand staffing patterns.

FTEs

A **full-time equivalent (FTE)** is a measure of the work commitment of a full-time employee. A full-time employee typically works 5 days a week, or 37.5 hours per week for 52 weeks a year, which amounts to 1,950 hours of work time (see Figure 12-1).

A full-time employee who works 37.5 hours a week is referred to as 1.0 FTE. A part-time employee who works 5 days in a 2-week period is considered a 0.5 FTE. The FTE calculation is used to mathematically describe how much an employee works (see Figure 12-2). Understanding FTEs is essential when moving from a staffing pattern to the actual number of staff required.

FTE hours are a total of all paid hours: worked hours plus benefit hours. Worked hours are the number of hours the employee is providing direct care to clients, or is participating in indirect care, such as documentation.

Benefit hours include the number of hours spent on vacation; sick time; education time; statutory holidays; orientation; and paid leave, such as bereavement. When considering the number of FTEs you need to staff a unit, you must count only the worked hours available for each staff member. Available productive time can be easily calculated by subtracting benefit time from the time a full-time employee would work (see Figure 12-3).

You are a new nurse manager of a 28-bed surgical unit that uses total client care as the care delivery model. You have 15 full-time employees and 20 part-time employees, with vacancies for an additional 4 full-time staff. The current schedule utilizes 8-hour shifts, but the majority of full-time staff would like to work 12-hour shifts. However, the most experienced nurses on the unit threaten to retire if you implement 12-hour shifts. Recent graduates will only work for you if you offer 12-hour shifts.

How can you accommodate the needs of both groups of nurses?

What effect will the 12-hour shifts have on your care delivery model?

The ability of a nurse to provide safe and effective care to a client is dependent on many variables, including the knowledge and experience of the staff, the severity of illness of the clients, the amount of nursing time available, the care delivery model, care management tools, and organizational supports in place to facilitate care. This chapter will explore these factors, how they affect planning for staffing, and the results of staffing plans. By the end of this chapter, you will understand how to plan staffing and how to measure the effectiveness of a staffing plan. You will also be able to articulate the models of care delivery that are applicable to your environment and client population.

5 days per week	× 7.5 hours per day	= 37.5 hours per week
37.5 hours per week	× 52 weeks per year	= 1,950 hours per year

Figure 12-1 Calculation of Full-Time Equivalent Hours.

> 1.0 FTE = 37.5 hours per week or five 7.5-hour shifts per week
>
> 0.8 FTE = 30 hours per week or four 7.5-hour shifts per week
>
> 0.6 FTE = 22.5 hours per week or three 7.5-hour shifts per week
>
> 0.4 FTE = 15 hours per week or two 7.5-hour shifts per week
>
> 0.2 FTE = 7.5 hours per week or one 7.5-hour shift per week

Figure 12-2 FTE Calculation for Varying Levels of Work Commitment.

Vacation hours	20 days	or	150 hours
Sick time (average)	6 days	or	45 hours
Statutory holidays	12 days	or	90 hours
Education	2 days	or	15 hours
Total benefit hours		=	300 hours

1,950 − 300 = 1,650 worked hours available for each staff member with these benefits

Figure 12-3 Calculation of Worked and Benefit Hours.

> 20 clients on the unit
>
> 5 staff × 3 shifts = 15 staff
>
> 15 staff each working 7.5 hours = 112.5 hours available in a 24-hour period
>
> 112.5 nursing hours ÷ 20 clients = 5.6 NHPPD
>
> FTE = 7.5 hours per week or one 7.5-hour shift per week

Figure 12-4 Calculation of Nursing Hours per Patient Day (NHPPD).

In this case, a full-time registered nurse (RN) would have 1,650 worked hours per year available to care for clients.

Employees who work with clients can be classified into two categories: those who provide direct care and those who provide indirect care. **Direct care** is time spent providing hands-on care to clients. **Indirect care** is time spent on activities that are client related but do not involve hands-on client care. documentation, consulting with other health care disciplines, and following up on outstanding issues. Even though RNs, licensed practical nurses (LPNs), and unregulated care providers (UCPs) engage in indirect care activities, the majority of their time is spent providing direct care; therefore, they are classified as direct care providers, and are considered **unit producing.** Nurse managers, clinical specialists, unit clerks, and other support staff are considered **non-unit producing** because the majority of their work is indirect in nature and supports the work of the direct care providers.

NURSING HOURS PER PATIENT DAY

Nursing hours per patient day (NHPPD) is a standard measure that quantifies the nursing time available to each client by available nursing staff. For example, a nursing unit that has 20 clients at a given point during a 24-hour period, usually the midnight census, and 5 nursing staff each shift would calculate into 5.6 nursing hours per patient day. NHPPD reflect only worked hours available (see Figure 12-4). This measure is useful, in quantifying nursing care, to both nurses and financial staff in an organization.

WORKLOAD MEASUREMENT SYSTEMS

To assess how many staff are needed at any given time, it is necessary to determine the clients' needs. Workload measurement systems first appeared during the 1960s, when they were called patient classification systems. Many nurses still refer to them as such. A **workload measurement system** is a measurement tool used to articulate the nursing workload for a specific client or group of clients over a specific period of time. The measure of nursing workload that is generated for each client is called the **client acuity.** Classification data can be used to predict the amount of nursing time needed based on the client's acuity. As a client becomes sicker, the acuity level rises, meaning the client requires more nursing care. As a client acuity level decreases, the client requires less nursing care. In most patient classification systems, each client is classified using weighted criteria that are used to predict the nursing care hours needed for the next 24 hours. The criteria reflect care needed for bathing, mobilizing, and eating; supervision; assessment; frequent observations; and so on. In most cases, clients are classified once a day. The ideal workload measurement system produces a valid and reliable rating of individual client care requirements, which is matched to the latest clinical technology and caregiver skill variables (Malloch & Conivaloff, 1999). These systems are generally applied to all inpatients in an organization. Systems to classify outpatients have been less prevalent because outpatients tend to be more stable and similar in care needs. There are two different types of classification systems: factor and prototype.

FACTOR SYSTEM

The factor system uses units of measure that equate to nursing time. Nursing tasks are assigned time or are weighted to reflect the amount of time needed to perform the task. These systems attempt to capture the cognitive functions of assessment, planning, intervention, and evaluation of client outcomes along with written documentation processes. Many factor systems have been homegrown or built for a specific organization, and many other factor systems are available for purchase on the open market. The factor system is the most popular type of classification system because of its ability to project care needs for individual clients as well as client groups. The time assigned or the weighted factor for different nursing activities can be changed over time to reflect the changing needs of the clients or the hospital system.

ADVANTAGES AND DISADVANTAGES   In the factor system, data are generally readily available to managers and staff for day-to-day operations. These data provide a base of information against which one can justify changes in staffing requirements.

Disadvantages to this system type include the ongoing workload for the nurse in classifying clients every day. Problems have also been documented with classification creep, whereby acuity levels rise as a result of misuse of classification criteria. Another, disadvantage is that these systems do not holistically capture the client's needs for psychosocial, environmental, and health management support. And finally, these systems calculate nursing time needed based on a typical nurse. A novice may take longer to perform activities than the average nurse or a more experienced nurse. If a majority of staff are novices, the recommended nursing times needed will be longer than the actual time needed, based on the actual expertise of the staff.

The prototype system allocates nursing time to large client groups based on an average of similar clients. For

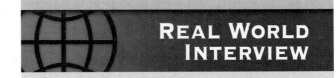

REAL WORLD INTERVIEW

Our hospital uses a workload classification system, and the nurses calculate the requirements daily, but we don't pay much attention to the data collected. Some of my colleagues deliberately "fudge" the numbers to determine if anybody is paying attention! The challenge with the system we use is that it doesn't anticipate demand, or adjust for the learning time necessary for new employees. In addition, it doesn't provide time for us to have relationships with our clients, it just gives us time to complete tasks. It also doesn't recognize the change in workload related to admissions and discharges throughout the 24 hours. Now, it isn't recognizing the fact that I am slower than I was 20 years ago!

Claire Stanfield, MScN
Prototype System

example, specific **case mix groups (CMGs)** have been used as groupings of clients to which a nursing acuity is assigned based on past organizational experience. CMGs are client groupings established by the Canadian Institute for Health Information (CIHI) group and describe types of clients discharged from acute care hospitals. To measure the expected use of hospital resources, CIHI developed weights, known as **resource intensity weights (RIWs),** based on U.S. charge data and Canadian length-of-stay data. Cost weights are relative resource values associated with specific grouping methodologies. In addition to CMGs and RIWs, day procedure group RIWs have been developed, based on the same scale as the in-resource allocation methodology developed for continuing care residents.[1]

RESOURCE AND FTE REQUIREMENTS

ADVANTAGES AND DISADVANTAGES   The distinct advantage of the prototype system is the reduction of work for nurses who are not required to classify clients daily. A major disadvantage of this system is the lack of ongoing measure of the actual nursing work required by individual clients. Also, no ongoing data is available to monitor the accuracy of the pre-assigned nursing care requirements. This type of system is much less common than the factor system.

UTILIZATION OF CLASSIFICATION SYSTEM DATA

A large body of literature is available on workload measurement systems, such as Baumann et al., (2001), Giovannetti

(1994), McGillis Hall et al. (2006), O'Brien-Pallas (2007), Shamian and El-Jardali (2007), and the Final Report of the Canadian Nursing Advisory Committee in 2002 (Canadian Nursing Advisory Committee, 2002). Although managers cannot rely entirely on the workload measurement system to predict staff requirements and produce a staffing plan, this system provides some useful information related to acuity.

CONSIDERATIONS IN DEVELOPING A STAFFING PATTERN

Developing a staffing pattern is a science and an art. The following sections will consider other areas in addition to the acuity data and NHPPD just discussed. Each of these areas should be reviewed and the findings incorporated into development of the staffing pattern.

BENCHMARKING

Benchmarking is a management tool for seeking out the best practices in one's industry so as to improve performance (Swansburg, 1996). When developing a staffing pattern that will lead to a budget, your planned NHPPD should be benchmarked against other organizations with similar client populations. Purchased workload measurement systems often offer both acuity and NHPPD benchmarking data from across the country as part of their system. Such data can be helpful in establishing a starting point for a staffing pattern or to help justify an increase or reduction in nursing hours. Use caution, however, because each organization has, at the unit level, varying levels of support in place for the nurse. For example, in a nursing unit where aides from the dietary department distribute and pick up meal trays, less nursing time is needed than in a unit that has no external support for this activity. Such factors contribute significantly to differences in hours of care from one organization to another.

REGULATORY REQUIREMENTS

In Canada, no regulatory requirements address staffing levels. However, in the United States, the situation is changing as the nursing shortage heightens. California has mandated nurse staffing levels in emergency departments and critical care units. Several other states have legislation pending, which has aroused considerable controversy within the nursing profession. Some nurses are adamant that they need to be protected by law with stipulated staffing levels. Some nurse leaders are concerned that the mandated staffing levels would soon become the maximum staffing levels rather than the minimum.

The Joint Commission on Accreditation of Healthcare Organizations (JCAHO) surveys hospitals on the quality of care provided. The JCAHO does not mandate staffing levels but does assess an organization's ability to provide the right number of competent staff to meet the needs of clients served by the hospital (Joint Commission on Accreditation of Healthcare Organizations, 2000). Part of this assessment asks how often a unit is staffed to the requirements of its staffing pattern and how the effectiveness of the staffing pattern is evaluated. If a staffing pattern calls for four RNs for twenty clients, the JCAHO will assess how often you meet your own standards by allocating one nurse for every five clients. As a rule, nurses in the United States pay close attention to the state and federal regulations related to their client population for any regulated staffing requirements.

In Canada, the Canadian Council on Health Services Accreditation surveys hospitals on the quality of care provided, but does not mandate the staffing levels. The human resources team may identify the number of overtime hours provided for client care, or the number of illness-related absent days. Indirectly, the surveyors assess whether the organization has met its standards with respect to staffing.

SKILL MIX

Skill mix is another essential element in nurse staffing. **Skill mix** is the percentage of one type of staff to the total staff complement. For example, an RN skill mix represents the percentage of RN staff to all staff, including other direct care staff, LPNs, and unregulated care providers (UCPs), and a professional skill mix represents the percentage of professional staff to all staff, including unregulated staff. In a unit that has 40 FTEs budgeted—20 RNs and 20 FTEs of other skill types—the RN skill mix is 50 percent. If the unit had 40 FTEs—30 RNs and LPNs—the professional skill mix would be 75 percent.

The skill mix of a unit should vary according to the care required and the care delivery model utilized. For example, in a critical care unit, the RN skill mix will be much higher than in a nursing home where the skills of an RN are required to a lesser degree. Although professional (RN and LPN) hours of care are more costly than those of unregulated providers, evidence shows that RNs and LPNs are a very productive and efficient type of labour. As nurses become scarcer, and clients are discharged earlier from acute care facilities, it will become even more important to evaluate the client care required and determine the most appropriate care provider to utilize. For instance, when many clients require assistance with daily living, an unregulated care provider may be most appropriate.

A note of caution: When you consider skill mix, make sure you clearly understand the activities each level of staff can engage in within the scope of practice in your province or territory. In some organizations, UCPs may catheterize clients or administer sliding scale insulin if they have received training and are competent. In other organizations, UCPs may not perform these functions, regardless of their training and expertise.

STAFF SUPPORT

Another important factor when developing a staffing pattern is the supports in place for the operations of the unit or department. For instance, does your organization have a systematic process to deliver medications to the unit or do unit personnel have to pick up client medications and narcotics? Does your organization have staff to transport clients to and from ancillary departments?

The less support available, the greater the number of nursing hours that need to be built into the staffing pattern. Nursing areas such as critical care that track and supply a significant amount of equipment may benefit greatly from adding a materials coordinator. This kind of support for staff allows staff to spend their precious available time with clients rather than looking for equipment or supplies.

An additional important unit-based need is clerical support. If the unit has admissions, discharges, and transfers, providing unit clerical support makes sense. In intensive care units (ICUs) and emergency departments (EDs), unit clerks are commonly scheduled around the clock to provide support for the unit staff as well as for other disciplines.

HISTORICAL INFORMATION

As you consider the many variables that affect staffing, it helps to ask, What has worked in the past? Were the staff able to provide the care that was needed? How many clients were cared for? What kind of clients were they? How many staff were utilized and what kind of staff were they? This information can help to identify operational issues that would not be apparent otherwise. For example, an older part of a facility may not have a pneumatic tube delivery system, a system that is available in most other parts of the facility. Because it is generally available, you may overlook its absence, but its absence means a significant amount of time will be required to collect needed items, affecting the staffing pattern you develop. It is also important to review any data on quality or staff perceptions regarding the effectiveness of the previous staffing pattern. This information will allow you to calculate previous NHPPD and outcomes for comparison to your staffing plan. History is a valuable tool that we often overlook as we plan for the future.

ESTABLISHING A STAFFING PATTERN

A **staffing pattern** is a plan that articulates how many and what kind of staff are needed per shift and per day to staff a unit or department. A staffing pattern can be developed in two basic ways: by determining the required ratio of staff to clients and then calculating nursing hours and total FTEs; or by determining the nursing care hours needed for a specific client or group of clients, and then generating the FTEs and staff-to-client ratio needed to

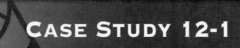

CASE STUDY 12-1

You are the manager of a 22-bed critical care unit. The nurse-to-client ratio is budgeted at one nurse to one client for 16 of the beds, and one nurse to two clients for six of the beds. Of the 22 clients in your unit, three are well enough to go to a general medical-surgical unit where the nurse-to-client ratio is one to five. You are planning the staff requirements for the next 12 hours. What factors should you consider? After consideration of key factors, what is your plan for staffing? What would you communicate to your staff?

provide that care. In most cases, you will use a combination of methods to validate your staffing plan. We will start with development of a plan from the staff-to-client ratio.

INPATIENT UNIT

An **inpatient unit** is a hospital unit that provides care to clients 24 hours a day, 7 days a week. Establishing a staffing pattern for an inpatient unit utilizes all the data discussed above. Using data from all your sources, you can build a staffing pattern that you believe will meet the needs of the clients, the staff, and the organization. Utilizing a staffing pattern template, plot out the number and type of staff needed during the week and weekend for 24 hours a day for the number of clients you expect to have (see Figure12-5). In this example, the number and type of staff are delineated as well the additional FTEs for weekend coverage, orientation and education, and benefit hours.

For example, on a 24-bed medical unit, you expect to have, on average, 22 clients per day. The ratio of one RN to five clients and one UCP for every twelve clients works well from 0700 to 1900 hours. From 1900 to 0700 hours, the ratio can go to one RN to eight clients. Two UCPs are needed from 1900 to 2300 hours; and then one UCP from 2300 to 0700 hours. A total of 131.25 staff hours per day are needed. The average number of clients on this unit is 22. To calculate the NHPPD see Figure 12-6.

In this example, the number of care hours available would be six NHPPD.

As you can see, the staffing pattern drives the NHPPD. The more staff available per client, the higher the NHPPD. Cost is associated with hours of care available and skill mix. Some staffing patterns have many hours of care available, but they may be lower-cost FTEs. The key is to have the right number and skill level of caregivers available to ensure safe, effective, and appropriate care.

Hospital Business Planning Brief/Accountability Agreement 2005/06

Hospital Site: Brantford General Site

Department Name:

Department No.::

NOTE: One shift equals 7.5 hours

WORKED TIME

Job Class-Descrip	Shifts	S	S	M	T	W	T	F	TOTAL	Worked Time
Job Code	D									
	E									
	N									

Weekly # of Shifts
F.T.E.'s (# Shifts divided by 5)
Paid Hours (FTE's X 1950 hours)

BENEFIT TIME

	F/T		# of Days	Total Days	Shifts Not Replaced	Shifts Replaced	Benefit Time
Statutory Holidays		X					
Paid Sick (Average)		X					
Education Leave		X					
Inservice		X					
Orientation		X					
Vacation							

Total # of Shifts
F.T.E.'s (# Shifts divided by 260 days)
Paid Hours (FTE's X 1950 hours)

NOTE: Worked time plus benefit time replaced equals Total Staff F.T.E.'s

NOTE: Shifts not replaced and shifts replaced equals Benefit Hours

NOTE: Worked time less shifts not replaced equals Worked Hours

For Premium Calculations Only

*Annual Shifts ***Weekly Shifts**

M.L.O.A. (# of Weeks)	Even. Prem.	
O/T Shifts - Annual	Night Prem.	
# Call Backs - Annual	Wkend Prem.	
Stats Worked - Annual	In Charge	
M.O.A. - U.I.C. Pymts.	Resp. Shifts	
Other:	Resp. Shifts	
Other:	Stdby. Shifts	

TOTAL STAFFING REQUIREMENTS

Staff Ratio	TOTAL F.T.E.'s	F.T.E.'s		TOTAL PD. HRS	Paid Hours	
		Worked	Benefit		Worked	Benefit
Full-Time						
Part-Time						
TOTAL						

*STAFF COUNT

Full-Time	Part-Time

Note: Staff Count should be actual number of bodies

Note: Annual Shifts are calculated by taking the number of shifts per day and multiplying by 7 (number of Days in a week) then multiplying by 52 (number of weeks in a year)

Note: Weekly Shifts are calculated by taking the number of shifts per day and multiplying by 7 (Number of days in a week)

Figure 12-5 Brant Community Healthcare System—Staffing Pattern Worksheet and Human Resources.

Hospital Business Planning Brief/Accountability Agreement 2005/06

HUMAN RESOURCE and FTE REQUIREMENTS

Site: _____ Brantford General Site

Dept. Name: _____

Dept. No.: _____

Job Classification Description	Status	Number of Staff						Full-Time Equivalents						Rationale for Increases/Decreases in Number of Staff or FTE's
		Current	Current Req'd PT Casual	Current Req'd Job Shares	05/06 Budget	Req'd PT Casual	Req'd Job Shares	03/04 Budget	03/04 Actual	04/05 Budget	Proj. 04/05 Actual	Changes to 04/05 Budget	2005/06 Budget	
	Full-Time													
	Part-Time													
	Full-Time													
	Part-Time													
	Full-Time													
	Part-Time													
	Full-Time													
	Part-Time													
	Full-Time													
	Part-Time													
Department Total														

Figure 12-5 (Continued)

Source: Brant Community Healthcare System, Brantford, ON. Reprinted with Permission.

Skill	Day	Evening	Night	Total
Direct				
UM				
RN	5.5	4.25	3	12.75
LPN				
Tech				
UCP	2	2	1	5
Subtotal				

12.5 staff	× 7.5-hour shifts	= 93.75 hours
5 staff	× 7.5-hour shifts	= 37.5 hours
Staff hours available per day		= 131.25 hours
131.25 hours ÷ 22 clients per day		= 6 hours of NHPPD
131.25 hours ÷ 7.5-hour shifts		= 17.5 FTEs to fill the staffing pattern

Figure 12-6 Staffing Plan for a 24-Bed Medical Unit.

To develop a staffing pattern using NHPPD, start with a target NHPPD. If your target NHPPD were 8, for example, and you expected to have 22 clients on your 24-bed unit, you would multiply 8 NHPPD times 22 clients to get 176 worked hours needed every day. Dividing 176 by 7.5-hour shifts worked by an FTE gives you 23.5 FTEs needed per day.

DETERMINING THE NUMBER OF FTES NEEDED TO MEET THE STAFFING PATTERN

You have determined a staffing pattern for your unit. The staffing pattern calculates the number of FTEs needed per day, but does not account for the benefit hours or replacement hours for staff days off. You must now calculate the number of additional staff that will be needed to provide for days off and benefit hours. Direct caregivers will need to be replaced, but the support staff may not need to be replaced for days off or benefit hours. Managers typically are not replaced on days off. Noting that each 7.5-hour shift for a FTE is equal to 0.2 FTE, to provide coverage for 2 days off a week multiply the number of staff needed per day by a 0.4 FTE. In the example in Figure 12-6, 17.75 FTEs per day multiplied by 0.4 FTE would be an additional 7.1 FTEs to cover 2 days off per week for a total of 24.8 FTEs.

The next step would be to provide additional FTEs for coverage of benefit hours, which includes vacation, educational time, orientation time, and so on. The amount of time away from work varies by organization. If every employee receives 4 weeks of vacation a year and

2 educational days, the benefit hours would equate to 1,785 hours of worked time per FTE (1,950 possible hours minus 165 hours). Total FTE hours divided by 1,785 hours gives you the total FTEs needed to provide coverage. In the previous example, 24.8 FTEs multiplied by 1,950 hours equals 48,360 hours, and 48,360 hours divided by 1,785 would be 27.1 FTEs or 2.3 additional FTEs to ensure that there are staff available to work when other staff are taking benefited time off. Thus, a total of 27.1 FTEs are needed to staff this 24-bed unit.

DETERMINING THE FTES NEEDED TO STAFF AN EPISODIC CARE UNIT

An **episodic care unit** refers to a unit that sees clients for defined episodes of care; for example, a dialysis unit or an ambulatory care unit. In these units, clients tend to be more homogenous and have a more predictable path of care. Determining staffing needs for an episodic unit starts with an assessment of the hours of care required by the clients. Using a dialysis unit as an example, to care for 16 clients receiving treatments, you determine you need 4 RNs for all 12 hours the unit is open, or 48 hours of RN care per day. The unit is open 12 hours a day, 6 days a week, or 312 days a year; 48 hours per day multiplied by 312 days = 14,976 total hours. As in the previous example, the number of FTEs needed to provide coverage for worked hours can be calculated by dividing the total number of hours needed by the actual number of worked hours an employee would work. This method provides coverage for days off and benefit hours for direct caregivers. Using our worked FTE hours of 1,650 from Figure 12-3 divided into the 14,976 hours required equates to a total of 9.1 RN FTEs.

The same calculation can be applied to other caregivers. In this same example, if two technicians were required for 12 hours a day of operation, that would mean 2 × 12 = 24 hours needed per day, and 24 × 312 days = 7,488 total hours needed.

The benefit package for technical staff is not as rich as the RN package. Their vacation allotment is 10 days or 75 hours per year, which increases their productive time to 1,875 hours per year; 7,488 divided by 1,875 = 4.0 technical FTEs. Any staff members who do not require coverage would simply be added to the overall FTEs for the unit as a 1.0 FTE. This situation might apply to a secretary, social worker, or nurse manager, who supports the unit but is not necessary to replace on their days off and benefited time off.

SCHEDULING

Scheduling of staff is the responsibility of the nurse manager, who must ensure that the appropriate staffs are scheduled on each day and on each shift for safe, effective

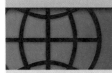

REAL WORLD INTERVIEW

One of the things that always amazed me was that managers tended to use different figures and assumptions when planning their staffing needs. As a result, I formed a committee of nurse managers and directors to see whether or not we could develop a template for them to use, which would ultimately save time and frustration. The spreadsheet template we developed afforded the managers an opportunity to accurately project the number of FTEs needed to meet the staffing pattern. This template included worked and benefit hours. The benefit hours included vacation, statutory holidays, sick time, education days, orientation days, and paid leave. In addition, the template included opportunities to budget for maternity leaves of absence (MLOA). One of the biggest benefits for the managers is that the template allowed them to develop what-if scenarios for planning purposes.

Peter Exford, C.A.
Director of Finance

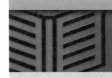

LITERATURE APPLICATION

Citation: Canadian Nursing Advisory Committee. (2002). Our health, our future: Creating quality workplaces for Canadian nurses: Final report of the Canadian Nursing Advisory Committee. Ottawa: Advisory Committee on Health Human Resources.

Discussion: The Canadian Nursing Advisory Committee (CNAC) was created in 2001 in response to the National Nursing Strategy. Because of concerns regarding the nursing shortage in the Canadian nursing workforce in the late 1990s, the Conference of Deputy Ministers and Ministers of Health directed the Advisory Committee on Health Human Resources (ACHHR) "to develop a pan-Canadian strategy for nursing" (Advisory Committee on Health Human Resources [ACHHR], 2000a, p. 2). The primary goal of the CNAC was to formulate recommendations "for policy direction to improve quality of nursing work life which would provide a framework and context for work life improvement strategies at the provincial/territorial level" (ACHHR, 2000b). The Committee made recommendations for changes in three key areas: 1) increasing the number of nurses; 2) improving the education and maximizing the scope of practice of nurses; and 3) improving working conditions of nurses.

Implications for Practice: It is clear that there is and will continue to be a nursing shortage for the next decade. In addition to devising global strategies to draw more people into the nursing profession, it is imperative for managers and nurse leaders to create environments that retain staff, including the planning of staff schedules that nurses find compatible with their personal lives. As the nursing workforce ages, we must also take measures to make accommodations for the older worker, including technology to simplify work and physical plant changes to make the work less physically taxing.

client care. Many issues need to be considered when you schedule staff: the client type and acuity, the number of clients, the experience of your staff, and the supports available to the staff. The combination of these factors should guide the number of staff scheduled on each day and shift. These factors must be reviewed on an ongoing basis as client types and client acuity drive different client needs and staff expertise.

CLIENT NEEDS

Clients' nursing needs are measured by the workload measurement system. Workload measurement systems, however, do not predict when, over the next 24 hours, the nursing activity will take place. In addition to planning for the acuity of the clients, the staffing pattern must support having staff at work when the work needs to be done. A good example is an oncology unit, where chemotherapy and blood transfusions typically occur on the evening shift. In this scenario, more staff may be needed in the evening to support these nurse-intensive activities. As client types change, so do clients' needs and staffing requirements. Adding a population of step-down clients from the ICU would likely require additional FTEs on a medical-surgical unit. When client populations change, staffing and NHPPD should be assessed.

EXPERIENCE AND SCHEDULING OF STAFF

Nurses differ regarding their knowledge base, experience level, and critical thinking skills. A novice nurse takes longer to accomplish a task than an experienced nurse. An experienced RN can handle more, in terms of workload and acuity of clients. If your area requires special skills or competencies of your staff, you will also want to plan for additional nursing hours, so that staff with the special skills are scheduled when the need for their skills is most likely to arise. Remember, the underlying principle of good

> Weekend staff working at $35 an hour $\times$ 24 hours = $840 per weekend
>
> Regular staff working at $20 an hour $\times$ 24 hours = $480 per weekend
>
> Difference in cost = $360 per weekend
>
> Six weekend staff members at $360 would cost $2,160 more than regular staff per weekend;
> $2,160 $\times$ 52 weekends a year would cost $112,320 more than regular staff annually.

Figure 12-7 Annual Cost of a Weekend Program for One Nursing Unit.

staffing is that those you serve come first. Following this principle may lead to some undesirable shifts, but your responsibility is to ensure both the appropriate number of staff and the appropriate mix of staff are on hand to care for the clients you serve. Figure 12-5 shows how the number of staff is plotted out across a staffing sheet.

NEW OPTIONS IN STAFFING PATTERNS   As the nursing shortage deepens, schedules will need to be developed to meet the needs of both clients and workers. In recent years, more new options in scheduling have been available to meet both of these needs. Twelve-hour shifts have become very popular across the country. In the future, it might be possible for nurses to work fewer than 37.5 hours per week and still be able to obtain full-time benefits. Some schedules allow nurses to work a rotation of four shifts on, five shifts off. These new scheduling options require flexibility in the wording of union contracts.

A popular option in the United States is to schedule shifts that work only on weekends. Weekend program staff work 24 hours in two 12-hour shifts every weekend and are paid a rate equal to 40 hours of work during the week. Some of these programs include full-time benefits as well. Such programs are designed to improve weekend staffing and to allow full-time staff members, who usually work 26 weekends a year, to work fewer weekends for staff retention purposes.

IMPACT ON CLIENT CARE   Any time you implement a scheduling plan, assessing the effect on the care of clients is essential. For example, workweeks made up of three 12-hour shifts have, in many units, disrupted the continuity of care, especially when the 12-hour shifts are not scheduled together. To mediate this impact, 12-hour staff can be paired so that the client has the same pair of nurses every day for 3 days, and then the client can be transitioned to a new pair of 12-hour staff. Units that have short client lengths of stay may have fewer continuity problems than units with longer lengths of stay. When implementing weekend programs, you must always ensure that the staff scheduled are familiar with the clients and the events that have transpired previously.

FINANCIAL IMPLICATIONS   New staffing patterns or program changes may have significant financial implications. Because of the nursing shortage, a number of new programs are being initiated to recruit staff and to encourage staff to work more hours. Weekend programs are more expensive than traditional staffing patterns because of the high rate of hourly pay, but they are a recruitment and retention tool for nursing leadership. For example, see the financial impact of the weekend program referred to earlier (see Figure 12-7).

Before implementing a similar program or other new programs, collaboration with the finance and human resources departments is necessary. This collaboration is needed to develop a financial analysis that measures the dollar and human resource impact of the program.

SELF-SCHEDULING

Self-scheduling is a process in which staff on a unit collectively decide and implement the monthly work schedule (Dearholt & Feathers, 1997). One of the issues that drives nurses from their place of employment is scheduling (Hill-Popper, 2000). Self-scheduling has been implemented to boost staff morale by increasing staff control over their work environment through self-governance activities (Dearholt & Feathers, 1997). It provides opportunities for staff to increase communication among themselves and promotes empowerment and professional growth. This form of scheduling provides maximum flexibility for staff and serves to increase their sense of ownership and shared responsibility in ensuring that their respective work areas are adequately staffed (Shullanberger, 2000). To ensure that client care needs are met, self-scheduling programs need to be structured.

BOUNDARIES OF SELF-SCHEDULING   To implement self-scheduling, responsibilities and boundaries need to clearly state the expectations of staff. These guidelines are best established by a unit committee of staff that reports to the nurse manager. The roles and responsibilities should be spelled out for everyone—the unit-based committee, the chairperson if there is one, the staff, and the manager. Generic boundaries need to be established regarding fairness, fiscal responsibility,

TABLE 12-1	ISSUES TO BE SPELLED OUT IN SELF-SCHEDULING GUIDELINES

1. **Scheduling period:** Is the scheduling period a 2-, 4-, or 6-week interval?

2. **Schedule timeline:** What are the time frames for staff to sign up for regular work commitments, special requests, and overtime?

3. **Staffing pattern:** Will 8- or 12-hour shifts be used, or a combination of both? What are the union contract requirements?

4. **Weekends:** Are staff expected to work every other weekend? If there are extra weekends available, how are they distributed?

5. **Holidays:** How are they allocated?

6. **Vacation time:** Are there restrictions on the amount of vacation during certain periods?

7. **Unit vacation practices:** How many staff from one shift can be on vacation at any time?

8. **Requests for time off:** What is the process for requesting time off?

9. **Short-staffed shifts:** How are short-staffed shifts handled?

10. **On call, if applicable:** How are staff assigned on-call time or how do they sign up for on-call time?

11. **Cancellation guidelines:** How and when are staff cancelled for scheduled time if they are not needed?

12. **Sick calls:** What are the expectations for calling in sick, and how are these shifts covered?

13. **Schedule changes:** What is the process for changing one's schedule after the schedule has been approved?

14. **Shifts defined:** When do available shifts begin and end?

15. **Committee time:** When does the self-scheduling committee meet and for how long?

16. **Seniority:** How does seniority affect staffing and request decisions?

17. **Staffing plan for crisis/emergency situations:** What is the plan when staffing is inadequate?

evaluation of the self-scheduling process, and the approval process. Table 12-1 spells out specific issues that must be addressed. During the self-scheduling process, the unit staff should be included and educated regarding the guidelines as they are being developed. For this process to be successful, all staff members must understand the process, their responsibilities, and the effect of their decisions on staffing. All personnel must also be committed to providing safe staffing on all shifts for their clients.

EVALUATION OF STAFFING EFFECTIVENESS

Many client outcomes are driven by the available hours of care delivered and the competence of staff delivering the care. The nurse manager and the organizational nurse leader have the ongoing responsibility to monitor the effectiveness of the staffing pattern. To ensure objectivity, staffing outcomes must be delineated, measured, and reviewed.

CLIENT OUTCOMES AND NURSE STAFFING

The Canadian Nurses Association has summarized, on its website, numerous research studies that highlight relationships between nurse staffing and client outcomes. All these studies confirm that there is a relationship. The outcomes found to be affected by nurse staffing are length of stay, incidence of pneumonia, postoperative infections, medication errors, falls, client satisfaction, and nurse satisfaction. These outcomes are negatively affected when nurse staffing or the skill mix is inadequate (Aiken et al., 2002; Aiken et al., 2003; McGillis Hall et al., 2004; O'Brien-Pallas et al., 2001, 2002; Sovie & Jawad, 2001). Tracking these outcomes over time will provide the data to judge whether your staffing pattern is adequate or inadequate.

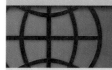

REAL WORLD INTERVIEW

As a staff nurse of a busy surgical unit, I can say that self-scheduling has greatly increased the staff's satisfaction with their schedules. I think the biggest factor in the success of our process was the initial buy-in from the staff. The staff originally requested that they be responsible for the schedule. Following discussion, and lengthy literature review, the staff voted 100 percent to try self scheduling. The next step was to establish an implementation committee made up of staff from the unit. One of the first tasks the implementation committee undertook was to establish clear guidelines for the process. These included time-lines for how and when staff can sign up for time and how time off is prioritized.

During implementation, the staff learned many things. One key factor they had not anticipated was that confrontation and nego-tiation skills were required in order for this process to work. Inevitably there were situations when staff had to change their schedule. When confrontation and negotiation didn't take place, there were periods of short staffing and of client care needs not being met. They also learned that scheduling is a time-consuming process. It takes about 16 hours per month for the self-scheduling committee to put the schedule together.

Another key element was the manager had to maintain accountability for staffing. She met with the scheduling committee regu-larly and provided any new staff with an orientation to the self-scheduling process. She approved and signed every schedule to ensure that the schedule maintained appropriate staffing levels at all times. She also needed to identify trends that may be affect-ing staffing and assist the staff to address those trends. And finally, the most important role she played was to be very clear about the expectations for all—the committee, the staff, and the manager. This scheduling process has been one of the most positive quality-of-work-life efforts for my staff.

Sharon Bilan, BScN
Staff Nurse, 3 West, Surgery

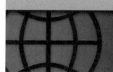

REAL WORLD INTERVIEW

In July of 2005, a practice change took place in the Children's Hospital Emergency Department (ED), which enabled nurses to order X-rays on children who presented with minor orthopedic injuries. Prior to this practice change, X-rays were exclusively ordered by physicians. A working group was established and after doing a process flowchart, it was hypothesized that if nurses could initiate X-rays before clients were seen by a physician, ED waiting times could be reduced. To determine whether this hy-pothesis was successful, a chart audit was conducted to compare waiting times before and after the practice change. Children with minor orthopedic injuries, prior to the practice change, waited an average of 1 hour, 22 minutes from the time they were triaged to the time they received an X-ray, whereas after the practice change, they waited an average of only 20 minutes. Having nurse-initiated X-rays also served to shorten the length of ED visits. Prior to the practice change, the average time between triage and discharge was 2 hours, 28 minutes. After nurse-initiated X-rays were implemented, the time between triage and discharge went down by 48.6 percent to 1 hour, 16 minutes. Statistical testing confirmed that the difference in ED waiting times between the sample of clients seen prior to the practice change and after the practice change was not due to chance alone. An audit has also shown that 55.5 percent of nurse-delegated X-rays indicate abnormalities, which suggests that this process change has not resulted in excessive use of X-rays.

Maggie Jugenburg, Quality Analyst
Child Health Quality Team
Winnipeg Health Sciences Centre

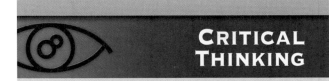

CRITICAL THINKING

Recently, you have been able to access data on your unit's decubitus ulcer rates. In researching further, you uncover that your unit's rates are significantly higher than those of other units. Your staffing has been stable and in accordance with your staffing plan. Your staff are experienced, and, in fact, you have the longest tenured staff in the hospital.

Why are your pressure ulcer rates higher than other units? What would you do?

NURSE STAFFING AND NURSE OUTCOMES

In the previous section, we reviewed outcome measures for clients directly affected by staffing. In addition to client outcomes, nurse outcomes should also be measured. Nurses should be able to communicate their staffing concerns in both written and verbal forms so that their perceptions of staffing adequacy can be tracked. Nurses have the obligation to report to their supervisor their concerns regarding staffing, and every manager has the responsibility to follow up on staffing issues identified by staff. Formalizing this communication process indicates that you take the issues seriously and also provides you with data to act on. In addition, actual staffing levels compared to the recommended staffing levels should be tracked to identify changes in client acuity and clues to other possible staffing issues. Medication error is another measure that has been linked with inadequate NHPPD. When resources are scarce, data are imperative to drive the needed changes. The outcomes of ineffective staffing patterns and nursing care can be devastating to both clients and staff.

MODELS OF CARE DELIVERY

To ensure that nursing care is provided to clients, the work must be organized. A **care delivery model** organizes the work of caring for clients. Over the history of nursing, many models of care delivery have been implemented. The decision of which care delivery model to use is based on the needs of the clients and the availability of competent staff in the different skill levels. The model of care delivery utilized is often determined by the nurse leader and applied across an organization. Managers have the responsibility to implement models and evaluate the outcomes in their area. Staff have the responsibility to engage in the implementation and evaluation process. Each model has strengths and weaknesses that should be considered when deciding which model to implement. Several different care delivery models are explored in the following sections.

CASE METHOD

The case method is the oldest model for nursing care delivery. When nurse training programs began to turn out educated nurses, these nurses were found working mainly in the homes of the sick, taking care of one individual client. In this model of care, the nurse cares for one client exclusively. Total patient care is the modern-day version of the case method.

TOTAL PATIENT CARE

In **total patient care,** nurses are responsible for the total care for their client assignment for the shift they are working. The RNs or LPNs have several clients that they are responsible for. They may have some support from UCPs, but the UCPs are not assigned to a specific group of clients. The RN or LPN's client assignment may change from day to day.

ADVANTAGES AND DISADVANTAGES

The advantage of total patient care and the case method for the client is the consistency of one individual caring for clients for an entire shift, which enables the client, nurse, and family to develop a relationship based on trust. This model provides a higher number of RN or LPN hours of care than other models. The nurse has more opportunity to observe and monitor progress of the client. One disadvantage is that the nurse may not have the same clients from day to day and therefore cares for the client on a shift-by-shift basis rather than on a continuum of care. Another disadvantage is that these models utilize a high level of professional nursing hours to deliver care and, thus, are more costly than other models of delivery.

FUNCTIONAL NURSING

This model of care delivery became popular during World War II when there was a significant shortage of nurses. This method allowed LPNs and UCPs to take on tasks that were previously carried out by the RN in the case method. **Functional nursing** divides the nursing work into functional units, which are then assigned to one of the team members. In this model, each care provider is responsible for specific duties or tasks. For instance, a typical division of labour for RNs is medication nurse or procedure nurse and so on. Decision making is usually at the level of the head nurse or charge nurse (see Figure 12-8).

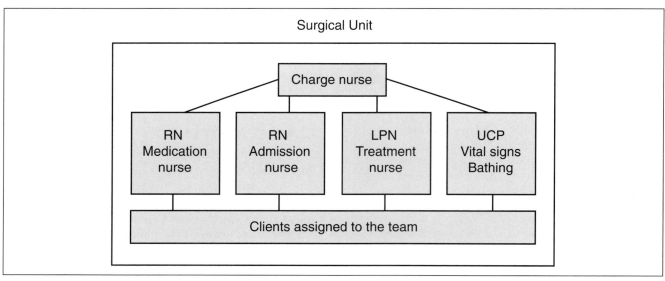

Figure 12-8 Functional Nursing Model.

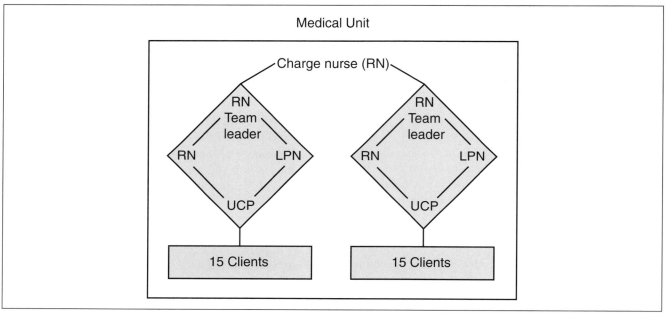

Figure 12-9 Team Nursing Model.

ADVANTAGES AND DISADVANTAGES

In this model, care can be delivered to a large number of clients. This system utilizes other types of health care workers when there is a shortage of RNs. Clients are likely to have care delivered to them in one shift by several staff members. To a client, care may feel disjointed. A risk of this model is that clients become the sum of the tasks of care they require rather than being regarded as an integrated whole.

TEAM NURSING

Team nursing is a care delivery model that assigns staff to teams that then are responsible for a group of clients. A unit may be divided into two teams, and each team is led by a registered nurse. The team leader supervises and co-ordinates all the care provided by those on the team. The team is most commonly made up of RNs, LPNs, and UCPs. Care is divided into the simplest components and then assigned to the appropriate care provider. In addition to supervision duties, the team leader also is responsible for providing professional direction to those on his team regarding the care provided (see Figure 12-9).

A **modular nursing** delivery system is a kind of team nursing that divides a geographic space into modules of clients, with each module cared for by a team of staff led by an RN. The modules may vary in size, but typically the team is made up of one RN with a LPN and UCP. In this case, the RN is responsible for the overall care of the clients in the module.

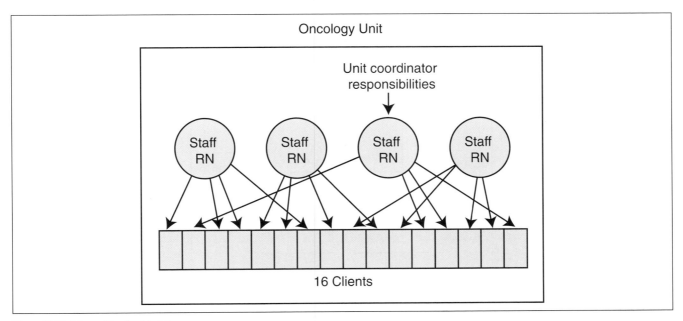

Figure 12-10 Primary Nursing Model.

ADVANTAGES AND DISADVANTAGES

In team nursing and modular nursing, the RN is able to accomplish work through others, but clients often receive fragmented, depersonalized care. Communication in these models is complex, requiring the RN to have good delegation and supervision skills. The shared responsibility and accountability can cause confusion and lack of accountability. These factors contribute to RN dissatisfaction with these models.

PRIMARY NURSING

Primary nursing is a care delivery model that clearly delineates the responsibility and accountability of the RN and designates the RN as the primary provider of care to clients. Primary nursing is a form of the case model that consists of four elements: 1) one individual allocates and accepts individual responsibility for decision making; 2) daily care is assigned by the case method; 3) direct person-to-person communication; and 4) one person is operationally responsible for the quality of care administered to clients on a unit 24 hours a day, 7 days a week (Manthey, 1980).

Clients are assigned a primary nurse, who is responsible for developing with the client a plan of care that is followed by other nurses caring for the client. Nurses and clients are matched according to needs and abilities. Clients are assigned to their primary nurse regardless of unit geographic considerations. In the primary nursing model, the role of the head nurse changes to one of leader by empowering the staff RNs to be knowledgeable about their clients and to direct the care of their primary clients. The primary nurse has the authority, accountability, and responsibility to provide care for a group of clients. Several associate nurses are assigned for each client to provide care when the primary nurse is not working (see Figure 12-10).

ADVANTAGES AND DISADVANTAGES

An advantage of this model is that clients and their families are able to develop a trusting relationship with their nurse. Defined accountability and responsibility allow the nurse to develop a plan of care with the client and family. This holistic approach to care facilitates continuity of care rather than a shift-to-shift focus. Nurses, when they have adequate time to provide necessary care, find this model professionally rewarding because it gives the authority for decision making to the nurse at the bedside. Disadvantages include a high cost because of a higher RN skill mix. The nurse who makes the assignments needs to be knowledgeable about both the clients and the staff to ensure appropriate matching of a nurse's skill to a client's needs. With no geographical boundaries within the unit, nursing staff may be required to travel long distances at the unit level to care for their primary clients. Nurses often perform functions that could be completed by other staff. And finally, nurse-to-client ratios must be realistic to ensure sufficient nursing time is available to meet the client care needs.

CLIENT-CENTRED OR CLIENT-FOCUSED CARE

Client-centred care or **client-focused care** is designed to focus on client needs rather than staff needs. In this model, required care and services are brought to the client. In the highest evolution of this model, all client services are decentralized to the client area, including radiology and pharmacy services. Staffing is based on client needs. In this

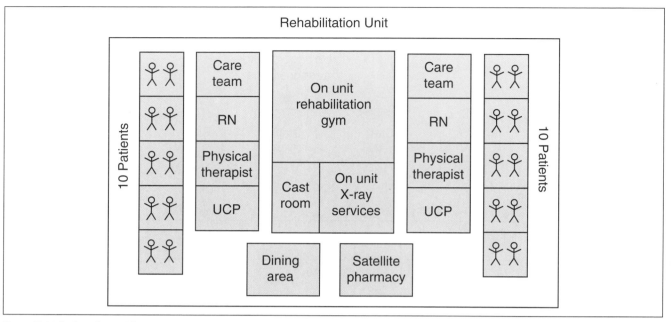

Figure 12-11 Patient-Centred Care Model.

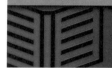

LITERATURE APPLICATION

Citation: McGillis Hall, L., Doran, D., & Pink, G. H. (2004). Nurse staffing mix models, nursing hours, and patient safety outcomes. *Journal of Nursing Administration, 34*(1), 41–45.

Discussion: This descriptive correlational study compared nursing staff mix models with a higher proportion of RNs and their client outcomes. The sample was composed of 77 adult medical, surgical, and obstetrical units in 19 urban teaching hospitals in Ontario, Canada. Nurse staffing was categorized into four models: an RN/RPN mix, an all-RN mix, a proportion of regulated to unregulated mix, and an RN/RPN/UCP mix. Client safety outcomes included the rate of medication errors, urinary tract infections, wound infections, and client falls.

When the proportion of RNs and RPNs was lower, the number of medication errors and wound infections increased, and the number of nursing hours increased. The less experienced the RNs and RPNs were, the higher the number of wound infections. Older and more complex clients used more RN and RPN hours.

Implications for Practice: This study showed that increasing the proportion of unregulated providers on medical-surgical units can influence client safety and increase nursing costs. Nurse managers need to consider the complexity of the client needs, the experience level of the nursing staff, and the mix of nursing staff when planning the staffing requirements of the unit. Less experienced RNs and RPNs need supports such as mentoring and unit-based orientation and education to improve their practice and increase client safety. In addition, strategies are required to recruit and retain experienced nurses.

model, effort is focused on having the right person doing the right thing. Care teams are established for a group of clients. The care teams may include other disciplines, such as respiratory or physical therapists. In these teams, all disciplines collaborate to ensure that clients receive the care they need. Staff work close to the clients in decentralized work stations. For example, on a rehabilitation unit, physical therapists may be members of the care team who work at the unit level rather than in a centralized physical therapy department (see Figure 12-11).

ADVANTAGES AND DISADVANTAGES

The pros of the system are that it is most convenient for clients and expedites services to clients. But it can be extremely costly to decentralize major services in an

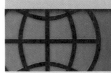

REAL WORLD INTERVIEW

In our organization, we have implemented a model of differentiated practice. Our purpose was to match individual competencies with job descriptions to maximize an individual's skills. Our model has one staff nurse title, but job descriptions and performance expectations are based on the nurse's level of education—associate degree, bachelor's degree, or master's degree. Pay is based on level of education and performance. Performance expectations were developed for each education level and organized using the nursing process as a framework. The nursing process statements for each level of education reflect nursing practice from novice to expert. In this model, all nurses may participate in activities such as discharge planning, but the performance expectations for a master's-prepared nurse would be different from the expectations for a diploma-prepared nurse. Each nurse has an individual performance plan to meet established performance expectations and to develop and meet individual goals. This performance plan is developed annually by the staff nurse with the nurse manager.

The outcomes of this model have been improved job satisfaction and reduced turnover of the nursing staff. We have noted that more staff have engaged in formal education and are accessing educational opportunities within the organization. Some of the lessons we learned were that we had to look at people as individuals. Staff did not fit into neat categories. We learned that some in the nursing administrative ranks feared how the staff would react to a differentiated practice model. In reality, the staff accepted the model and the message that everyone has value and brings different skills to the workplace. The goal of the model was to maximize those two messages. In communicating to the staff, hierarchy of any sort in the model was minimized.

In retrospect, I would have spent more time upfront with the managers and other leadership staff. It is key that leadership staff have a complete understanding of the model, how to communicate the key elements of the model, and how to implement the model at the unit level. Although implementing this model was a significant culture change for our organization, the outcomes for the staff have been positive and well worth the efforts put forth.

Kathleen Brodbeck, RN, MSN
Vice President for Patient Care

organization. A second disadvantage is that some staff have perceived the model as a way of reducing RNs and cutting costs in hospitals. In fact, this intention has been true in some organizations, but many other organizations have successfully used the client-centred model to ensure the right staff are available for the needs of the client population.

CARE DELIVERY MANAGEMENT TOOLS

In the 1980s and 1990s, several initiatives were introduced to improve care and reduce costs, many of which had positive effects. The Canadian Institute for Health Information (CIHI) established case mix groups (CMGs) and resource intensity weights (RIWs). Case mix groups are groups of cases that are clinically similar with respect to resource use. The CMG is a way of relating the type of client a hospital treats to the resources utilized by the hospital. Cases are categorized by type of data, such as clinical (e.g., diagnosis, procedure); demographic (e.g., age, gender); or resource consumption (e.g., costs, length of stay). CMGs are modelled after the DRG (diagnosis-related group) in the United States, and were implemented in 1983.

Resource intensity weights or RIW values are calculated using exclusively Canadian data. The RIW system is a relative resource allocation method for estimating a hospital's inpatient specific costs for both acute care and day procedure care. RIWs are used to standardize the expression of hospital case volumes, recognizing that not all clients require the same health care resources.

RIWs are used for the following purposes:

- To translate case mix data into cost data
- To determine unit costs for atypical cases
- To identify priorities by CMG for utilization management
- To plan new programs
- To evaluate program efficiency[2]

As hospitals looked for opportunities to reduce costs through reductions in clients' length of stay (LOS), clinical pathways and case management surfaced as significant strategies.

CLINICAL PATHWAYS (CARE MAPS)

Clinical pathways were a major initiative to emerge from the efforts to reduce LOS and are widely used to enhance outcomes and contain costs within a constrained length of stay (Lagoe, 1998). **Clinical pathways** are care management tools that outline the expected clinical course and outcomes for a specific client type. Clinical pathways take a different form in each organization that develops them. Typically they outline the normal course of care for a client. Pathways are often set up each day, with each day's expected outcomes being articulated. Client progress is then measured against the expected outcomes. In some facilities, pathways have physician orders incorporated into the pathway to facilitate care. In some organizations, the pathways include multidisciplinary orders for care, including orders from nursing; medicine; and other allied health professionals, such as physical therapy and dietary services. This approach serves to further expedite care for clients. Figure 12-12 provides an

---

Clinical Pathway: Lower Extremity Revascularization
Page 21 of 22

ADDRESSOGRAPH

DAILY ANTICIPATED OUTCOMES

POD2	Date/Time /Init When met	POD3	Date/Time /Init When met	POD4	Date/Time /Init When met	POD5	Date/Time /Init When met
Client rates pain 0-2 on pain scale 0-10 using po analgesia.		Graft signal present with doppler		Graft signal present with doppler		Graft signal present with doppler	
Graft signal present with doppler.		Incisional edges will be approximated without drainage.		Able to participate in self-care and adjunct therapies.		Ambulates independently	
Client will verbalize knowledge of plan of care, testing and treatment.		Site of invasive devices without signs of infection.		Patient viewed diet video.		Patient/significant other will verbalize understanding of activity/diet restrictions, medication use, wound management.	
Ambulate in hall Q I D		Ambulates in hall qid.				Completed nutrition post test.	
Tolerates po solids		Patient/significant other will describe appropriate problem solving skills to decrease anxiety.					
Voiding without difficulty		Rehab referral started: _yes _no					
		Family support available at discharge, specify _____ _____					

TO BE KEPT IN PROGRESS NOTE SECTION OF CHART AT ALL TIMES.

Figure 12-12 Example of a Clinical Pathway (Excerpt). (Courtesy of Albany Medical Center, Albany, NY.)

excerpt from a clinical pathway that identifies expected outcomes.

These pathways can be used by physicians, nurses, and case managers to care for the client and measure the client's progress against expected outcomes. Any variance in outcome can then be noted and acted upon to get the client back on track. Some organizations have up to 60 pathways implemented.

ADVANTAGES AND DISADVANTAGES

By articulating the normal course of care for a client population, clinical pathways are a powerful tool for managing care. They are very instructive for new staff, and they save a significant amount of time in the process of care. In most cases, the implementation of a clinical pathway will improve care and shorten the length of stay for the population on the pathway. Pathways also allow for data collection of variances to the pathway. The data can then be used to look for opportunities for improvement in hospital systems and in clinical practice.

An issue with development of pathways is that some physicians perceive pathways to be cookbook medicine and are reluctant to participate in their development; however, their participation is essential. Development of multidisciplinary pathways also requires a significant amount of work to gain consensus from the various disciplines on the expected plan of care. For client populations that are nonstandard, pathways are less effective because the pathway is constantly being modified to reflect the individual client's needs.

Clinical practice guidelines are evidence-based statements of best practice in the prevention, diagnosis, or management of a given symptom, disease, or condition for individual clients. The Canadian Medical Association (CMA) states that clinical practice guidelines provide better health care by clarifying which care is appropriate, promoting utilization or more beneficial care, and reducing liability. Clinical practice guidelines are an integral component of the CMA quality of care program. More than 40 organizations have been actively involved in guideline development, and Canada has more than 400 clinical practice guidelines.[3]

CASE MANAGEMENT

Case management is another strategy to improve client care and reduce hospital costs through coordination of care. Typically a case manager is responsible for coordinating care and establishing goals from preadmission through discharge (Del Togno-Armanasco, Hopkin, & Harter, 1995). In the typical model of case management, a nurse is assigned to a specific high-risk client population or service, such as cardiac surgery clients. The case manager has the responsibility to work with all disciplines to facilitate care. For example, if a post-surgical hospitalized client has not met ambulation goals according to the clinical pathway, the case manager would work with the physician and nurse to determine what is preventing the client from achieving this goal. If it turns out that the client is elderly and is slow to recover, they may agree that physical therapy would be beneficial. In other models, the case management function is provided by the staff nurse at the bedside. This approach works well if the population requires little case management, but if the client population requires significant case management services, sufficient RN time needs to be allocated for this activity. In addition to facilitating care, the case manager usually has a data function to improve care. In this role, the case manager collects aggregate data on client variances from the clinical pathway. The data are shared with the responsible physicians and other disciplines that participate in the clinical pathway and are then used to explore opportunities for improvement in the pathway or in hospital systems.

KEY CONCEPTS

- To plan nurse staffing, you must understand and apply the concepts of full-time equivalents (FTEs) and nursing hours per patient day (NHPPD).

- Workload measurement systems predict the nursing time required for a specific client and then whole groups of clients; the data can then be utilized for staffing, budgeting, and benchmarking.

- Determining the number of FTEs needed to staff a unit requires review of client classification data, NHPPD, regulatory requirements, skill mix, staff support, historical information, and the physical environment of the unit.

- The number of staff and clients in your staffing pattern drives the amount of nursing time available for client care.

- In developing a staffing pattern, additional FTEs must be added to a nursing unit budget to provide coverage for days off and benefit hours.

- Scheduling of staff is the responsibility of the nurse manager, who must consider client need and intensity, volume of clients, and the experience of the staff.

- When choosing a staffing variation, assessing the effect on client care and cost is essential.

- Self-scheduling can increase staff morale and professional growth but to be successful, it requires clear boundaries and guidelines.

- Evaluating the outcomes of your staffing plan on clients, staff, and the organization is an essential activity that should be done daily, monthly, and annually.

- Case management, clinical pathways, and clinical practice guidelines are care management tools that have been developed to improve client care and reduce hospital costs.

KEY TERMS

benchmarking	inpatient unit
care delivery model	modular nursing
case management	non-unit producing
case mix groups (CMGs)	nursing hours per patient day
client acuity	primary nursing
client-centred care	resource intensity weights
client-focused care	(RIWs)
clinical pathways	self-scheduling
clinical practice guidelines	skill mix
direct care	staffing pattern
episodic care unit	team nursing
full-time equivalent (FTE)	total patient care
functional nursing	unit producing
indirect care	workload measurement system

REVIEW QUESTIONS

1. Workload measurement systems assess the nursing workload needed by the client. The higher the client's acuity, the more care required by the client. Which of the following statements represents a weakness of workload measurement systems?
   A. Workload measurement data are useful in predicting the required staffing for the next shift and for justifying nursing hours provided.
   B. Workload measurement data can be utilized by the nurse making assignments to determine what level of care a client requires.
   C. Workload measurement systems typically focus on nursing tasks rather than a holistic view of a client's needs.
   D. Aggregate workload measurement data are useful in costing out nursing services and for developing the nursing budget.

2. To determine the number of FTEs required for a renal transplant unit, which of the following does *not* need to be reviewed?
   A. Regulatory requirements from your government
   B. The client population care needs and the impact on your skill mix
   C. Organizational structure or supports in place to enable care providers to care for clients.
   D. The chief financial officer's opinion on the number of staff needed for your unit

3. In calculating the number of FTEs needed to staff your medical-surgical unit, which of the following does *not* require the scheduling of additional FTEs?
   A. Benefit hours such as vacation and sick time
   B. Educational time for staff, including orientation of new staff
   C. Indirect client care staff that support the operation of the direct care staff 24 hours a day
   D. Coverage for other departments that do not staff to cover their own benefit hours.

4. If your RN staff members receive four weeks of vacation and six days of sick time per year, how many worked hours would each RN log in one year if all benefit hours were used?
   A. 1,950 worked hours
   B. 1,755 worked hours
   C. 1,905 worked hours
   D. 1,800 worked hours

5. In building your staffing plan, which of the following would *not* be a major consideration for determining how many staff you need each day and shift?
   A. The need for your staff to have more weekends off
   B. The volume of clients that you have at different times of the day
   C. The timing and volume of nurse-intensive activities such as administration of chemotherapy and blood
   D. The skill mix of your staff and the client care requirements throughout a 24-hour period

6. Client outcomes are the result of many variables, one being the model of care delivery that is utilized. From the following scenarios, select the worst fit between client needs and the care delivery model.
   A. Cancer clients cared for in a primary nursing model
   B. Rehabilitation clients cared for in a client-centred model
   C. Medical intensive care clients being cared for in a team nursing model
   D. Ambulatory surgery clients with a wide range of illnesses being cared for using a primary nursing model.

7. The care management tools of case management and clinical pathways have led to several improvements. Which of the following would *not* be considered an outcome of these care management tools?
   A. Increased public awareness of the nurse's role in health care
   B. Length-of-stay reductions
   C. Reduced cost of care in many populations
   D. Identification of opportunities for improvement in care or in hospital systems

REVIEW ACTIVITIES

1. How do you know whether the outcomes of your staffing plan are positive? What measures do you have available in your organization to indicate your staffing is adequate or inadequate?

2. You are a nurse manager of a new unit for psychiatric clients. What would you consider in planning for FTEs and staffing for this unit?

3. You are a new nurse and you have increasing concerns regarding the staffing levels on your unit. You are becoming increasingly anxious each time you go to work. What would you do?

EXPLORING THE WEB

- To get more information on mandated staffing levels, go to *http://www.ana.org*. Go to staffing issues on the menu and review the legislative agenda for the American Nurses Association (ANA) regarding staffing. Also review the data on the ANA's latest staff survey.

- Canada does not have mandated staffing levels; however, a recent Canadian Federation of Nurses Unions' report recommended a pilot project to test the use of standardized nurse-patient ratios in an appropriate setting. Read about it at *http://www.nursesunions.ca/extension.php?docex=56*.

- To get more information on nursing quality measures, go to *http://www.hc-sc.gc.ca/hcs-sss/pubs/nurs-infirm/2002-cnac-cccsi-final/index_e.html* and *http://www.cna-nurses.ca/CNA/practice/environment/worklife/default_e.aspx*. What are the quality indicators?

REFERENCES

Advisory Committee on Health Human Resources. (2000a). *The Nursing Strategy for Canada*. Ottawa, ON: Author. Retrieved from http://www.hc-sc.ca/english/nursing/, August 17, 2007.

Advisory Committee on Health Human Resources. (2000b). *The Canadian Nursing Advisory Committee*. Retrieved from http://www.hc-sc.gc.ca/english/nursing/cnac.htm, August 17, 2007.

Aiken, L. H., Clarke, S. P., Cheung, R. B., Sloane, D. M., & Silber, J. H. (2003). Educational levels of hospital nurses and surgical patient mortality. *Journal of the American Medical Association, 290*(12), 1617–1623.

Aiken, L. H., Clarke, S. P., & Sloane, D. M. (2002). Hospital staffing, organization and quality of care: Cross-national findings. *International Journal for Quality in Health Care, 14*(1), 5–13.

Baumann, A., O'Brien-Pallas, L., Armstrong-Stassen, M., Blythe, J., Bourbonnais, R., Camerson, S., et al. (2001). *Commitment and care: The benefits of a healthy workplace for nurses, their patients and the system*. Policy Synthesis. The Change Foundation.

Canadian Nursing Advisory Committee. (2002). *Our health, our future: Creating quality workplaces for Canadian nurses: Final report of the Canadian Nursing Advisory Committee*. Ottawa: Advisory Committee on Health Human Resources.

Dearholt, S., & Feathers, C. A. (1997). Self-scheduling can work. *Nursing Management, 28*(8), 47–48.

Del Togno-Armanasco, V., Hopkin, L. A., & Harter, S. (1995). How case management really works. *American Journal of Nursing, 5,* 24i, 24j, 24l.

Giovannetti, P. (1994). Measuring nursing workload. In J. M. Hibberd & M. E. Kylie (Eds.), *Nursing management in Canada* (pp. 331–349). Toronto: W.B. Saunders.

Hill-Popper, M. (2000, January). *Reversing the flight of talent*. Symposium at the Nursing Executive Center annual meeting, The Advisory Board Company, Washington DC.

Joint Commission on Accreditation of Healthcare Organizations. (2000). *2000 hospital accreditation standards*. Oakbrook Terrace, IL: Author.

Lagoe, R. J. (1998). Basic statistics for clinical pathway evaluation. *Nursing Economic$, 16*(3), 125–131.

Malloch, K., & Conivaloff, A. (1999). Patient classification systems, part 1. *Journal of Nursing Administration, 29*(7/8), 49–56.

Manthey, M. (1980). *The practice of primary nursing*. Boston: Blackwell Scientific.

McGillis Hall, L., Doran, D., & Pink, G. H. (2004). Nurse staffing mix models, nursing hours and patient safety outcomes. *Journal of Nursing Administration, 34*(1), 41–45.

McGillis Hall, L., Pink, L., Lalonde, M., Murphy, G., O'Brien-Pallas, L., Laschinger, H., et al. (2006). *Evaluation of nursing staff mix and staff ratio tools and models. Final report*. Ottawa: Canadian Nurses Association and Health Canada.

O'Brien-Pallas, L. (2007). Mapping out the territory. *Healthcare Papers, 7*(sp), 74–78.

O'Brien-Pallas, L., Doran, D. I., Murray, M., Cockerill, R., Sidani, S., Laurie-Shaw, B., et al. (2001). Evaluation of a client care delivery model, part 1: Variability in nursing utilization in community home nursing. *Nursing Economic$, 19*(6), 267–276.

O'Brien-Pallas, L., Doran, D. I., Murray, M., Cockerill, R., Sidani, S., Laurie-Shaw, B., et al. (2002). Evaluation of a client care delivery model, part 2: Variability in client care outcomes in community home nursing. *Nursing Economic$, 20*(1), 13–21, 36.

Shamian, J., & El-Jardali, F. (2007). Healthy workplaces for health workers in Canada: Knowledge transfer and uptake in policy and practice. *Healthcare Papers, 7*(Sp), 6–25.

Shullanberger, G. (2000). Nurse staffing decisions: An integrative review of the literature. *Nursing Economic$, 18*(3), 124–136.

Sovie, M. D., & Jawad, A. F. (2001). Hospital restructuring and its impact on outcomes: Nursing staff regulations are premature. *Journal of Nursing Administration, 31*(12), 588–600.

Swansburg, R. C. (1996). *Management and leadership for nurse managers* (2nd ed.). Sudbury, MA: Jones & Bartlett.

SUGGESTED READINGS

A brief history of pathways: From case management plans to care maps. (1998). *Hospital Case Management, 6*(4), 67, 84, 98.

Aiken, L. H., Sloane, D. M., & Sochalski, J. (1998). Hospital organization and outcomes. *Quality in Healthcare, 7*(4), 222–226.

American Hospital Association. (2002). *In our hands: How hospital leaders can build a thriving workforce.* Washington, DC: AHA Commission on Workforce for Hospitals and Health Systems.

Baker, C. M., Lamm, G. M., Winter, A. R., Robbleloth, V. B., Ransom, C. A., Conly, F., et al. (1997). Differentiated nursing practice: Assessing the state-of-the-science. *Nursing Economic$, 15*(5), 253–261.

Buckingham, M., & Coffman, C. (1999). *First break all the rules: What the world's greatest managers do differently.* New York: Simon & Schuster.

Falco, J., Wenzel, K., Quimby, D., & Penny, P. (2000). Moving differentiated practice from concept to reality. *Aspen Advisor for Nurse Executives, 15*(5) 6–9.

Ferguson-Paré, M. (2004). ACEN position statement: Nursing workload: A priority for healthcare. *Canadian Journal of Nursing Leadership, 17*(2), 24–26.

HayGroup. (2001). *The retention dilemma: Why productive workers leave—Seven suggestions for keeping them.* Working Paper. Philadelphia: Hay Group, Inc.

Lichtig, L. K., Knaug, R. A., Rison-McCoy, R., & Wozniak, L. M. (2000). *Nurse staffing and patient outcomes in the inpatient hospital setting.* Washington, DC: American Nurses Association.

Morash, R., Brintnell, J., & Rodger, G. L. (2005). A span of control tool for clinical managers. *Canadian Journal of Nursing Leadership, 18*(3), 83–93.

Nardone, P. L., Markie, J. W., & Tolle, S. (1995). Evaluating a nursing care delivery model using a quality improvement design. *Journal of Nursing Care Quality, 10*(1), 70–84.

Needleman, J., Buerhaus, P., Mattke, S., Stewart, M., & Zelevinsky, K. (2002). Nurse staffing levels and the quality of care in hospitals. *New England Journal of Medicine, 346*(22), 1715–1722.

Nelson, J. W. (2000). Consider this. . . Models of nursing care: A century of vacillation. *Journal of Nursing Administration, 30*(4), 156, 184.

Priest, A. (2006). *What's ailing our nurses? A discussion of the major issues affecting nursing human resources in Canada.* Ottawa: Canadian Health Services Research Foundation.

Seago, J. A. (1999). Evaluation of hospital work redesign: Patient focused care. *Journal of Nursing Administration, 29*(11), 31–38.

Tourangeau, A. E., Giovannetti, P., Tu, J. V., & Wood, M. (2002). Nursing-related determinants of 30-day mortality for hospitalized patients. *Canadian Journal of Nursing Research, 33*(4), 71–88.

Zander, K. (1996). The early years: The evolution of nursing case management. In D. L. Flarey, et al. (Eds.), *Handbook of nursing case management: Health care delivery in a world of managed care* (pp. 23–45). Gaithersburg, MD: Aspen.

CHAPTER ENDNOTES

1. Canadian Institute for Health Information, "Case Mix Groups." Retrieved from http://www.cihi.ca/cihiweb/dispPage.jsp?cw_page=casemix_e, July 14, 2006.

2. Canadian Institute for Health Information, "Resource Intensity Weights and Expected Length of Stay." Retrieved from http://secure.cihi.ca/cihiweb/dispPage.jsp?cw_page=casemix_riw_e, April 15, 2007.

3. CMA Infobase Clinical Practice Guidelines, "Foreward." Retrieved from http://mdm.ca/cpgsnew/cpgs/gccpg-e.htm, August 1, 2006.

CHAPTER 13

Delegation of Nursing Care

Maureen T. Marthaler, RN, MS
Adapted by: John P. Angkaw, RN, BScN, MEd(c)

If a procedure has been formally delegated to a nurse, the nurse is authorized to perform the procedure once it is determined that it is appropriate for a particular client or group of clients.
(College of Nurses of Ontario)

OBJECTIVES

Upon completion of this chapter, the reader should be able to:

1. Review the history of delegation.
2. Define delegation, accountability, responsibility, authority, and assignment making.
3. Identify responsibilities the health team members can perform.
4. List concepts associated with the delegation process.
5. Identify three potential delegation barriers.
6. List six cultural phenomena that affect transcultural delegation.

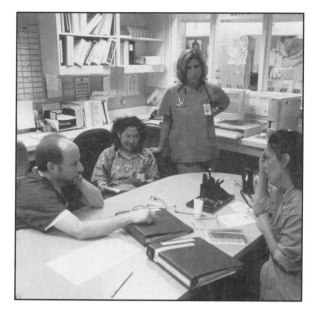

Delegation to the appropriate personnel is an important responsibility in nursing. Inappropriate delegation can be life threatening, as illustrated in the following example.

A client was admitted to the hospital for asthma exacerbation. The client also had a history of chronic obstructive pulmonary disease (COPD). The client was receiving Ventolin every four hours and Atrovent therapy via inhalation every hour as needed. She required respiratory assessments to be performed at the onset of every shift and whenever necessary as indicated by a change in the client's condition. The night nurse assessed the client at the beginning of her shift, noting that her respiratory status was stable. The client did not appear to be in any respiratory distress. During the night, the nurse periodically checked on the client every two hours but did not awaken the client. A sitter was in the room with the client and had assured the nurse that the client was "doing fine." The sitter did not report that when the client had been assisted to the bathroom initially, she had no difficulty. Upon assisting the client a second time, the sitter noted that the client became extremely short of breath and was becoming increasingly weak and becoming unstable. The sitter eventually required help from two unregulated care providers.

The incident and the change in the client's condition were not reported to the nurse. In the morning, the client's family became aware of the scenario and filed a formal complaint that their relative had not received any treatment during her distress.

How could this situation have been prevented?

Who is accountable?

What are the responsibilities of the nurse, the sitter, and the two unregulated care providers?

How could delegation have been appropriately performed in this situation?

On the Canadian Registered Nurse Examination (CRNE), students may encounter test questions that assess the ability of the nurse to delegate care. Safeguarding clients is a number-one care priority. To ensure that this responsibility is met, nurses are accountable under the law for care rendered by both themselves and other personnel.

Multiple levels of unregulated care providers (UCPs) give care to clients, including nurse aides, personal support workers, health care aides, unit assistants, attendants, home support workers, homemakers, and other non-licensed personnel (College of Nurses of Ontario, 2005). This wide use of UCPs is part of a response to changes in the structuring of health care delivery. Recent cost containment efforts have resulted in a variety of nurses being placed in new and innovative positions. Consequently, UCPs are often asked to consider performing duties that may not be within the scope of their education and abilities.

With increased opportunities to delegate care, nurses will be able to meet the duty of providing safe, quality care to their clients only by delegating properly. Without delegation skills, nurses caring for clients in today's health care community will not be able to complete the necessary duties, tasks, and responsibilities. They will find themselves stressed and exhausted by the many activities their nursing role requires. An inability to delegate can engender feelings of frustration, poor self-esteem, and lack of control. As nurses develop appropriate delegation skills, they become more productive and enjoy their work more.

PERSPECTIVES ON DELEGATION

As the history of nursing shows, Florence Nightingale had foresight regarding how nurses would function. Delegation in nursing was formally recognized in the 1800s, with Nightingale, and has continued to evolve as health care delivery models have developed.

Today, delegation is a must for the new nurse as well as the experienced nurse. Delegating to personnel with different educational levels from a variety of nursing programs requires nurses to be vigilant in ensuring that safety is maintained for the client.

According to Fisher (2000), delegation of certain tasks helps reduce health care costs by making more efficient use of nursing time and the facility's resources. Efficient delegation of care protects the client and provides desirable outcomes.

DELEGATION DEFINED

Different organizations and experts define delegation in different ways. According to the Canadian Nurses Association (CNA), delegation includes accepting accountability for actions and decisions when delegating, delegating health care activities to other health care providers consistent with levels of expertise and education, and evaluating the outcome of delegated health care activities (Canadian Nurses Association, 2002). **Delegation** is defined as the transfer of responsibility for a task when it is not part of the scope of practice of the care provider. The care provider performing the task must be accountable and competent in performing the delegated task. The safety of the client should not be compromised by substituting a less qualified worker to provide the care or perform the task (Saskatchewan Registered Nurses Association, 2004).

All delegation involves at least two individuals and specific duties to be accomplished with or through others via a transfer of authority. The authority needs to be delegated along with the ability to direct others. To be effective in accomplishing goals, the individual who is delegating must take on the leadership role. With successful delegation, the client's personal health needs are addressed and the nurse's professional goals are achieved. Communication techniques facilitate the delegation process for the registered nurse.

Registered nurses may be frustrated by having to accomplish all of their duties single-handedly. Many new graduate nurses become overwhelmed by the large number of duties to be learned and implemented. In nursing school, students typically perform total client care for one or two clients. Students might occasionally ask another student to help them, or they might pitch in to help others on their unit. Rarely will they have the opportunity to delegate to another nurse or to a UCP. Consequently, new nurses may be shocked to learn that delegation is now an expected part of their behaviour; however, delegation is required in the health care setting, and the CRNE tests nurse candidates on their ability to delegate.

Delegation is not meant to intimidate or isolate the new nurse. The sole purpose of delegation is to get the job done in the most efficient way, utilizing appropriate resources. The job must be delegated to staff who can handle it and who understand the goal. Delegation can spark interest and prevent individuals from becoming bored, nonproductive, and ineffective. Finding the duties or tasks that are most suitable can help people feel as if they are part of the team, regardless of their position. All staff want to feel they are making a difference in the well-being of the client, whether by giving a bath, dispensing medications, or even by sharing a simple smile. To delegate, the nurse takes into account other peoples' personal and professional positions within the health care team, including their abilities, education, and experience as well as the client's needs. Infection control and client safety are high priorities in making assignments. An RN Delegation Decision-Making Framework, originally adapted from the National Council of State Boards of Nursing (NCSBN) (1995), is available at its website (https://www.ncsbn.org/

delegationgrid.pdf). The NCSBN outlines five rights of delegation: the right task, the right circumstances, the right person, the right direction/communication, and the right supervision. The College of Nurses of Ontario has a decision tree for teaching or delegating the performance of a procedure. It can be found on its website (http://www.cno.org/docs/prac/41014_workingucp.pdf). In addition, the College of Nurses of Ontario also has guides to practise decision making for both entry-level licensed practical nurses and entry-level registered nurses.

ACCOUNTABILITY AND RESPONSIBILITY

Nurses are legally liable for their actions and are answerable for the overall nursing care of their clients. This is the definition of **accountability.** RNs and LPNs are accountable for their actions and related consequences, including the initiation and follow-through of the nursing process. Nurses are also accountable for following their provincial and territorial standards of practice and legislation, the policies of their health care organization, and for demonstrating professional conduct as reflected by attitudes, beliefs, and values espoused in the CNA *Code of Ethics for Registered Nurses* (Canadian Nurses Association, 2002). RNs and LPNs are accountable for monitoring changes in a client's status, noting and implementing treatment for human responses to illness, and assisting in the prevention of complications. The assessment, analysis, diagnosis, planning, teaching, and evaluation stages of the nursing process may not be delegated to UCPs. Delegated activities usually fall within the implementation phase of the nursing process.

Responsibility involves reliability, dependability, and the obligation to accomplish work. Responsibility also includes each person's obligation to perform at an acceptable level—the level to which the person has been educated. For example, a personal support worker (PSW) is expected to provide the client with a bed bath. The PSW does not administer pain medication or perform invasive or sterile procedures. After performing the assigned duties, the PSW provides, within a specified time frame, feedback to the nurse about the performance of the duties and the outcome of the actions. Note that feedback works two ways. The registered nurse has a responsibility to follow up with ongoing supervision and evaluation of activities performed by non-regulated nursing personnel. Although the nurse transfers responsibility and authority for the completion of a delegated task, the nurse retains accountability for the delegation process. Whenever nursing activities are delegated, the RN must follow the appropriate provincial or territorial nursing scopes of practices, nursing rules and regulations, and the standards of the hospital or health facility.

AUTHORITY

The responsibility to delegate duties and give direction to UCPs places the RN and LPN in a position of authority. **Authority** refers to a person's right to delegate, based on the provincial or territorial nursing scope of practice, and based on that person also receiving official power from an agency to delegate. According to Ellis and Hartley (2000), the concept of authority is often associated with power because authority given by an agency legitimizes the right of a manager or supervisor to give direction to others and to expect that they will comply. The best working environment is one in which staff members view authority with respect.

ASSIGNMENT MAKING

Assignment making is the process of delegating the duties and all aspects of client care to individual staff, including giving clear, concise directions and delegating the responsibility and the authority for the performance of the care. The RN or LPN retains accountability for the assignment, and must ensure that the education, skill, knowledge, and judgment levels of the personnel being assigned to a task are commensurate with the assignment. For example, administration of intravenous solutions to clients on a nursing unit would initially best be assigned to an RN or LPN who has received education about intravenous solutions and who has been performing these duties on a regular basis, rather than to someone who has little or no experience in administering intravenous solutions. When an assignment is made, the RN or LPN should specify the expected outcome of the assignment, the time frame for completion, and any limitations on the assignment.

RESPONSIBILITIES OF HEALTH TEAM MEMBERS

The new graduate nurse may feel overwhelmed by the amount of client care required and the lack of time to complete the care. The new graduate may be consumed by feelings of inadequacy and failure. Not knowing how to answer the phone or where to find a washcloth, and not having time to eat lunch can be exhausting. All of these feelings and behaviours may be a result of trying to do it all and not asking for help. New graduate nurses will quickly realize that if they do not delegate, the client's care will not be completed in a timely and effective manner.

Attention to the following six factors will improve both nursing delegation and nursing care:

1. The individual is adequately trained for the task.
2. The individual has demonstrated that the task has been learned.
3. The individual can perform the task safely in the given nursing situation.
4. The client's status is safe for the person to carry out the task.
5. Appropriate supervision is available during the task implementation.
6. The task is an established policy in the nursing practice setting and policy is written, recorded, and available to all (LSBN, 2003).

THE NURSE MANAGER'S RESPONSIBILITIES

The nursing manager is responsible for developing the staff members' ability to delegate. Guidance in this area is necessary because new graduates, who want to be regarded favourably, may not ask too much of other staff members. Delegation is a skill that requires practice.

The nurse manager will determine the appropriate mix of personnel on a nursing unit. The nurse manager may have staff with a variety of skills, knowledge, and educational levels. The acuity and needs of the clients usually determine the personnel mix. From this personnel mix, the new graduate nurse will begin to identify who can best perform the assigned duties. The non-nursing duties are shifted toward clerical personnel, UCPs, or housekeeping staff to make the best use of individual skills.

THE NEW GRADUATE'S RESPONSIBILITIES

New graduate nurses need to focus on the duties for which they are directly responsible. What duties can they delegate and to what extent? What do UCPs do? What do licensed practical nurses do? These questions need to be answered prior to the delegation of duties. Table 13-1 includes delegation suggestions for RNs.

THE REGISTERED NURSE'S RESPONSIBILITIES

The registered nurse is responsible and accountable for the provision of nursing care. According to the Canadian Nurses Association (2002), the registered nurse is always responsible for client assessment, diagnosis, care planning, and evaluation. Although unregulated care providers may measure vital signs, intake and output, or other client status indicators, the registered nurse or licensed practical nurse analyzes these data for comprehensive assessment, nursing diagnosis, and development of the plan of care. Unregulated personnel may perform simple nursing interventions

TABLE 13-1   DELEGATION SUGGESTIONS FOR RNs OR LPNs

1. Include all personnel in the delegation process when making assignments.

2. Assess which tasks are to be delegated and identify the staff to best complete the assignment.

3. Communicate the duty to be performed and identify the time frame for completion. The expectations for personnel should be clear and concise.

4. Avoid removing duties after they have been assigned. Removing duties should be considered only when the duty is above the level of the assigned staff member, such as when the client's care is in jeopardy because the client's status has changed.

5. Evaluate the effectiveness of the delegation of duties, check in frequently, and ask for a feedback report on the outcomes of care delivery.

6. Accept minor variations in the style in which the duties are performed. Individual styles are acceptable provided the duty is performed correctly within the scope of practice.

related to client hygiene, nutrition, elimination, or activities of daily living, but the registered nurse or licensed practical nurse remains responsible for the client outcome. Having UCPs perform functions outside their scope of practice is a violation of provincial and territorial nursing practice acts and is a threat to client safety.

Misusing UCPs is a practice common to many health care settings. According to the Canadian Nurses Association (2002), the use of UCPs has a great impact on the care provided to the clients, and therefore several factors have to be considered. Primary considerations include the complexity of the care required and the safety of the client. Secondary considerations are respect for personal autonomy and the rights of clients to participate in decision making. Research indicates that the use of UCPs instead of nurses poses a risk to the public, and as a result nurses must be alert to avoid such misuse of UCPs.

THE UCP'S RESPONSIBILITIES

The increase in the numbers of UCPs in acute care settings poses a degree of risk to the client. Many initiatives have been advanced to ensure safe staffing levels using an appropriate skills mix. Ideally, UCPs are to be trained to perform duties such as bathing, feeding, toileting, and ambulating clients (see Figure 13-1). UCPs are also expected to document and report information related to these activities. The RN or LPN will delegate to the UCP and is liable for those delegations. According to the CNA (2002), if the RN or LPN knows or reasonably believes that the UCP has the appropriate training, orientation, and documented competencies, then the RN or LPN can reasonably expect that the UCP will function in a safe and effective manner.

Reasons for using UCPs in acute care settings include controlling costs; freeing RNs or LPNs from duties that are primarily non-nursing in nature; and allowing time for RNs or LPNs to complete assessments of clients and their potential responses to treatments. UCPs cannot be assigned to assess or evaluate responses to treatment, which is the role of the RN or LPN. It is cheaper to have UCPs perform non-nursing duties than to have nurses perform them. UCPs can deliver supportive care, but they cannot practise nursing or provide total client care. The RN or LPN has an increased scope of liability when tasks are delegated to UCPs. The RN or LPN must be aware of the job description, skills, and educational background of the UCP prior to the delegation of duties.

Because the RN or LPN is accountable for the delegation of nursing care activities, the following questions need to be considered when considering utilizing a UCP to deliver effective, safe, and ethical delivery of care:

- Is it appropriate that a UCP perform this activity, considering the client's condition, the associated risks, and the environmental supports?
- Is there a UCP available with the potential to perform the procedure?
- Is there a mechanism to determine the ongoing competence of the UCP?

THE LICENSED PRACTICAL NURSE'S RESPONSIBILITIES

Licensed practical nurses have a different scope of practice from registered nurses. Most provinces and territories differentiate the role of the licensed practical nurse from the role of the registered nurse related to the

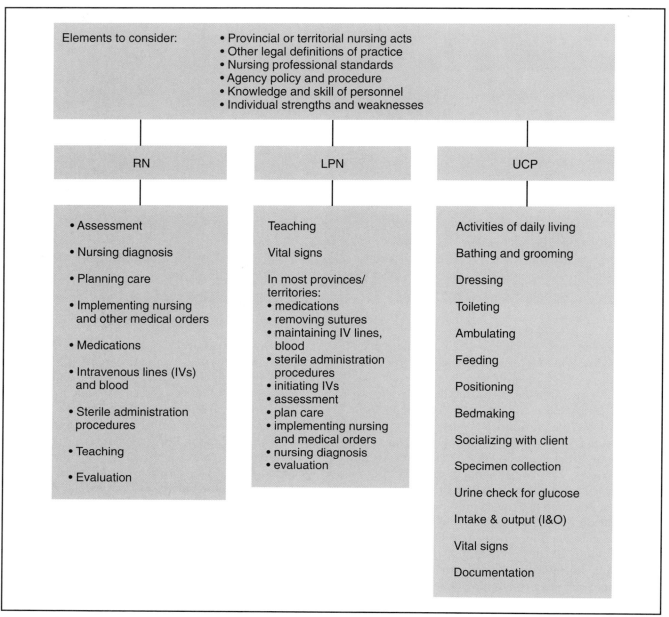

Elements to consider:
- Provincial or territorial nursing acts
- Other legal definitions of practice
- Nursing professional standards
- Agency policy and procedure
- Knowledge and skill of personnel
- Individual strengths and weaknesses

RN

- Assessment
- Nursing diagnosis
- Planning care
- Implementing nursing and other medical orders
- Medications
- Intravenous lines (IVs) and blood
- Sterile administration procedures
- Teaching
- Evaluation

LPN

Teaching

Vital signs

In most provinces/territories:
- medications
- removing sutures
- maintaining IV lines, blood
- sterile administration procedures
- initiating IVs
- assessment
- plan care
- implementing nursing and medical orders
- nursing diagnosis
- evaluation

UCP

Activities of daily living

Bathing and grooming

Dressing

Toileting

Ambulating

Feeding

Positioning

Bedmaking

Socializing with client

Specimen collection

Urine check for glucose

Intake & output (I&O)

Vital signs

Documentation

Figure 13-1 Considerations in Delegation.

LPN's breadth and depth of knowledge and the stability of the client the licensed practical nurse cares for. LPNs are held to the same standard of care as registered nurses and, similarly, are responsible and accountable for their actions. LPNs commonly have the most responsibilities of all regulated care providers in care facilities, particularly in the long-term care sector. In that environment, the LPN is primarily responsible for overall client assessment, nursing diagnosis, planning, implementation, and evaluation of the quality of care delegated. The five rights of delegation, as highlighted in *Delegation: Concepts and Decision-Making Process*, are

identified in Table 13-2. These rights can be used as a mental checklist to clarify elements in the decision-making process (National Council of State Boards of Nursing, 1997).

When considering delegating the right task to the right person, check the applicable provincial or territorial nursing practice acts, the policies and procedures of the agency, and the job descriptions of all staff involved (e.g., LPNs, UCPs, RNs, and so on). Also consider the training and competence of all staff. Is the task being delegated by the right person to the right person? Is it a task that can be delegated by a nurse?

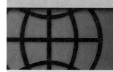

REAL WORLD INTERVIEW

I use delegation now that I have completed school. I began working as a new graduate nurse immediately after graduating. Prior to graduation, I worked as a personal support worker. I feel that I understand how it feels to be at both ends of the spectrum of client care delivery. I vowed that when I became a registered nurse, I would delegate appropriately and fairly to others.

As a registered nurse, I make it a point to delegate appropriately to personal support workers (PSWs). I delegate duties such as changing beds, bathing clients, feeding clients, and performing an accurate intake and output. I delegate these things after giving my PSW a complete report of my clients.

It is important to mention that I never delegate client assessments or client education. These duties are reserved for the registered nurse or licensed practical nurse. I will never delegate to a PSW to watch over clients while they take their medication. I never delegate the insertion or removal of Foleys. In short, I never delegate any tasks or responsibilities that are outside the PSW's scope of education and ability. I do believe my PSWs take me seriously as I do not delegate anything that I am not willing to do myself and have not done myself in the past. In essence, I do not give the impression that I am "beyond" or "better" than anyone else.

I am concerned when I see a nurse walk out of a client's room who has just requested a bedpan to look for a PSW to get that bedpan. I would never make my client wait to perform such a necessary and often immediate task. Like I said earlier, I have been on both ends of client care delivery, and I know what it feels like to be neglected and unappreciated. So far, I have stuck to my promise to delegate appropriately and fairly. I strongly believe my PSWs would agree.

Shelly A. Thompson
New Graduate Nurse

TABLE 13-2	FIVE RIGHTS OF DELEGATION

1. The right task
2. Under the right circumstances
3. Using the right person
4. With direction and communication
5. With the right supervision

When considering the right circumstance, determine whether the staff members understand how to administer a procedure safely and correctly, and whether the action requires staff competency to be documented.

When considering the right person, ascertain whether the client is stable with predictable outcomes and whether it is legally acceptable to delegate to this person, keeping in mind the setting and available resources.

When considering the right direction and communication, ensure the RN communicates the task with clear directions and that the steps of the task and its expected outcomes are carefully spelled out.

When considering the right supervision, ensure the RN answers all staff members' questions and is available to solve problems as needed. The UCP should report both task outcomes and the client's response to the RN who delegated the task. Thus, appropriate supervision and evaluation are maintained. The RN provides follow-up monitoring, intervention, feedback, evaluation, teaching, and guidance to the staff in an ongoing fashion.

DIRECT DELEGATION VERSUS INDIRECT DELEGATION

According to the CNA, direct delegation is usually verbal direction by the RN delegator regarding a procedure or task in a specific nursing care situation. Indirect delegation is performed using an approved listing of activities or tasks that have been established in the policies and procedures of the health care institution or facility.

The use of good professional judgment is vital when making the decision to delegate. Direct delegation gives the RN the opportunity to communicate clearly the duty to be completed, what to expect while completing the duty, and what the RN expects. The staff member then should have the opportunity to clarify the duty.

The process of indirect delegation begins at a variety of levels. The nurse manager prepares a list of duties that can be delegated, including those duties that are delegated from nurse manager to RN, RN to UCP, RN to LPN, LPN to UCP, nurse manager to unit clerk, RN to unit clerk. and so on. The duties are listed according to the hospital policy. The types of duties delegated reflect the ability of UCPs to complete the duties in a timely manner, according to their education and experience.

UNDERDELEGATION

People in a new job role, such as nurse manager, RN, LPN, or nursing graduate, often underdelegate. Believing that older, more experienced staff may resent having someone new delegate to them, new nurses may simply avoid delegation. Or, new nurses may seek approval from other staff members by demonstrating their capability to complete all assigned duties without assistance. In addition, new nurses may be reluctant to delegate because they do not know or trust individuals on their team or are not clear on the scope of the duties of the other staff or what they are allowed to do. New nurses can become frustrated and overwhelmed if they fail to delegate appropriately. They may fail to establish appropriate controls with staff or fail to follow up properly; they may fail to delegate the appropriate authority to go with certain responsibilities. Perfectionism and a refusal to allow mistakes can lead new nurses to be in over their head in client care responsibilities. More-experienced staff members can help new personnel by intervening early on and assisting in the delegation process, and by clarifying responsibilities.

INAPPROPRIATE DELEGATION

Inappropriate delegation of duties can place the client at risk. Delegating duties to others who have been inadequately educated is inappropriate and dangerous. The liability resting on the RN or LPN who has delegated professional duties to a UCP is clear. Although such inappropriate delegation is against provincial and territorial nursing standards of practice, the reasons for it are

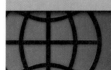

REAL WORLD INTERVIEW

Upon evaluating delegation on several, varied nursing units, I arrive at one conclusion: we as professional nurses just do not do it well. There is the exception, of course, that being the individuals who have developed an outstanding ability to delegate nearly all of their responsibilities to others in an authoritative or diplomatic manner with the recipients either loving or hating it.

On a nursing unit, the role of delegation and assigning tasks typically falls on the charge nurse. For this role, they are often criticized, most frequently behind the scenes, although at times, they are criticized openly. "What do you mean I am getting the next admission; I already have two!" One becomes apprehensive when assigning *anything*, from an admission to discharging a client. I wonder, if that is the fate of the charge nurse, just how well would one expect the staff RN to delegate?

I believe that the art of delegation and its related processes need to be taught and increasingly emphasized in nursing education, along with concepts of teamwork. The team becomes ineffective when proper delegation is neglected. The challenges in contemporary health care are tremendous, and will only become even more challenging in the future. Professional nurses would greatly benefit when they acquire advanced skills in delegation, team building, and diplomacy, as these are skills that will become essential tools to possess and utilize in the near future.

Andrea Chang, RN, MSN
Charge Nurse

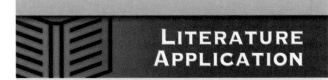

LITERATURE APPLICATION

Citation: Hansten, R., & Washburn, M. (2001, March). Delegating to UAPs: Making it work. *NurseWeek*, 21–23.

Discussion: As a result of the declining enrollment in nursing schools, Canada and other countries have resorted to filling in the gaps with UCPs. Partnering with UCPs and working effectively in a team-based system, RNs and LPNs can improve client care outcomes. Coercing UCPs to perform tasks beyond their capabilities, however, creates risk for the client and nurse. It is important to remember the "rights of delegation."

Implications for Practice: It is important for nurses to delegate correctly to ensure safe client care.

numerous. Staff may feel uncomfortable performing a duty with which they are unfamiliar, or they may be unorganized or inclined to either avoid responsibility or to immerse themselves in trivia. Inappropriately delegating duties can overwork some staff and underwork others, creating resentment among colleagues.

TRANSCULTURAL DELEGATION

Nurses and clients come from diverse cultural backgrounds. Transcultural delegation is the process of having staff perform duties while taking this cultural diversity into consideration. Poole, Davidhizar, and Giger (1995) suggest six cultural phenomena should be considered when delegating to a culturally diverse staff: communication, space, social organization, time, environmental control, and biological variations.

COMMUNICATION

Communication, the first cultural phenomenon, is greatly affected by cultural diversity in the workforce. Elements of communication, including communication patterns (i.e., the proximity of those communicating, such as different perceptions of personal space and tolerance of touching), body movements, paralanguage (i.e., inflections, silences, volume of voice, and pace of speaking), and density of language are among some of the characteristics that differ among cultures. All these elements influence how messages are sent and received (Grohar-Murray & DiCroce, 2003). For example, if a nurse were talking to a UCP in a loud voice, it could be interpreted as anger.

However, the nurse may be from a cultural background whose members always speak loudly—she may not be angry at all. Alternatively, a nurse, because of cultural upbringing, may speak in a quiet, nondirective way that could be wrongly perceived as lacking authority. All nursing programs teach basic communication skills, which are the basis of delegation.

SPACE

Cultural background influences the space that individuals maintain between themselves. Some cultures prefer physical closeness while other cultures prefer more distance to be maintained between people. Ineffective delegation can take place when an individual's space is violated. Some delegators stand too close when speaking. Conversely, some members of a group may feel left out if they are not sitting close to the delegator. They may not feel included or important.

SOCIAL ORGANIZATION

In different cultures, the social support in a person's life varies from support in one's own family to support from collegial relationships with coworkers. If a staff member looks to other staff for social support, those staff may have difficulty fulfilling any tasks delegated to them, which could threaten their social organization.

TIME

Another cultural phenomenon affecting delegation is the concept of time. How often have you heard people say, "They are on their own time schedule"? Some people tend to move slowly and are often late, whereas other people move quickly and are prompt in meeting deadlines.

Poole, Davidhizar, and Giger (1995) describe different cultural groups as being either past-, present-, or future-oriented. Past-oriented cultures focus on their tradition and its maintenance. For example, these cultures invest time into preparation of food that is traditional even though prepared food can be bought in a store. Present-oriented cultures focus on day-to-day activities. For example, our present-oriented culture works hard for today's wages and does not plan for the future. Future-oriented cultures worry about what might happen in the future and prepare diligently for a potential problem, which could be financial- or health-related. A nurse delegator should always be aware of duties to be completed and their deadlines so that appropriate personnel can achieve their responsibilities in a timely fashion. Otherwise, the people who meet deadlines in a timely fashion may be frustrated by those who do not.

ENVIRONMENTAL CONTROL

Environmental control refers to people's perception of their control over their environment, which is also called internal locus of control. Some cultures place a heavier

CASE STUDY 13-1

A new nursing graduate, Melody, has been assigned to work with Patrick, who is a UCP, and six clients. Melody introduces herself to Patrick and asks him what types of client care he usually performs. He tells Melody that he gives baths and takes vital signs. Melody asks Patrick to get all of the vital signs and give them to her written on a piece of paper. She asks Patrick if he ever documents them. He replies that he does document them, and he will provide her with the set of vital signs as soon as he obtains them.

Later that morning, Dr. Parinas is making rounds on his clients, two of whom are Melody's clients. He asks Melody for their most recent vital signs. She then asks Patrick for the vital signs on all her clients. Patrick tells her he has not taken them yet as he was busy engaging in other client care activities. Dr. Parinas then asks Melody to obtain the vital signs herself. By the time Melody returns with the recorded vital signs, Dr. Parinas has gone and has left written orders that she cannot read.

Several factors in this delegation situation should have been handled differently. Can you name any?

Do you think the new graduate was ready to delegate to the UCP? Why?

Were the duties delegated appropriate for the UCP?

weight on fate, luck, or chance, believing, for example, that a client is cured from cancer based on chance. They may believe the health care treatment had something to do with the cure but was not the sole cause of the cure. The way in which staff members perceive their control of the environment may affect how they delegate and perform duties. Staff with an internal locus of control are geared toward taking more initiative and not requiring assistance in decision making. They believe in taking action and not relying on fate. Staff with an external locus of control may wait for fate to determine their actions.

BIOLOGICAL VARIATIONS

The sixth and final cultural phenomenon is biological variations. Biological variations are the biopsychological differences between racial and ethnic groups, which include physiological differences, physical stamina, and susceptibility to disease. Such factors need to be considered when delegating tasks. For example, it would be problematic if the care of a comatose client who weighs more than 135 kilograms and needs frequent turning were delegated to a small nurse who cannot physically handle the client. Perhaps this client should be assigned to two nurses. A nurse who is pregnant would not be assigned to this particular client because of the potential injury to the baby and nurse. Likewise, a pregnant nurse would not be assigned to a client with radium implants because of the risks that the radium poses to the baby and mother. Biological variations must be considered, for the sake of both the health care providers and the client.

KEY CONCEPTS

- Delegation is a practised and learned behaviour.

- The RN must have a clear definition of what constitutes the scope of practice of all personnel.

- The five rights of delegation are the right task, the right circumstance, the right person, the right direction and communication, and the right supervision and evaluation.

- Accountability refers to nurses' legal liability for their actions, being answerable for the overall nursing care of their clients.

- Responsibility involves reliability, dependability, and the obligation to accomplish work. Responsibility also includes each person's obligation to perform at an acceptable level.

- Authority refers to a person's right to delegate based on the provincial or territorial standards of practice and based on that person also receiving official power from an agency to delegate.

- The RN is accountable for the delegation and performance of all nursing duties.

- There are several potential barriers to good delegation.

- Transcultural delegation is encouraged to provide clients with optimal care.

KEY TERMS

accountability   delegation
authority   responsibility

REVIEW QUESTIONS

1. Which of the following statements about RNs and UCPs is true?
    A. UCPs and RNs have equal responsibilities.
    B. UCPs are responsible for all client care.
    C. RNs are less accountable for client care when UCPs are assisting.
    D. The RN provides client care, delegating to other RNs or UCPs as necessary.

2. If a nurse has difficulty completing nursing duties on schedule, which of the following transcultural phenomenon should be considered?
    A. Biological variations
    B. Time
    C. Space
    D. Social organization

3. Which of the following is an inappropriate task for an LPN?
    A. Taking vital signs on a new client
    B. Completing a glucometer check and reporting it to the RN
    C. Completing a pain assessment that the UCP identified as being changed from an earlier assessment
    D. Discharging the client prior to obtaining doctor's orders

4. If a client being discharged requires teaching to be reinforced, which is the most appropriate caregiver to perform this task?
    A. A unit clerk
    B. An LPN
    C. A PSW
    D. A UCP

5. Which client is most appropriate to assign to the UCP for basic care?
    A. Client with acute peritonitis
    B. Client with stable congestive heart failure
    C. New post-op acute appendectomy client
    D. Recent head injury client

REVIEW ACTIVITIES

1. To determine your scope of practice, call your provincial or territorial nursing association for information on laws and regulations, or access the appropriate website.

2. Read the study in the April 14, 1999, *Journal of the American Medical Association*, by Dr. Peter Pronovost and colleagues at the John Hopkins University. They found that a decreased ICU nurse–client ratio during the day or evening was associated with increased ICU days and increased hospital length of stay. Could some of this high-acuity client care be safely delegated?

3. Observe delegation procedures at your institution. Is transcultural delegation considered? If so, which phenomena have you observed?

4. Take an informal survey of UCPs in the institution where you are serving your clinical practicum. Ask them what duties they are assigned. Are there any duties they are not comfortable performing? Discuss your findings.

5. Have you had any clinical opportunities to delegate duties? To whom did you delegate, and what did you delegate? Discuss how your delegating of duties affected the client and your work. What would you do differently next time?

EXPLORING THE WEB

- Log on to *http://www.cna-nurses.ca*. Note what policies, if any, consider delegation of care to UCPs and LPNs.

- The Province of Ontario outlines policies and standards of practice when working with UCPs. Log on to the College of Nurses of Ontario website at *http://www.cno.org* to view the policies.

REFERENCES

Canadian Nurses Association. (2002). Unregulated Health Care Workers Supporting Nursing Care Delivery. Retrieved from http://www.cna-nurses.ca/CNA/documents/pdf/publications/PS38_Unregulated_HCW_Supporting_NCD_March_1995_e.pdf, April 12, 2007.

College of Nurses of Ontario (2005). Working with unregulated care providers. *College of Nurses of Ontario: Compendium of Standards.* Toronto, ON: College of Nurses of Ontario.

Ellis, J. R., & Hartley, C. L. (2000). *Managing and coordinating nursing care.* Philadelphia: Lippincott.

Fisher, M. (2000). Do you have delegation savvy? *Nursing2000, 30*(12), 58–59.

Grohar-Murray, M., & DiCroce, H. (2003). *Leadership and management in nursing* (3rd ed.). New Jersey, NJ: Prentice Hall.

Hansten, R., & Washburn, M. (2001, March). Delegating to UAPs: Making it work. *NurseWeek,* 21–23.

National Council of State Boards of Nursing. (1997). Delegation: Concepts and decision-making process. *Issues,* 1–2.

Poole, V., Davidhizar, R., & Giger, J. (1995). Delegating to a transcultural team. *Nursing Management, 26*(8), 33–34.

Saskatchewan Registered Nurses Association. (2004). Practice of Nursing: RN Assignment and Delegation. Retrieved from http://findarticles.com/p/articles/mi_qa3980/is_200401/ai_n9421570, August 18, 2007.

SUGGESTED READINGS

American Association of Critical Care Nurses (AACN). (1990). *Delegation of nursing and non-nursing activities in critical care: A framework for decision making.* Irvine, CA: Author.

American Nurses Association (ANA). (1996). *Registered professional nurses and unlicensed assistive personnel* (2nd ed.). Washington, DC: American Nurses Publishing.

Barter, M., & Furmidge, M. L. (1994). Unlicensed assistive personnel: Issues relating to delegation and supervision. *Journal of Nursing Administration, 24*(4), 36–40.

Barter, M., & McLaughlin, F. E. (1997). Registered nurse role changes and satisfaction with unlicensed assistive personnel. *Journal of Nursing Administration, 27*(1), 29–38.

Bellack, J. P., & O'Neil, E. H. (2000). Recreating nursing practice for a new century: Recommendations and implications of the Pew Health Professions Commission's final report. *Nursing and Health Care Perspectives, 21*(1), 14–21.

Benner, P. (1984). *From novice to expert: Excellence and power in clinical nursing practice.* Menlo Park, CA: Addison-Wesley.

Bernreuter, M. E., & Cardona, M. S. (1997). Survey and critique of studies related to unlicensed assistive personnel from 1975 to 1997, part I. *Journal of Nursing Administration, 27*(6), 24–29.

Blouin, A. S., & Brent, N. J. (1995). Unlicensed assistive personnel: Legal considerations. *Journal of Nursing Administration, 25*(11), 7–8.

Boucher, M. A. (1998). Delegation alert. *American Journal of Nursing, 98*(2), 26–32.

Burns, J. P. (1998). Performance improvements with patient service partners. *Journal of Nursing Administration, 28*(1), 31–37.

Canadian Nurses Association. (1995). *Policy statement: Necessary support for safe nursing care.* Ottawa: Author.

Canavan, K. (1997, May). Combating dangerous delegation. *American Journal of Nursing, 97*(5), 57–58.

Gordon, S. (1997). What nurses stand for. *Atlantic Monthly, 279*(2), 80–88.

Johnson, S. (1996). Teaching nursing delegation: Analyzing nurse practice acts. *The Journal of Continuing Education in Nursing, 27,* 52–58.

Parkman, C. A. (1996, September). Delegation: Are you doing it right? *American Journal of Nursing 96*(9), 43–48.

Parsons, L. C. (1997). Delegation decision-making. *Journal of Nursing Administration, 27*(2), 47–52.

Princeton Research Survey Associates. (1996). *Nursing and the quality of patient care: 1996 survey.* Princeton, NJ: Author.

Shindul-Rothschild, J., Berry, D., & Long-Middleton, E. (1996, Nov.). Where have all the nurses gone? Final results of our Patient Care Survey. *American Journal of Nursing, 11,* 25–39.

Smith, J. (1998, July). RNs and UAPs: Not much difference? *RN, 62*(7), 37–38.

UNIT IV
Managing Care

CHAPTER 14

First-Line Unit Management

Kathleen Fischer Sellers, PhD, RN
Adapted by: Heather Crawford, BScN, MEd, CHE

Perhaps the single most critical factor in determining the success or failure of professional practice is the quality of the management and leadership at the unit level.

(Joyce Clifford, 1990)

OBJECTIVES

Upon completion of this chapter, the reader should be able to:

1. Define first-line unit management.
2. Discuss the elements of strategic planning—philosophy, mission, and vision.
3. Define nursing shared governance.
4. Identify Benner's concepts of novice, advanced beginner, competent, proficient, and expert nursing practice.
5. Identify accountability-based care delivery systems.
6. Identify measures of a unit's performance.

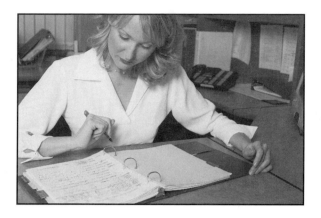

A first-line unit manager has been informed that plans are underway to merge the acute care surgical unit that she manages with an ambulatory surgery unit that currently cares for clients requiring 24-hour observation. As a visionary first-line unit manager with a great depth of experience, she has been recommended to oversee the development of the new work unit. The institution believes the creation of this new unit will enhance staff productivity and continuity of client care, and assist to balance the organization's budget. Therefore, resources are available to design and staff the new work unit in a manner that is congruent with the institution's mission, with the understanding that the investment will bring added value to the organization.

> *What structures and processes need to be put in place?*
>
> *What care delivery system would you put in place?*
>
> *How would you ensure the competency and continued professional growth of new staff?*
>
> *What outcomes would you hope to achieve? Within what time frames?*

First-line unit management utilizes the nursing process to plan, implement, and evaluate the outcomes of care for populations of clients rather than individual clients. First-line unit management is akin to conducting a large orchestra. Like the conductor, the first-line unit manager leads or coordinates a team of diverse individuals with varied talents and expertise toward a common goal (MacGregor-Burns, 1979). The orchestra creates beautiful music. The client care team provides an outcome of quality, cost-effective client care. Successful first-line unit management requires governance structures, client care delivery processes, and measures of the outcomes of care delivery that are consistent with the mission and vision of the organization and are built on a philosophy of professional practice. First-line unit management built on the tenets of professional nursing practice requires a structure of shared decision making or shared governance between nursing management and clinical nursing staff. Such a framework creates an environment in which the processes of client care delivery demand an accountability-based system, such as primary nursing, client-focused care, or case

management. In such an environment, the outcomes of care delivery, clinical quality, access, service, and cost can regularly be evaluated.

UNIT STRATEGIC PLANNING

Strategic planning is a process designed to achieve goals in dynamic, competitive environments through the allocation of resources (Andrews, 1990).

ASSESSMENT OF EXTERNAL AND INTERNAL ENVIRONMENT

As outlined in Figure 14-1, strategic planning involves clarifying the organization's philosophical values; identifying the mission of why the organization exists; articulating a vision statement; and then conducting an environmental assessment, or SWOT analysis, which examines the strengths, weaknesses, opportunities, and threats of the

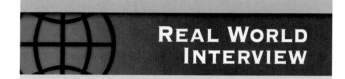

REAL WORLD INTERVIEW

At our academic health science centre, leaders in the organization, board members who represent the community, and customer stakeholders develop the strategic plan. Once the strategic plan is developed, it is published and reviewed at a centre-wide management meeting. It is then reviewed in divisional meetings and presented to staff through unit staff meetings, where the voice of the chief nursing officer has the most impact. I essentially interpret the rationale for the corporate strategic plan to my staff and glean their reactions. I then communicate the staff's feedback to the corporate level.

In our organizational newsletter for all staff, articles are published describing the plan and addressing points of clarification. Each division and department then undertakes the process of developing divisional and departmental plans that support the strategic plan. For example, a few years ago, the strategic plan articulated that our academic centre would become a major cardiac centre with a state-of-the-art cardiac catheterization laboratory. The department of cardiac services then included development of a state-of-the-art cardiac catheterization laboratory into its plan.

Anne L. Bernat, RN, MSN, CNAA
Chief Nursing Officer

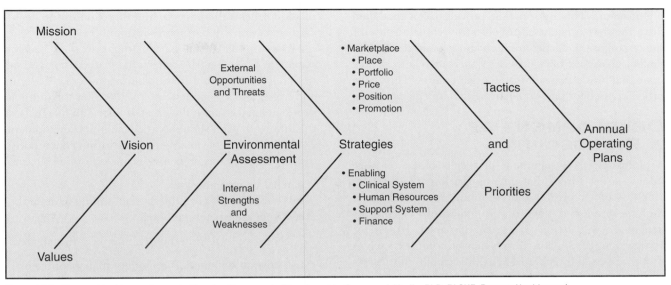

Figure 14-1a Bassett Healthcare Strategic Planning Framework. (Developed by Gennaro J. Vasile, PhD, FACHE, Bassett Healthcare.)

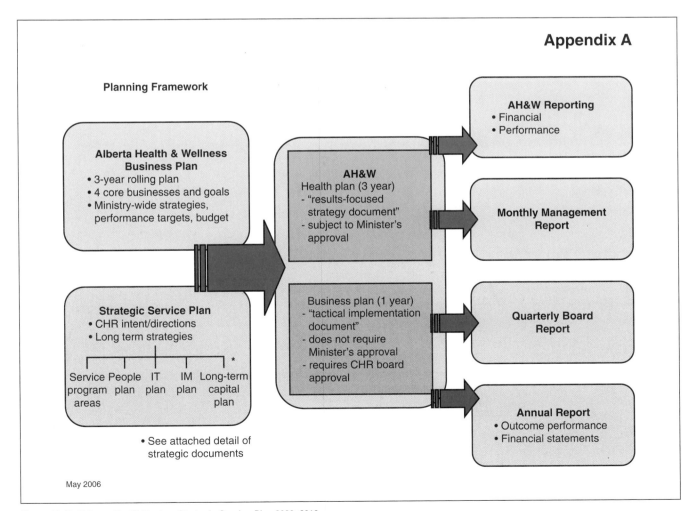

Figure 14-1b Calgary Health Region, Strategic Service Plan 2006–2010.

Source: Calgary Health Region, Retrieved from http://www.calgaryhealthregion.ca/communications/publications/strategic_Service_Plan-word_version.pdf, April 20, 2007. Reprinted with Permission.

organization. This information provides data that then drive the development of three- to five-year strategies for the organization. Tactics are then created and prioritized. Finally, goals and objectives are concretized into annual operating work plans for the organization. This same process is used for unit or departmental strategic planning.

DEVELOPMENT OF A PHILOSOPHY

A **philosophy** is a statement of beliefs based on core values—inner forces that give us purpose (Yoder-Wise, 1999). A unit's mission and vision are most authentic if they are developed based on the philosophy or core beliefs of the work team (Wesorick, Shiparski, Troseth, & Wyngarden, 1997). Core beliefs may be complex, such as those expressed in Table 14-1, or they can be short statements developed from a staff brainstorming session, such as "client centred," "partnering," "healing environment," and the like. A unit's core beliefs or values are then incorporated into the unit's mission and vision statements.

MISSION STATEMENT

A **mission** is a call to live out something that matters or is meaningful (Wesorick et al., 1997). An organization's mission reflects the purpose and direction of the health care agency or a department within it.

Covey (1990) states, "An organizational mission statement—one that truly reflects the shared vision and values of everyone within that organization—creates a unity and tremendous commitment" (p. 139). For the unit mission statement to have the greatest effect, all members of the unit work team should participate in its development.

Questions to be answered by the group charged with development of the unit mission include the following:

- What do we stand for?
- What principles or values are we willing to defend?
- Whom are we here to help?

There are three criteria for a unit mission statement:

1. A mission statement is no longer than a couple of sentences.
2. It states the unit's purpose using action words.
3. It should be simple and from the heart. (Jones, 1996)

Mission statements are so broad that units often adopt the organization's mission statement, as the surgical unit of Bassett Healthcare did. The mission statement shown in Figure 14-2 is that of both the organization and the unit.

TABLE 14-1	**CORE BELIEFS**

- Quality exists where shared purpose, vision, values, and partnerships are lived.
- Each person has the right to health care, which promotes wholeness in body, mind, and spirit.
- Each person is accountable to communicate and integrate his/her contribution to health care.
- Partnerships are essential to plan, coordinate, integrate, and deliver health care across the continuum.
- Continuing to learn and think in different ways is essential to improve health.
- A healthy culture begins with each person and is enhanced through self-work, partnerships, and systems supports.

Source: From "Mission and Core Beliefs," by B. Wesorick, *CPMRC Connections . . . for Continuous Learning,* December 2000, 3, p. 3.

BASSETT HEALTHCARE *Mission*

The mission of Bassett Healthcare is to provide excellence in patient care services, to educate physicians and other health care professionals and to pursue health research.

Figure 14-2 Bassett Healthcare Mission Statement. (Courtesy Patricia Roesch, BS, RN, Bassett Healthcare.)

TABLE 14-2	SURGICAL UNIT VISION STATEMENT

The work we do: Affects the outcomes that clients desire in their pursuit of wellness.

Why we do it: To provide a healing environment in which an individual's physical, mental, emotional, and spiritual well-being will be nurtured.

Who we are: Practising within partnering relationships that communicate respect while recognizing and valuing diversity.

How we do it: By committing to continued learning. Our knowledge fosters our growth; our mentoring nurtures our practice. (Roesch, 2000)

VISION STATEMENT

The unit vision statement reflects the organization's vision. A unit vision statement exemplifies how the mission and vision of the unit will be actualized within the organization's mission and vision.

Following are four criteria of a vision:

1. It is written down.
2. It is written in present tense, using action words, as though it were already accomplished.
3. It covers a variety of activities and spans broad time frames.
4. It balances the needs of providers, clients, and the environment. This balance anchors the vision to reality. (Wesorick et al., 1997)

The surgical unit vision statement in Table 14-2 exemplifies the core values of the unit: client centred, partnering, healing environment, and knowledge. The written statement tells the reader the work of the unit, why it is done, how, and for what reasons. In short, it delineates how the unit fulfills its mission.

GOALS AND OBJECTIVES

The next step in the strategic planning process is for the work unit to develop broad strategies that span the next three to five years and then develop annual goals and objectives to meet each of these strategies. A **goal** is a specific aim or target that the unit wishes to attain within the time span of one year. An **objective** is the measurable step to be taken to reach a goal.

THE STRUCTURE OF PROFESSIONAL PRACTICE

In an organization in which professional nursing practice is valued, strategic initiatives are developed and implemented most effectively through a structure of shared governance and shared decision making between management and clinicians.

SHARED GOVERNANCE

Shared governance is an organizational framework grounded in a philosophy of decentralized leadership that fosters autonomous decision making and professional nursing practice (Porter-O'Grady, 1992). Shared governance, by its name, implies the allocation of control, power, or authority (i.e., governance) among mutually (i.e., shared) interested vested parties (Stichler, 1992). In most health care settings, the vested parties in nursing fall into two distinct categories: (1) nurses practising direct client care, such as staff nurses; and (2) nurses managing or administering the provision of that care, such as managers. In shared governance, a nursing organization's management assumes the responsibility for organizational structure and resources. Management relinquishes control over issues related to clinical practice. In return, staff nurses accept the responsibility and accountability for their professional practice.

Unit-based shared governance structures are most successful when an organization-wide structure of shared governance is in place that unit-based functions can articulate with. Organizational shared governance structures are usually council models that have evolved from pre-existing nursing or institutional committees. In a council structure, clearly defined accountabilities for specific elements of professional practice have been delegated to five main arenas: clinical practice, quality, education, research, and management of resources (Porter-O'Grady, 1992). Figure 14-3 illustrates a shared governance model.

CLINICAL PRACTICE COUNCIL

The purpose of the clinical practice council is to establish the practice standards for the work group. Often, this council or committee is a unit-level committee that works in conjunction with the organizational committee accountable for determining policy and procedures related to clinical practice. Evidence-based practice fostered by

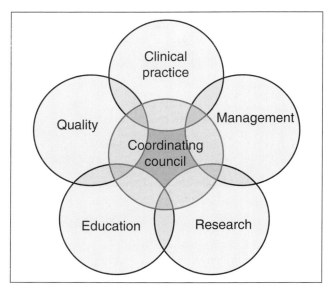

Figure 14-3 A Shared Governance Model.

research utilization initiatives ensures that practice standards are developed based on the state of the science of clinical practice and not merely on tradition.

QUALITY COUNCIL

The purpose of the quality council is twofold: (1) to credential staff and (2) to oversee the unit's quality management initiatives. In the role of credentialing staff, this committee is responsible for interviewing potential staff and reviewing their qualifications, or credentials. It then makes recommendations regarding hiring. The quality committee also serves as the body that reviews staff credentials on an ongoing basis and makes recommendations regarding promotion. Quality management initiatives for which the council is responsible can include review of indicators of the unit's overall clinical performance, such as medication errors, client falls, family satisfaction, and response time in answering call lights. At times, a unit will also participate in an organizational disease management study looking at the care of a specific client population, such as clients with diabetes.

EDUCATION COUNCIL

The purpose of the education council is to assess the learning needs of the unit staff and develop and implement programs to meet these needs. This council usually works closely with organizational education and training departments. Unit orientation programs and training programs related to new clinical techniques and new equipment are examples of programs sponsored by the education council.

RESEARCH COUNCIL

At the unit level, the research council advances research utilization with the intent of incorporating research-based

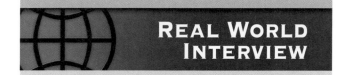

REAL WORLD INTERVIEW

We plan every year, but I'd say we look at our unit philosophy based on our core values and re-evaluate the strategic plan every two to three years. We had three core values that guided us, and then this year, with all the external pressures, we added a fourth. We keep these core values in the forefront when we do our annual planning. The process we used to develop and re-evaluate the core values was really very powerful and staff driven.

SPAN—Staff Planning Action Network—is our unit-based shared governance organization. SPAN met and developed draft mission and vision statements from our philosophy, which is based on our current core values—a client centred, partnering, and healing environment. They then transcribed these draft statements onto three flip charts and for 15 minutes per shift circulated these terms throughout the unit and got staff's re-action and feedback to the statements. Revisions were made from the feedback received. These revisions were then presented at a staff meeting. What was emerging from the feedback was a focus on the need for continuing education and training related to the rapidly changing environment. So we added a fourth value—knowledge.

Our unit philosophy, stemming from our core values, is what we believe in. We've expanded these core values into a vision statement that demonstrates what it is to practice on this unit.

Pat Roesch, BSN, RN
First-Line Unit Manager

findings into the clinical standards of unit practice. Research utilization is the process of staff critiquing available research literature and then making recommendations to the practice council so that clinical policies and procedures can be based on evidence-based research findings. The research council may also coordinate research projects if advanced practice nurses are employed at the institution.

MANAGEMENT COUNCIL

The purpose of the management council is to ensure that the standards of practice and governance agreed upon by unit staff are upheld and that adequate resources are available to deliver client care. The first-line unit manager

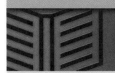

LITERATURE APPLICATION

Citation: Sellers, K. F. (1996). The meaning of autonomous nursing practice to staff nurses in a shared governance organization: A hermeneutical analysis. Unpublished doctoral dissertation, Adelphi University, Garden City, New York.

Discussion: Sellers conducted a study looking at autonomous nursing practice in an acute care hospital that was part of an integrated rural health network in upstate New York. She wished to know the impact of implementing a shared governance structure on autonomous nursing practice. She reviewed recent literature (Ludemann & Brown, 1989; Welsch & LaVan, 1981; Westrope, Vaughn, Bott, & Taunton, 1995) that had found that this model fostered recruitment and retention of nurses. However, she was interested in its effect on the autonomous practices of nurses in a hospital setting.

Sellers found that autonomous nursing practice was an everyday occurrence and to some extent had always existed within this organization. However, it had not always been recognized and legitimized by the larger organizational culture. Therefore, the staff nurses had not always had the opportunity to practise authentically, that is, with recognition. In the past, when the nursing organization was more traditional and centralized, autonomous nursing practice was informal. Often actions were performed at the risk of receiving an administrative reprimand. Despite this potential threat, autonomous actions were performed because they were appropriate actions to take for the client. The catalyst for autonomous nursing practice had always been client advocacy or doing what is right for the client.

Today, autonomous nursing practice within the context of a shared governance organization manifests itself in everyday patterns of action determined by decisions that staff nurses make themselves, based on knowledge gained from their experience. These actions are determined through the process of collaboration and shared decision making with colleagues within and outside the profession. These patterns of action include everyday practices of responding to clients' clinical needs and coordinating systems of care to meet the needs of clients. These practices are legitimized in collaboratively negotiated, written protocols and standards that are recognized by the larger community. As such, the shared governance culture has created the opportunity for legitimate or authentic nursing practice within the nursing organization of this hospital setting. The findings of this study indicate that as this institution shifted from a hierarchical nursing organization to a shared governance culture, the autonomous nursing practices of staff nurses were recognized, acknowledged, and legitimated. Therefore, the autonomous professional identity of nursing is now valued in this organization.

Implications for Practice: A culture of shared governance on a nursing unit helps develop the autonomous professional identity of nursing.

is a standing member of this council. Other members include the assistant nurse managers and the charge or resource nurses from each shift.

COORDINATING COUNCIL

Shared governance structures also include a coordinating council, whose purpose is to facilitate and integrate the activities of the other councils. This council is usually composed of the first-line unit manager and the chairpersons of the other councils. This council usually facilitates the annual review of the unit mission and vision and develops the annual operational plan (Sellers, 1996).

Unit-based shared governance structures may be less diverse. Often, some of the councils are combined into one council, for example, education and research. Or a council may contain subcommittees whose purposes are

to perform very specific tasks, for example, to credential and promote staff or to recruit and retain staff. Unit-based structures are varied, with the primary purpose being to empower staff by fostering professional practice while meeting the needs of the work unit.

ENSURING COMPETENCY AND PROFESSIONAL STAFF DEVELOPMENT

Professional practice through the vehicle of shared governance requires competent staff. Competency is defined as possession of the required skill, knowledge, qualification, or capacity (*Webster's Encyclopedic Unabridged Dictionary*, 1996) and is best determined in practice by a group of one's peers. Alspach (1984) defines competency as a determination of an individual's capability to perform to defined expectations (p. 656). Competency of professional staff can be ensured through credentialing processes developed around a clinical or career ladder staff promotion framework. A **clinical ladder** acknowledges that staff members have varying skill sets based on their education and experience. As such, depending on skills and experience, staff members may be rewarded differently and

carry differing responsibilities for client care and the governance and professional practice of the work unit.

BENNER'S NOVICE TO EXPERT

Benner's (1984) model of novice to expert provides a framework that, when developed into a clinical or career promotion ladder, facilitates professional staff development by building on the skill sets and experience of each practitioner. Benner's model acknowledges that practitioners can be expected to have acquired tasks, competencies, and outcomes that are based on five levels of experience.

Benner's model of novice to expert is based on the Dreyfus and Dreyfus (1980) model of skill acquisition applied to nursing. Benner's model has five stages: novice, advanced beginner, competent, proficient, and expert. Novice nurses are recognized as being task-oriented and focused. After they have mastered most tasks required to perform their ascribed roles, they move on to the phase of advanced beginner. The nurse who can demonstrate marginally acceptable independent performance illustrates the advanced beginner.

A competent nurse is one who has been in the same role for two to three years. These nurses have developed the ability to see their actions as part of the long-range goals set for their clients. The conscious, deliberative planning that is characteristic of this skill level helps achieve efficiency and organization.

Proficient nurses characteristically perceive situations as wholes rather than as series of tasks. They develop a plan of care and then guide the client from point A to point B. They draw on their past experiences and know that in a typical situation, a client must exhibit specific behaviours to meet specific goals. They realize that if

CRITICAL THINKING

As a nurse practising in a shared governance organization, you remember a decade ago when the organization decentralized, made a commitment to nursing professional practice, and implemented shared governance. Everywhere you went, people were talking about it and displaying posters and other signs of nursing's importance to the organization. That was years ago, before managed care and all its changes and before this latest nursing shortage. Now you do not hear people talking about it so much. You wonder, Does professional practice still exist? How can you tell? How does your organization compare with other organizations that do not have shared governance? Is it possible that professional practice has become the culture and so there is no need to talk about it anymore?

CASE STUDY 14-1

You are a competent nurse who is a member of the credentialing committee of the quality council. A fellow peer has presented his credentials for review in hopes of being promoted to the next level on the clinical ladder. You review the packet and make the recommendation that he be promoted. However, at the credentialing committee meeting, you learn that the first-line unit manager and the individual's preceptor, another member of the committee, have not recommended promotion.

You wonder whether your colleague is aware of concerns about his performance.

Are there guidelines and standards that you are not aware of that have not been met?

What is the next course of action for the committee?

What should your response be at this meeting?

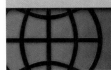

REAL WORLD INTERVIEW

There are five levels of our clinical ladder, which is similar to Benner's novice to expert model. The RN Is, or novices, are the new graduates and people in orientation. The experts are the clinical specialists. A lot of them have also become nurse practitioners so that the organization can receive some reimbursement for their client care services. This is a good thing because otherwise I'm afraid we wouldn't have these expert nurses anymore. They are the true mentors for nursing staff, especially when you are working with a very complex or difficult client situation.

Staff nurses also mentor each other. During orientation, your preceptor guides you along the path from RN I to RN II. When you decide you'd like to advance to RN III, you can choose another mentor. RN IIIs provide much more clinical leadership for staff and for the overall unit. I decided I was ready to be promoted to that level when other staff consistently were coming to me for clinical guidance and with client care questions. Now, as an RN III, I am the chairperson of our unit-credentialing committee, which is part of the quality council of our shared governance model.

Our clinical ladder uses a portfolio as the main tool to evaluate the nurse's readiness to advance. When you are an RN I in orientation, you are first introduced to the idea of a portfolio and how to put it together. It is difficult at first, because people do not know what is expected. However, after that first time when you are promoted from an RN I to an RN II, it becomes easier. You just build on what is already in the portfolio.

A portfolio should include the following:

Registrations

Your résumé

Letters of reference

Evaluations

Clinical documentation of client care

Validations for competencies related to technical skills (medication administration, IV therapy)

Examples of participation in development of the team plan of care

Exemplars

CEU certificates

Presentations

Publications

The portfolio tells the story of your practice. When a group of people are ready for promotion, the members of the credentialing committee meet. We review the portfolios and make recommendations related to advancement. The nurse manager is a member of this committee. She always reviews the portfolio and gives us her feedback even if she is unable to attend the credentialing meeting. I enjoy reading the exemplars the best. Exemplars are mini-stories that paint the pictures of each nurse's practice, and they are all so different.

Stacey Conley, RN, BS
Staff Nurse

those behaviours are not demonstrated within a certain time frame, then the plan needs to be changed.

The experts are those nurses who intuitively know what is going on with their clients. Their expertise is so embedded in their practice that they have been heard to say, "Something's wrong with this client. I'm not sure what's going on, but you had better come and evaluate this." Not heeding the call derived from the intuitive sense of an expert nurse has resulted in a client's cardiac arrest. These expert nurses often seek advanced education and become clinical specialists.

The Colorado Differentiated Nursing Practice Model (see Figure 14-4) builds on the work of Benner (1984) regarding career ladder stages. Stage I is characterized as the entry/learning stage. Stage II is characterized by the individual who competently demonstrates acceptable performance adapting to time and resource constraints. Stage III is characterized by the individual who is proficient. And stage IV is characterized by the individual who is an expert. The stages in this model are specifically defined by behaviours that are consistently exhibited or practiced over a defined period of time.

Colorado Differentiated Practice Model

The Colorado Differentiated Practice Model for Nursing has a separate clinical ladder for the six preparatory backgrounds depicted on the conceptual model (Diagram 1). A nurse selects the education clinical ladder according to the nursing credential s/he has attained.

The framework for each educational ladder has four distinct stages. These stages allow nurses to self-pace their advancement. A nurse is placed in a stage according to his or her own competency and experience.

Each nursing ladder has four weighted components as follows:
- Competency Statements 60%
- Skills 10%
- Institutional Goals 15%
- Professional Activities 15%

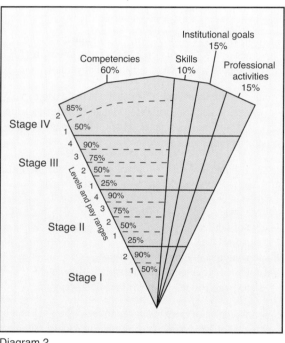

Conceptual model — Diagram 1

Sample ladder — Diagram 2

Figure 14-4 Colorado Differentiated Nursing Practice Model. (Courtesy Marie E. Miller, Colorado Nursing Task Force.)

THE PROCESS OF PROFESSIONAL PRACTICE

Ongoing professional staff development is part of the regular performance feedback that staff can expect from the first-line unit manager or the credentialing committee. The first-line unit manager also provides ongoing professional development of staff in their daily interactions on the unit and identifies projects and activities that meet a staff member's readiness for leadership development and advancement.

SITUATIONAL LEADERSHIP

The leadership framework developed by Hersey and Blanchard (1993) can be combined with an individual's position on a clinical/career ladder to assist the first-line unit manager in discerning the best approach for developing the potential of staff members. **Situational leadership** maintains that there is no one best leadership style, but rather that effective leadership lies in matching the appropriate leadership style to the individual's or group's level of task-relevant readiness. Readiness refers to how able and motivated an individual is to perform a particular task. A basic assumption of situational leadership is that a leader should help followers grow in their readiness to perform new tasks as far as they are able and willing to go. This development of followers is accomplished by adjusting leadership behaviour through four styles along the leadership curve.

According to Hersey and Blanchard's (1993) model, individual followers with low task readiness, such as novice nurses, require a telling style on the part of the leader. They need to be told what to do and to be given strong direction if they are to be successful and productive. As these followers grow in readiness, the leader should shift to a selling style,

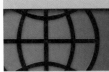

REAL WORLD INTERVIEW

I have a particularly touching story to tell you. D.T. was a 44-year-old man who was admitted from our ear, nose, and throat clinic with a large mass at the base of his tongue. Upon arrival on the unit, the client appeared very anxious, not knowing what he would face in the next few days. The client and his wife had been told that he would have a tracheostomy placed, which was quite a shock to them. They were both feeling overwhelmed with the situation.

As it happened, I was present for every major event that occurred with this family during that admission. I can recall the day when the client was told that the mass was cancerous. He and his family were devastated. I went to talk with the family and proceeded to tell them I could not begin to imagine what they must be going through, but that if they needed to talk, I was a good listener. I could tell that they very much appreciated that.

During the next few days, the family began to accept what was going on, and we began working together to teach them all they needed to know about tracheostomies and how to care for them. D.T. and his wife learned quickly how to be independent with tracheostomy care. In the coming days, the client underwent a feeding tube placement so that he could get some nutrition. I taught him and his wife how to care for the feeding tube and how to hang tube feedings. They learned so quickly that toward the end of the hospital stay, they were doing all his care independently. The client was informed that he would need to undergo radiation and chemotherapy. In preparation for the treatment, the client needed to have a complete dental extraction. Considering all that D.T. and his wife went through in such a short time, they both responded quite well to the situation.

Upon discharge, I set the client up with Lifeline (an emergency response service), nursing services, and equipment for the tracheostomy and tube feedings. This was no easy task because they did not have much money and their insurance company was quite difficult to deal with. As their primary nurse, I spent days on the phone in preparation for their discharge. It was quite challenging but rewarding when all was accomplished. It was both a happy and a sad day when the client and his wife were discharged. Since the client has left, I have kept in touch through writing, and I've talked to him in person when he has been readmitted to the medical floor for his chemotherapy treatment. I am glad to report that thus far D.T. is doing well.

This was a particularly touching experience for me. This family was very special to me, and I am glad for the opportunity I had to get to know them and be a special part of their lives. As an unknown author has said, in the end, we will not remember the years we spent nursing, we will only remember the moments.

Stacey Conley, RN, BS
Staff Nurse

with more positive reinforcement and socio-emotional support. Once individuals reach higher levels of readiness, as a proficient or expert nurse, the leader should respond by decreasing control. The leader moves first to a participatory style characterized by a high degree of relationship with staff and a lower need to give task direction, and then, with expert staff, the leader moves to a style of delegating, communicating a sense of confidence and trust because highly competent individuals respond best to greater freedom.

Individuals' readiness to learn and accept new tasks may change for a variety of reasons. When first-line managers discern a change, they must readjust their style of interaction with the nurse—moving forward or backward through the leadership curve—to provide the appropriate level of support and direction to facilitate that individual's continued development, productivity, and success as a member of the client care team. Development of staff based on their innate readiness to accept new tasks and responsibilities facilitates their promotion along a continuum of novice to expert and ensures a professional client care team that is able to consistently deliver accountability-based client care.

ACCOUNTABILITY-BASED CARE DELIVERY

Accountability-based care is essential in today's value-driven workplace. Individuals who are accountable are, by definition, able to report, explain, or justify their actions (*Webster's Encyclopedic Unabridged Dictionary,* 1996). Accountability is about achieving outcomes and is the foundation for evaluation (Porter-O'Grady, 1995). The following care delivery systems are built on the tenet of accountability to the clients who are the receivers of nursing care. As such, they provide systems or processes of care congruent with professional practice.

CASE STUDY 14-2

You are a primary nurse working as part of the interdisciplinary orthopedic team. You notice that an increasing number of diabetic clients are being admitted for elective total hip surgery. Because the length of stay is so short and your team has such a surgical focus in caring for clients, the clients' underlying chronic diseases have not been a focus on the unit. However, you are aware that the larger organization is beginning to evaluate how different populations of clients, such as diabetics, are cared for across the continuum of care.

What should you do to improve care for your clients?

PRIMARY NURSING

Primary nursing is a system of care that was founded in the 1960s, at a time when nurses were searching for more independence and autonomy in their practice. In a **primary nursing** model, one nurse is accountable for the care a client receives during a given episode of care. Primary nurses function through associate nurses during the hours when they are not present in the workplace. Communications occur through a written plan of care. The primary nurse assumes responsibility for the client's admission to the site of care, development of the care plan, major communications with other care providers, and overseeing the client's discharge to home or to another level of care. The hallmark of primary nursing is that one nurse maintains 24-hour accountability for a specific client's care. In this model, the role of the first-line unit manager is to manage the staff not the client care, ensure that systems work for the caregivers, and ensure that caregivers work for their clients.

The advantages of primary nursing include continuity of client care, as well as nurse and client satisfaction. Primary nursing is, however, an expensive system of care delivery because it requires a higher proportion of registered nurses. As such, in recent years, health care delivery systems have had difficulty continuing to support the model.

CLIENT-FOCUSED CARE

Client-focused care is a model of differentiated nursing practice that emphasizes quality, cost, and value (Reisdorfer, 1996). In this model, first-line unit managers assume an expanded role. They assume accountability to manage nurses and staff from other departments, such as staff from radiology, physical therapy, and so on. Their focus is more sophisticated and has expanded to include overseeing the coordination of all care activities required by clients and their support systems.

CASE MANAGEMENT

Nursing case management is another accountability-based care delivery system that evolved in the late 1980s and early 1990s in response to spiraling health care costs. The primary goal of **case management** is to deliver high-quality client care in the most cost-effective way by managing human and material resources. Other goals are to manage the delivery of care within a given time frame, to decrease length of stay for inpatient care, to ensure appropriate utilization of services and resources, to improve continuity of care, to standardize the care delivered for a given diagnosis, and to improve client outcomes from a given episode of care (Satinsky, 1995). Nursing case management has used critical paths, care mapping (Zander, 1995), and interdisciplinary care protocols to achieve its objectives. The indicators of care embedded in these tools are used to measure the outcomes of care delivery.

MEASURABLE QUALITY OUTCOMES

An important component of first-line unit management is regular evaluation of a unit's performance to ensure that the outcomes of care delivery are meeting the objectives of professional practice as outlined in the unit's annual operational plan. The development of process improvement measures in today's health care organizations is driven by the multiple domains of quality required by the Canadian Council on Health Services Accreditation (CCHSA).

UNIT-BASED PERFORMANCE IMPROVEMENT

To develop a comprehensive unit-based continuous quality improvement program to meet the requirements of today's health care system, the first-line unit manager should track outcomes from four domains: access, service, cost, and clinical quality (G. Vasile, Cooperstown, NY, Bassett Healthcare, personal communication, August 16, 2000). See Figure 14-5 for the performance improvement plan.

INPATIENT SURGICAL UNIT

2000 PERFORMANCE IMPROVEMENT PLAN

As part of Bassett's commitment to quality, the Surgical Unit will strive to improve performance through a cycle of planning, process design, performance measurement, assessment and improvement. There will be ongoing assessment of important aspects of care and service and correction of identified problems. Problem identification and solution will be carried out using a systematic intra- and interdepartmental approach organized around patient flow or other key functions, and in concert with the approved visions and strategies of the organization. Priorities for improvement will include high risk, high volume and problem-prone procedures.

The Surgical Unit will:

• promote the Plan-Do-Check-Act methodology for all performance improvement activities
• provide staff education and training on integrated quality and cost improvement
• collect data to support objective assessment of processes and contribute to problem resolution

In identifying important aspects of care and service, the Surgical Unit will select performance measures in the following operational categories:

A. Clinical Quality
1. Patient safety

• Patient falls
• Indicator: # of patient falls per month/# of patient days with upper control limits set by the research department based on statistical deviation

• Medication and IV errors
• Indicator: # of patient IV/medication errors per month/# of patient days with upper control limits set by the research department based on statistical deviation

• Restraint use
• Indicator: % of compliance with policy for use of restraints and overall rate of restraint use

2. Pressure ulcer prevention
• Indicator: Rates of occurrence-quarterly tracking report

3. Surveillance, prevention and control of infection
• Indicator: Infection control statistical report of wound and catheter associated infections
• Indicator: Quarterly monitoring of compliance with standards for Acid Fast Bacilli (AFB) room use; evidence of staff validation in AFB practice

4. Employee safety
• Injuries resulting from
• Back and lifting-related injuries
• Morbidly obese patients
• Orthopedic patients
• Indicators: # of injuries sustained by employees and any resultant workmen's compensation (Human Resources quarterly report)
• 100% competency validation in lifting techniques and back injury prevention
• Respiratory fit testing
• Indicator: competency record of each employee

5. Documentation by exception
Indicators:
• 100% validation of RN/LPN staff
• Monthly chart audit (10% average daily census or 20 charts) meeting compliance with established standards

B. Access:
• Maintenance of the 30 minute standard for bed assignment of ED admissions
• Indicator: Quarterly review of ED tracking record

C. Service:
Patient Satisfaction
Indicator: Patient Satisfaction Survey: 90% or above response to, "Would return", and "Would recommend"

D. Cost:
• Nursing staff productivity will remain at 110% of target of 8.5 worked hours per adjusted patient day within a maximum variance range of 10%

For each of the above performance measures, this performance improvement plan will:

• address the highest priority improvement issues
• require data collection according to the structure, procedure and frequency defined
• document a baseline for performance
• demonstrate internal comparisons trended over time
• demonstrate external benchmark comparisons trended over time
• document areas identified for improvement
• demonstrate that changes have been made to address improvement
• demonstrate evaluation of these changes; document that improvement has occurred or, if not, that a different approach has been taken to address the issue

The Inpatient Surgical Unit will submit biannual status reports to the Bassett Improvement Council (BIC) through the Medical Surgical Quality Improvement Council (MSQIC).
I

Approved by:_____**Date:**_____

(Chief or Vice President)

Figure 14-5 Performance Improvement Plan.

Outcomes of unit continuous quality improvement programs can be succinctly displayed using the Quality Compass (Nelson, Mohr, Batalden, & Plume, 1996). The Bassett Quality Compass in Figure 14-6 measures quality from four domains: functional status, clinical outcomes, cost and utilization, and client (patient) satisfaction. This Quality Compass depicts the outcomes of an organization-wide disease management asthma study prior to an asthma disease management intervention. The Quality Compass tells us that functionally 30 per cent of the population has moderately severe asthma and that the majority of asthmatics have little documented teaching in use of a peak flow metre or metred-dose inhalers (MDIs), which is the current standard of care. More than 30 per cent of the client visits for asthma are urgent visits, indicating that a large portion of the asthma population will benefit from the disease management intervention of increased client teaching and development of individual specific asthma care plans. The Quality Compass provides a framework to guide the development of a unit-based quality improvement program and

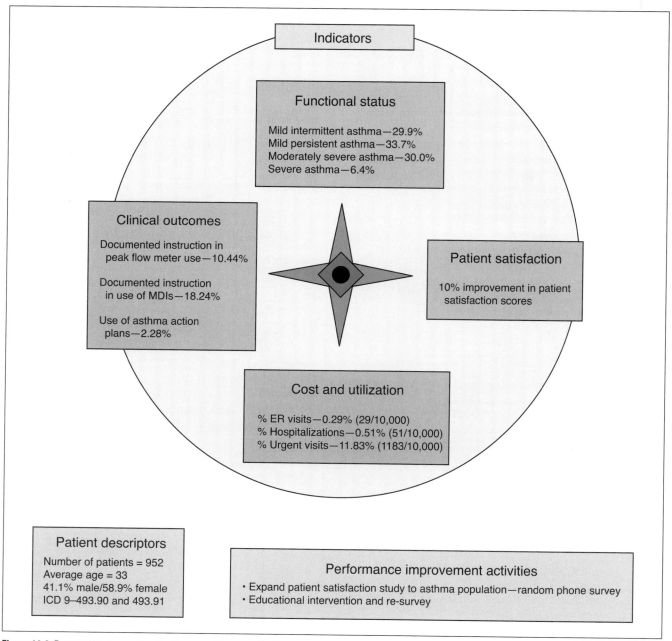

Figure 14-6 Bassett Healthcare Quality Compass. (Courtesy Kathleen F. Sellers, PhD, RN, Bassett Healthcare.)

provides a tool with which to present the outcomes of quality improvement in the succinct visual format of an executive summary.

The first-line unit manager is the fundamental operations person in the health care system. Successful orchestration of a client care unit in today's health care system is achieved through vision-driven professional practice. Implementing this vision is achieved through a unit governance structure of shared decision making, an accountability-based client care delivery system, and regular evaluation of performance based on the tenets of performance improvement.

KEY CONCEPTS

■ Successful orchestration of a client care unit in today's health care environment is achieved through vision-driven professional practice.

■ Strategic planning is a process designed to achieve goals in dynamic, competitive environments through the allocation of resources (Andrews, 1990).

■ Shared governance is an organizational framework grounded in a philosophy of decentralized leadership that fosters autonomous decision making and professional nursing practice.

■ A clinical or career promotional ladder provides a framework that facilitates professional staff development by building on the skill sets and experience of each practitioner.

■ Situational leadership maintains that there is no one best leadership style, but rather that effective leadership lies in matching the appropriate leadership style to the individual's or group's level of task-relevant readiness.

■ Individuals who are accountable are, by definition, able to report, explain, or justify their actions.

■ Accountability-based care delivery systems include primary nursing, client-focused care, and case management.

■ A comprehensive unit-based quality improvement program should include outcomes that are tracked from four domains: access, service, cost, and clinical quality.

KEY TERMS

case management
client-focused care
clinical ladder
goal
mission
objective

philosophy
primary nursing
shared governance
situational leadership
strategic planning

REVIEW QUESTIONS

1. Shared governance
   A. is an accountability-based care delivery system.
   B. is a tested framework of organizational development.
   C. is a competency-based career promotion system.
   D. implies the allocation of control, power, or authority (i.e., governance) among interested parties.

2. Which of the following is *not* one of the five levels of a clinical promotion ladder built on Benner's theoretical framework?
   A. proficient.
   B. competent.
   C. orientee.
   D. expert.

3. Case management, client-focused care, and _____ are accountability-based nursing care delivery systems.
   A. functional nursing
   B. team nursing
   C. primary nursing
   D. case finding

4. Which of the following areas is *not* considered when developing a unit-based Quality Compass?
   A. client satisfaction.
   B. cost.
   C. administrative satisfaction.
   D. clinical outcomes.

REVIEW ACTIVITIES

1. You have been asked by your first-line unit manager to participate in a performance improvement team looking at care of the diabetic client. What areas other than clinical quality will you evaluate? Identify indicators for each area to measure. What is it you are seeking to improve?

2. You have been practising now for three years. This summer you have been precepting a new graduate who is having difficulty mastering changing a sterile dressing. You need to give some feedback, but you are uncertain how to do this effectively and wonder whether you are part of the reason this new graduate is having difficulty. Review the section on situational leadership (pages 258–259). At what level of readiness is this new graduate? Has your leadership style been appropriate for that level of experience and motivation?

3. You have been practising as a new graduate for a little over a year. You are feeling more confident about your

clinical practice and think you might want to expand your leadership experience. Your unit governance framework is shared governance. Review the common councils of shared governance. Given your education and experience, which council would you like to join?

EXPLORING THE WEB

- You have been asked by your unit manager and members of the credentialing committee to revamp the current clinical promotion ladder so that it more clearly differentiates and rewards nurses for their education level and their expertise. Go to *http://www.uchsc.edu/ahec/cando/nursing/diffpractice97.htm*

- What does the University of Colorado's clinical ladder incorporate that yours does not?

- Go to the magnet hospitals site *(http://nursecredentialing.org/magnet/)* and see whether the information there would help your organization foster professional nursing practice. Striving for magnet hospital designation increases an organization's ability to recruit and retain nurses.

- Go to *http://www.nursingsociety.org*. This site provides weekly literature updates from Sigma Theta Tau International, the nursing profession's honour society. What new books and periodicals are available that may be helpful to you in your practice?

REFERENCES

Alspach, J. (1984). Designing a competency-based orientation for critical care nurses. *Heart and Lung, 13,* 655–662.

Andrews, M. (1990). Strategic planning: Preparing for the 21st century. *Journal of Professional Nursing, 6*(2), 103–112.

Benner, P. (1984). *From novice to expert.* Menlo Park, CA: Addison-Wesley.

Clifford, J., & Horvath, K. J. (1990). *Advancing professional nursing practice: Innovations at Boston's Beth Israel Hospital.* New York: Springer.

Covey, S. R. (1990). *The seven habits of highly effective people.* New York: Fireside.

Dreyfus, S. E., & Dreyfus, H. L. (1980). *A five stage model of the mental activities involved in directed skill acquisition.* Unpublished report supported by the Air Force Office of Scientific Research, USAF (Contract F49620-79-C-0063), University of California at Berkeley.

Hersey, R. E., & Blanchard, T. (1993). *Management of organizational behavior.* Edgewood Cliffs, NJ: Prentice-Hall.

Jones, L. B. (1996). *The path: Creating your mission statement for work and for life.* New York: Hyperion.

Ludemann, R. S., & Brown, C. (1989). Staff perceptions of shared governance. *Nursing Administration Quarterly, 13*(4), 49–56.

MacGregor-Burns, J. (1979). *Leadership.* New York: Harper & Row.

Nelson, E., Mohr, J. J., Batalden, P. B., & Plume, S. K. (1996, April). Improving health care, part 1: The clinical value compass, *Journal of Quality Improvement, 22*(4), 243–258.

Porter-O'Grady, T. (1992). *Implementing shared governance: Creating a professional organization.* St. Louis, MO: Mosby-Year Book.

Porter-O'Grady, T. (1995). *The leadership revolution in health care.* Gaithersburg, MD: Aspen.

Reisdorfer, J. T. (1996). Building a patient-focused care unit. *Nursing Management, 27*(10), 38, 40, 42, 44.

Roesch, P. (2000, October). Surgical unit practice. *Nursing Matters, 7*(3), 1. Bassett Healthcare, Cooperstown, NY.

Satinsky, M. A. (1995). *An executive guide to case management strategies.* Chicago: American Hospital.

Sellers, K. F. (1996). *The meaning of autonomous nursing practice to staff nurses in a shared governance organization: A hermeneutical analysis.* Unpublished doctoral dissertation, Adelphi University, Garden City, New York.

Stichler, J. F. (1992). A conceptual basis for shared governance. In N. D. Como & B. Pocta (Eds.), *Implementing shared governance: Creating a professional organization* (pp. 1–24). St. Louis, MO: Mosby.

Webster's encyclopedic unabridged dictionary of the English language (2nd ed.). (1996). New York: Random House.

Welsch, H., & LaVan, H. (1981). Inter-relationships between organizational commitment and job characteristics, job satisfaction, professional behavior, and organizational climate. *Human Relations, 24*(12), 1079–1089.

Wesorick, B., Shiparski, L., Troseth, M., & Wyngarden, K. (1997). *Partnership council field book: Strategies and tools for co-creating a healthy work place.* Grand Rapids, MI: Practice Field.

Westrope, R. A., Vaughn, L., Bott, M., & Taunton, R. L. (1995, December). Shared governance: From vision to reality. *Journal of Nursing Administration, 25*(12), 45–54.

Yoder-Wise, P. S. (1999). *Leading and managing in nursing* (2nd ed.). St. Louis, MO: Mosby.

Zander, K. (1995). *Managing outcomes through collaborative care: The application of care mapping and case management.* Chicago: American Hospital.

SUGGESTED READINGS

Aiken, L. H., Havens, D. S., & Sloane, D. M. (2000, March). The magnet nursing services recognition program. *American Journal of Nursing, 100*(3), 26–35.

Bell, C. (1996). *Managers as mentors.* San Francisco: Berrett-Koehler.

Bridges, W. (2000). *Managing transitions: Making the most of change.* New York: Perseus Books Group.

Hirsh, S. K., & Kummerow, J. M. (1990). *Introduction to type in organizations.* Palo Alto, CA: Consulting Psychologists Press.

Kaplan, R. S., & Norton, D. P. (2001). *The strategy focused organization.* Boston, MA: Harvard Business School.

Loverage, C., & Cummings, S. H. (1996). *Nursing management in the new paradigm.* Gaithersburg, MD: Aspen.

Manion, J. (1996). *Team based health care organizations.* Gaithersburg, MD: Aspen.

McClure, M. L., Poulin, M. A., Sovie, M. D., & Wandelt, M. A. (1983). *Magnet hospitals.* Kansas City, MO: American Nurses Publishing.

Myers, I. B. (1993). *Introduction to type.* Palo Alto, CA: Consulting Psychologists Press.

Sellers, K. F., Hargrove, B., & Jenkins, P. (2000). Asthma disease management programs improve clinical and economic outcomes. *MEDSURG Nursing, 9*(4), 201–203, 207.

Senge, P. (1990). *The fifth discipline.* New York: Doubleday.

Senge, P. (1994). *The fifth discipline fieldbook* (p. 49). New York: Doubleday.

Silvetti, C., Rudan, V., Frederickson, K., and Sulivan, B. (2000, April). Where will tomorrow's nurse managers come from? *Journal of Nursing Administration, 30*(4) 157–159.

Wesorick, B. (1998). *The way of respect in the workplace* (p. 15). Grand Rapids, MI: Practice Field.

Zemke, R., Raines, C., & Filipczak, B. (2000). *Generations at work: Managing the clash of veterans, boomers, xers and nexters in your workplace.* New York: AMACOM.

CHAPTER 15

Change and Conflict Resolution

Margaret M. Anderson, EdD, RN-C, CNAA
Adapted by: Heather Crawford, BScN, MEd, CHE

Quantum theory has taught us that change is not a thing or an event but rather a dynamic that is constitutive of the universe. People cannot avoid change, since it is everywhere, but they can influence its circumstances and consequences. In short, they can give it direction.
(Porter-O'Grady & Malloch 2003)

OBJECTIVES

Upon completion of this chapter, the reader should be able to:

1. Define change from personal, professional, and organizational perspectives.
2. Identify the change theorists.
3. Discuss the concept of the learning organization.
4. Identify driving and restraining forces of change within a structured setting context.
5. Discuss change strategies.
6. Discuss the role and characteristics of a change agent in the change process.
7. Utilize the change process to plan, implement, and evaluate a change project.
8. Identify conflict situations.
9. Identify steps in the conflict resolution process.

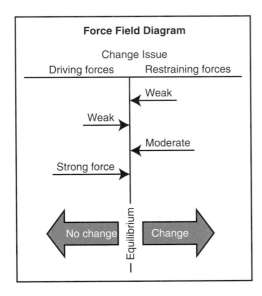

Force Field Diagram

Change Issue

Driving forces | Restraining forces

Weak

Weak

Moderate

Strong force

Equilibrium

No change | Change

JoAnne has been a nurse manager for five years. During that time, she has had no fewer than five directors. In addition, she has had two different medical directors for her unit, two different methods of care delivery, and the amalgamation of two nursing units, resulting in a change of culture and mission. JoAnne has just started her master of science in nursing (MScN) degree, and wonders whether she can make it through another change. She shuts her desk drawer, looks in the mirror, and says to her reflection, "You can do it. You know you love a challenge. The only thing that is constant is change, and this will give you an opportunity to apply your education to the current exciting change initiatives!" JoAnne immediately straightened her shoulders, put her head up, and walked out of her office. She smiled at her staff and said, "Hello."

What do you think JoAnne is feeling?

How should JoAnne go about introducing yet another change to her staff?

In health care, is change inevitable, pervasive, and exciting?

This chapter is designed to introduce the concepts of change and conflict resolution. Change is an inevitable and frequent occurrence in health care and in life. Technology, biomedical discoveries, and advances in disease treatment and medications cause revolutions in the treatment and course of illness. These advances also make changes in wellness and health promotion rapid and sweeping. Along with change, conflict is also inevitable. The resolution of that conflict is necessary for the good of the client and the organization. Although conflict in itself is not a bad thing, unresolved conflict can thwart the efforts of the best-intentioned change agent and cause stagnation and tension in a work team.

This chapter will help to alleviate the anxiety surrounding change and conflict as well as teach the importance of embracing change and confronting conflict.

Change is frightening only when you are not a part of it or you have no input into it. The staff nurse has a responsibility to provide input, even if it is not invited, and to become involved in the planning and implementation of change. Equally important is the evaluation of change. Evaluating honestly and making necessary modifications are as important to the success of a change project as the planning and orderly implementation. If nothing else is learned, learn to embrace change as an opportunity to improve client care and to advance the profession of nursing. Look at conflict resolution as an opportunity to learn something new or as the opportunity to persuade others.

CHANGE

There are many definitions of change, and there are many types of change. For simplicity, **change** can be defined as "the act, process, or result of altering or modifying" (*Nelson Canadian Dictionary*, 1997, p. 233). The outcome may be the same, but the actions performed to reach the outcome may be different. For instance, because of road closures, how you get to work may be different. The goal of getting to work remains the same, but the method may be different, perhaps by driving a different route or by taking the bus rather than driving. In the professional nursing setting, new client admission forms may require a different method of assessing the client or may change the number of people involved in the admission process. Rather than one registered nurse conducting the entire admission process, the process may be broken down so that individuals with different skill levels conduct different parts of the process. The goal is still the admission of the client to a unit; how it is done may be different. Most change is implemented for a good or reasonable purpose. Most organizational change is planned. The change is intentional and goal-oriented, with activities that are proactive and purposeful (Robbins & Langton, 2002). If employees do not understand the reason behind change, they should ask.

For purposes of discussion, **personal change** is a change made voluntarily for one's own reasons, usually for self-improvement. Personal change may include altering your diet for health reasons, taking classes for self-improvement, or removing yourself from a destructive or unhealthful environment or situation. **Professional change** may be a change in position or job, such as obtaining education or credentials that will benefit your current position or allow you to be prepared for a future position. Professional change is often planned and can involve extensive change in both your personal and professional lives. Although either personal or professional change may be stressful, if it is voluntary and carries intrinsic or extrinsic rewards, it is often considered important and worth the stress.

Organizational change is the type of change that often causes the most stress or concern. **Organizational**

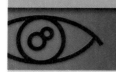

CRITICAL THINKING

Think about a time you were determined to make a personal change in your life. What emotions did you experience? Did you have support for this change? Did you set a realistic goal for yourself?

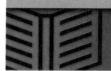

LITERATURE APPLICATION

Citation: Ingersoll, G. L., Kirsch, J. C., Merk, S. E., & Lightfoot, J. (2000). Relationship of organizational culture and readiness for change to employee commitment to the organization. *Journal of Nursing Administration, 30*(1), 11–20.

Discussion: This research article discusses the relationship of organizational culture and readiness for change to employee commitment to the organization. The authors found that employee readiness for change often lagged behind the need for change within the organization.

Implications for Practice: Both employers and employees should recognize that change is inevitable. In these times of rapid health care change, employee readiness and commitment are important, but they cannot be the deciding factor in whether to change. The employer must change to keep up with the economic climate. The employee has a responsibility to change as necessary to help the employer maintain fiscal health.

Unfortunately, when organizational change is planned, the employees who are often the last to know about the anticipated change are frequently the ones most affected by it. The staff nurse who is expected to implement the new care delivery system may be the last one to know about the change until it is to be implemented. For example, in an organization in which primary nursing has been the care delivery system for several years, the implementation of modified team nursing is a major change in philosophy and thinking. If proper care and planning of the change process is not used, the staff will resist the change and make the implementation much more stressful than necessary.

change can be defined as "an alteration of an organization's environment, structure, technology or people" (Robbins, DeCenzo, & Stuart-Kotze, 2002, p. 183). Sometimes a lot of preparation and prior discussion precedes organizational change. Sometimes it is a surprise to the employees and causes a great deal of consternation and stress. Organizational change can affect five different aspects of an organization: its culture, structure, technology, physical setting, and human resources. Changing an organization's culture may be one of the most difficult changes because the underlying values and goals of the organization need to change. Changing structure involves altering authority relations, job redesign, or similar structure variables. Changing technology includes modification in the way work is processed, or in the methods and equipment used. Changing the physical setting involves altering the space and layout arrangements. Changing human resources refers to changes in employee skills, expectations, or behaviour (Robbins & Langton, 2002, p. 187).

TRADITIONAL CHANGE THEORIES

The change theories discussed here are Lewin's Force-Field Model (1951), Lippitt's Phases of Change (1958), Havelock's Six-Step Change Model (1973), and Rogers' Diffusion of Innovations Theory (1983). These are classic change theories and are based on Lewin's original model.

Lewin's model has three simple steps. The steps are unfreezing, movement, and refreezing. Unfreezing refers to a thawing of the current or old way of doing things. Individuals begin to be aware of the need for doing things differently, that change is needed for a specific reason. In the next step, the intervention or change is introduced and explained. The benefits and disadvantages are discussed, and the change—the move to a new level—is implemented. In the third step, refreezing occurs, meaning that the new way of doing is incorporated into the routines or habits of the affected people. Although these steps sound simple, the process of change is, of course, more complicated (Flower & Guillaume, 2002).

Lippitt's Phases of Change are built on Lewin's model. Lippitt defined seven stages in the change process: (1) diagnosis of the problem, (2) assessment of the motivation and capacity for change, (3) assessment of the change agent's motivation and resources, (4) the selection of progressive change objectives, (5) choosing an appropriate role for the change agent, (6) maintenance of the change once it has been started, and (7) termination of the helping relationship. Lippitt emphasized the participation of key personnel and the change agent in designing and planning the intended change project.

Lippitt also emphasized communication during all phases of the process (Sullivan & Decker, 2001).

Havelock designed a six-step model of the change process. This model is based on Lewin's model, but Havelock included more steps in each stage. The planning stage includes (1) building a relationship, (2) diagnosing the problem, and (3) acquiring resources. This planning stage is followed by the moving stage, which includes (4) choosing the solution and (5) gaining acceptance. The last stage, the refreezing stage, includes (6) stabilization and self-renewal. Havelock emphasized the planning stage. He believed that resistance to change can be overcome with careful planning and inclusion of the affected staff. Havelock also believed that the change agent, the person responsible for planning and implementing the change, should encourage participation of the affected employees. The more the people affected by the change participate in the change, the more they are likely to make the change successful and to support the necessity for the change (Sullivan & Decker, 2001; Tappen, Weiss, & Whitehead, 2004).

In 1983, Rogers published his Diffusion of Innovations Theory. Although based on Lewin's model, this theory is much broader in scope and approach. He developed a five-step innovation/decision-making process. Rogers believed that change can be rejected initially and then adopted at a later time. He believed that change is a reversible process and that initial rejection does not necessarily mean the change will never be adopted. This theory also works in reverse—the change may initially be adopted and then rejected at a later time. Rogers' approach emphasized the capriciousness of change. In his theory, timing and format take on new meaning and importance—as the time involved in change implementation grows longer, the more the change process takes on a life of its own and the original change and reasons for it may be lost. The change process must be carefully managed and planned to ensure that it survives mostly intact. Table 15-1 is a comparison chart of these change models.

The theories described in Table 15-1 are linear in nature, meaning they more or less proceed in an orderly

TABLE 15-1 — **COMPARISON CHART OF CHANGE THEORIES AND THEIR USES**

Theorist and Year	Lewin (1951)	Lippitt (1958)	Havelock (1973)	Rogers (1983)
Title of Model	Force-Field Model	Phases of Change	Six-Step Change Model	Diffusion of Innovations Theory
Steps in Model (The steps in the models are spaced to indicate their correlation to Lewin's model.)	1. Unfreeze 2. Move 3. Refreeze	1. Diagnose problem 2. Assess motivation and capacity for change 3. Assess change agent's motivation and resources 4. Select progressive change objective 5. Choose appropriate role of change agent 6. Maintain change 7. Terminate helping relationship	1. Build relationship 2. Diagnose problem 3. Acquire resources 4. Choose solution 5. Gain acceptance 6. Stabilization and self-renewal	1. Awareness 2. Interest 3. Evaluation 4. Trial 5. Adoption

Source: Adapted from *Introductory Management and Leadership for Nurses* (2nd ed., p. 327) by R. C. Swansburg and R. J. Swansburg (1998), Boston: Jones & Bartlett Publishers.

manner from one step to the next. This linearity and the fact that they are all based on Lewin's theory make them similar in complexity and in use. These theories work well for low-level, uncomplicated change. They do not work well in highly complex and nonlinear situations. Health care organizations are very complex and require more sophisticated theories of change.

EMERGING THEORIES OF CHANGE

Much more complex in breadth and depth than the theories previously discussed are two often-used and emerging theories of change: the chaos theory and the learning organization theory. According to Wagner and Huber (2003), "organizations can no longer rely on rules, policies, and hierarchies, or afford to be inflexible; and small changes in the initial conditions of a system can drastically affect the long-term behaviour of that system." Chaos theory hypothesizes that chaos actually has an order. That is, although the potential for chaos appears, at first glance, to be random, further investigation reveals some order to the chaos.

Health care organizations have experienced chaos in the past 10 to 15 years, which, according to chaos theory, is normal. Most organizations go through periods of rapid change and innovation and then stabilize before chaos erupts again. Even though each chaotic occurrence is similar to the one that occurred before, each is different. The political, scientific, and behavioural components of the organization are different from before, so the chaos looks different. Order emerges through fluctuation and chaos. Thus, the potential for chaos means that the organization must be able to organize and implement change quickly and forcefully. Little time is available for orderly linear change. Leaders in these organizations are expected to act quickly and be flexible to meet the challenge of the potentially chaotic forces. Organizations today are required to deal with highly unstable environmental conditions, and are compelled to change in a manner that allows for constant fluidity and continuous renewal (Ayers, 2002).

Peter Senge (2006) first described learning organization theory. Learning organizations demonstrate responsiveness and flexibility. Senge believed that because organizations are open systems, they can best respond to unpredictable changes in the environment by using a learning approach in their interactions and interdisciplinary workings with one another. The whole cannot function well without a part regardless of how small that part may seem. For example, a well-equipped stove cannot work without a source of either electricity or gas. It does not matter how new, innovative, or energy efficient the stove is, it cannot function without an energy source. An example in health care is that the laboratory department cannot complete an accurate test and assessment without the cooperation of the physician, nurse, nurse assistant, or unit clerk. If the physician does not order the appropriate test, and the nurse does not adequately prepare the client for the test, then the laboratory cannot prepare an accurate report. Without the proper requisition, the laboratory cannot perform the appropriate test on the specimen. The learning organization understands these interrelationships and responds quickly to improve relationships. This response may be through dialogue or team problem solving, but all parties must understand what is at stake for cooperation to occur.

Senge developed five disciplines that he believed are necessary for organizations to achieve the "learning organization status" to deal effectively with chaos: systems thinking, personal mastery, mental models, building shared vision, and team learning. Senge defined a discipline as "a body of theory and technique that must be studied and mastered to be put into practice"(Senge, 2006, p. 10). In the learning organization, each individual has something to offer that melds with what others have to offer to determine the right steps to take in sorting out the causes of chaos and responding positively to it. The goals of the organization and individual are mutually related so that quick response to chaos occurs, with positive results for both the organization and the individual. The key to development of Senge's five disciplines is two-way communication or open discussion, dialogue, and being a lifelong learner (Senge, 2006). Most experts agree that few, if any, health care organizations have evolved to the learning organization status. Although this is a goal to work toward, health care itself has not evolved to the point of quick reaction to chaos and a rapidly changing environment.

THE CHANGE PROCESS

Planned change in the work organization is not much different from planned change on a personal level. The major difference is that more people are involved, the scale is larger, and more opinions must be considered. There are three basic reasons to introduce a change: (1) to solve a problem, (2) to improve efficiency, or (3) to reduce unnecessary workload for some group (Marquis & Huston, 2006). To plan change, one must know what has to be changed. Change for the sake of change is unnecessary and stressful (Bennis, Benne, & Chin, 1969).

STEPS IN THE CHANGE PROCESS

The change process can be related to the nursing process. Using the nursing process as a model, the first step in the change process is assessment.

ASSESSMENT   In assessment, one identifies the problem or the opportunity for improvement through change, by collecting and analyzing data. The data collection and analysis should be from several perspectives: structural, technological, and people.

A structural perspective is one of physical space or the configuration of physical space. For instance, a medical-surgical unit in a hospital may plan to move to the space vacated by the obstetrics unit. The space is large enough but is not configured to be conducive to the care of medical-surgical clients. Assessment of the structural components may include examination of the location of elevators, supply stations, client charts, telephones, call lights, and other physical or structural components. Structural components often mandate how the work is done or the process of doing the work. Poor structural configuration may require the work team to perform extra steps to accomplish its goals.

A technological perspective may address a lack of wall outlets for necessary equipment, poorly situated computer locations, and lack of computer system interface ability. Sometimes, technology lags behind the goals of a work team and therefore slows down the team. The team spends more time troubleshooting technology than in providing care.

A perspective on people may bring to light personnel with inadequate training to accomplish the goals, an unwillingness to meet the goals, a lack of commitment to the organization, or a lack of understanding for the need for change.

Assessment data are collected from internal and external sources. Lewin identified forces that were supportive of change as well as forces that were barriers to change. He called these driving and restraining forces. If the restraining forces outweigh the driving forces, then the change must be abandoned because it cannot succeed. Driving and restraining forces include political issues, technology issues, cost and structural issues, and people issues. The political issues include the power groups in favour of or in opposition to the proposed change, and may include physicians, administrators, civic and community groups, or provincial and federal restrictions. The technology issues include whether to update old equipment, computer systems, or methods for accounting for supply use. Cost and structural issues include the costs, desirability, and feasibility of remodelling or building new construction for the change project. People issues include the commitment of the staff, their level of education and training, and their interest in the project. The most common people issue is fear of job loss or fear of not being valued. It bears repeating that if the restraining forces outweigh the driving forces, the change will not succeed, and it should be abandoned or rethought.

During data analysis, potential solutions may be identified, sources of resistance may come to light, determination of strategies may become apparent, and some areas of consensus may become evident. Statistical analysis is an important component of analysis, which should be conducted whenever possible to provide persuasive information in favour of the change, especially when the issue is either meeting the cost objectives or the mission objectives. The goal of data analysis is to support the need to change and to offer data to support the potential solution selected. The people who are potentially most affected by the change need to be involved in the assessment, data collection, and data analysis. They have a vested interest in the change and must not only support the change but also be willing to implement change (Bennis, Benne, & Chin, 1969).

PLANNING The next step is to plan. This step determines who will be affected by the change and when change will occur. All the potential solutions are examined. The driving and resisting forces are again examined and strategies determined for implementing the change. The target date for implementation and the outcomes or goals are clearly delineated and stated in measurable terms. Again, the most successful plan for change is one in which the individuals who will be most affected are involved, satisfied, and committed.

The plan should also address how the change will be implemented, although it may require modification as the implementation begins. For instance, how many work groups or units will implement the change at once? Will the change implementation be staggered from month to month or week to week? Will the supports that are necessary to manage the change be implemented first? Just how will this change be implemented? Finally, the overall plan includes strategies for evaluation. It is crucial that evaluation be built in. Expected outcomes must be identified in measurable terms, and the plan to evaluate those outcomes and a timetable for evaluation must be evident. Unevaluated change will not succeed.

IMPLEMENTATION OF CHANGE STRATEGIES
Bennis, Benne, and Chin (1969) identified three strategies to promote change in groups or organizations: the power-coercive strategy, the normative-reeducative strategy, and the rational-empirical strategy. Different strategies work in different situations. The power or authority of the change agent influences the strategy selected. Most change agents use a variety of strategies to promote successful change.

The power-coercive strategy is very simple—"do it or get out." This strategy is based on the application of power by a legitimate authority, economic sanctions, or the political clout of the change agent (Marquis & Huston, 2006). Little effort is required to encourage participation of employees, and little concern surrounds their acceptance or resistance to the proposed change. An example of this strategy would include implementation of the Canadian government's privacy legislation across the nation. This group of strategies is generally reserved for situations in which resistance is expected but not important to the power group.

The second group-change strategy is normative-reeducative. This strategy is based on the assumption that group norms are used to socialize individuals. This strategy focuses on using the individual's need for satisfying social relationships in the workplace. Very few individuals can withstand social isolation or rejection by the work group. Compliance and support for a change are garnered by focusing on the perceived loss of social relationships in the workplace. Although some resistance to change may be expected, this strategy assumes people are interested in preserving relationships and will go along with the majority. The change agent does not necessarily require a legitimate power base, but gains power by skill in interpersonal relationships (Marquis & Huston, 2006).

The third group of strategies is rational-empirical. This group assumes that humans are rational people and will use knowledge to embrace change. It is assumed that once the self-interests of a group are evident, the group will see the merit in a change and embrace it. Knowledge and training are the components used to encourage compliance with change. This strategy is very successful when little resistance is anticipated. Table 15-2 summarizes the three strategies for change.

EVALUATION OF CHANGE   In the evaluation step, the effectiveness of the change is evaluated according to the outcomes identified during the planning phase. Evaluation is the most overlooked component, although it is considered by some experts to be the most important aspect of change. Usually, not enough time is allowed for the change to become effective or stable, which is a grave error. The time intervals for evaluation should be identified and allowed to elapse before modifications are made and declarations of failure are asserted. A certain period of confusion and turmoil accompanies all changes, whether large or small. If the outcomes are achieved, then the change was a success. If not, then some revision or modification may be necessary to achieve the outcomes that were anticipated.

STABILIZATION OF CHANGE   After effectiveness has been determined, then stabilization of the change is complete. The project is no longer a pilot or experiment but is a part of the culture and function of the organization. Although there is no magical time frame for stabilization to occur, it should be encouraged as soon as possible to make the change project complete. Often, reevaluation is planned after the first six months or year of implementation to ensure that stabilization of the change has occurred.

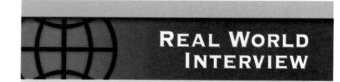

REAL WORLD INTERVIEW

One of the things I have learned about change is to include everyone affected by the change in the plan from the beginning. Everyone is encouraged to voice an opinion regarding the change and the change process. It is understood that if their ideas are not realistic, the rationale would be explained and not ignored. This encourages everyone to be committed to the process.

Sheila Joseph, BScN
Unit Manager

TABLE 15-2	STRATEGIES FOR CHANGE
Strategy	**Description**
Power-coercive approach	Uses authority and the threat of job loss to gain compliance with change.
Normative-reeducative approach	Uses social orientation and the need to have satisfactory relationships in the workplace as a method of inducing support for change. Focuses on the relationship needs of workers.
Rational-empirical approach	Uses knowledge as a power base. Once workers understand the organizational need for change or understand the meaning of the change to them as individuals and the organization as a whole, they will change.

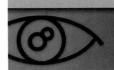

CRITICAL THINKING

Consider one of the changes you have experienced in a personal or work setting. Was there any plan for evaluation of the change? Was any thought given to making some modification in the change when it was obvious the change could not be implemented as designed? What could have been done differently?

RESPONSES TO CHANGE

People do respond to change. The most typical response to change is resistance. Humans like order and familiarity; they enjoy routine and the status quo. The more the relationships or social mores are challenged to change, the more resistance there is to change. Marquis and Huston (2006) point out that nurses are more likely to accept a change in an intravenous pump rather than a change in who can administer the intravenous fluid. This finding suggests that the social mores of a group are more important than technology in a change. The social mores dictate the roles and responsibilities of groups of workers, such as registered nurses, licensed practical nurses, unregulated care providers, and so on. Registered nurses are often less concerned with technology and more concerned with maintaining traditional roles and responsibilities.

Several factors affect resistance to change. The first is trust. The employee and employer must trust that each is doing the right thing and that each is capable of producing successful change. In addition to capability, predictability is important. The employee wants a predictable work environment and security. When change is introduced, then that predictable environment—and, therefore, the employee's comfort zone—begins to come into question (Lapp, 2002). Another factor is the individual's ability to cope with change. Silber (1993) points out four factors that affect an individual's ability to cope with change:

1. Flexibility for change, that is, the ability to adapt to change
2. Evaluation of the immediate situation, that is, if the current situation is unacceptable, then change will be more welcome
3. Anticipated consequences of change, that is, the impact change will have on one's current job
4. Individual's stake or what the individual has to win or lose as an effect of the change, that is, the more individuals perceive they have to lose, the more resistance they will offer.

Change is a scary prospect for those who have not had much experience with change or who have had only negative experiences with change. It is important to help people remember that change is inevitable and ever present. Developing an attitude of embracing and accepting change is desirable.

Bushy (1993) has identified six behavioural responses to planned change. These behavioural responses are usually apparent in every health care facility and every nursing unit:

1. Innovators: Change embracers. Enjoy the challenge of change and often lead change.
2. Early adopters: Open and receptive to change but not obsessed with it.
3. Early majority: Enjoy and prefer the status quo but do not want to be left behind. They adopt change before the average person.
4. Late majority: Often known as the followers. They adopt change after expressing negative feelings and are often skeptics.
5. Laggards: Last group to adopt a change. They prefer tradition and stability to innovation. They are suspicious of change.
6. Rejectors: Openly oppose and reject change. May be surreptitious or covert in their opposition. They may hinder the change process to the point of sabotage.

Other responses to change have been identified, including grief, denial, anger, depression, and bargaining (Marquis & Huston, 2006). Regardless of the importance and necessity of change, the human response is very important and cannot be dismissed. So often, in one's zeal to respond to a need, the change agent forgets that the human side of change must be dealt with. People have a right to their feelings and a right to express them. The important point is the change agent helps people respond and then move on to the goal of implementing the change. Gently but firmly, people must be guided toward acceptance.

THE CHANGE AGENT

Throughout this discussion of change, the term **change agent** has been used instead of manager, leader, or administrator. The change agent is the person responsible for implementation of a change project. This person may be from within or outside an organization, and is often a leader or manager because leaders and managers are usually innovators and therefore are likely to enjoy change. A change agent is ultimately responsible for the success of the change project, large or small. The role of the change agent is to manage the dynamics of the change process, which requires knowledge of the organization, knowledge of the change process, knowledge of the participants in the change process, and understanding of the feelings of the group undergoing change.

TABLE 15-3 ROLES AND CHARACTERISTICS OF THE CHANGE AGENT

- Lead the change process by example
- Manage process and group dynamics and show others how to adapt to change
- Demonstrate that the change is critical and inspire response from others
- Understand feelings of the group experiencing the change; engage them in the process
- Maintain momentum and enthusiasm

- Maintain vision of change
- Communicate change, progress, and feelings
- Knowledgeable about the organization
- Honest and direct
- Respected
- Intuitive

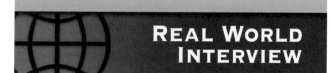

REAL WORLD INTERVIEW

I have always enjoyed trying new things and developing to my potential. However, I have no patience for a manager who is not truthful. Once she pretends to have the answers, and makes up her plan as she goes, I lose all respect, and trust is destroyed. It's okay to say, "I don't know," *but* you need to find the answer, and report back to me. Don't lie to me.

Margaret Mary Chester, RN
Staff Nurse

Probably the most important role of the change agent is to maintain communication, momentum, and enthusiasm for the project while still managing the process. Table 15-3 summarizes the roles and characteristics of the change agent.

The recipients of change must trust the change agent's interpersonal skills to provide information and manage change but also the agent's personal integrity and honour as an honest, principled individual. The executives in the organization must trust that the change agent will accomplish the established goals, given the proper support. The change agent also needs to recognize that those developing the project have some definite inclusion concepts that must be folded into the vision for success. Inclusion concepts are those ideas or concepts that the affected parties believe are absolutely necessary for their peace of mind or moral value. When these concepts are included, people feel ownership and value— a piece of them or their idea is in the plan.

Finally, the change agent must use some intuition during the evaluation steps to be able to bow out of the change, and to allow those affected to accept ownership. This decision is a matter of timing and insight into when the staff is ready to accept and incorporate the change as its own. Bennis (1989) warns that not stepping away from the project and cutting the ownership bonds means that it is the change agent's project for many years to come, even after that person leaves the organization. During evaluation, the change agent must support modifications and revisions that help transfer project ownership.

CHANGE AGENT STRATEGIES

Following are some strategies the change agent can use in managing the process:

1. Begin by articulating the vision clearly and concisely. Use the same words over and over. Constantly remind people of the goals and vision.
2. Map out a tentative timeline and sketch out the steps of the project. Have a good idea of how the project should go.
3. Plant seeds or mention some ideas or thoughts to key individuals from the first step through the evaluation step so that an idea of what is expected is under consideration.
4. Select the change project team carefully. Make sure it is heavily loaded with those who will be affected and other experts as needed. Select a variety of people. For example, an innovator, someone from the late majority group, a laggard, and a rejector are probably good to include. These people provide insight into what others are thinking.
5. Set up consistent meeting dates and keep them. Have an agenda and constantly check the timeline for target activities.
6. For those not on the team but affected by the project, give constant and consistent updates on

progress. If the change agent does not update staff, someone on the project team will, and the change agent wants to control the messages.

7. Give regular updates and progress reports both verbally and in writing to the executives of the organization and those affected by the change.

8. Check out rumours and confront any conflict head on. Do not look for conflict, but do not back away from it or ignore it.

9. Maintain a positive attitude and do not get discouraged.

10. Stay alert to political forces both for and against the project. Reach consensus on important issues as the project goes along, especially if policy, money, or philosophy issues are involved. Obtain consensus quickly on major issues or potential barriers to the project from both executives and staff.

11. Know the internal formal and informal leaders. Create a relationship with them. Consult them often.

12. Having self-confidence and trust in oneself and one's team will overcome a lot of obstacles. (Lancaster, 1999).

Leaders/managers must act as role models during the change process. It is important that change is presented in a positive light, particularly because change frightens most people. Remember the phrase "fear of the unknown." Does it apply to change? One can never over-communicate when it comes to change, particularly to those affected by the change. The only thing really constant about change is change itself! Porter-O'Grady and Malloch (2003) suggest that "change is . . . a never-ending journey" (p. 12). Every point of arrival is also a point of departure. As a result, leaders must carefully balance periods of effort and action with periods of rest and celebration so that the stakeholders will be regularly refreshed and reenergized to meet future challenges."

CONFLICT

An important part of the change process is the ability to resolve conflict. Conflict resolution skills are leadership and management tools that all registered nurses should have in their repertoire. Conflict itself is not bad. Conflict is healthy. Like change, conflict allows for creativity, innovation, new ideas, and new ways of doing things. It allows for the healthy discussion of different views and values and adds an important dimension to the provision of quality client care. Conflict can occur in almost any situation about almost anything. Conflict can arise over a matter as trivial as the size of an earring allowed in the dress code or as serious as who has the final authority on client care policy. Without some conflict, groups or work teams tend to become stagnant and routinized. Nothing new is

allowed to penetrate the "way we have always done it" mentality. The change agent and the nurse manager quickly become targets if they introduce new ideas or new systems of operating.

There are a variety of definitions of conflict. Conflict can be defined as two or more parties holding differing views about a situation (Tappen, 2001); or as the dynamic content of diversity, with human conflict as the diversity being worked out in the human community (Porter-O'Grady & Malloch, 2003). As can be surmised from these definitions, **conflict** can be defined as a disagreement about something of importance to each person involved. Not all disagreements become conflicts, but all disagreements have the potential for becoming a conflict, and all conflicts involve some level of disagreement. The astute manager can determine which disagreements might become conflicts and which ones will not. This discussion of conflict resolution does not include professional communication skills, which are discussed in Chapter 6.

SOURCES OF CONFLICT

Whenever there is an opportunity for disagreement, there is a potential source of conflict. The common sources of conflict in the professional setting include disputes over resource allocation or availability, personality differences, differences in values, threats from inside or outside an organization, cultural differences, and competition. In recent years, organizational, professional, and unit goals have served as major sources of conflict. Nurses frequently see financial goals and client care goals as being in direct conflict. In many organizations, this issue is the most frequently mentioned source of emotionally charged conflict (Sullivan & Decker, 2001).

Sources of conflict in personal arenas include differences in values, threats to security or well-being, financial problems, and cultural problems. Family relationships are often sources of conflict because of the complexity of these relationships.

TYPES OF CONFLICT

There are three broad types of conflict: intrapersonal, interpersonal, and organizational. Intrapersonal conflict occurs within the individual. For example, if Marilyn is not granted her requested day off, she may have an internal conflict about whether to call in sick or to take the day off without pay or to go to work. Or Marilyn may have conflict about priorities: should she attend her daughter's softball game or write her paper for school?

An interpersonal conflict occurs between two people or between groups or work teams. A disagreement may arise in philosophy or values, or policy or procedure. It may be a personality conflict; for example, two people just irritate each other. This type of conflict is not unusual in work situations. People new to a team may have ideas that are not totally acceptable to the team members

TABLE 15-4	SOURCES OF CONFLICT

Environmental Sources	Individual Sources
Cultural	Ego
Nationality	Personality
Religion	Identity
Class	Intimate relationships
Economics	Beliefs
Politics	Perceptions
Society	Perspectives
Resources	Education
Race	Position and role

Source: Porter-O'Grady & Malloch. (2003). *Quantum Leadership: A Textbook of New Leadership.* Mississauga: Jones and Bartlett Publishers Canada. p. 81.

already in place. Individuals who transfer from one unit to another often create a certain amount of conflict over processes and procedures. For example, the nurse transferring from the intensive care unit (ICU) to the coronary care unit (CCU) may be comfortable with one way of making assignments and then try to encourage the new peers to adopt that methodology without sharing the rationale for why the new way is better.

Organizational conflict can be a healthy way of introducing new ideas and encouraging creativity. Competition for resources, organizational cultural differences, and other sources of conflict help organizations identify areas for improvement. Conflict helps organizations identify legitimate differences among departments or work teams based on corporate need or responsibility. When organizational conflict is highlighted, corporate values and differences are aired and resolved.

THE CONFLICT PROCESS

Before attempting to intervene in a conflict situation, the conflict's five stages should be accurately assessed. The five stages are "latent conflict, which implies the existence of antecedent conditions; perceived conflict, which often involves issues and roles; felt conflict, which occurs when the conflict is emotionalized; manifest or overt conflict, when action is taken; and conflict aftermath" (Marquis & Huston, 2006). Conflict always has consequences, whether they are positive or negative. If the conflict is managed effectively, the people involved will believe their issues have been heard, and the situation

was dealt with appropriately. If the conflict was handled poorly, the conflict issues are unresolved and are almost guaranteed to resurface at a later date and will cause further conflict (Marquis & Huston, 2006).

CONFLICT RESOLUTION

The ideal goal when attempting to resolve conflict is to create a win-win solution. Such a solution is not always possible, but the manager is responsible for controlling the conflict so that individual differences are minimized. There are essentially seven methods of conflict resolution that dictate the outcomes of the conflict process.

Although some methods are more desirable or produce more successful outcomes than others, all the methods have a place in conflict resolution, depending on the nature of the conflict and the desired outcomes.

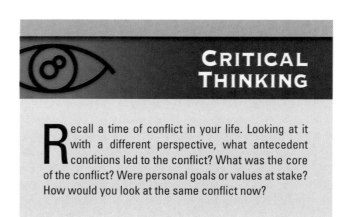

CRITICAL THINKING

Recall a time of conflict in your life. Looking at it with a different perspective, what antecedent conditions led to the conflict? What was the core of the conflict? Were personal goals or values at stake? How would you look at the same conflict now?

TABLE 15-5   SUMMARY OF CONFLICT RESOLUTION TECHNIQUES

Conflict Resolution Technique	Advantages	Disadvantages
Avoiding—ignoring the conflict	Does not make a big deal out of nothing; conflict may be minor in comparison to other priorities	Conflict can become bigger than anticipated; the source of conflict might be more important to one person or group than others
Accommodating—smoothing or cooperating. One side gives in to the other side	One side is more concerned with an issue than the other side; stakes are not high enough for one group and that side is willing to give in	One side holds more power and can force the other side to give in; the importance of the stakes is not as apparent to one side as the other; can lead to parties feeling used if they are always pressured to give in
Competing—forcing; the two or three sides are forced to compete for the goal	Produces a winner; good when time is short and stakes are high	Produces a loser; leaves anger and resentment on the losing side
Compromising—each side gives up something and gains something	No one should win or lose but both should gain something; good for disagreements between individuals	May cause a return to the conflict if what is given up becomes more important than the original goal
Negotiating—high-level discussion that seeks agreement but not necessarily consensus	Stakes are very high and solution is permanent; often involves powerful groups	Agreements are permanent, even though each side has gains and losses
Collaborating—both sides work together to develop the optimal outcome	Best solution for the conflict and encompasses all important goals to each side	Takes a lot of time; requires a commitment to success
Confronting—immediate and obvious movement to stop conflict at the very start	Does not allow conflict to take root; very powerful	May leave the impression that conflict is not tolerated; may make something big out of nothing

Table 15-5 is a summary of these methods, highlighting some of their advantages and disadvantages.

Avoiding is a very common technique. The parties involved in the conflict ignore it, either consciously or subconsciously.

Accommodating is often called cooperating. In this technique, one side of the disagreement decides or is encouraged to adjust or adapt to the other side by ignoring or sidestepping their own feelings about the issue. People often accommodate when the stakes are not that high and the need to move on is pressing. Frequent use of this method, however, can lead to feelings of frustration or being used—one person is "used" to get the cooperation of another. Sullivan (2004) suggests that losing this conflict is advisable, if the payoff assists you to win in the long-term.

Competing is a conflict resolution technique that produces a winner and loser. The concept is that there is an all-out effort to win at all costs. This technique may be used when time is too short to allow other techniques to work or when a critical, though unpopular, decision has to be made quickly. This technique is often called forcing because the winner forces the loser to accept the winner's stance on the conflict.

Compromising is a method used to achieve conflict resolution in situations in which neither side can win and neither side should lose. Compromise is rampant in our society and is useful for goal achievement when the stakes are important but not necessarily critical. Compromise is often seen as appeasement—each side gives up something and each side gains something. Compromise is a good technique for minor conflicts or conflicts that cannot be resolved satisfactorily for both sides. Both parties win and lose.

Collaboration occurs in conflict resolution when both sides work together to develop a mutually acceptable outcome. It is an assertive and cooperative means of achieving important goals, which results in a win-win solution. This technique requires both sides to seek an acceptable solution to the conflict so all parties feel their goals or objectives have been achieved.

Negotiating requires careful communication techniques and highly developed skills. The optimum solution for the conflict may not be reached, but each side has some wins and some losses. The term *negotiation* is often used in reference to collective bargaining or politics; however, it is a very useful technique for conflict resolution at all levels. Negotiating is used when the stakes are considerably higher or when return to the conflict cannot occur. Return to the conflict may not be possible for a variety of reasons, such as a union contract, a permanent change in policy or governance, or career or life changes. The idea of negotiation is that each party will gain something, so general agreement is reached, but consensus—that is, agreement in concept—is not necessarily the goal.

According to Lewicki, Hiam, and Olander (1996), there are five basic approaches to negotiating: collaborative (win-win), competitive (win at all costs), avoiding (lose-lose), accommodating (lose to win), and compromise (split the difference). These five approaches to negotiation are influenced by the importance of maintaining the relationship relative to the importance of achieving one's desired outcomes (see Figure 15-1).

Sometimes, agreement cannot be met through negotiation. In these situations, alternative dispute resolution may be utilized in order to keep privacy in the dispute and to avoid expensive litigation. The College of Nurses of Ontario has an alternative dispute resolution called the Participative Resolution Program (PRP). The Participative Resolution Program is an alternative to the complaint investigation process. It allows the complainant, nurse, and the College to work together to create solutions that satisfy everyone involved. The PRP attempts to bring an effective solution to the complaint that will continue to protect the public interest. This process supports the College's efforts to encourage quality improvement in nursing practice and at the same time reflects the trend toward utilization of non-adversarial ways of dealing with conflict.

One other technique used in conflict resolution is *confronting*. This technique heads off conflict as soon as the first symptoms appear. Both parties are brought together, the issues are clarified, and some outcome is achieved.

Success of the techniques presented here depends on several factors. The importance of the issue in the

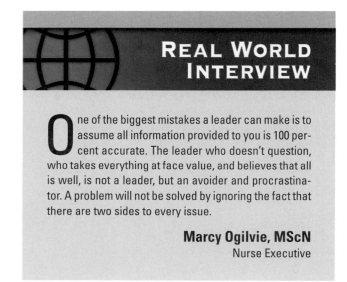

REAL WORLD INTERVIEW

One of the biggest mistakes a leader can make is to assume all information provided to you is 100 percent accurate. The leader who doesn't question, who takes everything at face value, and believes that all is well, is not a leader, but an avoider and procrastinator. A problem will not be solved by ignoring the fact that there are two sides to every issue.

Marcy Ogilvie, MScN
Nurse Executive

	Importance of OUTCOME	
High Importance of **RELATIONSHIP** **Low**	Accommodating	Collaborative
	Compromise	
	Avoiding	Competitive
	Low	**High**

Figure 15-1 Negotiation Strategies.

conflict to the various sides has an enormous impact on the technique selected and the degree of success that will be achieved. Conflict resolution is never really permanent because new issues will always arise. The challenge for the leader/manager is to determine which conflicts require intervention and which techniques stand the best chance of success. If one technique does not work, try another. Conflicts should be suppressed or avoided only under special circumstances that are dependent on the issues involved and the importance of the issues to the parties. Keep in mind that little problems become big problems later if the stakes are high and the issue is important to someone.

STRATEGIES TO FACILITATE CONFLICT RESOLUTION

Open, honest, clear communication is the key to successful conflict resolution. The nurse manager/leader and all parties to the conflict must agree to communicate with one another openly and honestly. Courtesy in communicating is to be encouraged, which includes listening actively to the other side.

The setting for the discussions for conflict resolution should be private, relaxed, and comfortable. If possible, external interruptions from phones, pagers, overhead speakers, and other personnel should be avoided or kept to a minimum. The setting should be on neutral territory so that no one feels overpowered. The ground rules, such as not interrupting, who speaks first, time limits, and so on, should be agreed upon in the beginning. Adherence to ground rules should be respected.

In the conflict resolution process, both sides in the conflict are expected to comply with the results. If one party cannot agree to comply with the decisions or outcomes, there is no point to the process. In such cases, disciplinary action should be considered if the employee is disrupting the team's function or interfering with goal achievement. In the rare cases of noncompliance or nonadherence to an agreed-upon conflict resolution, the leader/manager should seek expert legal counsel within the organization. In most conflicts, the parties are more than willing to comply with the results, and the outcomes prove to be positive. A tool for assessing conflict is identified in Figure 15-2. This tool can be used to determine interpersonal or intergroup conflict within an organization and whether a given conflict is functional or dysfunctional.

LEADERSHIP AND MANAGEMENT ROLES

Marquis and Huston (2006) have identified the importance of integrating leadership skills and management functions in managing conflict. The manager must be able to discern constructive conflict from destructive conflict. Constructive conflict will result in creativity, innovation, and growth for the individuals concerned. When conflict is destructive, managers must deal appropriately with the conflict or risk follow-up activity that may be more destructive than the original conflict (Marquis & Huston, 2006). Leadership roles include the role modelling of conflict resolution methods as soon as the conflict is evident. This strategy demonstrates awareness and works to resolve intrapersonal or interpersonal conflict and sets the goal of conflict resolution so that both parties win. The leader also works to reduce the perceptual differences of the conflicting parties about the conflict and tries to encourage each side to see the other's view. The nurse manager/leader assists the conflicting parties to identify techniques that may resolve the conflict and accepts differences between the parties without judgment or accusation. The leader fosters open and honest communication.

The manager role includes the creation of an environment conducive to conflict resolution. The manager uses authority to solve conflicts, including the use of competition for immediate or unpopular decisions. The manager facilitates conflict resolution in a formal manner when necessary. The manager competes and negotiates for available resources for the unit's needs when necessary. The manager can compromise unit goals when necessary to achieve another more important unit goal. The manager negotiates consensus or compliance to conflict resolution outcomes or goals. Although the roles of leader and manager often appear in the same person, the leadership roles in conflict resolution are often more important to resolution and compliance. The manager has formal power that can be used when necessary, but it should be reserved for important issues that are truly irresolvable.

CONFLICT MANAGEMENT AND CHANGE

Conflict management and resolution are important parts of the change process. Change can often threaten individuals and groups; thus, conflict is an inevitable part of the process. Keep in mind that some conflicts resolve themselves, so the change agent should not be too quick to jump into an intervention mode. Figure 15-3 provides a guide for assessment of the level of conflict. If the level of conflict is too high, the nurse manager must apply conflict resolution strategies.

Interpersonal or intergroup?

1.   Who?
     - Who are the primary individuals or groups involved? What are their characteristics (values; feelings; needs; perceptions; goals; hostilities; strengths; past history of constructive conflict management; self-awareness)?
     - Who, if anyone, are the individuals or groups that have an indirect investment in the result of the conflict?
     - Who, if anyone, is assisting the parties to manage the conflict constructively?
     - What is the history of the individuals' or groups' involvement in the conflict?
     - What is the past and present interpersonal relationship between the parties involved in the conflict?
     - How is power distributed among the parties?
     - What are the major sources of power used?
     - Does the potential for coalition exist among the parties?
     - What is the nature of the current leadership affecting the conflicting parties?

2.   What?
     - What is (are) the issue(s) in the conflict?
     - Are the issues based on facts? Based on values? Based on interests in resources?
     - Are the issues realistic?
     - What is the dominant issue in the conflict?
     - What are the goals of each conflicting party?
     - Is the current conflict functional? Dysfunctional?
     - What conflict management strategies, if any, have been used to manage the conflict to date?
     - What alternatives exist for managing the conflict?
     - What are you doing to maintain the conflict?
     - Is there a lack of stimulating work?

3.   How?
     - What is the origin of the conflict? Sources? Precipitating events?
     - What are the major events in the evolution of the conflict?
     - How have the issues emerged? Been transformed? Proliferated?
     - What polarizations and coalitions have occurred?
     - How have parties tried to damage each other? What stereotyping exists?

4.   When/Where?
     - When did the conflict originate?
     - Where is the conflict taking place?
     - What are the characteristics of the setting within which the conflict is occurring?
     - What are the geographic boundaries? Political structures? Decision-making patterns? Communication networks? Subsystem boundaries?
     - What environmental factors exist that influence the development of functional versus dysfunctional conflict?
     - What resource persons are available to assist in constructive conflict management?

Functional or dysfunctional?	**YES**	**NO**
Does the conflict support the goals of the organization?	[ ]	[ ]
Does the conflict contribute to the overall goals of the organization?	[ ]	[ ]
Does the conflict stimulate improved job performance?	[ ]	[ ]
Does the conflict increase productivity among work group members?	[ ]	[ ]
Does the conflict stimulate creativity and innovation?	[ ]	[ ]
Does the conflict bring about constructive change?	[ ]	[ ]
Does the conflict contribute to the survival of the organization?	[ ]	[ ]
Does the conflict improve initiative?	[ ]	[ ]
Does job satisfaction remain high?	[ ]	[ ]
Does the conflict improve the morale of the work group?	[ ]	[ ]

A yes response to the majority of the questions indicates that the conflict is probably functional. If the majority of responses are no, then the conflict is most likely a dysfunctional conflict.

Figure 15-2 Guide for the Assessment of Conflict.

Is conflict too low?	YES	NO
Is the work group consistently satisfied with the status quo?	[ ]	[ ]
Are no or few opposing views expressed by work-group members?	[ ]	[ ]
Is little concern expressed about doing things better?	[ ]	[ ]
Is little or no concern expressed about improving inadequacies?	[ ]	[ ]
Are the decisions made by the work group generally of low quality?	[ ]	[ ]
Are no or few innovative solutions or ideas expressed?	[ ]	[ ]
Are many work-group members "yes-men"?	[ ]	[ ]
Are work-group members reluctant to express ignorance or uncertainties?	[ ]	[ ]
Does the nurse manager seek to maintain peace and group cooperation regardless of whether this is the correct intervention?	[ ]	[ ]
Do the work-group members demonstrate an extremely high level of resistance to change?	[ ]	[ ]
Does the nurse manager base the distribution of rewards on "popularity" as opposed to competence and high job performance?	[ ]	[ ]
Is the nurse manager excessively concerned about not hurting the feelings of the nursing staff?	[ ]	[ ]
Is the nurse manager excessively concerned with obtaining a consensus of opinion and reaching a compromise when decisions must be made?	[ ]	[ ]

A yes response to the majority of these questions can be indicative of a too-low conflict level in a work group.

Is conflict too high?	YES	NO
Is there an upward and onward spiraling escalation of the conflict?	[ ]	[ ]
Are the conflicting parties stimulating the escalation of conflict without considering the consequences?	[ ]	[ ]
Is there a shift away from conciliation, minimizing differences, and enhancing goodwill?	[ ]	[ ]
Are the issues involved in the conflict being increasingly elaborated and expanded?	[ ]	[ ]
Are false issues being generated	[ ]	[ ]
Are the issues vague or unclear?	[ ]	[ ]
Is job dissatisfaction increasing among work-group members?	[ ]	[ ]
Is the work-group productivity being adversely affected?	[ ]	[ ]
Is the energy being directed to activities that do not contribute to the achievement of organizational goals (e.g., destroying opposing party)?	[ ]	[ ]
Is the morale of the nursing staff being adversely affected?	[ ]	[ ]
Are extra parties getting dragged into the conflict?	[ ]	[ ]
Is a great deal of reliance on overt power manipulation noted (threats, coercion, deception)?	[ ]	[ ]
Is there a great deal of imbalance in power noted among the parties?	[ ]	[ ]
Are the individuals or groups involved in the conflict expressing dissatisfaction about the course of the conflict and feel that they are losing something?	[ ]	[ ]
Is absenteeism increasing among staff?	[ ]	[ ]
Is there a high rate of turnover among personnel?	[ ]	[ ]
Is communication dysfunctional, not open, mistrustful, and/or restrictive?	[ ]	[ ]
Is the focus being placed on nonconflict relevant sensitive areas of the other party?	[ ]	[ ]

A yes response to the majority of these questions can be indicative of a conflict level in a work group that is too high.

Figure 15-3 Guide for the Assessment of Level of Conflict.

CASE STUDY 15-1

Jane's supervisor has just appointed her to the role of coordinator. However, the current coordinator, Gwen, will remain working in the same department with Jane. Gwen tends to be negative about change and the organization, but she has excellent clinical knowledge.

What do you think Jane should do to help Gwen adjust to the change? Should Jane explore Gwen's feelings about the change? Which situation will be more stressful for Jane—being the coordinator or working with Gwen? Should Jane's supervisor have done something to prepare either Jane or Gwen for this change? What should have been done?

KEY CONCEPTS

- Change is inevitable, exciting, and anxiety provoking.

- Change is defined as making something different from what it was.

- Major change theorists include Lewin, Lippitt, Havelock, and Rogers.

- Senge's model of five disciplines describes the learning organization. This model describes organizations undergoing continuous and unrelenting change.

- The change process is similar to the nursing process.

- Strategies for change include the power-coercive approach, the normative-reeducative approach, and the rational-empirical approach.

- The change agent plays an important role in the change process. The change agent is responsible and accountable for the project.

- Conflict is a normal part of any change project.

- Conflict comes from many sources, including value differences, fear, and goal disagreement.

- The techniques for conflict resolution include avoiding, accommodating, compromising, competing, confronting, collaborating, negotiating, and alternative dispute resolution.

- There are several strategies for conflict resolution. Clear, open communication is key.

- Conflict can move the change process along if it is handled well. Conflict can stop the change process if it is handled poorly or allowed to get out of control.

KEY TERMS

change
change agent
conflict

organizational change
personal change
professional change

REVIEW QUESTIONS

1. What is the most desirable conflict resolution technique?
   A. Avoiding
   B. Competing
   C. Negotiating
   D. Collaborating

2. What is the most common source of conflict in today's health care organization?
   A. Goals
   B. Values
   C. Resource allocation disputes
   D. Competition

3. Which of the following characteristics describe both the change agent and the person responsible for conflict resolution?
   A. Secretive and willful
   B. Trustworthy and a good communicator
   C. Ambitious and avoiding
   D. Powerful and dictatorial

REVIEW ACTIVITIES

1. Select a change project that you have either personally achieved or experienced in a clinical situation. Discuss with your classmates how you felt and how the change agent maintained momentum and enthusiasm for the project. If you chose a personal change, how did you maintain enthusiasm?

2. Recall a conflict you have been involved with in the clinical setting. Discuss each of the methods of conflict resolution identified in the chapter. Identify which methods would have helped. Did the conflict ever get resolved? How?

3. Discuss with a nurse manager how to determine whether a conflict is occurring. What steps does the nurse manager take to bring it out in the open? Share the information with your classmates.

4. Discuss with a nurse manager what it feels like on a personal level to have constant change? How did the nurse manager present an impending change to the staff? Did the nurse manager use any of the techniques discussed in this chapter? Was the change successful?

EXPLORING THE WEB

- Look up this journal and describe its purpose. Would this journal be useful to the new nurse manager? A new nurse? Anyone else in health care?

- Journal of Conflict Resolution: *http://jcr.sagepub.com/*

- The College of Nurses of Ontario has an alternative dispute resolution called the Participative Resolution Program (PRP): *http://www.cno.org/ih/prp_intro.html*. Describe the PRP's resolution process.

REFERENCES

Ayers, D. F. (2002). Developing climates for renewal in the community college: A case study of dissipative self-organization. *Community College Journal of Research and Practice, 26*(2), 165–185.

Bennis, W. (1989). *On becoming a leader.* Reading, MA: Addison-Wesley.

Bennis, W., Benne, K., & Chin, R. (Eds.). (1969). *The planning of change* (2nd ed.). New York: Holt, Rinehart, Winston.

Bushy, A. (1993). Managing change: Strategies for continuing education. *The Journal of Continuing Education in Nursing, 23,* 197–200.

Flower, J., & Guillaume, P. (March/April 2002). Surfing the edge of chaos. *Health Forum Journal,* 17–20.

Havelock, R. G. (1973). *The change agent's guide to innovation in education.* Englewood Cliffs, NJ: Educational Technology.

Ingersoll, G. L., Kirsch, J. C., Merk, S. E., & Lightfoot, J. (2000). Relationship of organizational culture and readiness for change to employee commitment to the organization. *Journal of Nursing Administration, 30*(1), 11–20.

Lancaster, J. (1999). *Nursing issues in leading and managing change.* St. Louis, MO: Mosby.

Lapp, J. (2002). Thriving on change. *Caring Magazine,* 40–43.

Lewicki, R. J., Hiam, A., & Olander, K. W. (1996). *Think before you speak.* New York: John Wiley & Sons.

Lewin, K. (1951). *Field theory in social science.* New York: Harper & Row.

Lippit, R., Watson, J., & Westley, B. (1958). *The dynamics of planned change.* New York: Harcourt, Brace.

Marquis, B. L., & Huston, C. J. (2006). *Leadership roles and management functions in nursing: Theory and application* (5th ed.). Philadelphia: Lippincott

Nelson Canadian dictionary of the English language. (1997). Toronto: ITP Nelson.

Porter-O'Grady, T., & Malloch, K. (2003). *Quantum leadership: A textbook of new leadership.* Mississauga: Jones and Bartlett Publishers Canada.

Robbins, S., DeCenzo, D. A., & Stuart-Kotze, R. (2002). *Fundamentals of management: Essential concepts and applications* (3rd Canadian ed.). Toronto: Prentice-Hall.

Robbins, S., & Langton, N. (2002). *Organizational behaviour: Concepts, controversies, applications* (2nd Canadian ed.). Toronto: Prentice-Hall.

Rogers, E. M. (1983). *Diffusion of innovations* (3rd ed.). New York: Free Press.

Senge, P. M. (2006). *The fifth discipline: The art and practice of the learning organization.* New York: Doubleday.

Silber, M. B. (1993). The "C"s in excellence: Choice and change. *Nursing Management, 24*(9), 60–62.

Sullivan, E. J. (2004). *Becoming influential: A guide for nurses.* Upper Saddle River, NJ: Pearson/Prentice Hall.

Sullivan, E. J., & Decker, P. J. (2001). *Effective leadership & management in nursing* (5th ed.). Menlo Park, CA: Addison-Wesley.

Tappen, R. M. (2001). *Nursing leadership and management: Concepts and practice* (4th ed.). Philadelphia: F. A. Davis.

Tappen, R. M., Weiss, S. A., & Whitehead, D. K. (2004). *Essentials of nursing leadership and management* (3rd ed.). Philadelphia: F. A. Davis Company.

Wagner, C. M., & Huber, D. L. (2003). Catastrophe and nursing turnover: Nonlinear models. *Journal of Nursing Administration, 33*(9), 486–492.

SUGGESTED READINGS

Bennis, W., & Biederman, P. W. (1997). *Organizing genius: The secrets of creative collaboration.* Reading, MA: Addison-Wesley.

Bennis, W., & Nanus, B. (1985). *Leaders: The strategies for taking charge.* New York: Harper & Row.

Curtin, L. L. (1995). Blessed are the flexible. . . . *Nursing Management, 26*(3), 7–8.

Duck, J. D. (1993, November/December). Managing change: The art of balancing. *Harvard Business Review,* 109–118.

Entine, J., & Nichols, M. (1997, January/February). Good leadership: What's its gender? *Female Executive,* 50–52.

Heifetz, R. A., & Linsky, M. (June 2002). A survival guide for leaders. *Harvard Business Review,* 65–74.

Heim, P. (1995). Getting beyond "she said, he said." *Nursing Administration Quarterly, 19*(2), 6–18.

Johnson, S. (1998). *Who moved my cheese?* New York: G.P. Putnam.

Jost, S. G. (2000). An assessment and intervention strategy for managing staff needs during change. *Journal of Nursing Administration, 30*(1), 34–40.

Keenan, M. J., & Hurst, J. B. (1999). Conflict: The cutting edge of change. In P. S. Yoder-Wise, *Leading and managing in nursing* (2nd ed., pp. 318–334). St. Louis, MO: Mosby.

Kotter, J. P. (1996). *Leading change.* Boston: Harvard Business School Press.

Marriner-Tomey, A. (2000). *Guide to nursing management and leadership* (6th ed.). St. Louis, MO: Mosby.

McDaniel, R. R. (1997). Strategic leadership: A view from quantum and chaos theories. *Health Care Management Review, 22*(1), 21–37.

McFarland, G., Leonard, H., & Morris, M. (1984). *Nursing leadership and management.* New York, NY: Wiley.

Menix, K. D. (1999). Leading change: Nurse manager as innovator. In P. S. Yoder-Wise, *Leading and managing in nursing* (2nd ed., pp. 73–89). St. Louis, MO: Mosby.

Rosswurm, M. A., & Larrabee, J. H. (1999). A model for change to evidence-based practice. *Image: Journal of Nursing Scholarship, 31*(4), 317–322.

Schweikhart, S. B., & Smith-Daniels, V. (1996). Reengineering the work of caregivers: Role redefinition, team structures, and organization redesign. *Hospital & Health Services Administration, 41*(1), 19–36.

Shortell, S. & Kaluzny, A. D. (1994). *Health care management: Organization design and behavior* (3rd ed.). Clifton Park, NY: Delmar Learning.

Silber, M. B. (1993). The "C"s in excellence: Choice and change. *Nursing Management, 24*(9), 60–62.

Simms, L. M., Price, S. A., & Ervin, N. E. (2000). *The professional practice of nursing administration* (3rd ed.). Clifton Park, NY: Delmar Learning.

Thietart, R. A., & Forgues, B. (1995). Chaos theory and organizations. *Organization Science, 6*(1), 19–31.

Zukowski, B. (1995). Managing change—before it manages you. *Medical Surgical Nursing, 4*(4), 325–326.

CHAPTER 16

Power

Terry W. Miller, PhD, RN
Adapted by: Sandra Trubyk, MSA, BN, BA

Significant progress has occurred over the years toward advancing nursing's presence, role, and influence in the development of health care policy. However, more nurses need to learn how to identify issues strategically; work with decision makers; understand who holds the power in the workplace, communities, provincial, territorial and federal level organizations; and understand who controls the resources for health care services. (Stephanie L. Ferguson, 2001)

OBJECTIVES

Upon completion of this chapter, the reader should be able to:

1. Define the concept of power.
2. Identify the various sources of power—coercion, reward, legitimacy, expertise, reference, information, and connection.
3. Recognize power at a personal level, a professional level, and an organizational level.
4. Describe how a nurse's perception of power affects client care.
5. Describe the association of connection power and relationships.
6. Explain why nurses are faced with a paradox within the context of information power.

2004). However, nursing has a rich history, and many of its leaders have overcome the prejudicial challenges confronting them. This chapter will discuss power and how nursing power affects client care.

DEFINITIONS OF POWER

Power has been defined in multiple ways, some not so positive. Commonly, **power** is described as the ability to create, acquire, and use resources to achieve one's goals. When the goals are self-determined, even greater power is implied than when the goals are made either by others or with others. Power can be defined at various levels: personal, professional, or organizational. Power, regardless of level, comes from the ability to influence others or to affect others' thinking or behaviour.

Power at the personal level is closely linked to how an individual perceives power, how others perceive the individual, and the extent to which an individual can influence events. Nurses who feel empowered at a personal level are likely to manifest a high level of self-awareness. They are more likely to understand nursing as a profession because it represents a group to which they belong. They also understand the structure and operations of health care because it represents their work environment.

People who are perceived as experts in health care have a significant amount of authority and influence, which makes them more effective than those not perceived as experts. The influence of an expert can be wielded in at least two ways. The first way is to be introduced and promoted to a group as an expert, which validates one's expertise; the second way is to actually become an expert based on knowledge, skills, and abilities that are consistently demonstrated in practice settings. Remarkably, nurses are often reluctant to be identified as experts to clients, physicians, administrators, other nurses, other health care workers, and the public in general. This lack of awareness must be addressed if the nursing profession is to achieve the status and degree of empowerment it seeks. As Disch (2000) stated, "In today's health care environment, what is valued, preserved, and receives resources is that which is visible" (p. 189).

The personal power of nurses is evident in the decisions they make on a daily basis to organize their lives and their work so that they can accomplish what they want and obtain what they need for themselves and their clients. The more that nurses believe they can influence events through personal effort, the greater their sense of power. Many accept the idea that if individuals believe they can make a difference and influence events in their lives, they are likely to participate actively in trying to achieve what they want. This participation will make them feel more powerful even if their efforts are not all that successful. Similarly, if

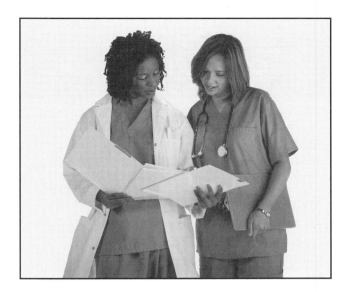

The facility manager, Bryan, has been heard boasting about the authority he has over the nursing staff. Bryan's background is in social work. The hospital has several part-time facility managers with backgrounds in various fields other than nursing. Bryan is demanding to make bed changes on the medical ward 2A. The unit nurse, Sara, looks over the 2A clients' charts but feels all her clients are appropriate for the ward's program and should not be moved in order to make accommodations for a surgical client from the day surgery area.

What would you do if you were Sara?

How would you approach the facility manager, Bryan?

Effective nurses are powerful. They show objectivity, creativity, and knowledge throughout their practice and regardless of their work setting. They have power and exert it appropriately by understanding the concept of power from multiple perspectives. They use this understanding to motivate others; accomplish organizational goals; and provide safe, competent care. Yet the nursing profession has been criticized for not accepting this fact and for not knowing enough about the power that nursing holds.

Nurses have struggled with the concept of power throughout the profession's history. Many outside the profession continue to challenge the nurse's role in wielding power at any level, including the bedside. In Canada, in 2005, women still dominated the nursing occupation with male nurses accounting for only approximately 5.5 percent of all nurses.[1] Nurses do have great responsibility, and linked to that responsibility is power. In some countries, such as Iran and Iraq, women have a restricted role, low status, and little or no access to power in government policymaking. Therefore, the nursing profession has little or no power as it tries to obtain acceptance and recognition as a profession (Nasrabadi, Lipsion, & Emami,

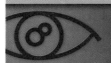

CRITICAL THINKING

The work and contributions of some nurses are so significant that they change the world. To be effective, these nurses define themselves as something far more powerful than what others may want them to be. When we ignore the relevance and significance of nursing history, we discount the contributions nurses have made to improve the lives of others. Our lack of historical awareness empowers others to discount the value of nursing. Ultimately, we limit our own future as nurses by hindering our potential for making even greater contributions to the future of health care.

Name two nurses who represent powerful figures in modern history. (If you need some help, see this chapter's Exploring the Web, page 293.) Why are their contributions are so significant?

Can you identify some obstacles they experienced because they were nurses?

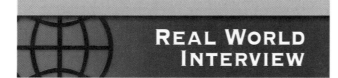

REAL WORLD INTERVIEW

In my years of clinical experience, I found the best nursing managers were the ones who gave away some of their power to the nursing staff. These were the managers that did not hover over you on the ward, but let you manage your workload and team. These managers knew when to delegate, to whom they could delegate, and they provided the right tools to perform the job. That is, I was recognized as a professional with sound nursing knowledge, organizational skills, and a caring attitude. This recognition enabled me to grow in my profession and heightened my self-esteem, which I conveyed to the clients I cared for. New graduates need a role model to assist them in improving their skills and knowledge. New graduates also need a leader who will guide but not take away their self-confidence. Managers who hold tightly onto the reins of managing are probably less confident in their own skills and knowledge, and that has an impact on the nurses they manage.

Sandra Martin, MS, RN

individuals believe themselves to be powerless to influence events and do not even try to exert any influence, they will feel even more powerless (Rowland & Rowland, 1997).

POWER AND ACCOUNTABILITY

Nurses have a professional obligation not to view power merely as a negative concept so that they can avoid both power struggles and those who seem to savour power.

Effective nurses view their ability to understand and use power as a significant part of their responsibilities to clients, their coworkers, the nursing profession, and themselves.

Traditionally, accountability has been considered one of the major hallmarks of the health care professions. Nursing is a profession and, as such, nurses have the primary responsibility for defining and providing nursing services. Yet some nurses appear to have a difficult time understanding the underlying accountability that comes with this powerful claim. Inherent in the role of the nurse are professional accountability and direct responsibility for decisions made and actions rendered.

SOURCES OF POWER

What sources of power do you use in your nursing? Chances are you use several types of power and at times may not be cognizant that you are using power. Most researchers agree that **sources of power** are a combination of conscious and unconscious factors that allow an individual to influence others to think or act in a certain way (Fisher & Koch, 1996). Power can be used to influence subordinates, as in the use of legitimate power, or to influence peers and superiors, as when expert power could be used. Most people would choose not to use coercive power because it lowers their referent power. Other nurses earn an informative power due to up-to-date knowledge on specific areas of health care.

Power derived from the knowledge and skills nurses possess is referred to as **expert power.** However, special considerations should be kept in mind regarding expertise and power. The geometric explosion of knowledge has made expertise more valuable, and technological advances for accessing information have enabled more people to acquire expertise on any given subject. Knowing more about a subject than others, combined with the legitimacy of holding a position, gives an individual a decided advantage in any situation. But the less acknowledged that experts are in a group, the less effective their expert powers become. Visible reciprocal acknowledgment of expertise among group members balances power and enhances productivity, whereas lack of reciprocal acknowledgment has the opposite effect. Combining expertise with high position is most powerful if the person consistently demonstrates expertise.

Legitimate power is power derived from the position a nurse holds in a group, which also indicates the nurse's degree of authority. The more comfortable nurses are with their legitimate power as nurses, the easier it is for them to fulfill their role. Nurses in legitimate positions are expected to use the authority they have and may be punished for not doing so. Sometimes, too little legitimacy or authority is delegated to nurses who are given the responsibility for leading. People generally follow legitimate leaders with whom they agree. Although legitimacy is a significant part of influence and control, it is not universally effective and is not sufficient as one's only source of power.

Power derived from the degree to which others respect and like an individual, group, or organization is referred to as **referent power,** or charismatic power. Nurses who are trusted and respected by others are most able to exert their influence. People want to agree with and follow referent leadership. Such leaders tend to be charismatic, and followers often rationalize or explain away any incongruent behaviours to maintain their high level of trust in the referent. It is erroneous to assume that only people who are less intelligent than the charismatic or referent leader will follow that leader. The referent leader who inspires trust and confidence also makes other people feel valuable.

The ability to reward or punish others, as well as to create fear in others to influence them to change their behaviour, is commonly termed **reward power and coercive power.** Meaningful rewards exist other than money, such as formal recognition before one's nursing peers at an awards ceremony. The manner in which rewards are distributed is important. Rewards seldom motivate as effectively as a vision that unifies the members of the group; thus, reward power is an uncertain instrument for long-term change. Rewards are not likely to permanently change attitudes. Withholding rewards or achieving a goal by instilling fear in others often results in resentment.

People who have the ability to administer punishment or take disciplinary actions against others have coercive power. Wielding this type of power is often considered the least desirable tactic used by people in positions of authority. Typically, people do not enjoy being coerced into doing something other than what they choose to do, and often perceive punishment as humiliating.

All types of power may be used to influence a peer or subordinate but attempting to influence superiors may meet with counter power and leave little choice other than to comply with their wants (Greenberg & Baron, 2000).

The extent to which nurses are connected with others having power is called **connection power.** Leaders can dramatically increase their influence by understanding that people are attracted to those with power and their associates. As a new nurse, when you go to the office of the director of nursing services, or the chief nursing officer or the president of the health care facility, do not forget that the clerical workers in the outside office have relationships with their boss—thus they have connection power. If you try to go around them and take their power lightly, or insult or patronize them, you have risked your own power base in relation to the director, or chief nursing officer, or president. Similarly, if a nurse bypasses a person who is directly responsible for a situation, the attempted circumvention reflects negatively on the nurse. Nurses should work to resolve issues at the appropriate level before they take their concerns to a higher level of authority. Nurses are expected to understand the structure and policies of the organizations in which they provide services.

Nurses who influence others with the information they provide to the group are using **information power.** Regardless of a nurse's leadership style, information plays an increasingly critical role. Legitimate power, reward power, and coercive power tend to be bestowed on individuals by their organizations. These forms of power tend to be effective only for a short period of time unless they are accompanied by another form of power, such as information power. Information power is especially important because, to be functional, health care teams and organizations require accurate and timely information that is shared. To be seen by others as having information power, nurses must share knowledge that is both accurate and useful. Information sharing can improve client care, increase collegiality, enhance organizational effectiveness, and strengthen one's professional connections. See Table 16-1 for a summary of the different types of power.

Effective nurses use the sources of power covered thus far: expertise, legitimacy, reference, reward, coercion, connection, and information. For example, nurse managers have legitimate power due to their position in a health care facility. As well, nurse managers may have several other forms of power, such as expertise and charisma. Nurse managers must decide which sources of power to use with each participant in their objectives in order to gain the most towards their goals. Nurse managers are then using power strategy, which is a plan to use sources of power on key individuals and groups in order to have similar sources of power on both sides of an argument (Hibberd and Smith, 2006).

TABLE 16-1	PRINCIPLES FOR UNDERSTANDING AND USING DIFFERENT TYPES OF POWER

Concept	How It Works
Expert Power	The power nurses obtain due to their knowledge and skills base in a particular area of nursing (Hibberd and Smith, 2006).
Legitimate Power	Legitimate power is the authority within a nursing position that is acknowledged and received by others in the health care facility, such as a nursing unit manager (Hibberd and Smith, 2006). Legitimacy as a nurse is based on several factors, including registration (Fisher & Koch, 1996), academic degrees, certification, and experience in the role.
Referent Power	This power is derived from desirable personal qualities. People with referent power are liked and respected by their peers and others (Greenberg & Baron, 2000). Nurses with referent power can influence the actions of others because of their charisma. The referent person has the ability to inspire confidence. In any situation, strong referent leaders are considered people of great vision, which may or may not be the reality.
Reward and coercive	The ability to reward or punish others as well as to create fear in others to influence them to change their behaviour is commonly termed reward power and coercive power.
Connection	Both personal and professional relationships are part of a nurse's connections. People who are strongly connected to others, both personally and professionally, have enhanced resources, a capacity for learning and information sharing, and an ability to increase their overall sphere of influence. Teamwork, collaboration, networking, and mentoring are some of the ways in which nurses can become more connected and therefore more powerful.
Information	Information power is based on the information that any person can provide to the group (Bower, 2000). Authoritarian leaders attempt to control information. Charismatic leaders provide information that is seductive for many people. Information leaders provide a sense of stability with the use and synthesis of information. If one knows how to get it and what to do with it, the greatest power may be in information.

PERSONAL ORIENTATION AND THE INTERNET

In the simplest terms, a person's desire for power, whether it is for impact, strength, or influence, takes one of two forms. The first form is an orientation toward achieving personal gain and self-glorification. The second form is an orientation toward achieving gain for others or the common good. Orientation to power as corruptive or evil is reflected in the 19th-century quote attributed to Lord Acton:

"All power corrupts, but absolute power corrupts absolutely" (Bothamley, 1993). People having this orientation tend to believe that those wielding or afforded power ultimately should not have power because of their potential to misuse it, that people desiring power should not be trusted because their motivation for acquiring power is inherently wrong—they want power for personal gain at any cost.

Many believe the Internet will level the playing field of power for all humanity. The free flow of information will empower nurses and other people, that is, all those who have access to the Internet and have the ability to use it effectively.

EMPOWERMENT AND DISEMPOWERMENT

Empowerment is a popular term in the nursing literature related to management, leadership, and politics. Kelly (Kelly & Joel, 1996) defined **empowerment** as the "process by which we facilitate the participation of others in decision making and take action within an environment where there is an equitable distribution of power" (p. 420). By empowering others, the nursing manager has passed on responsibility and with it, authority. For empowering to be effective, the manager should share the appropriate information and knowledge with the staff nurse in order to meet the planned goals (Greenberg & Baron, 2000).

Nurses empower themselves and others in many ways. At the most basic level, they empower others because they perceive them to be powerful. If an individual, a group, or an organization is perceived as being powerful, that perception can empower that individual, group, or organization. Some health care provider groups are viewed as more powerful than others because of the alliances they have formed with associations that are known to be powerful, such as the Canadian Medical Association (CMA). Similarly, nurses disempower themselves if they see nurses or nursing as powerless.

ROLE OF THE MEDIA

People who work in the media recognize the relationship between power and perception. Those who work in advertising, marketing, and public relations understand how the public's perception can be created or changed through advertising and marketing campaigns, damage control, timely press releases, and well-orchestrated media events.

The way the media present nursing to the public will empower or disempower nursing. Nurses have not been able to consistently use the media as effectively as other more powerful occupational groups. To date, the media have failed to recognize nursing as one of the largest groups in health care. It is hoped that the media's presentation of the rapidly growing nursing shortage over the next decade will improve the public's perceptions of nursing as a career and human service. The media need to show nurses as decision-makers, coordinators of care, and primary care providers as well as order followers in health care. Too often the media has presented a stereotypical, insignificant view of nurses, and too often nurses fail to view nursing as the honourable profession it is.

One strategy for empowering nursing is to employ the media to create a stronger, more powerful image of nursing. This strategy would require more nurses to become active participants in some formal part of their profession—the Canadian Nurses Association (CNA); their provincial or territorial regulatory body and professional association; or one of the nursing specialty organizations, such as the Canadian Association of Critical Care Nurses (CACCN) or the Canadian Hospice Palliative Care Association (CHPCA).

A PLAN FOR PERSONAL EMPOWERMENT

Understanding power helps the novice nurse to become more effective, to make better decisions, and to better help others. Understanding power from a variety of perspectives is not just important for nurses professionally, it is important

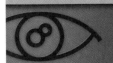

CRITICAL THINKING

Are you interested in becoming the best nurse possible? Do you enjoy meeting and associating with people who are successful? Do you feel most comfortable when you are in control over personal situations? Do you feel uncomfortable when you have little or no influence over the actions of others? Responding yes to these questions suggests that you have motives for personal achievement, being affiliated with others, and having power. **Achievement** (i.e., accomplishment of goals through effort), **affiliation** (i.e., associations and relationships with others), and power are interrelated from a behavioural perspective. All three can be positive attributes of one's personality, or they can lead to highly destructive behaviour. Affiliation and power needs are predominantly interpersonal, whereas the need for achievement is predominantly intrapersonal, that is, motivated by a personal conviction to be capable and competent. People with high achievement needs tend to rely on themselves to get things done. They activate their intrapersonal motivation. Consequently, they expend a high degree of energy and focus on improving their personal skills and learning new things. Depending on their past experiences and current interests, nurses engage in a variety of behaviours that reflect their needs for achievement, affiliation, or power Can you think of two nurses who are highly motivated in terms of their achievements, position, and power? Would these two nurses be role models for you? Why, or why not?

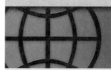

REAL WORLD INTERVIEW

Ms. Cox is 38 years old and has been hospitalized four times. She underwent surgery this past spring and has encountered nursing care and nurses in various roles throughout the health care system. Ms. Cox is articulate and reflective. She earned a degree in English and currently holds a position at a selective liberal arts university as an admissions counsellor. She states, "I don't think nurses know they are powerful....Nurses can take on more than they think they can. They have the power to change the system in which they work. Yet I see nurses as the most overworked, underpaid, and underachieving professions also. There is so much more they could be doing if they didn't spend so much time railing against the machine. They are telling the wrong people—each other—that they are frustrated. They should be telling the ones with real power, or better yet, more of them should become the ones in power. Instead, they suffer with each other and stay angry. It appears almost passive-aggressive how nurses deal with power. My concern is that it can affect client care in such a negative way. Believe me when I say clients value nurses, but the people writing the paycheque for nurses must value nurses. Clients need nursing far more than they need anything else. The better nurses who have cared for me have been instrumental in my healing. Beyond knowing when I need medication or doing some procedure, it is the smile, the touch, and the well-placed word of encouragement that has gotten me through. This is where nurses have power because no one but a real nurse can provide it. It comes from the heart."

Audrey Cox (Client)

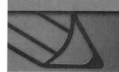

CASE STUDY 16-1

Maria and Haley work on the same nursing unit in a large, metropolitan hospital. Both predominantly work the evening shift and have less than one year's experience since graduating from nursing school. Maria has been offered increasingly difficult client assignments, entrusted with charge duties, and recently was selected for a two-week leadership training program.

Haley has not adapted as well and has withdrawn from what was once a close friendship with Maria. Haley seeks consolation with the nurses she and Maria claimed they would never emulate. Haley takes her breaks and eats dinner with two nurses who complain that the best nurses are undervalued in the organization, yet these same nurses were not supportive of Maria or Haley or any other new nurses oriented to their unit.

Maria seeks out others she perceives to be knowledgeable and more satisfied in their professional roles. She strives to participate in non-mandatory meetings as well as clinical rounds, using them as an opportunity to ask questions. Thus, she is beginning to increase her personal level of power by connecting with the other staff and gathering information.

One night after a difficult shift, Haley accuses Maria of abandoning her and playing up to administration, and says that Maria is being used by the unit's nurse manager. Haley tells Maria that the other nurses are planning to file a complaint against the unit supervisor for selecting Maria to attend the leadership training program over the nurses that have been on the unit longer.

How should Maria respond to Haley?

for them personally as well. Nurses are able to gain more control of their work lives and their personal lives.

The future can be imagined in three ways: (1) what is possible, (2) what is probable, and (3) what is preferred.

Nurses who want to experience a preferred future should think about what is happening to them as a person and as a nurse, the possibilities they face as a person and as a nurse, and what they are going to do about it.

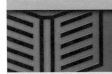

LITERATURE APPLICATION

Citation: Laschinger, H. K. S., & Wong, C. (1999). Staff nurse empowerment and collective accountability: Effect on perceived productivity and self-rated work effectiveness. *Nursing Economic$, 17*(6), 308–316.

Discussion: The findings of this survey supported empowerment, collective decision-making authority, productivity, accountability, formal and informal power, and political and social alliances in the workplace. Shared governance was criticized because the authority for client care was not shifted to nurses. The study reported that an essential strategy for fostering high-quality professional practice was creating environments that offered staff nurses free access to empowering structures and to information and resources, along with appropriate support. Nurses reported their accountability to each other and their contribution to the organization as moderate, their overall work effectiveness high, but their productivity lower than expected. Recommendations included essential changes in the manager role to exclude traditional control and include support for nurses in their performance.

Implications for Practice: Assumption of greater power by nurses as primary service providers requires far-reaching changes in organizational operations, administrative structures, budget processes, individual service planning procedures, and professional cross-disciplinary relationships. The findings of this study offer more insight into what staff nurses expected to be more effective in providing client care services.

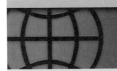

REAL WORLD INTERVIEW

Power is the ultimate responsibility to care for the client. Our assessment and subsequent actions can determine whether a client will live or die. I feel confident in my abilities for the future, but as a new nurse, it is difficult to feel powerful because there is so much to learn. I believe that nurses tend to perceive power as being able to stand up to those above or higher up in the work setting. I think nursing is changing for the better because of the power gained with nurses having more autonomy. There is more trust put into the nurse's judgment because women's roles in society have changed and more men are entering the profession. Equal opportunity programs have created the structure to protect women and others who have been vulnerable to those in positions of greater power. I have learned that you do not have to be afraid to advocate for your client. If you need to call the attending physician during the night, then you do it. I have come to realize that power is not abusing the people working under you. Also, to understand power, it is important to understand people's roles and where they are coming from.

Julie Bergman
New Nursing Graduate

POWER AND THE LIMITS OF INFORMATION

Even if nurses could fully trust the completeness and accuracy of information they have in their practice, they would have insufficient data. Things are always changing; therefore, information always needs to be updated. Nurses should never stop assessing and gathering information. To make good decisions, nurses must be able to gather enough data and realistically interpret its value, as well as share and apply information in a safe, competent manner. Effective nurses understand time constraints and set priorities to ensure that what is most important receives the most attention. These nurses are willing to take the inherent risk of making a decision, while understanding there will always be more information to gather and analyze. They recognize that choosing to make no decision is a decision in itself and that information is never complete. Table 16-2 presents a framework for becoming empowered using information.

TABLE 16-2   A FRAMEWORK FOR BECOMING EMPOWERED USING INFORMATION

Background	As an empowered nurse, you have the ability to discover important information and to use it to your advantage, as well as to the advantage of your clients.
Steps	■ Find and maintain good sources of information. ■ Get involved beyond direct client care. ■ Ask questions. ■ Listen to and analyze the answers. ■ Make a plan with the information acquired. ■ Evaluate the plan.
Information for providing care	■ Assess the client's condition using relevant, objective measurements. ■ Consult with other nurses, physicians, and other health care workers involved in the care of your clients. ■ Consult with the client's significant others, family members, and friends.

Information for becoming more effective in the work setting	■ Get involved beyond direct client care.
	■ Volunteer for committee assignments that will challenge you to learn and experience more than what is expected of you in a staff nurse role.
	■ Think about the following when involved with committees:
	  1. What is the committee trying to do?
	  2. What specific information does the committee use to make decisions?
	  3. How does the committee's work apply to my practice, my colleagues, my clients, my organizational unit, and the organization as a whole?
	■ Assess the strength of the information you have in relation to your clients, your colleagues, your organizational unit, the organization as a whole, and the profession of nursing.
	■ Readily share information with others who will value it and use it to a good end.

Evaluation	Periodically, re-examine your plans. Did you achieve your expected outcomes? If not, why not? Were there staffing problems or client crises? Were the activities that were necessary for outcome achievement carried out? What have you learned from this evaluation that you can apply to the future?

MACHIAVELLI ON POWER

Machiavelli wrote in his political treatise, *The Prince*,

There is nothing more difficult to try, nor more doubtful of success, nor more dangerous to deal with, than to take it upon oneself to introduce new institutions, because the introducer makes enemies out of all those who benefit from the old institutions and is feebly defended by all those who might benefit from the new ones (Machiavelli, 1532/1996, p. 51).

KEY CONCEPTS

■ Effective nurses are powerful. They show objectivity, creativity, and knowledge throughout their practice and regardless of their work setting.

■ Effective nurses have power and exert it appropriately by understanding the concept of power from multiple perspectives. They then use this understanding to motivate others; accomplish organizational goals; and provide safe, competent care.

■ Power has been described as the ability to create, acquire, and use resources to achieve one's goals.

- Power can be defined at a personal level, a professional level, and an organizational level.

- The personal and information power of nurses is evident in the decisions they make.

- Hibberd and Smith (2006) help the nurse to understand how different people perceive power by describing sources of power as coercion, rewards, legitimacy, expertise, reference, information, and connection.

KEY TERMS

achievement
affiliation
connection power
empowerment
expert power
information power

legitimate power
power
referent power
reward power and
    coercive power
sources of power

REVIEW QUESTIONS

1. The most effective nurses use power
   A. in one primary way.
   B. to influence others or affect others' thinking or behaviour.
   C. predominantly at an organizational level.
   D. only to gain the necessary resources to be a better nurse.

2. Power has been described in the literature
   A. consistently as a negative concept.
   B. most often as a manifestation of personal ambition.
   C. as maintained through one's position in society, a work setting, or family.
   D. in multiple ways, some not so positive.

3. When people fear another person enough to act or behave differently from how they would otherwise, the source of the other person's power is called
   A. coercive power.
   B. reward power.
   C. expert power.
   D. connection power.

4. What source of power has become increasingly important because of technological innovation in the past decade?
   A. Expert power
   B. Information power
   C. Connection power
   D. Legitimate power

5. Nurses disempower themselves by
   A. facilitating the participation of others in decision making.
   B. taking action within an environment where there is an equitable distribution of power.

C. believing they are empowered.
D. discounting the role the media plays in the public's perception of nursing.

6. A nurse's personal power can be enhanced by
   A. collaborating with colleagues on special projects outside the work setting.
   B. developing skills that do not apply directly to client care.
   C. volunteering to serve on organizational committees led by people who are not nurses.
   D. all of the above

REVIEW ACTIVITIES

1. Identify a nursing leader. Observe this person and note the type of power this leader uses to meet objectives.

2. Watch a television show that portrays nurses. Note how nurses use or do not use the different types of power available to them. What do you observe?

3. Observe our national leaders. What examples of the use of power do you see? Is power used in helpful or unhelpful ways? Explain.

EXPLORING THE WEB

- Which sites can you visit for information on nursing leaders and nursing history?

  http://www.cna-nurses.ca/CNA/practice/advanced/dialogue/default_e.aspx

  http://www.chsrf.ca/research_themes/pdf/NLOP_e.pdf

  http://www.longwoods.com/home.php?cat=252

  www.chsrf.ca/research_themes/nlop_e.php

- Which sites can you visit for information on power, leadership, and women?

  http://www.guide2womenleaders.com/

  http://www.elcinfo.com/initiatives_senior_wallst.htm

  http://www.atkinson.yorku.ca/~dce/Programs/Certificates/CTLW/CTLW_Desc.html

- What sites support political power for clients?

  http://www.nursingworld.org/ojin/topic32/tpc32_4.htm

  http://nursingworld.org/AJN/2002/sept/wawatch.htm

  http://www.i2i.org/main/article.php?article_id=1112

  http://www.healthcarereform.net

- Which sites discuss a variety of nursing resources and issues, including collective power?

http://www.cna-nurses.ca/cna/default_e.aspx

http://www.nursingworld.org

- Go to the site for the Ontario Training Centre for Health Services and Policy

http://www.otc-hsr.ca/

- Note the onsite and online courses offered to nurses interested in health policy.

- What are some other sites related to health policy?

http://www.cihr-irsc.gc.ca/e/13733.html

http://chspr.queensu.ca/

http://www.chspr.ubc.ca/

http://www.msfhr.org/sub-health.htm

REFERENCES

Bothamley, J. (1993). *Dictionary of theories*. London: Gale Research International.

Bower, F. L. (2000). *Nurses taking the lead: Personal qualities of effective leadership*. Philadelphia: Saunders.

Disch, J. (2000). Nurse executive: Make the glue red. *Journal of Professional Nursing, 16*(4), 189.

Ferguson, S. L. (2001). An activist looks at nursing's role in health policy development. *Journal of Obstetric, Gynecologic, and Neonatal Nursing, 30*(5), 546–551.

Fisher, J. L., & Koch, J. V. (1996). *Presidential leadership: Making a difference*. Phoenix, AZ: American Council on Education and The Oryx Press.

Greenberg, J., & Baron, R. (2000). *Behavior in organizations* (7th ed.). Upper Saddle River, NJ: Prentice Hall.

Hibberd, J. M., & Smith, D. L. (2006). *Nursing leadership and management in Canada* (3rd ed.). Toronto: Elsevier Canada.

Kelly, L. Y., & Joel, L. A. (1996). *The nursing experience: Trends, challenges, and transitions* (3rd ed.). New York: McGraw-Hill.

Laschinger, H. K. S., & Wong, C. (1999). Staff nurse empowerment and collective accountability: Effect on perceived productivity and self-rated work effectiveness. *Nursing Economic$, 17*(6), 308–316.

Machiavelli, N. (1996). *The prince* (P. Sonnino, trans.). Atlantic Highlands, NJ: Humanities Press International, Inc. (Original work published 1532.)

Nasrabadi, A. N., Lipsion, J. G., & Emami, A. (2004). Professional nursing in Iran: An overview of its historical and sociocultural framework. *Professional Nurse, 20*(6), 396–402.

Rowland, H. S., & Rowland, B. L. (1997). *Nursing administration handbook*. Rockville, MD: Aspen.

SUGGESTED READINGS

Anderson, M. A. (2001). *Nursing leadership, management, and professional practice for the LPN/LVN* (2nd ed). Philadelphia: F. A. Davis Company.

Belle, F. (2002). Women managers and organizational power. *Women in Management Review, 17*(3/4), 151–156.

Benner, P. E. (2000). *From novice to expert: Excellence and power in clinical nursing practice* (commemorative edition). Upper Saddle River, NJ: Prentice Hall.

Denis, J. L., Lamoth, L., & Langley, A. (2001). The dynamics of collective leadership and strategic change in pluralistic organizations. *Academy of Management Journal, 44*(4), 809–837.

Government Technology (any recent issue). (Available free online at www.govtech.net or by writing to Government Technology at 100 Blue Ravine Road, Folsom, CA 95630.) Addresses the information age and the power of information.

Hanna, L. A. (1999). Lead the way. *Nursing Management, 30*(11), 36–39.

Laschinger, H. K. S., & Shamian, J. (1994). Staff nurses' and managers' perceptions of job-related empowerment and managerial self-efficacy. *Journal of Nursing Administration, 24*(10), 38–47.

Leddy, S., & Pepper, J. M. (1998). *Conceptual bases of professional nursing* (4th ed.). Philadelphia: Lippincott.

Mason, D. J., Talbott, S. W., & Leavitt, J. K. (1993). *Policy and politics for nurses: Action and change in the workplace, government, organizations and community*. Philadelphia: Saunders.

Short, P. M. (1998). Empowering leadership. *Contemporary Education, 69*(2), 70–72.

Spitzer, K. L., Eisenbery, M. B., & Lowe, C. A. (1998). *Information literacy essential skills for the information age*. Syracuse, NY: ERIC Clearinghouse on Information & Technology.

Stelter, N. (2002). Gender differences in leadership: Current social issues and future organizational implications. *Journal of Leadership and Organizational Studies, 8*(4), 88–99.

Wilson, B., & Laschinger, H. S. (1994). Staff nurse perceptions of job empowerment and organizational commitment: A rest of Kanter's theory of structural power in organizations. *Journal of Nursing Administration, 24*(4S), 39–47.

CHAPTER ENDNOTE

1. Health Canada, Health Care System, "Findings from the 2005 National Survey of the Work and Health of Nurses." Retrieved from http://www.hc-sc.gc.ca/hcs-sss/pubs/care-soins/2005-nurse-infirm/index_e.html, April 2, 2007.

CHAPTER 17

Managing Performance and Outcomes Using an Organizational Quality Improvement Model

Mary McLaughlin, RN, MBA
Karen Houston, RN, MS
Adapted by: Heather Crawford, BScN, MEd, CHE

Opportunity is missed by most people because it is dressed in overalls and looks like work.
(Thomas Edison)

OBJECTIVES

Upon completion of this chapter, the reader should be able to:

1. Articulate the major principles of quality and continuous quality improvement (CQI), including customer identification; the need for participation at all levels; and a focus on improving the process, not criticizing individual performance.

2. Describe how quality improvement affects the client and the organization.

3. Identify how data are utilized for CQI (e.g., time series data, Pareto charts).

4. Describe the difference between risk management and CQI.

5. Describe how the principles of CQI are implemented in an organization.

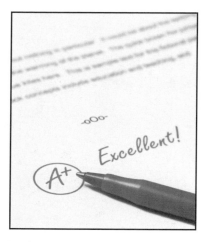

We Survived Accreditation! ... What Did They Say?

The surveyors reported that the Child Health Program is thriving and CCHSA's [Canadian Council on Health Services Accreditation] ratings were higher than our self-assessment ratings. They gave particular kudos to DERCA [Diabetes Education Research for Children and Adolescents], The Maestro Project, and Asthma care, by listing these as a "Good Practices." Good Practices will be listed in the next CCHSA Annual Report as an example for centres across Canada to strive for.

Is It All Over?

It's never over—Quality Improvement is continuous! The accreditation survey visit will be in November 2008, but there is much work to be done in the meantime. We need to keep doing what we do best—monitoring indicators, making continuous quality improvements, and including expert parents on working groups and committees. The surveyors identified some specific areas for improvement: increasing timely access to MRI's including access to procedural sedation, strengthening the consent process for the administration of chemotherapy or blood products, increasing pharmacy support for the St. Boniface Hospital NICU [neonatal intensive care unit] and Women's Hospital Intermediate Care Nursery (IMCN), working with Public Health to increase vaccination coverage for preventable diseases, providing clearer information to parents, developing a comprehensive infection prevention and control surveillance program, and considering a redevelopment that would locate the HSC [Winnipeg Health Sciences Centre] NICU closer to the labour floor and IMCN. Many of these improvements will require leadership from the top and collaboration with other programs. The Accreditation Survey has been a very worthwhile exercise to help guide and focus us on specific quality improvements initiatives while at the same time maintaining the high level of care and service we currently provide. It has also reminded us of the value of the work we do and how much our patients and their families appreciate it. Let's continue to "Work Together for Healthier Children"!

Source: Hoare, K., & Cronin, G. (2006). We survived accreditation! ... What did they say? Child Health Quality Team, *Quality for Kids Newsletter, 5*(1), 1. Reprinted with Permission.

Continuous quality improvement has been shown to be a powerful tool to help make health care organizations more effective. Rondeau and Wagar (2002) report that it is generally believed that the failure of most total quality management (TQM) and continuous quality improvement programs is not the result of flaws in either the philosophy or the principles of quality improvement but the result of ineffective implementation systems. These sources of failure include a lack of commitment and understanding on the part of organizational leaders and ineffective management of the change process. The improvement philosophies of quality experts, such as Deming (1986) and Crosby (1989), also emphasize the commitment of management.

Quality improvement is described as both a science and an art. The science of improvement is the development of new ideas, the testing of those ideas, and the implementation of change. As Langley, Nolan, Norman, Provost, and Nolan (1996) described, W. Edwards Deming has provided an important contribution to the science of improvement. Deming's components of appreciating a system, understanding variation, and applying knowledge and psychology are fundamental improvement principles. Quality improvement is also described as an art that taps into creative, out-of-the-box ideas. It is about systematically testing new ideas to improve customer care. Health care customers are clients, families, staff, community, and agencies, to name a few. If the change is planned, measured, and does not negatively affect the quality of customer care, there are limitless boundaries to what can be achieved.

Adapting the concepts of science and art in improving health care can create an enthusiasm for change and a passion for results. This chapter will discuss and provide examples of the application and implementation of quality improvement principles in a health care setting.

HISTORY OF QUALITY ASSURANCE

Berwick et al. (1991) suggested a tremendous amount of waste and rework were a result of process complexity. Some studies suggest the amount of waste and rework can amount to 25 to 30 percent of total costs of production. Consider Berwick and Plsek's red bead example (1992):

In a group of beads in a bag, there are 90 blue beads and 10 red beads. There are four workers whose job it is to take blue beads out of a bag. They cannot see what colour bead they are taking. The supervisor watches to see how many red beads are pulled out of the bag. The first day, worker A has 1 red bead, worker B has 4 red beads, worker C has 3 red beads, and worker D has 2 red beads. The supervisor states that worker A has done a great job

CRITICAL THINKING

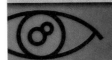

Children with cancer, who present to an Emergency Department (ED), with a fever and who have a low white blood cell count (Febrile Neutropenia) require timely assessment and administration of antibiotics. In December, 2003, a Child Health Standards audit indicated the average time from triage to antibiotic administration was 5 hours. Opportunities for improvement were identified.

A working group, established in June 2004, developed a physicians' standard order sheet that was implemented in the Children's Hospital ED in December 2004. During the next year, twenty-four children were admitted from the ED to the inpatient oncology unit with Febrile Neutropenia. An analysis of the charts has shown that the average time from triage to antibiotic administration has decreased to 1.46 hours—a significant improvement in providing safe and timely care (see Figure 17-1).

Congratulations to the ED staff for all their support of and interest in this initiative. Thank you to the members of the Febrile Neutropenia Working Group.

What would you have done to improve the quality of care? How could you bring your ideas to other staff members without making them feel that the quality of their care was being criticized? What measures would you use to ensure that while you were improving some aspects of care, you were not decreasing other critical outcome measures?

Source: Galloway, L. (2006). Improving timeliness of care. *Quality for Kids Newsletter, 5*(1), 2. Reprinted with Permission.

and worker B has done a terrible job. He tells them they have to improve. The beads go back in the bag and they start over the next day. This day, worker A has 4 red beads, worker B has 0 red beads, worker C has 2 red beads, and worker D has 4 red beads. The supervisor praises worker B for the improvement and yells at workers A and D for not doing a good job. The truth is these workers do not have any ability to change the number of red beads that they pull out of the bag.

This example demonstrates random variation. Using inspection in systems to reward or punish random variation results in tampering with the system rather than quality improvement. Instead of improving the process, the tampering encourages staff to look for someone to blame rather than to change the process to improve outcomes. So the question is, how much variability do we expect? Variability can be calculated on a time series chart, which is discussed in more detail later in the chapter (see p. 309).

Quality assurance (QA) emerged in health care in the 1950s. It began as an inspection approach to ensure that health care institutions—mainly hospitals—maintained minimum standards of care. For example, nurses remember completing chart audits to determine whether or not bowel movements had been documented on the graphic vital signs sheet! The use of QA grew over time. QA departments became the organizational mechanism for measuring performance against standards and reporting incidents and errors, such as mortality and morbidity rates. This approach was reactive and fixed the errors after a problem was

noted. QA's methods consisted primarily of chart audits of various client diagnoses and procedures. The method was thought to be punitive, with its emphasis on "doing it right," and did little to sustain change or proactively identify problems before they occurred. The culture was one of blame versus learn. It did, however, accomplish the task of monitoring minimum standards of performance.

TOTAL QUALITY MANAGEMENT

Total quality management (TQM), also referred to as continuous quality improvement (CQI) and **performance improvement (PI),** began in the manufacturing industry with W. Edwards Deming and Joseph Juran in the 1950s. The total quality management approach revolutionized the industrial world with the search for manufacturing excellence through higher productivity, lower cost and a competitive edge. Deming is credited with being the main generating force in Japan's post–World War II rise to manufacturing excellence as a world industrial leader. The lessons learned from Deming's strategy for quality are applicable to the achievement of excellence and quality in health care management.[1]

Seeman and Brown (2006) reviewed Peter Drucker's most significant writings, including his prediction, in the 1940s, of the rise of the knowledge worker. They conducted an empirical review of his impact on contemporary quality improvement principles in health care by examining academic citations to his work and ideas. In their article, Seeman and Brown cited Drucker's 1988

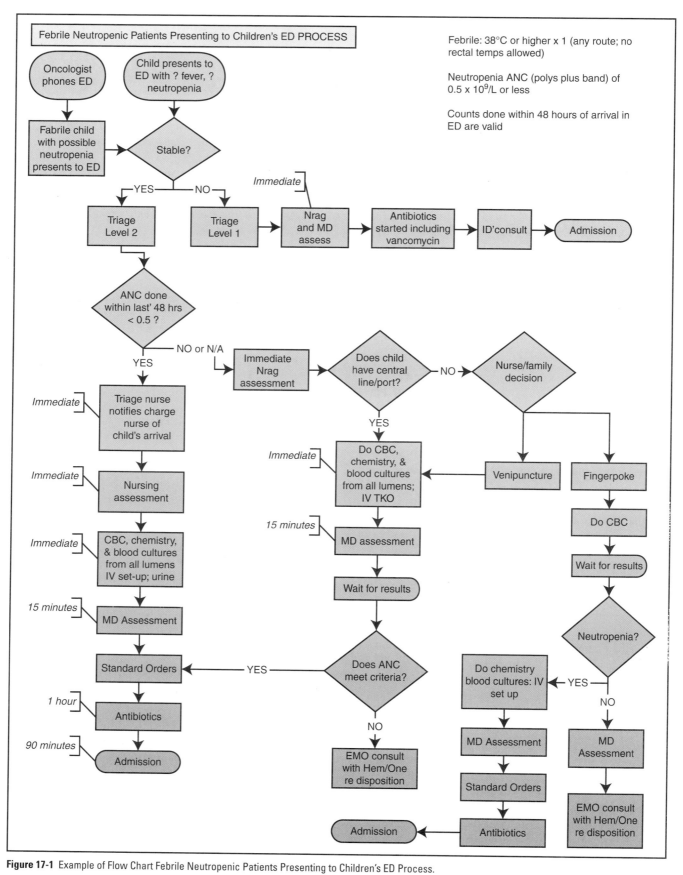

Figure 17-1 Example of Flow Chart Febrile Neutropenic Patients Presenting to Children's ED Process.

Source: Galloway, L. (2006). Improving timeliness of care, *Child Health Quality Team, Quality for Kids Newsletter, 5*(1), 2. Reprinted with Permission.

TABLE 17-1	DIFFERENCE IN FOCUS BETWEEN QUALITY ASSURANCE AND CONTINUOUS QUALITY IMPROVEMENT

Focus of Quality Assurance (doing it right)

1. Assessing or measuring performance

2. Determining whether performance conforms to standards

3. Improving performance when standards are not met

Focus of Continuous Quality Improvement (doing the right thing)

1. Meeting the needs of the customer

2. Building quality performance into the work process

3. Assessing the work process to identify opportunities for improved performance

4. Employing a scientific approach to assessment and problem solving

5. Improving performance continuously as a management strategy, not just when standards are not met

article, "The Coming of the New Organization" published in the *Harvard Business Review* (Drucker, 1988). According to Drucker, efficiencies could be achieved through formalizing communication and information-sharing across the organizations, and he identified hospitals specifically as knowledge-based organizations.

TQM, CQI, and PI are terms that are frequently interchanged. For the purposes of this chapter, **continuous quality improvement (CQI)** will be referred to as a systematic process used to improve outcomes based on customers' needs. This proactive approach emphasizes "doing the right thing" for customers, and the end result of this method is to satisfy customers. The goal of CQI is to consistently meet or exceed the needs of clients, families, staff, health professionals, and community. This approach was integrated into the health care industry in the 1980s when cost and quality of care pressures were steadily increasing. Movement into QI is thought to be more an overall management approach than a single program. Integrating concepts of quality into daily organizational operations are key to successful outcomes. Table 17-1 notes the difference in focus between quality assurance and quality improvement.

GENERAL PRINCIPLES OF QUALITY IMPROVEMENT

Quality improvement is a structured system for creating organization-wide participation and partnership in planning and implementing continuous improvement methods to understand and meet or exceed customer needs and expectations. Quality principles include the following:

1. The priority is to benefit clients and all other internal and external customers.
2. Quality is achieved through the participation of everyone in the organization.
3. Improvement opportunities are developed by focusing on the work process.
4. Decisions to change or improve a system or process are made based on data.
5. Improvement of the quality of service is a continuous process.
6. Committed leadership is necessary to make it happen.
7. Both education and long-term commitment are required.

Early QA literature focused on fixing problems, "doing it right," and having zero defects. Over time, a gap was found between theory and practice. It was determined that quality is not about being perfect. First, it is about being better, doing things right the first time. This approach increases an organization's chances of survival during highly turbulent and competitive times.

Second, quality is about health care professionals seeing themselves as having customers or clients. The notion of "customer" or "client" requires major shifts in mind-set for the health care professional. These terms are frequently used in business, and referring to a patient as a customer or a client was initially thought to undermine the professional care provided to patients. Designing health care processes from the customer's point of view versus the professional's point of view is a challenge and requires changes in thinking and redesign of health care processes. Health care involves work processes in which one step leads to the next step. Improving these steps in the work process is an important part of improving care and customer satisfaction. Customer satisfaction is rooted in the way health professionals treat their clients/ customers and in the quality of their outcomes. Having the goal of astounding clients with quality in every interaction is key to achieving satisfaction and loyalty.

Third, quality directs health professionals to give their customers more than the basics so that they will recommend and demand these services. This goal is achieved by proactively seizing opportunities to perform better, driving for quality consistently and continuously, and not waiting for a problem to be pointed out or for pressure from an external stakeholder to improve. Improvements are sustained over time when interdisciplinary teams collaborate and decisions about change are supported by data.

The primary benefits of adopting quality concepts and principles include discovering performance issues more quickly and efficiently by looking at every problem as an opportunity for improvement; involvement of staff in how the work is designed and carried out to improve staff satisfaction; and empowering staff to identify and implement change. Other quality concepts are increasing the customer's perception that you care by designing health care work processes to meet the customer's needs, rather than the health care provider's needs, and decreasing unnecessary costs from waste and rework, lost time, and not meeting provincial requirements. These quality concepts should be emphasized until they become work habits and part of an organization's daily operations.

CUSTOMERS IN HEALTH CARE

A customer is anyone who receives the output of your efforts. There are internal and external customers. An internal customer is anyone who works within the organization and receives the output of another employee. Internal customers include health care staff, such as physicians, nurses, pharmacists, physical therapists, respiratory therapists, occupational therapists, pastoral caregivers, and so on. An external customer is anyone who is outside the organization and receives the output of the organization. Clients are external customers, but they are not the only external customers. Other external customers include private physicians; insurance companies, such as Blue Cross; government departments, such as Health Canada; the Canadian Council on Health Services Accreditation (CCHSA); and the community you serve.

PARTICIPATION OF EVERYONE IN THE ORGANIZATION

CQI is achieved through the participation of everyone in the organization at all levels. A participation and empowerment initiative must be built by first offering employees the opportunity for appropriate involvement. An organization that encourages empowerment promotes a culture of employee ownership, characterized by employees who do the following:

■ Take responsibility for the success or failure of an organization
■ Take an active part in developing new ways of doing things
■ Trust that their efforts are valued

A new staff member can participate in the design and improvement of daily work practices and processes on an individual, unit, or organizational level. For example, as an individual, a nurse could change the organization of her day to spend more time with clients' families. On a unit level, a nurse could work with others on the unit to make the client report more time efficient. On an organizational level, a nurse could suggest that the process for notifying the pharmacy about a missing medication could be improved, and the nurse could participate on a team to find a solution.

All members of the staff are encouraged to participate in quality improvement processes, including physicians, registered nurses, physical therapists, occupational therapists, speech language technologists, pharmacists, community case management workers, social workers, medical technologists, and any member of the health care team who cares for clients or contributes to the care of clients. The goal of CQI efforts, as well as the process being worked on, determines who participates on the team.

For example, if you were trying to decrease the time a client waits outside the radiology unit for a test, your CQI efforts would need to include the client transportation staff, unit clerks, unit registered nurses, and radiology staff. If you were trying to ensure that clients with congestive heart failure are discharged understanding the importance of weighing themselves daily, you would need the participation of the cardiac unit's registered nurse, the clinical dietician, home care association staff, the primary care physician, the cardiologist, the pharmacist, and a client and a client's family.

The key to determine who participates is including the point-of-care staff: the workers on the front line who do the direct care involved in the work process you are trying to change. These people have the most knowledge of the work process so they can look for potential areas of improvement. Staff should have a clearly identified way to suggest improvement opportunities that they see in

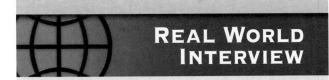

REAL WORLD INTERVIEW

I am more excited every day as I see nurses, physicians and others embrace the concept of quality improvement. Initially, the process was tedious, because there was skepticism, but as ideas were introduced, implemented, and were successful, the enthusiasm rose exponentially. Our decisions are based on clinically relevant data. It is important to gain support from key players who have to deal with the implementation of any change.

Sharon Townsend, BScN
Quality Officer

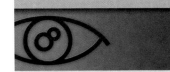

CRITICAL THINKING

In the original scenario at the start of this chapter, the Child Health Team had successfully completed an accreditation review. Although commendations were made, some areas for improvement were noted. One of the areas for improvement was to strengthen the consent process for the administration of chemotherapy or blood products.

What suggestions would you make to the team? What processes would be involved? How could the processes be improved? Who would participate with you to identify ways to strengthen the consent process?

their day-to-day work. For example, an X-ray technologist may note steps in the process of scheduling and transporting clients that create a long wait time for X-ray testing. A mechanism for suggesting improvement in the radiology department would encourage the technologist to suggest and test ideas for change.

FOCUS ON IMPROVEMENT OF THE HEALTH CARE WORK PROCESS

Improvement opportunities are focused on the process of work that the health care team delivers. The dictionary defines a **process** as a series of actions, changes, or functions bringing about a result. All work processes have inputs, steps, and outputs. An example of a work process is a client attending a preoperative clinic. All the steps of the preoperative visit can be measured. These steps are then reviewed, applying evidence-based principles, as appropriate, to improve client care. Steps may be eliminated or changed and then standardized so that all staff use the improved work process.

IMPROVEMENT OF THE SYSTEM

A **system** is an interdependent group of items, people, or processes with a common purpose (Langley et al., 1996). In a system, the processes as well as the relationships among the processes lead to the outcome. You can improve the outcome by examining these processes and relationships. In a system, every step of a process affects the following step. For example, if the X-ray staff members place the client who has had a chest X-ray in the hall and call transportation to take the client back to his room but do not consider the transportation process, they may decrease the total time a client is in radiology but

increase the client's time in the hall waiting for transportation. You cannot improve care unless you review all the steps in the system's process.

A CONTINUOUS PROCESS

Improvement of quality of service is a continuous process. Walter Shewhart, the director of Bell Laboratories in the mid-1920s, is credited for the concept of the cycle of continuous improvement. This concept suggests that products or services are designed and made based on knowledge about the customer. Those products or services are marketed to and judged by the customer. As the customer makes judgments, changes are made to improve the product or service (Al-Assaf & Schmele, 1997). Hence, the process of QI is continuous, because it is linked to changing customer needs and judgments.

IMPROVEMENT BASED ON DATA

Decisions to change or improve a system or process are made based on data. When someone says, "the clients are waiting too long to return from radiology," it is time to look at the data. Review the wait time data to see whether wait times are increasing. The data will clarify these claims.

Using data correctly is important. Data should be used for learning, not for judging. It is critical to look at work processes rather than people for improvement opportunities. In the radiology example, if we jumped to the conclusion that someone was not doing his job correctly, we might criticize the transportation staff person who returned the client from radiology. This approach would not foster improvement ideas. By not analyzing the process (e.g., the client has a chest X-ray, is put in hall, a clerk calls transportation, the transportation clerk pages transportation aide, and so on) and the relationships among the processes (e.g., waiting times between calls, transportation phone process, page system, and so on), we could miss finding where the real improvement opportunity lies. Perhaps it has nothing to do with the transportation person who returned the client to the room. The actual root cause may be a long delay in the paging system. Reviewing the wait time data is an example of examining the process, not the people carrying out the process.

IMPLICATIONS FOR CLIENT CARE

The implications of quality improvement for client care can be measured by the overall value of care. Value is a function of both quality outcomes and cost.

Outcomes can be a client's clinical or functional outcomes. For example, did the client live, can the client go back to work? Outcomes can also be measured by client satisfaction. For example, would the client recommend this health care facility to someone else?

Cost is the cost of both direct and indirect client care needs. Direct cost is the cost of the care of the client: for example, cost of medications, operating room equipment, and direct client caregiver salaries. **Indirect costs** are the costs of other care activities, including utility costs, such as electricity, and salaries of those who are not involved in direct client care, such as secretaries, unit clerks, and human resource staff.

$$Value = \frac{Quality\ of\ outcomes}{Cost}$$

In most QI efforts, as quality is improved by standardizing care delivery processes and applying evidence-based principles, the cost of care decreases.

METHODOLOGIES FOR QUALITY IMPROVEMENT

Several models outline methodologies for quality improvement. One is reviewed here: the FOCUS-PDSA quality improvement model [Plan Do Study Act (PDSA) Cycle and the FOCUS methodology]. Improvement comes from the application of knowledge (Langley et al., 1996). Thus, any approach to improvement must be based on building and applying knowledge. (This acronym is also known as FOCUS-PDCA—Plan Do Check Act (PDCA) Cycle and the FOCUS methodology).

THE PLAN DO STUDY ACT CYCLE

The PDSA Cycle starts with three questions:

1. What are we trying to accomplish?
2. How will we know that a change is an improvement?
3. What changes can we make that will result in improvement?

As these questions are being answered, testing needs to be done to evaluate the effect of a proposed change and to learn about different alternatives (see Figure 17-2). The goal is to increase the ability to predict the effect that one or more

---

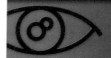

CRITICAL THINKING

Winnipeg Children's Hospital has joined a Canadian Collaborative on Medication Reconciliation. The Collaborative was a joint initiative of the Canadian Association of Pediatric Health Centres and the Canadian Patient Safety Institute's Safer Healthcare Now! campaign. Medication reconciliation is a formal process of obtaining a complete and current list of each client's current home medications, including name, dosage, frequency, and route, and comparing it to the physician's admission, transfer and/or discharge orders. Discrepancies are brought to the attention of the prescriber, and if appropriate, changes are made and documented. There are three types of discrepancies: intentional discrepancy, where the physician makes an intentional change and the choice is clearly documented; undocumented intentional discrepancy, where the physician makes an intentional choice to change, but it is not clearly documented; and unintentional discrepancy, where the physician unintentionally changed, added, or omitted a medication that the client was taking prior to admission. The second and third choices put the clients at risk of a medication error.

What kind of process can you envision implementing to determine the rate of discrepancy? What potential recommendations can you make regarding the care provided to the clients?

(Adapted from Galloway, L., Caligiuri, C., & Epp, G. (2006). Medication reconciliation, *Child Health Quality Team, Quality for Kids Newsletter, 5*(1), 3)

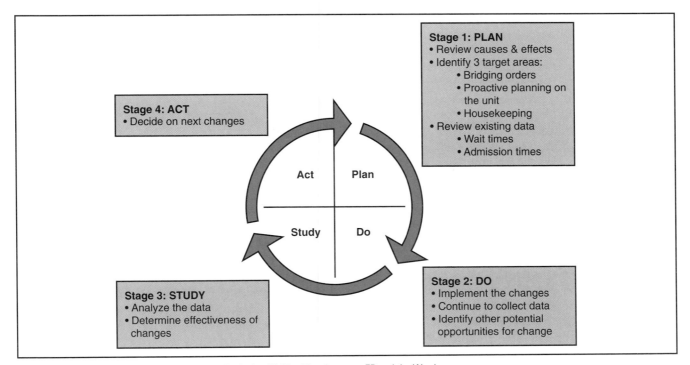

Figure 17-2 Plan/Do/Study/Act (PDSA) Example: Reducing Waiting Time between ER and the Ward.

Source: Hoare, K. (2003). What is PDSA? Child Health Quality Team, *Quality for Kids Newsletter, 2*(2), 1. Reprinted with Permission.

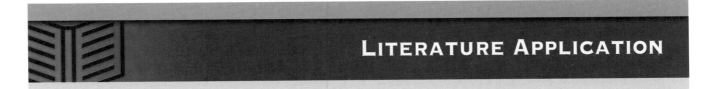

LITERATURE APPLICATION

Citation: Aldarrab, A. (2006). Application of Lean Six Sigma for patients presenting with ST-elevation myocardial infarction: The Hamilton Health Sciences experience. *Healthcare Quarterly, 9*(1), 56–61.

Discussion: The Hamilton Health Sciences (HHS), a three-site tertiary/quaternary care facility, with thrombolysis available at all three sites, and percutaneous coronary intervention available at only one site during limited hours, combined the principles of the FOCUS-PDCA quality improvement model with a Lean Six Sigma approach, to apply the American College of Cardiology and American Heart Association guidelines to their clinical setting.

Implications for Practice: The systemic application of a continuous quality improvement model using evidence-based guidelines can successfully optimize a process to create a new model of health care delivery. In addition, cooperative links throughout the organization were developed and strengthened.

changes would have if they were implemented (Langley et al., 1996). The plan for testing should cover who will do what, when they will do it, and where they will do it. Using the PDSA cycle encourages ongoing quality improvement.

THE FOCUS METHODOLOGY

The FOCUS methodology describes in a stepwise process how to move through the improvement process (see Figure 17-3).

F: Focus on an improvement idea. This step asks the question, Is there a problem? During this phase, an improvement opportunity is articulated and data are obtained to support the hypothesis that an opportunity for improvement exists.

O: Organize a team that understands the process. Identify a group of staff members (i.e., key players) who are direct participants in the process to be examined—the point-of-care staff. A team leader is identified who will appoint team members.

Table 1 FOCUS-PDCA model for AMI project	
F	Find a process for improvement opportunity (purpose, determine if there is a problem)
O	Organize a team who understands the process (key players)
C	Clarify the current knowledge of the process (process mapping)
U	Uncover the root cause of variation and poor quality (root cause analysis) Use data analysis
S	Select the process improvement and clarify the aim of goal
P	Plan the process improvement and data collection
D	Do the improvement data collection and analysis
C	Check/study the result of improvement and lessons learned
A	Act to hold the gain by adopting, adjusting or abandoning the change

Figure 17-3 FOCUS-PDCA model for AMI (acute myocardial infarction) project.

Source: Aldarrab, A. (2006). Application of Lean Six Sigma for patients presenting with ST-elevation myocardial infarction: The Hamilton Health Sciences experience. *Healthcare Quarterly, 9* (1), 56–61. Reprinted with Permission.

C: Clarify what is happening in the current process. A flow diagram (see Figure 17-4) is very helpful for identifying and understanding the current flow of events, and for determining where standardization might be possible. A detailed flowchart can be analyzed in two ways to uncover possible problems—at a macro level and at a micro level.

At the macro level, scan the flowchart for any indication that the process is broken. Red flags include the following:

- Many steps that represent quality checks or inspections for errors. Too many boxes in your flow diagram that describe similar steps could indicate rework or a lack of clarity in roles.
- Areas in the process that are not well understood or cannot be defined. If the process cannot be defined well, you can be certain it is not being performed efficiently, with maximized outcomes.
- Many wait times between processes. Wait times should always be minimized to improve efficiency of the process.
- Multiple paths that show lots of people involved in the activity or delivering the service to the customer. The involvement of too many staff is wasteful and confusing to the client.

    If the process seems reasonable, with one or two areas needing improvement, then a micro-level analysis of your flow diagram is needed.

- Examine decision symbols (i.e., diamonds) that represent quality inspection activities. Can these activities be eliminated? Do some errors go

undetected? Is the check redundant? This examination will ensure limited rework and maximum clarity.

- Examine each process in the diagram for redundancy and value. If a step is repeated or does not have any value for the customer, it should be eliminated.
- Examine processes for waiting time areas. The process should be changed to eliminate these wait times.
- Examine all processes for rework loops. A step should not be repeated. Resources are always limited, especially in hospitals today.
- Check that handoffs are smooth and necessary. Handoffs are times when a process is passed from one staff person or department to another. Handoffs always leave room for error. They are also common times for wait areas. During this phase, cause-and-effect diagrams and Pareto charts can be helpful. These tools are discussed on pages 309–311.

U: Understand the degree of change needed. In this stage, the team reviews what it knows and enhances its knowledge by reviewing the literature, available data, and competitive benchmarks. How are other health care organizations doing the process?

S: Solution: Select a solution for improvement. The team can brainstorm and then choose the best solution. It can then use the PDCA Cycle to test this solution. An implementation plan should be used to track progress and the steps required. This implementation plan can be in the

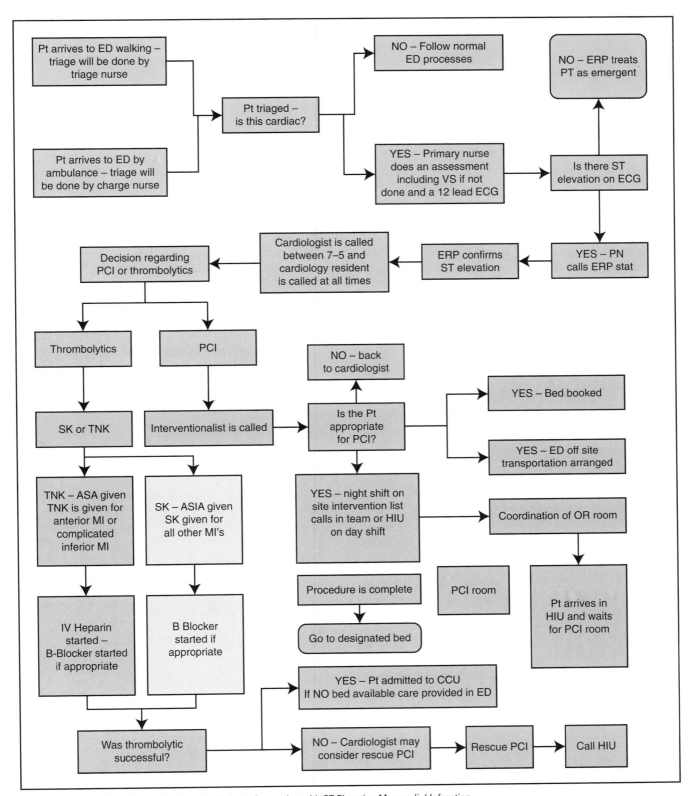

Figure 17-4 Application of Lean Six Sigma for Patients Presenting with ST-Elevation Myocardial Infarction.

Source: Aldarrab, A. (2006) Application of Lean Six Sigma for patients presenting with ST-elevation myocardial infarction: The Hamilton Health Sciences experience. *Healthcare Quarterly, 9*(1), 56–61. Reprinted with Permission.

TABLE 17-2 — CAUSES AND BRAINSTORMED SOLUTIONS OF DELAY FROM DOOR TO ECG TIME

Causes	Brainstormed Solutions
▪ Level of skill of new nurses	▪ Buddying with experienced nurses and education
▪ Availability of primary nurse	▪ ECG technician to do all ECGs
	▪ To look at nurse: patient ratio
	▪ Retention of staff
	▪ Healthy work environment
▪ Availability of bed	▪ Designated bed for ECGs
	▪ To always have one bed ready for the next patient arriving in the ED (12)
	▪ ECG technician to do all ECGs
	▪ EMS to do prehospital 12 lead ECG
▪ ECG machines/supplies	▪ Need for new/more machines with 15 lead capability
	▪ Use medical diagnosis unit machines during night time hours to add resources
	▪ Synchronization of clocks and ECG machines (digitalized clocks)
▪ Triage assessment	▪ Standard scales to ensure consistent triage
	▪ Triage nurses not to be pulled to regular nurse relief duties
	▪ Clarification of triage/charge nurse roles
	▪ Central bed manager on days
	▪ Use more experienced nurses in the triage role
	▪ Feedback loop to the ED nurses and MDs regarding meeting the timeline goals
	▪ Continuous education

Source: Aldarrab, A. (2006) Application of Lean Six Sigma for Patients presenting with ST-elevation myocardial infarction: The Hamilton Health Sciences experience. *Healthcare Quarterly, 9*(1), 56–61. Reprinted with Permission.

Activity	Responsible	July	Aug	Sept	Oct	Nov
Discuss move with staff	Manager	X				
Form an ad hoc planning group	Team Leader	X				
Receive report from group re: order of move	Team Leader and Manager		X			
Discuss report with staff	Manager, Team Leader and Staff		X			
Notify other departments			X	X		
Prepare offices in new building	Staff		X	X		
Pack office contents	Staff			X		
Move into new space and unpack	Staff				X	
Evaluate the moving process	Staff, Manager, Team Leader				X	
Make recommendations re: future moves	Staff, Manager, Team Leader					X

Figure 17-5 Example of a GANTT Chart: Preparation for an Office Move.

form of a work plan or Gantt chart. A Gantt chart is a chart in the form of a table that identifies what activity is to be completed, who is responsible for it, and when is it going to be completed (see Figure 17-5). It outlines the steps needed to implement the change.

Improvement strategies identified at the organizational level involve benchmarking, meeting government requirements, identifying opportunities for system changes following sentinel event review, using a balanced scorecard, and using a storyboard.

OTHER IMPROVEMENT STRATEGIES

BENCHMARKING

Benchmarking is the continual and collaborative discipline of measuring and comparing the results of key work processes with those of the best performers. Learning how to adapt these best practices can help to achieve breakthrough process improvement and build healthier communities (Gift & Mosel, 1994). Benchmarking focuses on key services or processes; for example, length of time in the operating room for a total hip replacement or length of stay in hospital post-procedure. A benchmark study will identify gaps in performance and provide options for selection of processes to improve, ideas for redesign of care delivery, and ideas for better ways of meeting customer expectation (Youngberg, 1998).

REGULATORY REQUIREMENTS

The Canadian Council on Health Services Accreditation (CCHSA) assists health organizations across the country to examine and improve the quality of care and the service they provide to their clients. The AIM Project (achieving improved measurement) was implemented in 2000. See Chapter 1, page 19, for further discussion on the AIM Project and the CCHSA accreditation process.

Accreditation is an ongoing cycle. It starts when a health care organization first applies to become accredited and subsequently prepares for an accreditation visit and review, by setting objectives and building teams. The purpose of establishing the teams is not only to prepare for the accreditation survey but also to assist with ongoing processes related to quality improvement and operations. The organization then assesses whether it complies with the national standards, submits its self assessment, and is evaluated by an external team of independent peer reviewers when the CCHSA survey team visits. Following conclusion of the site visit, the facility

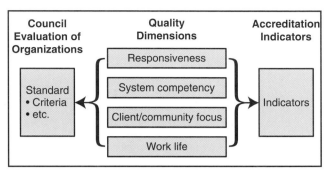

Figure 17-6 Link between CCHSA Standards, Quality Dimensions and Indicators.

Source: Health Canada. (2000). Link between indicators, quality dimension and accreditation standards. *Quest for quality in Canadian health care: Continuous quality improvement*, p. 162. Retrieved from http://www.hc-sc.gc.ca/hcs-sss/pubs/care-soins/2000-qual/indicat_e.html, March 15, 2007. Reprinted with permission from the Minister of Public Works and Government Services Canada, 2007.

receives a brief verbal summary of the findings. A formal written report, highlighting strengths and offering suggestions for improvement, is received within a few months. The survey results can be utilized as ideas for future CQI strategies.

CCHSA has four quality dimensions: responsiveness, system competency, client/community focus, and work life.[2] See Figure 17-6 for an example of the link between CCHSA standards, quality dimensions, and indicators; and Figure 17-7 for an example of the interactions between a standard, quality dimension and indicator.

SENTINEL EVENTS

A **sentinel event** is an unexpected incident, related to system or process deficiencies, which leads to death or major and enduring loss of function for a recipient of health care services. The major and enduring loss of function refers to sensory, motor, physiological impairment not present at the time services were sought or begun. The impairment lasts for a minimum period of two weeks and is not related to an underlying condition.[3] Events are called sentinel because they require immediate investigation. During analysis of these sentinel events, opportunities for improving the system will arise and should be taken advantage of. Linkage of sentinel event review to the organization's performance improvement system will identify strategies for prevention of future sentinel events. An example of a sentinel event is surgery performed on the wrong side of a client. Reviewing the surgical process and developing a system to mark the appropriate site is a change in process to prevent future harmful occurrences.

BALANCED SCORECARD

To ensure value in care, measurement of progress has to be balanced. Effective measurement must be an integral part of the management process. The balanced scorecard

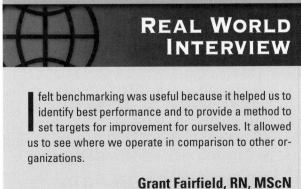

REAL WORLD INTERVIEW

I felt benchmarking was useful because it helped us to identify best performance and to provide a method to set targets for improvement for ourselves. It allowed us to see where we operate in comparison to other organizations.

Grant Fairfield, RN, MScN
Clinical Nurse Specialist, Rehabilitation

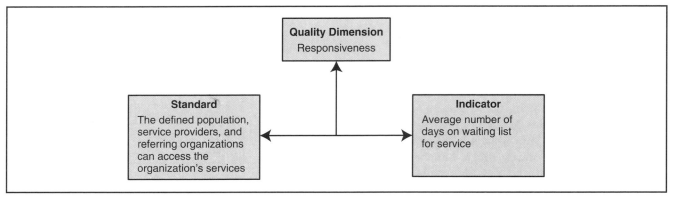

Figure 17-7 Example of a Standard, Quality Dimension and Indicator.

Source: Health Canada. (2000). Link between indicators, quality dimension and accreditation standards. *Quest for quality in Canadian health care: Continuous quality improvement,* p. 162. Retrieved from http://www.hc-sc.gc.ca/hcs-sss/pubs/care-soins/2000-qual/indicat_e.html, March 15, 2007. Reprinted with permission from the Minister of Public Works and Government Services Canada, 2007.

provides individuals with a framework that translates an organization's objectives into a set of linked performance measures (Kaplan & Norton, 1993). It provides answers to four basic questions:

How do customers see us? (i.e., customer perspective); What must we excel at? (i.e., internal perspective); Can we continue to improve and create value? (i.e., innovation and learning perspective); and How do we look to funders? (i.e., financial perspective). Generally, four cardinal domains of outcomes are measured: functional status of client, clinical outcomes, satisfaction, and costs (Caldwell, 1998).

Such an approach allows those reviewing data to examine all aspects of care. For example, client outcomes are reflected in a client's functional status and clinical status, which are balanced by client satisfaction and cost to ensure value. Data can be arranged to create a balanced scorecard, in an approach that uses the organization's priorities as categories for indicators. For example, three priorities might be customer service, cost-effectiveness, and positive clinical outcomes. These priorities help determine which indicators should be measured to give a balanced view of whether a strategy is working. Indicators are selected based on what they have in common, so that if a change occurs in the cost-effectiveness category, it will affect the data in another category. For example, the number of client referrals to home care is increased, is the client's satisfaction affected positively or negatively? If the length of stay for these clients is decreased, are complication rates increased or decreased? After indicators are selected, data are tracked over time at regular intervals (e.g., every month or every quarter). See Figure 11-1 (page 203) to see a balanced scorecard for a neonatal intensive care unit patient care team.

STORYBOARD: HOW TO SHARE YOUR STORY

Process improvement teams share their work with others through a storyboard. The storyboard usually takes the

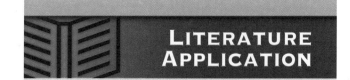

LITERATURE APPLICATION

Citation: Lesar, T., Briceland, L., & Stein, D. (1997). Factors related to errors in medication prescribing. *Journal of the American Medical Association, 277*(4), 312–317.

Discussion: Adverse drug events occur in up to 6.5 percent of hospitalized patients and account for almost one-fifth of all adverse patient events. Errors in the prescribing and management of drug therapy are common and have been identified as a major cause of adverse drug events. Understanding the many factors contributing to errors should assist in implementation of more effective error-prevention strategies. Several easily identified factors are associated with a large proportion of medication prescribing errors.

Implications for Practice: Nurses and doctors can help in identifying ways to improve processes to decrease medication errors. To help focus their efforts, they should review the information available about what factors have the greatest association with errors.

major steps in the improvement methodology and visually outlines the progress in each step. Displaying the storyboard in a high-traffic area of the organization will inform other staff of the QI efforts under way. Storyboarding can be done when a process is complete, or used during the process to communicate information.

CLIENT SATISFACTION DATA

Client satisfaction data can be obtained in several ways. Most health care facilities have clients complete a

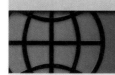

REAL WORLD INTERVIEW

Why is Jason in the hospital? Because he has a bad infection in his leg.

But why does he have an infection? Because he has a cut on his leg and it got infected.

But why does he have a cut on his leg? Because he was playing in the junkyard next to his apartment building and there was some sharp, jagged steel there that he fell on.

But why was he playing in a junkyard? Because his neighbourhood is run down. A lot of kids play there and there is no one to supervise them.

But why does he live in that neighbourhood? Because his parents can't afford a nicer place to live.

But why can't his parents afford a nicer place to live? Because his Dad is unemployed and his Mom is sick.

But why is his Dad unemployed? Because he doesn't have much education and he can't find a job.

But why......?

Gerarda Cronin, Director Child Health Quality Team
Winnipeg Regional Health Authority

Source: Federal, Provincial and Territorial Advisory Committee on Population Health. (1999). *Toward a healthy future: Second report on the health of Canadians.* Ottawa: Minister of Public Works and Government Services Canada. Retrieved from http://www.phac-aspc.gc.ca/ph-sp/phdd/pdf/toward/toward_a_healthy_english.PDF, July 23, 2007.

questionnaire that asks how they felt about their health care encounter. It is most helpful if this data can be compared or benchmarked with other organizations' data, which requires that several organizations use the same data collection tools. All client responses are entered into a database so the results can be compared. Another method to obtain client satisfaction information is via a focus group or a post-care interview, which requires meeting with one or more clients after their discharge and asking for feedback on their perceptions of their stay.

USING DATA

Several different types of charts are used to examine data in QI efforts: time series charts, Pareto charts, histograms, flowcharts, fishbone diagrams, pie charts, and check sheets.

TIME SERIES DATA

Time series data (see Figure 17-8) allow individuals to see changes in data over time. A time series chart allows the user to view a number of observations for a particular subject at regular intervals over time. An example of a time series chart is life expectancy at birth by sex.[4]

Tracking data over time allows you to see how a process is behaving, which a time series graph is able to illustrate. Graphs or charts—rather than tables of numbers—are used to display data because graphs are faster to interpret. The time series chart is used to look for trends, shifts, and unusual data.

CHARTS: PARETO, HISTOGRAM, FLOWCHARTS, FISHBONE DIAGRAMS, PIE CHARTS, AND CHECK SHEETS

In addition to time series data graphs, information can be displayed in several different ways to enhance decision making: Pareto diagrams, pie charts, flowcharts, and histograms. Figure 17-9 is an example of a fishbone diagram. (Fishbone diagrams are also

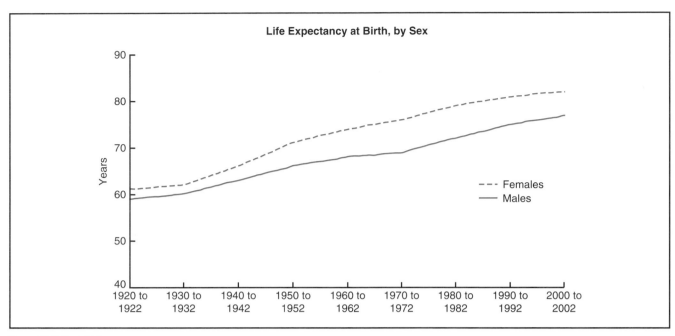

Figure 17-8 Time Series.

Source: Statistics Canada, "Life Expectancy at Birth, by Sex," CANSIM table 102-0511; Catalogue nos. 89-506-XPB1981001, B4-537-79E.

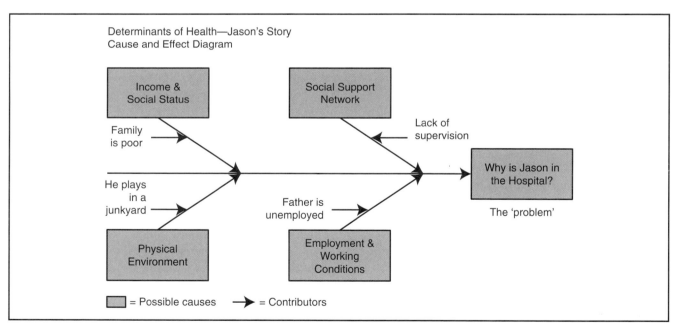

Figure 17-9 Root Cause/Fishbone Diagram/Cause and Effect Diagram/Ishikawa Diagram.
Source: Child Health Team, *Quality for Kids Newsletter,* Winnipeg Regional Health Authority. Reprinted with Permission.

referred to as root cause diagrams, cause-and-effect diagrams, or Ishikawa diagrams.) Note that many factors contribute to a problem. Review of a cause-and-effect chart encourages staff to look for all the causes of a problem, not just one cause. Figure 17-10 shows a check sheet, a Pareto chart, and a control chart. A full discussion of these tools is outside the scope of this chapter.

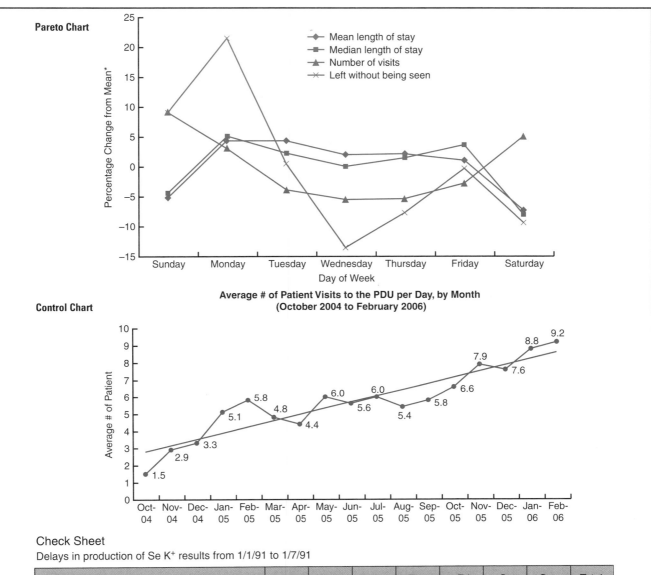

Figure 17-10 Pareto Chart. *Source:* Saunders et al. (2004). Variations in the use of emergency departments in Alberta's Capital Health Region, 1998–2000. *Healthcare Management Forum, 17*(2), 20. **Control Chart.** *Source:* Child Health Quality Team. (2006). Children's Hospital's newest unit is taking off! *Quality for Kids Newsletter, 5*(2), 1. **Check Sheet.** *Source: Clinical Laboratory Management Review,* November/December 1991, 5[6]:448–462. © Clinical Laboratory Management Association, Inc. All rights reserved.

PRINCIPLES IN ACTION IN AN ORGANIZATION

How are these principles and tools of quality management actually used on a day-to-day basis in a health care facility? An appropriate structure is set up for the organization, using a process for quality and monitoring outcomes.

ORGANIZATIONAL STRUCTURE

Most organizations today are structured to maximize QI efforts, which allows an organization to be flexible and nimble in a very turbulent health care environment. This organizational structure encourages accountability and communication and by focusing all staff on the priorities of the organization.

Figure 17-11 is an organizational chart that shows a structure for quality improvement. Note that it includes a range of people, from board members to staff on individual quality improvement teams (QITs). Communicating

priorities at all levels in the organization is key. Staff members must realize how their day-to-day work influences the accomplishment of strategic goals. Mission, vision, and value statements help accomplish this clarity of focus (see Chapter 14, pp. 252–253).

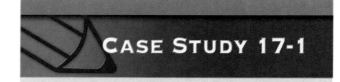

CASE STUDY 17-1

You work in a busy emergency department, where you have a good working relationship with your nursing colleagues and with the emergency physicians. You believe that the care delivery in the department could improve, thereby increasing client satisfaction and reducing the length of time clients wait to be seen. How would you proceed? Whose support would you enlist first? Who should be involved? What quality indicators could be measured?

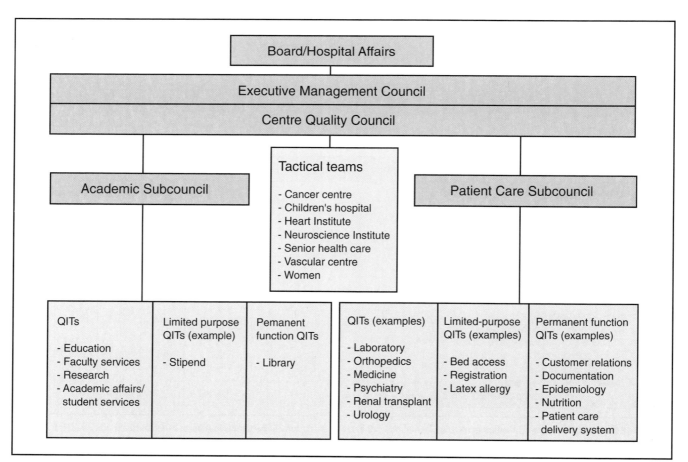

Figure 17-11 Structure for quality improvement (Courtesy of Albany Medical Center, Albany, NY).

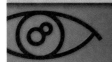

CRITICAL THINKING

At times, some care providers, particularly physicians, see clinical pathways and other standardized guidelines as cookie-cutter medicine. All health care providers like to think they give their clients the best care possible. Standardization and evidence-based clinical guidelines are intended to communicate the latest evidence as to the best practice for a given client problem. Using these guidelines allows care providers to focus on specific individual client needs rather than spending their energy on determining the best evidence-based strategy according to the current research.

In developing a clinical pathway or other standardized guideline, evidence-based practice guidelines should be incorporated. In the absence of evidence-based practices, consensus of the team should be used to develop the clinical pathway. In the absence of consensus, the client's health care provider should make an independent decision, which is not included in the clinical guideline.

A group that was developing a clinical pathway for the care of clients with acute myocardial infarction noted evidence showing that these clients should receive acetylsalicylic acid (ASA) on admission. The research in this area was very clear, and most providers believed this practice was being followed. When a chart audit was performed to determine whether it was, in fact, the practice on the unit, it was discovered that only 48 percent of clients were receiving ASA within eight hours of admission. The team added this practice to the clinical pathway. After it was implemented, 85 percent of clients received ASA within the first eight hours of admission.

What practices on your unit are based on an evidence-based clinical pathway? How can you participate in improving the care of more clients using evidence-based clinical pathways? Do you use clinical practice guidelines?

OUTCOMES MONITORING

Outcomes are a measurement of the client response to structure and process. Outcomes measure actual clinical progress. Outcomes can be short term, such as the average length of stay (ALOS) for a client population, or long term, such as a measure of clients' progress over time (e.g., survival rate for a transplant client at one, two, and three years after treatment). Outcomes can be studied to identify potential areas of concern, which may lead to an investigation of structure and process to determine any root causes. For example, when a postoperative infection rate was used as an outcome measure, an increase in the number of infections per month was noted. This finding led the team to review the client care process being used. The team discovered that preoperative prophylactic antibiotics were not given to the client because the order was not written. The team added this order to the initial order set, and all clients received prophylactic antibiotics. The number of postoperative infections decreased.

KEY CONCEPTS

- Quality improvement is a continuous process focused on improving client care processes and outcomes.

- Client care needs should drive improvement opportunities.

- Decisions should be driven by data.

- Improvement initiatives should be linked to the organization's mission, vision, and values.

- Organizational goals and objectives should be communicated up and down the organization.

- There should be a balance in improvement goals focused on client clinical and functional status, cost, and client satisfaction outcomes.

KEY TERMS

benchmarking
continuous quality improvement
indirect costs
performance improvement

process
quality assurance
sentinel event
system

REVIEW QUESTIONS

1. Which of the following describes the benchmarking process?
   A. Reviewing your own unit's data for opportunities
   B. Collecting data on an individual client
   C. Reviewing data in the literature
   D. Comparing your data to that of other organizations to identify opportunities

2. Identifying opportunities in the health care arena is the responsibility of which group?
   A. Administration
   B. Physicians
   C. Clients
   D. Everyone

3. Following a sentinel event, which step would be initiated first?
   A. No action
   B. Corrective action of personnel
   C. Reporting to health department/root cause analysis
   D. Immediate investigation

4. What document defines the purpose of an organization?
   A. Mission
   B. Fishbone diagram
   C. Balanced scorecard
   D. Process flowchart

5. What tool could be used to track a change in a process over time?
   A. Flowchart
   B. Histogram
   C. Time series chart
   D. Pie chart

REVIEW ACTIVITIES

1. Risk management, infection control practitioners, and a benchmark study have revealed that your unit's utilization of Foley catheters is above average. Brainstorm reasons why the use is so high. Create a fishbone (root cause) diagram to help determine all the possible causes.

2. After you have identified the root causes for the above-average use of Foley catheters, use the PDCA Cycle to identify improvement strategies.

3. Think about your last clinical rotation. Identify one process that you believe could be improved. How would you begin improving the process? Use the FOCUS methodology in your analysis.

EXPLORING THE WEB

- Use these sites for potential benchmark data:

  Cochrane Collaboration:
  http://www.cochrane.org/index.htm

  Canadian Institute for Health Information:
  http://www.cihi.ca

- The following sites are recommended when looking for evidence-based guidelines or research studies for a particular diagnosis:

  Institute for Clinical Evaluative Sciences:
  http://www.ices.on.ca

Health Information Research Unit:
http://hiru.mcmaster.ca/

Canadian Medical Association Clinical Practice Guidelines: *http://mdm.ca/cpgsnew/cpgs/index.asp*

Health Evidence Applications and Linkage Network:
http://www.nce.gc.ca/nces-rces/healnet_e.htm

REFERENCES

Al-Assaf, A. F., & Schmele, J. (1997). *Total quality in healthcare.* Boca Raton, FL: St. Lucie Press.

Aldarrab, A. (2006). Application of Lean Six Sigma for patients presenting with ST-elevation myocardial infarction: The Hamilton Health Sciences experience. *Healthcare Quarterly, 9*(1), 56–61.

Berwick, D., & Plsek, P. (1992). *Managing medical quality videotape series.* Woodbridge, NJ: Quality Visions.

Berwick, D. M., Blanton Godfrey, A., & Roessner, J. (1991). *Curing health care: New strategies for quality improvement.* San Francisco: Jossey-Bass Inc. Publishers.

Caldwell, C. (1998). *Handbook for managing change in health care.* Milwaukee, WI: ASQ Quality Press.

Crosby, P. B. (1989). *Let's talk quality.* New York: McGraw-Hill.

Deming, W. E. (1986). *Out of the crisis.* Cambridge, MA: Center for Advanced Engineering Study.

Drucker, P. F. (1988). The coming of the new organization. *Harvard Business Review, 66*(1), 45–53.

Gift, R. G., & Mosel, D. (1994). *Benchmarking in health care: A collaborative approach.* Chicago: American Hospital Publishing.

Kaplan, R., & Norton, D. (1993) Putting the balanced scorecard to work. *Harvard Business Review.* Sept/Oct, 134–147.

Langley, G. J., Nolan, K. M., Norman, C. L., Provost, L. P., & Nolan, T. W. (1996). *The improvement guide.* San Francisco: Jossey-Bass.

Lesar, T., Briceland, I., & Stein, D. (1997). Factors related to errors in medication prescribing. *Journal of the American Medical Association, 277*(4), 312–317.

Rondeau, K. V., & Wagar, T. H. (2002). Implementing CQI while reducing the work force: How does it influence hospital performance? *Healthcare Management Forum, 17*(2), 22–29.

Seeman, N. & Brown, A. D. (2006). Remembering Peter Drucker: Inspiring the quality revolution in healthcare. *Healthcare Quarterly, 9*(1), 50–52.

Youngberg, B. (1998). *The risk manager's desk reference.* Gaithersburg, MD: Aspen.

SUGGESTED READINGS

Duffy, J. R. (2000). Cardiovascular outcomes initiative: Case studies in performance improvement. *Outcomes Management in Nursing Practice, 4*(3), 110–116.

Harrigan, M. L. (2000) *Quest for quality in Canadian health care: Continuous quality improvement* (2nd ed.). Ottawa: Health Canada. Available at http://www.hc-sc.gc.ca/hcs-sss/pubs/care-soins/2000-qual/index_e.html.

Henry, S. B. (1995). Informatics: Essential infrastructure for quality assessment and improvement in nursing. *Journal of the American Medical Information Association, 2*(3), 169–182.

Kaplan, R., & Norton, D. (1996). *The balanced scorecard: Translating strategy into action.* Boston: Harvard Business School Press.

Kelly-Heidenthal, P., & Heidenthal, P. R. (1995). Benchmarking. *Nursing Quality Connections, 4*(5), 4.

King, K. M., & Teo, K. K. (2000). Integrating clinical quality improvement strategies with nursing research. *Western Journal of Nursing Research, 22*(5), 596–608.

Kipp, J., McKim, B., Zieber, C., & Neumann, I. (2006). What motivates managers to coordinate the learning experience of interprofessional student teams in service delivery settings? *Healthcare Management Forum, 19*(2), 42–48.

Kitson, A. (2000). Towards evidence-based quality improvement: Perspectives from nursing practice. *International Journal of Quality in Health Care, 12*(6), 459–464.

Koivula, M., Paunonen, M., & Laippala, P. (1998). Prerequisites for quality improvement in nursing. *Journal of Nursing Management, 6*(6), 333–342.

Maleyeff, J., Kaminsky, F. C., Jubinville, A., & Fenn, C. (2001). A guide to using performance measurement systems for continuous improvement. *Journal of Healthcare Quality, 23*(4), 33–37.

McGowan, J., Straus, S. E., & Tugwell, P. (2006). Canada urgently needs a national network of libraries to access evidence. *Healthcare Quarterly, 9*(1), 72–74.

Meisenheimer, C. G. (1997). *Improving quality: A guide to effective programs* (2nd ed.). Gaithersburg, MD: Aspen.

Mor, V., Morris, J., Lipsitz, L., & Fogel, B. (1998) Benchmarking quality in nursing homes: the Q-Metrics system. *Canadian Journal of Quality in Health Care, 14*(2), 12–17.

Patrick, L. (2004). Building an effective risk management program in a healthcare setting. *Healthcare Management Forum, 17*(3), 27–29.

Pink, G. H., Brown, A. D., Daniel, I., Hamlette, M. L., Markel, F., McGillis Hall, L., et al. (2006). Financial benchmarks for Ontario hospitals. *Healthcare Quarterly, 9*(1), 40–45.

Plsek, P. E. (1993). Tutorial: Quality improvement project models. *Quality Management in Health Care, 1*(2), 69–81.

Rantz, M. J., Petroski, G. F., Madsen, R. W., Scott, J., Mehr, D. R., Popejoy, L., et al. (1997). Setting thresholds for MDS (Minimum Data Set) quality indicators for nursing home quality improvement reports. *Joint Committee Journal on Quality Improvement, 23*(11), 602–611.

CHAPTER ENDNOTES

1. Health Canada, "Quest for Quality in Canadian Healthcare: Continuous Quality Improvement, The Focus of CQI (background)." Retrieved from http://www.hc-sc.gc.ca/hcs-sss/pubs/care-soins/2000-qual/intro_e.html, August 24, 2006.

2. "Canadian Council on Health Services Accreditation." Retrieved from http://www.cchsa.ca/default.aspx?section=FosterQuality&group=1, August 24, 2006.

3. Canadian Council on Health Services Accreditation, "Reference Guide on Sentinel Events." Retrieved from http://www.cchsa.ca/upload/files/pdf/Patient%20Safety/GuideForSentinelEvents_e.pdf, April 2, 2007.

4. Child Health Quality Team. (2006). "Incidence of Nosocomial Infection." Progress Report 2004–2006. Winnipeg Regional Health Authority.

CHAPTER 18

Decision Making

Sharon Little-Stoetzel, RN, MS
Adapted by: Eric Doucette, RN
Ined Parmar, RN, BScN, MA GNC (C)

Nurses have an important contribution to make in health services planning and decision-making, and in development of appropriate and effective health policy. They can and should contribute to public policy on the determinants of health. (International Council of Nurses, 2000)

OBJECTIVES

Upon completion of this chapter, the reader should be able to:

1. Apply effective decision making to clinical situations, incorporating critical thinking and problem solving.
2. Facilitate group decision making by using various techniques.
3. Apply technology, as appropriate, to decision making.
4. Examine the nurse's role in client decision making.
5. Examine strategies to improve decision making and to build self-confidence.
6. Describe the nature of decision making and the resulting cascades.
7. Identify their personal style in decision making.
8. Identify a minimum of three intrinsic factors that influence decision making in a health care environment.
9. Articulate the link between climate, culture, and locus of control.

You are a staff nurse on the medical cardiology unit, and you have just come from a unit meeting, where your nurse manager reported the results of the most recent client care score card. The incidence of client falls has increased by 75 percent. In addition, 35 percent of the clients have had repeat falls within 48 hours of their initial fall. Second and subsequent falls have a high correlation to the rate of injury and result in increased diagnostic testing and extended lengths of stay. The manager has selected a task force to investigate potential solutions to this problem, and you have been appointed chairperson. The unit action council has been trending falls for the past year and has identified some reasons for the undesirable fall rate: inconsistent admission assessments, client demographics inconsistent with the cardiac population, and a lack of a fall risk assessment tool.

> *What is your emotional connection to the problem?*
>
> *Is there enough information known?*
>
> *Which is the focus: problem solving the situation to identify the root cause or making a decision about the use of a fall predictive tool?*
>
> *Are you excited about the opportunity to assume a leadership role?*
>
> *What should be the first step of the task force?*
>
> *Can the decision-making process help the group solve the situation?*

This chapter explores the decision-making process and factors that promote or impede clinical and professional practice decision making. Strategies to facilitate both the frequency and quality of decision making are explored. Decision making is presented as an associated process within the problem-solving cycle. Critical thinking is essential when making decisions and solving problems. Application of decision-making models to clinical and management decisions are presented. The chapter examines advantages and limitations to group decision

making as well as the use of technology in decision making. Finally, it discusses the nurse's role in client decision making and strategies for improving the decision-making process.

CRITICAL THINKING

A buzzword or a concept? The words **critical thinking** have found their way into the mainstream of nursing language among nurses and across organizations. However, too many nurses use the term as a buzzword with little understanding of what critical thinking entails, how their own thinking differs from someone else's, and how to think critically in various situations (Alfaro-LeFevre, 2006). Critical thinking is essential when making decisions and solving problems. The Pew Health Professions Commission asserted that nurses must "demonstrate critical thinking, reflection, and problem-solving skills" to thrive as effective practitioners in the 21st century (Bellack & O'Neil, 2000. p. 16).

What does it mean to be a critical thinker? Scriven and Paul (2004), in a statement on critical thinking prepared for the National Council for Excellence in Critical Thinking Instruction, define critical thinking as "a mode of thinking—about any subject, content, or problem—in which the thinker improves the quality of their thinking by skillfully taking charge of the structures inherent in thinking and imposing intellectual standards upon them." Scriven and Paul also suggest that critical thinking can be seen as having two components: 1) a set of information and beliefs generating and processing skills; and 2) the habit, based on intellectual commitment, of using those skills to guide behaviour. Alfaro-LeFevre (2006) adds that critical thinking is contextual in that it changes depending on circumstances. Consequently, critical thinking needs to be viewed from three perspectives, namely: a) thinking ahead, b) thinking in action, and c) thinking back.

Thinking ahead is the ability to be proactive and anticipate what might happen. Novice nurses or novice nurse managers, as a result of their limited experience, may have to tap into the expertise of others, or refer to procedure manuals or texts to enhance their skills in order to be proactive. Nurses caring for clients in a pediatric setting might anticipate that separation anxiety will alter the sleeping pattern of a child and might plan with the parents a schedule that includes frequent visits. A nurse manager might anticipate the need for a critical incident debriefing session following a sentinel event on the unit (e.g., a client death via suicide).

Alfaro-LeFevre describes thinking in action as the ability to think on your feet. It "represents rapid, dynamic reasoning that considers several cues and priorities at once." She cautions that this type of critical thinking is more prone to "knee-jerk" responses and decisions than the other types of thinking. For example, in cardiac arrest situations, the nurse makes the following decisions: a) call for help, b) access Airway, Breathing, Circulation, c) initiate CPR, and once the cardiac arrest team arrives, ensure an IV is initiated. Another example of thinking on your feet, as a manager, would be responding to a situation of a witnessed threatened client assault of a nurse. Thinking back is the process of reflective thinking, and is described by Alfaro-LeFevre as the ability to recall and analyze the reasoning process to look for flaws or omissions, gain increased understanding, and correct and improve thinking.

Paul (1992) is quick to point out the many accurate definitions of critical thinking, most of which are consistent with each other. A good critical thinker is able to examine decisions from all sides and take into account varying points of view. A good critical thinker does not say, "We've always done it this way," and refuse to consider alternate ways. The critical thinker generates new ideas and alternatives when making decisions. The critical thinker asks "why" questions about a situation to arrive at the best decision. Four basic skills—critical reading, critical listening, critical writing, and critical speaking—are necessary for the development of critical thinking skills. These skills are part of the process of developing and using thinking for decision making. Ability in these four areas can be measured by the extent to which one achieves the universal intellectual standards illustrated in Table 18-1.

As you begin to apply critical thinking to nursing, use these universal intellectual standards when you are reading

material from a textbook, listening to an oral presentation, writing a paper, answering test questions, or presenting ideas in oral form. Ask yourself whether the ideas are clear or unclear, precise or imprecise, specific or vague, accurate or inaccurate, and so forth. You will improve your critical thinking skills over time. Scriven and Paul (2004) conclude that "no one is a critical thinker through-and-through, and for this reason the development of critical thinking skills and dispositions is a life-long endeavor."

REFLECTIVE THINKING

John Dewey, as cited in Teekman (2000), was possibly one of the first and most influential educational theorists to initiate the process of reflective thinking. Dewey believed that reflective thinking occurred due to doubt, uncertainty, and/or mental obscurity that encouraged the person to inquire and find the material that would help to overcome doubt and uncertainty. He recognized the importance of past experiences for reflection and argued that results and recommendations are dependent on one's past experiences because they do not arise out of nothing.

Pesut and Herman (1999) describe **reflective thinking** as watching or observing ourselves as we perform a task or make a decision about a particular situation, followed by thinking about what we have done, and how we could have done it better. We have two selves: the active self and the reflective self. The reflective self watches the active self as it engages in activities. The reflective self acts as

TABLE 18-1	**THE SPECTRUM OF UNIVERSAL INTELLECTUAL STANDARDS**	
Clear		Unclear
Precise		Imprecise
Specific		Vague
Accurate		Inaccurate
Relevant		Irrelevant
Consistent		Inconsistent
Logical		Illogical
Deep		Superficial
Complete		Incomplete
Significant		Insignificant
Adequate		Inadequate
Fair		Unfair

Source: Adapted from the Foundation for Critical Thinking, Dillon, CA. http://criticalthinking.org/university/unistan.html

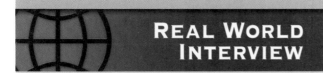

REAL WORLD INTERVIEW

To retain our staff and to improve the quality of our client care, we must provide support to our novice nurses by implementing a mentorship program in our hospital to provide an ongoing support to develop their skills in problem solving, decision making, and prioritization.

Terry Kuula
Director

DECISION MAKING

AN INTRODUCTION

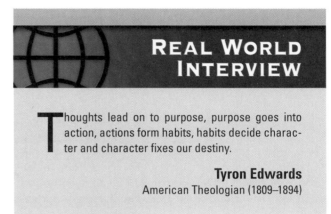

REAL WORLD INTERVIEW

Thoughts lead on to purpose, purpose goes into action, actions form habits, habits decide character and character fixes our destiny.

Tyron Edwards
American Theologian (1809–1894)

observer and offers suggestions about the activities. To be a good critical thinker, one must practise reflective thinking. Reflection upon a situation or problem after a decision is made allows the individual to evaluate the decision. Nurse educators assist students to become better reflective thinkers through the use of clinical journals. Using journals helps students reflect on clinical activities and improve their clinical decision-making abilities.

Donaghy and Morss (2000) describe a process of guided reflection as a structured approach within the context of a reflective practice framework that facilitates the individual's reflection because it is linked more closely with systematic critical enquiry, problem solving, and clinical reasoning. In Canada, the regulatory colleges for nurses have implemented continuing competence programs, which are designed to ensure ongoing competence and overall practice quality across the profession. Reflective thinking is becoming mainstream in all domains of practice (e.g., direct practice, administration, education, and research).

PROBLEM SOLVING

Problem solving is an active process that starts with a problem and ends with a solution. LeStorti et al. (1999) define a problem as the difference between the actual state and the desired state. The problem-solving process consists of five steps: identify the problem, gather and analyze data, generate alternatives and select an action, implement the selected action, and evaluate the action. Note the similarities to the nursing process steps of assessment, diagnosis, outcome identification, planning, implementation, and evaluation. The nursing process is applied to client situations or problems, whereas the problem-solving process may be applied to a problem of any type.

The mythology and legends of many different cultures include mythological creatures of human appearance but of extraordinary size and strength. *Giant* is the English word commonly used for such beings. The term *sleeping giant* has been coined to describe a calm, yet powerful force that is not to be disturbed for fear of the negative, unknown, or uncontrollable consequences that the force (i.e., the giant) can unleash.

Nursing in Canada is much like the sleeping giant, yet to be truly awakened. Described as the backbone of the health care system (Canadian Nursing Advisory Committee [CNAC], 2002), nursing comprises the largest number of health care professionals in Canada with the current estimate at 300,000 (CNAC, 2002). The active ingredient needed to awaken the giant is consistent and effective decision making that moves individual nurses and the profession as a whole in a trajectory, focused on nursing as a leader in the delivery of health care.

Imagine the health care system in Canada if nursing's voice were even more influential than it currently is perceived. The impacts on current issues in nursing practice would be phenomenal, especially in the areas of defining and measuring workload, scope of practice and non-nursing tasks, the quality of the practice environment, autonomy and respect, as well as leadership and education. Empowerment, competence, and self-confidence are enhanced through effective decision making. And success in decision making builds further success and awakens the sleeping giant to achieve greatness.

Rapid changes in the health care environment (e.g., the contracting of resources, changes in the skill mix, staffing challenges, and more informed consumers) provide opportunities for expanded decision making for nurses at all levels. Government requirements for accountability for positive client outcomes and fiscal responsibility have led to an increase in decision making by nurses, which is pivotal to an agency's strategic and operational success. Shrinking budgets and other constraining factors require that nurse managers and direct practice nurses be more innovative and creative than ever before. As a result, decision making has rapidly become a core competency for all nurses. It is generally understood that client care is more complex given co-morbidities and the number of social and cultural factors. Client acuity (i.e., severity of illness) is generally perceived to be higher than in the previous decades. Because clients are being discharged from acute care institutions earlier, and with higher acuity, effective decisions regarding treatment must be made in a timely manner.

So what, then, is **decision making?** Decision making is the cognitive process leading to the selection of a course of action among alternatives. Every decision-making process results in a final outcome that can take the form of an opinion or an action. Decision making is a process of reasoning that begins when there is a perceived need to do something but we are not sure of what to do.

Clinical decision making occurs within the context of a health care environment and a therapeutic practitioner relationship or professional relationship. Health care personnel apply their foundational knowledge on a daily basis, to the information gained about clients through history, examination and integration of diagnostic test results, and dialogue with individual clients in making important decisions about effective treatment. Despite the fact decision making seems so commonplace, Stanford School of Medicine's Center for Immersive Simulation-Based Learning asserts "decision making is very complicated and hard to learn."[1] Further, Stanford suggests that decision making is more difficult to learn in situations in which decisions are complex and involve substantial discussion with clients, or in settings such as critical care units or the operating room, where time is a major factor.[2]

NATURE OF DECISION MAKING IN NURSING

Decision making can either be daunting or exciting to the new graduate nurse or to the nurse who has achieved expert status in practice. That response can be influence by a number of individual and environmental factors (O'Reilly, 1993), which will be explored later in this chapter. Peter Block, author of *The Empowered Manager: Positive Political Skills at Work,* (1990) claims that we "walk the tightrope between advocating our own position and yet not increasing resistance against us by our actions (p. 7). In many cases, this tightrope is the juxtaposition that nurses in direct practice experience in often autocratic, hierarchical practice environments. Block claims that the decision path we take in our organizational situations is essentially influenced by one of two factors. Namely, we are influenced by our individual choices, which are focused on adaptation, and secondly, by the norms and values of the organizations we find ourselves embedded within.

Nurses begin their careers making essentially two types of decisions. Nurses are involved in making clinical decisions within the context of a therapeutic relationship with a client. They also make decisions that relate to the context and system of care delivery. Finally, decisions are made about their own professional development and the career path they choose to follow. In each of these areas, nurses have the opportunity to choose maintenance versus greatness, caution versus courage or dependency versus autonomy. Block (1990) describes these opportunities as the fundamental choices we make. Interestingly enough, these same fundamental choices are made by individual nurses, nursing managers, nursing executives within an organization, and by nursing as a discipline.

How does maintenance differ from greatness? Maintenance choices typically are those that permit us to hold on to what we have created or inherited; in other words, the status quo. This choice, repeated over time, although safe, does not result in forward direction. This type of decision making is characteristic in bureaucratic organizational cultures (Block 1990). Personal safety is a strong driver in this key decision. Based on learned behaviour, staff in bureaucratic situations may have learned that their achievements are rewarded less and that their errors in decision result in personal repercussion or punishment. Block states that the choice for maintenance is the choice to be led by others. Reflect, here for a moment on the current state of professional nursing within your clinical setting. Is nursing leading or being led by others outside of the discipline?

The alternative to maintenance is greatness. Block asserts that we tend to think of greatness as being something beyond our personal abilities because greatness is reserved for the Albert Schweitzers, the Bishop Tutus, or the Nelson Mandelas of the world. Yet these great people are ordinary individuals doing extraordinary things, all of which involved decision making at critical moments that were focused on greatness. Block defines greatness as giving up pessimism and the need for the insulation that comes with corporate structure and predictability. Choosing greatness requires knowledge, courage, and energy. All nurses have an opportunity to choose the status quo (i.e., maintenance) or positive change (i.e., greatness) in their daily practice and over the course of their careers. Choosing to accept the problem of ongoing staffing shortages is an example of accepting the status quo. Moving forward with a decision to explore a different skill mix, a change in staffing patterns, or to promote a full scope of practice would constitute making a decision of greatness.

What distinguishes caution from courage? Caution is a reflection of organizational values around risk-taking, autonomous decision making at the point of care, and organizational management style. Cautious decisions are often apparent in organizations in which staff feel a strong presence of supervision and management control. Language often heard is couched in caution, such as, "Be careful of so and so, who can be fatal if you get on his/her wrong side" or "You have to be politically astute to survive in this organization." The opposite of caution is to choose courage. "In our culture, moving forward and creating an organization we believe in always requires an act of courage," (Block, 1990, p. 15). To act courageously is to take an unpopular position or chart an unpopular path. The most solid example of courageous decision making by the nursing profession in Canada is illustrated in the fundamental change to degree education as an entry-to-practice requirement for all registered nurses. In the example above, the courage decision is to choose an unpopular path and examine staffing pattern changes or entertain revised skill mix. As the experienced decision-maker has learned, often through trial and error, the hard part of choosing courage over caution is learning to avoid suicide.

The importance of professional nurse autonomy has been extensively addressed in the nursing literature over the past two decades. Nurse autonomy is a key indicator of quality work environments, yet definition, measurement, and interpretation of research findings have complicated the effective integration and promotion of this key indicator into nursing work environments (Tranmer, 2004).

Block claims the third type of choice we make as individuals is to choose between dependency and autonomy. He suggests that in many organizations a gap exists between articulating the value of autonomy and living it. In the nursing context, autonomy is a complex, multidimensional phenomenon—an interactive, relational process that occurs within the context of one's being and work. Wade (1999) differentiated among three types of autonomy: (a) structural and work autonomy as the worker's freedom to make decisions based upon job requirements; (b) attitudinal autonomy as the belief in one's freedom to exercise judgment in decision making; and (c) aggregate autonomy, which encompasses attitudinal and structural dimensions, the socially and legally granted freedom of self-governance and control of the profession without influence from external sources. Keenan (1999) and Scott, Sochalski, and Aiken (1999) identified two dimensions of nurses' work autonomy: organizational and clinical practice. The capacity of nurses to be involved as participants in the decision-making process provides direction and stewardship of work at the unit and organizational level. Macdonald (2002) described professional autonomy as the right to exercise clinical and organizational judgment within the context of an interdependent health care team in accordance with the socially and legally granted freedom of the discipline. Choosing autonomous decision making over dependency puts us in charge of what is happening at the moment, a very useful concept given the nature of nursing care and the frequency of decision making.

Block indicates that autonomous decision making helps us to understand that we are the cause and not the effect. He also asserts that the fundamental vulnerability in the way most large organizations are managed is the pervasive feeling of dependency that is engendered. Language that might suggest a dependency environment may include "I was waiting for approval to do that" or "I'm counting on direction from above, or when top management gets its act together." This type of language is very much upward looking and is reflective of dependency. Is there a cost to individual nurses, managers, nurse executives and to the discipline as a whole for choosing the dependency approach? Absolutely, and it gets paid in the form of a sense of helplessness in which we wait for clear instructions before acting, despite our inherent intuition that courage, greatness, and autonomy are required to change the trajectory of nursing leadership.

FACTORS INFLUENCING DECISION MAKING

As nurses, we need to have working knowledge of what drives individuals (i.e., our peers and our clients) to make choices that set up the cascade of courage, greatness, and autonomy versus caution, maintenance, and dependency.

The research literature reports numerous factors that influence decision making (Pardue, 1987). These factors include individual variables, such as experience and knowledge (Benner, 1984; Benner & Tanner, 1987), creative thinking ability, education (Pardue, 1987), and self-concept (Joseph, 1985), as well as environmental and situational stressors (Cleland, 1967, Evans, 1990). These factors, either intrinsic or extrinsic, may serve to enhance or impede decision making in the area of clinical practice or professional development.

Examination of the intrinsic factors provides insight for all nurses into the factors, which, to borrow from the Heart and Stroke Foundation, are considered to be "controllable." Being controllable infers that we can make a conscious choice to alter or modify our behaviour to have an impact on the factor. Intrinsic factors include personal perception and preference, knowledge and experience, competence, self-confidence, and stress. Extrinsic factors that influence decision making include organizational climate and culture, client rights and choice, and legal legislative frameworks.

PERSONAL PERCEPTION AND PREFERENCE

Understanding how we perceive problems in clinical practice or in our professional lives helps us to see how we can influence our personal preference in decision making. ChangingMinds.org suggests that we have either subjective or objective perceptions.[3]

Objective perception is characterized by seeing the problem or decision point from the perspective of standing outside of our body. This viewpoint does not suggest any level of dispassion or disengagement, rather it simply represents an objective viewpoint, which is a comfortable place to be for many nurses. In this space of comfort, nurses can see things from a more impersonal, rational, and unemotional viewpoint. Typically, people who perceive opportunities for decision making in the objective view also tend to make thinking decisions. Thinking decisions are based on logic, an exploration of black and white tangible facts, and the use of clear rules. In organizations, these types of decision-makers may be perceived as cold and heartless by people who perceive opportunities for decision making on a more emotional basis.

Feelers tend to make decisions by considering the social context, listening to their heart, and considering the feelings of others. Feelers value harmony and use tact in their interactions with others.[4] Feelers are usually relationship-oriented and use a values base for decision making. As a result, feelers see the opportunity for decision making through the subjective lens, which tends to make them more empathetic and intuitive. Typically, thinkers, who are also objective, tend to be left-brain dominant, whereas feelers, who are subjective, tend to be right-brain dominant. The good news is that evidence now exists that shows that neither right- nor left-brain thinking is better than the other. Murphy (1985) asserts that each side is important, but each side also lacks something. In practical terms, both in a clinical and professional sense, we would never contemplate making a decision using only one-half of our brain.

KNOWLEDGE AND EXPERIENCE

Tanner, Padrick, Westfall, and Putzier (1987) studied the diagnostic reasoning approaches of nurses and nursing students and reported that increased knowledge and experience yielded more systematic data acquisition and greater diagnostic accuracy. Benner and Tanner (1987) also found that the difference in diagnostic accuracy was attributed to the ability of the expert nurse to intuitively determine the correct region for the assessment, select relevant data, and recognize the changing relevance of cues as the situation evolves. Picking up on these cues and intervening before a cascade of negative sequalae has given rise to a critical nurse-sensitive indicator first reported by Aiken et al.,(2002), called "failure to rescue." Benner and Tanner (1987) define intuition as "understanding without rationale" (p. 23). This level of expertise represents the hallmark of expert nursing judgment derived from the synergy of knowledge and experience. Evans (1990) suggests that ability to use intuition to rapidly identify important facts, and thereby limit the number of alternatives to be evaluated, reduces decisional conflict and stress, and therefore is seen as a factor that enhances decision making.

On the flip side, Correnti (1992) dismisses intuition as irrational guessing. Given the heavy and appropriate focus on evidence-based nursing in today's curriculum of undergraduate nursing programs, many nurses are reluctant to follow their so-called gut feelings and reject the use of intuition in decision making.

O'Reilly (1993) suggests the attitude of dismissing intuitive judgment as irrational guessing will generate decisional conflict, and create a barrier to expert nursing judgment. Given the current escalation of the client safety agenda by the new required organizational practices as defined by the Canadian Council on Health Services Accreditation (2006), it is critical that all nurses possess and maintain honed intuitive decision-making skills. Such skills will ensure that nurses are in a position to activate the decision-making threshold and act sooner rather than later, thereby minimizing client safety risks. Correnti (1992) also supported the strategy of nurse educators teaching the application of intuitive skills, cultivating intuitive knowledge, and promoting the development of creating thinking abilities for problem solving.

Knowledge and experience are also influenced by past experience that includes education and decision-making experience (Marquis & Huston, 2006). Life experience plays a significant role in decision making. Maturity helps individuals to see a problem from more perspectives, based on their life experiences, which can yield a rich bank of alternatives. Possessing knowledge of the theories that underpin decision making and the process and tools involved also influence the knowledge and experience factor. Dwyer, Schwartz, and Fox (1992) found that nurses' desire for autonomy varies widely across the profession, and they postulate that nurses seeking autonomy are more likely to have experience with decision making than those nurses who fear autonomy.

COMPETENCE

The Canadian Nurses Association (CNA) provides the following definition of competencies: The specific knowledge, skills, judgment and personal attributes required for a registered nurse to practise safely and ethically in a designated role and setting (Canadian Nurses Association, 2000, p. 6). Campbell and Mackay (2001) have a different interpretation of competence, and they identify three concepts: (a) the ability to practise in a specific role; (b) the influence of the practice setting on competence; and (c) the integration of knowledge, skills, judgments, and abilities. Despite these definitions, no single universal definition exists of nursing competence. Nurses practise individually, and in groups, in a wide array of clinical, nonclinical, and nontraditional settings. What is common to all nurses is the need to make clinical and professional decisions in their practice. To be effective decision-makers, nurses must have a solid anchoring in the core competencies related to entry to practice and must possess knowledge and abilities related to problem solving and decision making, which have been integrated into professional practice.

Hagbaghery, Salsali, and Ahmadi (2004) reported that effective clinical decision making depends on one's ability to gather, understand, and integrate the data with a focus on the clients' needs and clinical situation. The best way for nurses to develop competence in decision making is to make decisions.

SELF-CONFIDENCE

Joseph (1985) claims that perceptions of being less intelligent, less educated, and less competent result in relinquished authority to those perceived as being better. This observation plays itself out on many units within health care facilities on a day-to-day basis. In nursing, one has to "earn one's stripes" by gaining the confidence and the respect of one's peers. New graduates and new nurses joining an established team often feel that there is a need to prove themselves in order to be accepted by the more senior staff. Joseph also reports that an individual's locus of control (i.e., the extent to which people believe they can control events and outcomes), plays an important role in an individual person's perception of self-efficacy and self-concept. Individuals with an external locus of control, often the "upward lookers," believe that events and outcomes are dependent on the action of others (Lazarus & Folkman, 1984).

Self-confidence is a term used to describe how secure people are in their own decisions and actions. This definition can be applied generally, or to specific situations or tasks. Nurses who possess a high degree of confidence believe they have the competence (i.e., the knowledge, judgment, and skill) to perform an action correctly or achieve some specific goal. Confident and competent nurses usually have little difficulty making clinical decisions, such as starting an intravenous in urgent/emergent situations, referring a client to social work, or ordering a pressure-reduction overlay mattress. Self-confidence is learned through repeated successful application of the decision-making process. Decisions that require courage, autonomy, and greatness, and result in positive client outcomes become strong motivators to support decision making. Decisions that illustrate caution, dependency, and maintenance have less intrinsic reward for the nurse, and therefore such decisions have little ability to motivate continued decision making. The outcome can be a lack of self-confidence, which is reinforced with every missed opportunity for decision making.

A lack of self-confidence is created when an individual holds a belief that a specific action or decision will not generate the desired results. This belief is reinforced when the outcome is less than desirable or results in repercussion from peers or the immediate supervisor. Making staffing decisions in the absence of the manager is an example of a decision that may not generate the desired results. The nurse may decide that the sick staff nurse does not need to be replaced because client acuity and complexity is aligned with currently available staff. However, this decision can lead to negative feedback from peers. On the other hand, staff replacement, particularly when it incurs overtime costs, may not be welcomed by the manager, and will require the nurse to justify the decision with endless rationale. A lack of self-confidence is often coupled with self-consciousness, especially when someone is performing an action while being observed by others. Any mistake, however small, can be amplified by this preoccupation that someone is watching, and this perception will create an erosion of self-confidence and a heightening of self-consciousness. New graduates launching their professional careers need to be cautious not to fall into this trap.

STRESS

Stress arises when individuals perceive the environment to be demanding, because it exceeds their resources and threatens their personal well-being (Lazarus & Folkman, 1984). Bailey, Steffen, and Grout (1980) and Wakefield (1992) suggest that situations can be anxiety-provoking for some and stimulating for others, depending on how people perceive the environment. Generally speaking, nurses with an internal locus of control in a clinical setting perceive opportunities to influence outcomes for their clients, other nurses, and the organization. This approach leads to a greater sense of personal job satisfaction and reduction of stress. Staff with an external locus of control believe that external events and people are in control, and that they have very little choice over deciding their future.

Cleland (1967) studied the effects of stress upon nurses' thinking and concluded that moderate amounts of stress are required for optimal thinking. However, she also concluded that the long-term effects of functioning within highly stressful environments, such as today's health care settings, include stereotypical, unimaginative thinking, overgeneralization, and loss of interest. Bailey, Steffen, and Grout (1980) found that nurses identified the following factors as producing the greatest stress: interpersonal conflict, inadequate staffing, lack of support when dealing with death, and physical environment.

In 2007, the nursing profession found that stress is a constant and results in higher rates of job strain, lack of job satisfaction, and higher illness rates among nurses (Aiken et al., 2002). These results do not bode well for the future of nursing. Consequently, nurses and employers need to collaborate to create and maintain practice environments that support effective decision making at the point of care and thereby contribute to a high sense of job fulfillment and autonomy for nurses.

EXTRINSIC FACTORS

ORGANIZATIONAL CLIMATE AND CULTURE

Organizational climate and culture provide the context in which nursing practice occurs and can have a profound impact on the efficacious and effective application of that practice. Carman et al. (1996) and Doran et al. (2002)

conclude that organizational climate and culture are increasingly recognized as important variables in the success or failure of change initiatives, including quality improvement. Affonso and Doran (2000) add patient safety to the areas affected by an organization's climate and culture.

Hofstede (1998) notes that "culture is a characteristic of the organization, *not of individuals*" (p. 469). This description suggests that the culture in any organization is illustrated and measured through the language (i.e., verbal and nonverbal) being used and the behaviours being exhibited by individuals and groups at the organizational level. Organizational culture can be influenced by individuals, organizational features, and external factors. Shein (1991) reported that individuals can facilitate cultural change through leadership that clarifies values and develops a common organizational vision. Organizational structures, routines, command and control expectations, and operational norms influence the organization's culture (Langfield-Smith, 1995).

Cultural factors have an impact on decision making. For example, a conservative organization that is risk-averse, with a top-down bureaucratic operational style, is not likely to embrace a decentralized decision-making model in which nurses, nursing leaders, and nurse managers are encouraged to make pivotal decisions at the point of care. Block (1990) states that "if we sit on top of the pyramid we can have a very broad impact [i.e., influential decision making] on structure, policy, strategy and procedures" (p. 189). The opposite is true if nurses find themselves at the bottom of the pyramid. In this situation, nurses may only have impact on decisions that affect personal actions. Block asserts that regardless of the staff position, "the challenge is to pursue our vision with as much courage and intensity as we can generate" (p. 189).

CLIENT CHOICE AND RIGHTS

The Canadian Healthcare Association indicates that there is no national bill of client rights approved for use in Canada. However, various interest groups have adopted a bill of rights for the people they represent; for example, the Arthritis Society of Canada has a bill of rights for people with arthritis. Typically, a bill of rights is organizationally driven and reflects the following principles: the client's right to self-determination, respect, privacy, confidentiality, continuity in care delivery, and financial billing rights. In every interaction, nurses, nurse leaders, and nurse managers must respect the client's rights to self-determination, which might mean accepting the client's decision to refuse treatment or to live at risk. Nurses also must be aware that a client may reach a point of being unable to make treatment decisions. Consequently, nurses must have an understanding of the role of advanced directives; powers of attorney for care and finance; and substitute decision making, by either a substitute decision-maker of the client's choice or a court-appointed guardian. Nurses need to understand the legislative frameworks in which these various client representatives gain their power to act on behalf of the client. Above all, the client's wishes, directives, choices, and needs must be considered in the clinical decision-making process.

LEGISLATION AND REGULATION

External influences can include government legislation (e.g., Ontario's Regulated Health Professions Act, 1991), professional standards (e.g., the CNA Code of Ethics, various provincial regulators' standards of practice, and best practice guidelines), and various provincial government accountability agreements that outline performance standards. A classic example of the legislative and regulatory impact on decision making is the transfer of a controlled act from one discipline to another. In all provinces, nursing regulators have specific frameworks outlining how this transfer must occur. A nurse implementing a medical directive approved for use in the organization needs to use professional judgment in deciding whether to implement the directive. The nurse's actions within the directive are influenced by provincial legislation and professional regulation. This type of decision making in clinical practice is intense because of the speed of the decision and the consequences of indecision (e.g., deciding on whether to implement a medical directive on the management of chest pain).

REAL WORLD INTERVIEW

One of my clients at night on the medicine unit was complaining of a vague chest pain. I assessed him and was not sure what caused his discomfort. I phoned the physician-on-call and was advised that he was busy in emergency and would come to see the client as soon as possible. Then I called the Rapid Response Team (RRT) to assess the client. The RRT arrived and completed an ECG; it showed minor ischemic changes. The RRT informed the physician-on-call of the changes in the ECG. The client was prescribed nitro for his angina. I was glad that I listened to my gut instinct and decided to call the RRT, instead of waiting for the physician to see the client. The problem was diagnosed early enough to prevent further damage to the client's heart. I felt I made the right decision by calling the Rapid Response Team.

Mara Lopez, RN
New Graduate

TABLE 18-2	REVIEW OF DECISION MAKING AND CRITICAL THINKING
Decision making	Decision making is making a selection and implementing a course of action from a group of alternatives. It may or may not involve a problem.
Critical Thinking	Critical thinking is analyzing the way one thinks. It should be incorporated into all steps of problem solving and decision making.

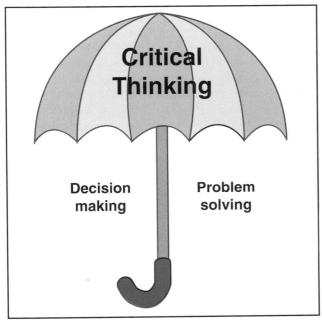

Figure 18-1 Critical Thinking Is Used in Both Problem Solving and Decision Making.

Consideration of regulatory legislation, professional standards, best practice guidelines, and organizational policies and procedures is foundational to effective clinical decision making. Thus, nurses must have knowledge and understanding of the regulatory framework that governs their practice, and they must understand other regulatory practice requirements defined in other types of federal and provincial legislation (e.g., the Personal Information Protection and Electronic Documents Act [PIPEDA], the Narcotic Control Act, acts governing consent and substitute decision-makers, and health information protection acts).

STEPS IN THE DECISION-MAKING PROCESS

In everyday practice, nurses make decisions about client care. As nurses gain experience in clinical practice, decision making becomes more automatic, but the complexity of many decisions remains. Huber (2000) defines

decision making as a "behaviour exhibited in making a selection and implementing a course of action from alternatives. It may or may not be the result of an immediate problem" (p. 378). Both decision making and problem solving use critical thinking. Table 18-2 reviews decision making and critical thinking. Figure 18-1 highlights the use of critical thinking in both problem solving and decision making.

Although decisions are unique to different situations, the decision-making process can be applied to each situation. The decision-making process is similar to the steps in problem solving. In the decision-making process, there are also five steps:

Step 1. Identify the need for a decision.
Step 2. Determine the goal or outcome.
Step 3. Identify the alternatives or actions along with the benefits and consequences of each action.
Step 4. Decide which action to implement.
Step 5. Evaluate the action.

In the following clinical application, the decision-making process is applied to a clinical situation.

CLINICAL APPLICATION

Your client is on droplet precautions because he has been diagnosed with tuberculosis. As per hospital policy, only two visitors are allowed at a time to see the client. No children under 12 years of age are allowed. The client does not speak English, and his family speaks very little English. You have noticed on two occasions that his visitors were not wearing masks. You inform the family about the importance of infection control practices and remind them of the hospital's policy regarding visitors. The family indicates to you that their grandfather really wants to see his 4-year-old grandson, who came to visit him from another province. Use your decision-making and problem-solving skills to help you decide what to do.

■ Step 1: Identify the need for a decision. Should you allow the grandson to visit? Consider all the information (e.g., the hospital policy, professional practice standards, the client's wishes, and the client's anxiety level).

- Step 2: Determine the outcome. What is the goal? Consider the following questions: Can an exception to hospital policy be made? Is the goal to allow the client to see his grandson? Will the client and his family be satisfied?
- Step 3: Identify all alternative actions and the benefits and consequences of each. If you enforce hospital policy, the benefits are that all clients are treated equally and the written policy supports the decision. The consequences are that the client and his family may not be satisfied, and the grandson and grandfather may be upset. In addition, the grandson's health may be at risk. The alternative is to allow the grandson to visit. The benefits are that the client's level of anxiety will decrease, and the client and his family will be satisfied. The consequence is that a precedent is set that may make it difficult to enforce the existing hospital policy.
- Step 4: Arrive at the decision. Consider the two alternatives and the benefits and consequences of each. Make the decision and implement it.
- Step 5: Evaluate the decision. Was the goal achieved?

From the beginning of their careers, new graduate nurses are faced with the responsibility of making decisions regarding client care. Beginning nurses commonly have more questions than answers. When nurses are faced with a difficult clinical decision, Marquis and Huston (2006) recommend consulting with others, such as other RNs on the unit or supervisors, as early as possible. Depending on the situation, recognize that you have knowledge and intuition that are valuable. With more experience comes greater trust in your decision making.

MANAGEMENT APPLICATION

Nurse managers sometimes face complex decisions. Decisions related to budget are common in our current health care environment with its emphasis on cost containment and quality maintenance. Disciplining an employee also creates a complex situation in which managers must make decisions regarding the employee's future. A decision-making grid may help to separate the multiple factors that surround a situation. Figure 18-2 illustrates use of a decision-making grid by managers who were told they had to reduce their workforce by two full-time equivalents (FTEs). This grid is useful to visually separate the factors of cost savings, effect on job satisfaction of remaining staff, and effect on client satisfaction. The manager needs to determine the priorities when developing a grid.

A decision-making grid is also useful when a nurse is trying to decide between two choices. Figure 18-3 is an example of a decision grid used by a nurse deciding between working at hospital A or hospital B.

The Program Evaluation and Review Technique (PERT) is useful in determining the timing of decisions. The flowchart provides a visual picture depicting the sequence of tasks that must take place to complete a project. Jones and Beck (1996) provide an example of a PERT flow diagram depicting a case management project (see Figure 18-4). The chart shows the amount of time taken to complete the project and the sequence of events to complete the project. An advantage of the PERT diagram is that participants can visualize a complete picture

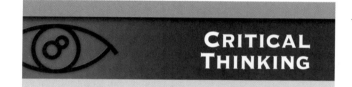

CRITICAL THINKING

You are a new nurse manager and have been in your position for two months. You are working on the holiday schedule, and the unit secretary with the most seniority comes to you and says that she needs both the week of Christmas and the week of New Year's Day off because she will be out of town. You remind her that hospital policy does not allow employees to have both holidays off. The secretary tells you that the previous manager always approved her request and that she has already bought plane tickets. Apply the steps of decision making to this situation.

Methods of Reduction	Cost Savings	Effect on Job Satisfaction	Effect on Client Satisfaction
Lay off the two most senior full-time employees	$93,500	Significant reduction	Significant reduction
Lay off the two most recently hired full-time employees	$63,200	Significant reduction	Moderate reduction
Reduce by staff attrition	$78,000	Minor reduction	Minor reduction

Figure 18-2 Sample Decision-Making Grid.

Elements	Importance Score (out of 10)	Likelihood Score (out of 10)	Risk (multiply scores)
If I work at hospital A			
Learning experience	10	10	100
Good mentor support	8	8	64
Financial reward	6	6	36
Growth potential	8	8	64
Good location	10	10	100
Total			364
If I work at hospital B			
Learning experience	8	8	64
Good mentor support	7	7	49
Financial reward	8	8	64
Growth potential	9	9	81
Good location	6	6	36
Total			294

Figure 18-3 Sample Decision-Making Grid for Weighing Options.

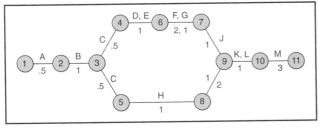

Figure 18-4 PERT Diagram with Critical Path for Implementation of Case Management.

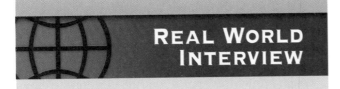

REAL WORLD INTERVIEW

I often find decisions about disciplinary action the most difficult ones to make. But, when I use a decision-making model, it helps me make the best decision. My goal in the decision-making process is often twofold—to help the nurse to learn from the experience and to provide the nurse with appropriate tools to prevent similar mistakes happening in the future.

Erica
Nurse Manager Intensive Care Unit

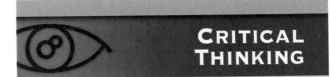

CRITICAL THINKING

You are working for a home health agency that employs 17 registered nurses. As the agency's census has increased, concerns have arisen about the staffing and scheduling. The manager has said that until more staff can be hired, there will be an increased need for on-call and overtime scheduling. The manager has given the responsibility to the entire group to figure out the best way to cover the client assignments.

What would be the best group decision-making strategy to use? What should the group do first?

of the project, including the timing of decisions from beginning to end.

DECISION TREE

A decision tree can be useful in making the alternatives visible. Figure 18-5 is a decision tree for choosing whether to go back to school.

Figure 18-6 identifies a decision analysis tree for a client who smokes.

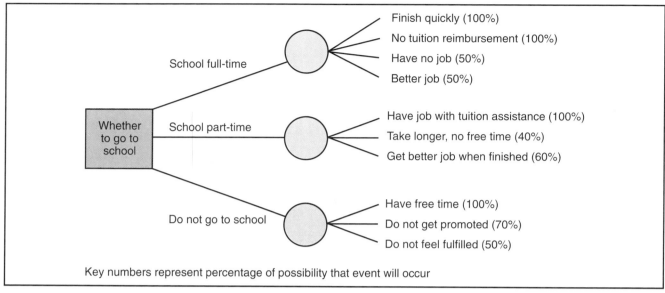

Figure 18-5 Decision Tree for Choosing Whether to Go Back to School.

GANTT CHART

A Gantt chart can be useful for decision-makers to illustrate a project from beginning to end. Figure 18-7 illustrates a Gantt chart used to show the progression of a nursing unit's pilot project.

GROUP DECISION MAKING

Certain situations call for group decision making. Vroom and Yetton (1973) identified certain questions managers should ask themselves before making a decision alone. In some situations, it is more appropriate for a group to make the decision rather than the individual manager. Each situation is different, and an effective manager adopts the appropriate mode of decision making—group or individual. The eight questions in Table 18-3 may assist the manager in determining which mode to use.

Today's leadership and management styles include people in the decision-making process who will be most affected by the decision. Decisions affecting client care should be made by those groups implementing the decisions.

The effectiveness of groups depends greatly on the group's members. The size of the group and the personalities of group members are important considerations when choosing participants. More ideas can be generated with groups, thus allowing for more choices, which increases the likelihood of higher-quality outcomes. Another advantage of groups is that when followers participate in the decision-making process, acceptance of the decision is more likely to occur. Additionally, groups may be used as a medium for communicating the decision and its rationale.

A major disadvantage of group decision making is the time involved. Without effective leadership, groups can waste time and be nonproductive. Group decision making can be more costly and can also lead to conflict. Groups can be dominated by one person or become the battleground for a power struggle among assertive members. See Table 18-4 for a listing of the advantages and disadvantages of groups.

TECHNIQUES OF GROUP DECISION MAKING

Various techniques can be used in group decision making. Nominal group technique, Delphi technique, and consensus building are different methods to facilitate group decision making.

NOMINAL GROUP TECHNIQUE

The nominal group technique was developed by Delbecq Van de Ven and Gustafson in 1971. The word *nominal* refers to the nonverbal aspect of this approach (Cawthorpe & Harris, 1999). In the first step, no discussion occurs: group members write out their ideas or responses to the identified issue or question posed by the group leader. The second step involves presentation of the ideas of the group members along with the advantages and disadvantages of each. These ideas are presented on a flipchart or a whiteboard. The third phase may offer an opportunity for discussion to clarify and evaluate the ideas. The fourth phase includes private voting on the ideas. Those ideas receiving the highest rating are the solutions implemented.

DELPHI GROUP TECHNIQUE

Delphi technique differs from nominal technique in that group members are not meeting face to face. Questionnaires are distributed to group members for their opinions,

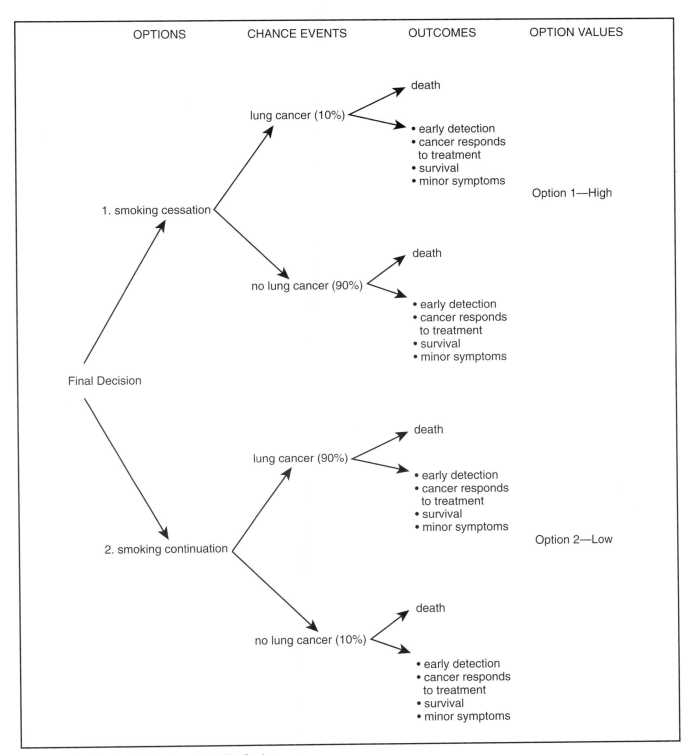

OPTIONS   CHANCE EVENTS   OUTCOMES   OPTION VALUES

lung cancer (10%) → death
• early detection
• cancer responds to treatment
• survival
• minor symptoms

1. smoking cessation

no lung cancer (90%) → death
• early detection
• cancer responds to treatment
• survival
• minor symptoms

Option 1—High

Final Decision

lung cancer (90%) → death
• early detection
• cancer responds to treatment
• survival
• minor symptoms

2. smoking continuation

Option 2—Low

no lung cancer (10%) → death
• early detection
• cancer responds to treatment
• survival
• minor symptoms

Figure 18-6 Decision Analysis Tree for a Client Who Smokes.

and the responses are then summarized and disseminated to the group members. This process continues for as many times as necessary for the group members to reach consensus. An advantage of this technique is that it can involve a large number of participants and thus a greater number of ideas.

CONSENSUS BUILDING

Consensus is defined by *The American Heritage Dictionary* (2000) as "an opinion or position reached by a group as a whole; general agreement or accord" (p. 391). A common misconception is that consensus means everyone agrees with the decision 100 percent. Contrary to this

A nurse manager has agreed to have her unit pilot a new care delivery system within six months. The Gantt chart can be used to plan the progression of the project.

Activities	Sept	Oct	Nov	Dec	Jan	Feb	Mar	Apr	May
Discuss project with staff	------ X								
Form an ad hoc planning committee	------	―― X							
Receive report from committee			------ X						
Discuss report with staff			------ ―― X						
Educate all staff to the plan				------ ―― X					
Implement new system						------	――――――		
Evaluate system and make changes							------	――	X

Key
------ Proposed Time
――― Actual Time
X   Complete

Figure 18-7 Gantt Chart: Implementation of Care Delivery System.

TABLE 18-3   INDIVIDUAL VS. GROUP DECISION-MAKING QUESTIONS

1. Does the manager have all the information needed?
2. Do the subordinates have supplementary information needed to make the best decision?
3. Does the manager have all the resources available to obtain sufficient information to make the best decision?
4. Is it absolutely critical that the team accept the decision prior to implementation?
5. Will the team accept the decision I make by myself?
6. Does the course of action chosen make a difference to the organization?
7. Does the team have the best interest of the organization foremost when considering the decision?
8. Will the decision cause undue conflict among the team?

Source: Adapted from *Leadership and Decision-Making* (pp. 21–30), by V. Vroom and P. Yetton, 1973, Pittsburgh, PA: University of Pittsburgh Press.

misunderstanding, **consensus** means that all group members can live with and fully support the decision regardless of whether they totally agree. This strategy is useful with groups because all group members participate and can realize the contributions each member makes to the decision (Sullivan & Decker, 2001). A disadvantage to the consensus strategy is that decision making requires more time. This strategy should be reserved for important decisions that require strong support from the participants who will implement them. Consensus decision making

TABLE 18-4	ADVANTAGES AND DISADVANTAGES OF GROUPS

Advantages

- Easy and inexpensive way to share information
- Opportunities for face-to-face communication
- Opportunity to become connected with a social unit
- Promotion of cohesiveness and loyalty
- Access to a larger resource base
- Forum for constructive problem solving
- Support group
- Facilitation of esprit de corps
- Promotion of ownership of problems and solutions

Disadvantages

- Individual opinions influenced by others
- Individual identity obscured
- Formal and informal role and status positions evolve—hierarchies
- Dependency fostered
- Time-consuming
- Inequity of time given to share individual information
- Existence of nonfunctional roles
- Personality conflicts

LITERATURE APPLICATION

Citation: Brooks, E. M., & Thomas, S. (1997). The perception and judgment of senior baccalaureate student nurses in clinical decision making. *Advances in Nursing Science, 19*(3), 50–69.

Discussion: One purpose of this study was to identify factors that affect decision making of senior baccalaureate student nurses. The authors used Brooks's Theory of Intrapersonal Awareness (BTIPA), which was based on the nursing theory of King's interacting systems framework. This framework includes perception and judgment as being integral to the nurse–client relationship. Decisions are influenced by nursing judgment, which, in turn, is influenced by values and perceptions. A structured interview and a written, simulated vignette of a clinical situation were given to 18 senior baccalaureate nursing students. The vignette consisted of a man injured in a motor vehicle accident in which his best friend was killed. The family of the injured man did not want him told of his friend's death. The most prominent intrapersonal characteristic affecting how the students made decisions regarding this vignette was experience. Experience was defined as work experience, clinical experience, personal experience, or lack of experience. The second most prominent intrapersonal characteristic was the student's personal values and beliefs. For example, the student would ask herself, "What would I want in this situation?" If someone believes in always telling the truth, then that individual would have a difficult time keeping the client's death from the other client.

Implications for Practice: Nurses need to recognize that people make decisions based on their own intrapersonal perceptual awareness. Prior experiences and personal values affect a person's decision making. The authors concluded that students need to be prepared to understand themselves and how their experiences and values will affect the decisions they make.

works well when the decisions are made under the following conditions: all members of the team are affected by the decision; implementation of the solution requires coordination among team members; and the decision is critical, requiring full commitment by team members. Although consensus can be the most time-consuming strategy, it can also be the most gratifying.

GROUPTHINK

Groupthink and consensus building are different. In consensus, the group members work to support the final decision, and individual ideas and opinions are valued. In groupthink, the goal is for everyone to be in 100 percent agreement. Groupthink discourages questioning and divergent thinking. It hinders creativity and usually leads to inferior decisions (Jarvis, 1997). The potential for groupthink increases as the cohesiveness of the group increases.

An important responsibility of the group leader is to recognize symptoms of groupthink. Janis (as cited in Jarvis, 1997) described examples of these symptoms. One symptom is that group members develop an illusion of invulnerability, believing they can do no wrong. This problem has the greatest potential to develop when the group is powerful and group members view themselves as invincible. The second symptom of groupthink is stereotyping outsiders, which occurs when the group members rely on shared stereotypes—such as, all Democrats are liberal or all Republicans are conservative—to justify their positions. People who challenge or disagree with the decisions are also stereotyped. A third symptom is that group members reassure one another that their interpretation of data and their perspective on matters are correct regardless of the evidence showing otherwise. Old assumptions are never challenged, and members ignore what they do not know or what they do not want to know.

Strategies to avoid groupthink include appointing group members to roles that evaluate how group decision making occurs. Group leaders should encourage all group members to think independently and verbalize their individual ideas. The leader should allow the group some time to gather further data and reflect on data already collected. A primary responsibility of the managers or the group leader is to prevent groupthink from developing.

LIMITATIONS TO EFFECTIVE DECISION MAKING

Useem and Useem (2005) suggest that as individuals, we are not lemmings heading over a cliff, because our decision-making processes are sound. Yet decision making in clinical practice or management can be flawed when nurses encounter classic pitfalls and are unable to recognize their impact.

What are obstacles to effective decision making? Past experiences, values, personal biases, and preconceived ideas affect the way people view problems and situations. Incorporating critical thinking into the decision-making process helps to prevent these factors from distorting the process. Hammond, Keeney, and Raiffa (1998) have identified pitfalls to effective decision making:

- Making the decision based upon the first available information
- Being comfortable with the status quo or not wanting to rock the boat
- Making decisions to justify previous decisions even if those decisions are no longer satisfactory

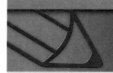

LITERATURE APPLICATION

Citation: Bucknall, T., & Thomas, S. (1997). Nurses' reflections on problems associated with decision-making in critical care settings. *Journal of Advanced Nursing, 25,* 229–237.

Discussion: A questionnaire was sent to 230 practising critical care nurses to collect data about the problems they experience when making clinical decisions. Lack of time to implement decisions was cited as the most frequent problem. Another problem that frequently was associated with decision making was staying current with the ever-changing treatments and technology. Nurses reported concerns about their abilities to make decisions based on a lack of current knowledge. Other areas of decision-making problems included nurses and physicians having different values about end-of-life treatment. The extent of nurses' autonomy in making decisions was also problematic. Working relationships between nurses and resident physicians were also cited as a frequent problem.

Implications for Practice: Recognizing frequently occurring problems with decision making is an important first step in stopping the problems from recurring. Solutions can also be found by collaborating with colleagues and researching the nursing literature for information related to the identified problems.

- Pursuing supporting evidence that verifies the decision while ignoring evidence to the contrary
- Presenting the issue in a biased manner or with a leading question
- Assigning inaccurate probabilities to alternatives.

USE OF TECHNOLOGY IN DECISION MAKING

The best source of clinical decision making and judgment is still the professional practitioner; however, computer technology can be used to support information systems, including decision making, for managers (Tomey, 2000). Patient classification systems, inventory control, scheduling staff, documentation of client care, order entry for tests, appointments, and changes in policies and procedures are but a few examples of how computers can assist managers with tracking the information needed in a management role. Computer software for the clinical practitioner is available for clinical decision making and should be carefully critiqued prior to use.

NURSES' ROLE IN CLIENT DECISION MAKING

In today's world, clients are taking a more active role in treatment decisions. Consumers of health care are more knowledgeable and have more options than in previous years. Nurses must be aware of clients' rights in making decisions about their treatments, and they must assist clients in their decision making. When clients are active participants, compliance with prescribed treatments is more likely to follow. Empowering the client in this manner ultimately promotes a more positive outcome.

STRATEGIES TO IMPROVE DECISION MAKING

Comfort with decision making improves with experience. Early in the nurse's career, the nurse is commonly indecisive or uncomfortable with decisions. Alfaro-LeFevre (1995) has identified several strategies that help to improve critical thinking, which, in turn, will also help to improve decision making. Do you have all the information needed to make a decision? At times, delaying a decision

until more information is obtained may be the best approach. Asking "why," "what else," and "what if" questions will help you arrive at the best decision. When more information becomes available, decisions can be revised. Very few decisions are set in stone. Another helpful strategy for improving decision making is to anticipate questions and outcomes. For example, when calling a physician to report a client's change in condition, the nurse will want to have pertinent information about the client's vital signs, lab values, and current medications readily available.

Nurses who practise strategies to promote their own critical thinking will, in turn, be good decision-makers. A foundation for good decision making comes with experience and learning from those experiences. Table 18-5 shows some additional tips to consider when making decisions. By turning decisions with poor outcomes into learning experiences, nurses will enhance their decision-making ability in the future.

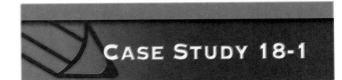

CASE STUDY 18-1

The manager has identified a problem for a group: Shortage of staff, high turnover, lack of experienced nurses on the unit, low staff satisfaction, and low morale. How will the group solve this problem?

TABLE 18-5	DOS AND DON'TS OF DECISION MAKING
Do	**Don't**
Make only those decisions that are yours to make.	Make snap decisions.
Write notes and keep ideas visible about decisions to utilize all relevant information.	Waste your time making decisions that do not have to be made.
Write down pros and cons of an issue to help clarify your thinking.	Consider decisions a choice between right and wrong but a choice among alternatives.
Make decisions as you go along rather than letting them accumulate.	Prolong deliberation about decisions.
Consider those affected by your decision.	Regret a decision; it was the right thing to do at the time.
Trust yourself.	Always base decisions on the "way things have always been done."

Source: Adapted from The Small Business Knowledge Base, 1999. Retrieved February 19, 2002, from http://www.bizmove.com.

KEY CONCEPTS

- The ever-changing health care system calls for nurses to be effective decision-makers. The ability of nurses to make appropriate decisions will affect their employer's ability to survive.

- A good critical thinker is able to examine decisions from all sides and take into account varying points of view. Use of the universal intellectual standards will improve a nurse's critical thinking.

- Practising reflective thinking helps individuals become better critical thinkers.

- Problem solving involves five steps: (1) identify the problem, (2) gather and analyze data, (3) generate alternatives and select action, (4) implement the selected action, and (5) evaluate the selected action.

- The decision-making process has five steps: Step 1— identify the need for a decision; Step 2—determine the goal or outcome; Step 3—identify alternatives or actions, along with their benefits and consequences; Step 4— decide on the action and implement it; Step 5—evaluate the action.

- Decision-making grids may be helpful to separate multiple factors during the decision-making process.

- The PERT model is useful for determining the timing of decisions.

- In some situations the nurse manager makes an individual decision. Other situations call for group decision making.

- Consensus is a strategy utilized when using group decision making.

- To be an effective decision-maker, individuals must identify and avoid certain traps during the decision-making process.

- Groupthink occurs when individuals are not allowed to express creativity, question methods, or engage in divergent thinking. Managers must be able to identify the symptoms of groupthink.

- The nurse must recognize the importance of empowering clients in making their own treatment decisions. The nurse needs to provide the client with information and assist the client to explore all possible options.

- Many strategies can be used to improve your decision making. Obtaining all the information, asking yourself "why" and "what if" questions, and developing good habits of inquiry are a few of the strategies that will help improve your decision-making skills.

KEY TERMS

consensus
critical thinking
decision making
Delphi technique
problem solving
reflective thinking

REVIEW QUESTIONS

1. Decision making is best described as the process one uses to
   A. solve a problem.
   B. choose between alternatives.
   C. reflect on a certain situation.
   D. generate ideas.

2. Which of the following is the best description of consensus?
   A. Everyone in the group agrees with the decision 100 percent.
   B. All members of the group vote on the selected action.
   C. Every group member compromises.
   D. Every group member fully supports the decision, once it is made.

3. Which of the following is a symptom of groupthink?
   A. The group members continually disagree with one another.
   B. The group members cannot come to a decision.
   C. The group members stereotype outsiders.
   D. The group members share a common bond.

4. Occasionally, making a decision is difficult because of the multiple factors that surround certain situations. To separate these factors, the nurse manager may utilize a
   A. decision grid.
   B. nominal group technique.
   C. Delphi group technique.
   D. consensus strategy.

REVIEW ACTIVITIES

1. You are the manager of a 12-bed surgical unit. Your supervisor informs you that 12 more beds will be opened for neurosurgical clients, and you are to be the manager. Draw a PERT diagram to depict the sequence of tasks necessary for the completion of the project.

2. The education forms are not being filled out correctly or in a timely manner on new admissions in your medical-surgical unit. Decide on your own the best action to take in this situation. Then, form a group and attempt to reach consensus on the best action to take. Compare the differences between individual and group decision making. What did you learn about developing consensus?

3. Identify a problem that you have been considering. Using the decision-making grid below, rate the alternative solutions to

	Cost	Quality	Importance	Location	Other
Alternative A					
Alternative B					
Alternative C					

the problem that you have been considering on a scale of 1 to 3 on the elements of cost, quality, importance, location, and any other elements that are important to you.

Did this exercise help you in thinking through your decision?

4. Identify a current problem in health care. Use the problem-solving process in a group to find a solution. Employ the nominal group technique and the Delphi technique.

EXPLORING THE WEB

- Test your critical thinking in critical care by reviewing the scenarios in "Leeches in PICU? (Critical Thinking in Critical Care)," an article by Marilu Dixon in the May 2003 issue of *Pediatric Nursing*. Access this article through your school library.

- Note the universal intellectual standards at the Foundation for Critical Thinking: *http://www.criticalthinking.org/ page.cfm?PageID=527&CategoryID=68*

- Visit this critical thinking site: *http://www. criticalthinking.org/*

- Note the following site for clinical decision–making. This site includes software for clinical decision making: *http://www.apache-msi.com/*

- *http://www.york.ac.uk/healthsciences/centres/ evidence/decrpt.pdf*

- Review this site on applying artificial intelligence to clinical situations: *http://groups.csail.mit.edu/medg/*

REFERENCES

Affonso, D., & Doran, D. M. (2002). Cultivating discoveries in patient safety research: A framework. *The Journal of Nursing Perspectives, 2*(1), 33–47.

Aiken, L. H., Clarke, S. P., Sloane, D. M., Sochalski, J., & Silber, J. H. (2002). Hospital nurse staffing and patient mortality, nurse burnout and job dissatisfaction. *Journal of the American Medical Association, 288*(10), 1987–1993.

Alfaro-LeFevre, R. (1995). *Critical thinking in nursing.* Philadelphia: Saunders.

Alfaro-LeFevre, R. (2006). *Critical Thinking Indicators™.* Stuart, FL: Author.

American heritage dictionary of the English language (4th ed.). (2000). Boston, MA: Houghton Mifflin.

Bailey, J. T., Steffen, S. M., & Grout, J. W. (1980). The stress audit: Identifying the stressors of ICU nursing. *Journal of Nursing Education, 19*(6), 15–25.

Bellack, J. P., & O'Neil, E. H. (2000). Recreating nursing practice for a new century: Recommendations and implications of the Pew Health Professions Commission's final report. *Nursing and Health Care Perspectives, 21*(1), 14–21.

Benner, P. (1984). *From novice to expert.* Menlo Park, CA: Addison Wesley.

Benner, P., & Tanner, C. A. (1987). How expert nurses use intuition. *American Journal of Nursing, 87*(1), 23–31.

Block, P. (1990). *The empowered manager: Positive political skills at work.* San Francisco: Jossey-Bass.

Brooks, E. M., & Thomas, S. (1997). The perception and judgment of senior baccalaureate student nurses in clinical decision making. *Advances in Nursing Science, 19*(3), 50–69.

Bucknall, T., & Thomas, S. (1997). Nurses' reflections on problems associated with decision-making in critical care settings. *Journal of Advanced Nursing, 25,* 229–237.

Campbell, B., & Mackay, G. P. (2001). Continuing competence: An Ontario nursing regulatory program that supports nurses and employers. *Nursing Administration Quarterly, 25*(2), 22–30.

Canadian Council on Health Services Accreditation. (2006). *CCHSA patient safety and required organizational practices.* Ottawa: Author.

Canadian Nurses Association (2000). *A national framework for continuing competence for registered nurses.* Ottawa: Author.

Canadian Nursing Advisory Committee (CNAC). (2002). *Our health, our future: Creating quality workplaces for Canadian nurses.* Ottawa: Author.

Carman, J. M., Shortell, S. M., Foster, R. W., Hughes, E. F., Boerstler, H., O'Brien, J. L. et al. (1996). Keys for successful implementation of total quality management in hospitals. *Health Care Management Review, 21*(1), 48–60.

Cawthorpe, D., & Harris, D. (1999). Nominal group technique: Assessing staff concerns. *Journal of Nursing Administration, 29*(7/8), 11, 18, 37, 42.

Cleland, V. (1967). Effects of stress on thinking. *The American Journal of Nursing, 67*(1), 108–111.

Correnti, D. (1992). Intuition and nursing practice implications for nurse educators: a review of the literature. *Journal of Continuing Nursing Education, 23*(2), 91–94.

Donaghy, M. E., & Morss, K. (2000). Guided reflection: A framework to facilitate and access reflective practice with the discipline of physiotherapy. *Physiotherapy and Practice, 16*(1), 3–14.

Doran, D. M., Baker, G. R., Murray, M., Bohnen, J., Zahn, C., Sidani, S. et al. (2002). Achieving clinical improvement: An interdisciplinary intervention. *Health Care Management Review, 27*(4), 42–56.

Dwyer, D. W., Schwartz, R. H., & Fox, M. L. (1992). Decision making autonomy in nursing. *Journal of Nursing Administration, 22*(2), 107–112,

Evans, D. (1990). Problems in the decision making process: a review. *Intensive Care Nursing, 6*(4), 179–184.

Hagbaghery, M. A., Salsali, M., & Ahmadi, F. (2004). The factors facilitating and inhibiting effective decision-making in nursing: a qualitative study. *BMC Nursing, 3*(1), 2.

Hammond, J. S., Keeney, R. L., & Raiffa, H. (1998). The hidden traps in decision making. *Harvard Business Review, 76*(5), 47–58.

Hofstede, G., (1998). Attitudes, values and organizational culture: Disentangling the concepts. *Organization Studies, 19*(3), 477–492.

Huber, D. (2000). *Leadership and nursing care management.* Philadelphia: Saunders.

Marquis, B. L., & Huston, C. J. (2006). *Leadership roles and management functions in nursing: Theory and application* (5th ed.). Philadelphia: Lippincott, Williams and Wilkins.

International Council of Nurses. (2000). *Position statement: Participation of nurses in health services decision making and policy development.* Geneva, Switzerland: Author.

Jarvis, C. (1997). *Groupthink.* Retrieved from http://www.bola.biz/communications/groupthink.html, July 27, 2007.

Jones, R. A. P., & Beck, S. E. (1996). *Decision making in nursing.* Clifton Park, NY: Delmar Learning.

Joseph, D. H. (1985). Sex-role stereotype, self concept, education and experience: Do they influence decision making? *International Journal of Nursing Studies, 22*(1), 21–32.

Keenan, J. (1999). A concept analysis of autonomy. *Journal of Advanced Nursing, 29*(3), 556–562.

Langfield-Smith, K. (1995). Organizational culture and control. In A. Berry, J. Broadbent & D. Otley (Eds.). *Management control theories, issues and practices* (pp. 179–202). London: Macmillan.

Lazarus, R. S., & Folkman, S. (1984). *Stress, appraisal and coping.* New York: Springer Publishing Company.

LeStorti, A., Cullen, P., Hanzlik, E., Michiels, J. M., Piano, L., Ryan, P. L. et al. (1999). Creative thinking in nursing education: Preparing for tomorrow's challenges. *Nursing Outlook, 47*(2), 62–66.

MacDonald, C. (2002). Nurse autonomy as relational. *Nursing Ethics, 9*(2), 194–201.

Murphy, E. C. (1985). Whole brain management: Part 1. *Nursing Management, 16*(3), 66.

Niadu, S., Oliver, M., & Koronious, A. (1999). Approaching clinical decision-making in nursing practice with interactive multimedia and case-based reasoning. *Interactive Multimedia Electronic Journal of Computer Enchanced Learning, 1*(2).

O'Reilly, P. (1993). Barriers to effective clinical decision making in nursing. *St Vincent's Nursing Monograph: 1993 Selected Works* (pp. 34–43). Sydney, Australia: Author.

Pardue, S. (1987). Decision-making skills and critical thinking ability among associate degree, diploma, baccalaureate, and master's-prepared nurses. *Journal of Nursing Education, 26*(9), 354–361.

Paul, R. (1992). *Critical thinking: What every person needs to survive in a rapidly changing world.* Santa Rosa, CA: Foundation for Critical Thinking.

Paul, R., & Elder, L. (2005). *The nature and functions of critical and creative thinking.* Dillon Beach, CA: The Foundation for Critical Thinking.

Pesut, D. J. & Herman, J. (1999). *Clinical reasoning: The art and science of critical and creative thinking.* Clifton Park, NY: Delmar Learning.

Scott, J. G., Sochalski, J., & Aiken, L. (1999). Review of magnet hospital research: Findings and implications for professional practice. *Journal of Nursing Administration, 29*(1), 9–19.

Scriven, M., and Paul R. (2004) *Defining critical thinking.* Santa Rosa, CA: Foundation for Critical Thinking. Retrieved from http://www.criticalthinking.org/aboutCT/definingCT.shtml, December 3, 2004.

Shein, E. (1991). *Organizational culture and leadership.* San Francisco: Jossey-Bass.

Tanner, C. A., Padrick, K. P., Westfall, U. E., & Putzier, D. J. (1987). Diagnostic reasoning strategies of nurses and nursing students. *Nursing Research, 36*(6), 358–363.

Teekman, B, (2000). Exploring reflective thinking in nursing. *Journal of Advanced Nursing, 31*(5), 1125–1135.

Sullivan, E., & Decker, P. (2001). *Effective leadership and management in nursing.* Menlo Park, CA: Addison Wesley Longman.

Tomey, A. (2000). Guide to nursing management and leadership. St. Louis, MO: Mosby.

Tranmer, J. (2004). Autonomy and decision making in nursing. In McGillis-Hall, L. (Ed.), *Quality work environments: Nurse and patient safety.* Sudbury, MA: Jones and Bartlett.

Useem, M., & Useem, J. (2005). Great escapes: Nine decision-making pitfalls and nine simple devices to beat them. *Fortune, 151*(13), 97–100.

Vroom, V. H., & Yetton, P. W. (1973). *Leadership and decision-making.* Pittsburgh: University of Pittsburgh Press.

Wade, G. H. (1999). Professional nurse autonomy: Concept analysis and application to nursing education. *Journal of Advanced Nursing, 30*(2), 310–318.

Wakefield, M. (1992). Stress control for nurses. *The Canadian Nurse, 88*(4), 24–25.

SUGGESTED READINGS

Aiken, L. H., Clarke, S.P., & Sloane, D. M. (2002). Hospital staffing, organization, and quality of care: Cross-national findings. *International Journal for Quality in Health Care, 14* (1), 5–13.

American Philosophical Association. (1990). *Critical thinking: A statement of expert consensus for purposes of educational assessment and instruction, recommendations prepared for the Committee on Pre-college Philosophy.* ERIC Doc. No. ED 315-423. p. 2.

Biafore, S. (1999). Predictive solutions bring more power to decision makers. *Health Management Technology, 20*(10), 12–14.

Boblin-Cummings, S., Baumann, A., & Deber, R. (1999). Critical elements in the decision-making process: A nursing perspective. *Canadian Journal of Nursing Leadership, 12*(1), 6–13.

Bryons, A., & McIntosh, J. (1996). Decision making in community nursing: An analysis of the stages of decision making as they relate to community nursing assessment practice. *Journal of Advanced Nursing, 24*(1), 24–30.

Crandall, S. (1993). How expert clinical educators teach what they know. *Journal of Continuing Education in the Health Professions, 13*(1), 85–98.

Duchscher, J. (1999). Catching the wave: Understanding the concept of critical thinking. *Journal of Advanced Nursing, 29*(3), 577–583.

Girot, E. A. (2000). Graduate nurses: critical thinkers or better decision makers? *Journal of Advanced Nursing, 31*(2), 288–297.

Goleman, D., (1998). What makes a leader? *Harvard Business Review*, November-December, 93–102.

Huston, C. J., & Marquis, B. L. (1995). Seven steps to successful decision-making. *Amercian Journal of Nursing, 95*(5), 65–68. Kontryn, V. (1999). Strategic problem solving in the new millennium. *AORN Journal, 70*(6), 1035–1044.

Marquis, B. L., & Huston, C. J. (1998). *Management decision making for nurses: 124 case studies* (3rd ed.). Philadelphia: Lippincott.

Martinez de Castillo, S. L. (1999). *Strategies, techniques, and approaches to thinking: Case studies in clinical nursing.* Philadelphia, PA: Saunders.

Parsons, L. (1999). Building RN confidence for delegation decision-making skills in practice. *Journal for Nurses in Staff Development, 15*(6), 263–269.

Radwin, L. (1995). Conceptualizations of decision making in nursing: Analytic models and "knowing the patient." *Nursing Diagnosis, 6*(1), 16–22.

Recker, D., Bess, C., & Wellens, H. (1996). A decision-making process in shared governance. *Nursing Management, 27*(5), 48A, 48B, 48D.

Schon, D. A. (1987). *Educating the reflective practitioner.* San Francisco: Jossey-Bass.

Schon, D. A. (1989). A symposium on Schon's concept of reflective practice: Critiques, commentaries, illustrations. *Journal of Curriculum and Supervision, 5*(1), 6–9.

Scordo, K. (1997). Reaching consensus through electronic brainstorming. *Computers in Nursing, 15*(2), 33–37.

Simms, L. M., Price, S. A., & Ervin, N. E. (2000). *Professional practice of nursing administration* (3rd ed.). Clifton Park, NY: Delmar Learning.

Swansburg, R. C., & Swansburg, R. J. (2002). *Introductory management and leadership for nurse managers* (3rd ed.). Boston: Jones and Bartlett.

Tabak, N., Bar-tal, Y., & Cohen-Mansfield, J. (1996). Clinical decision making of experienced and novice nurses. *Western Journal of Nursing Research, 18*(5), 534–547.

CHAPTER ENDNOTES

1. Stanford University School of Medicine, "Decision-making," Retrieved from http://cisl.stanford.edu/what_is/learning_types/decision_mkng.html, July 24, 2007.

2. Ibid.

3. ChangingMinds.org, "Subjective vs. Objectivity Preferences." Retrieved from http://changingminds.org/explanations/preferences/subjective_objective.htm, April 21, 2007.

4. ChangingMinds.org, "Thinking vs. Feeling." Retrieved from http://changingminds.org/explanations/preferences/thinking_feeling.htm, April 21, 2007.

CHAPTER 19

Legal Aspects of Client Care

Judith W. Martin, RN, JD, Sister Kathleen Cain, OSF, JD

Adapted by: Heather Crawford, BScN, MEd, CHE

The Sinclair Report was the inquest report that told the story of 12 children who died and the health care providers who worked with them, during 1994, in the pediatric cardiac surgery program at the Winnipeg Health Sciences Centre. I chaired the Winnipeg Health Sciences committee that examined the recommendations and identified an implementation plan. The Sinclair Report raised many legal issues that continue to concern and affect nurses across Canada on a daily basis. (Heather Crawford, former Vice-President and Chief Nursing Officer, Winnipeg Health Sciences Centre)

OBJECTIVES

Upon completion of this chapter, the reader should be able to:

1. Discuss the effect of law on nursing practice.
2. Describe the importance of the Canadian Constitution and the Canadian Charter of Rights and Freedoms to health care.
3. Describe the requirements of informed consent.
4. Name the most common areas of nursing practice cited in malpractice actions, and list actions a nurse can take to minimize these risks.
5. Describe the various forms of advanced directives and how these are commonly implemented.
6. Identify the lessons that can be learned from coroner's inquests.
7. Describe risk management and how it is used in the health care setting.
8. Discuss the rights of the nurse as an employee.

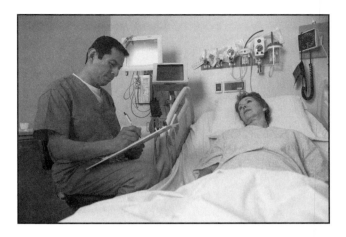

You are working on a medical-surgical unit when you admit an 82-year-old female, Mrs. Perkins. She has a medical diagnosis of abdominal pain and is admitted for further investigation. She is accompanied by her daughter, who leaves the room while you complete your admission nursing assessment. During your assessment, you notice bruises and welts across Mrs. Perkins' back, approximately two centimetres wide and the same distance apart. You ask Mrs. Perkins about these marks, but she tells you that she doesn't know how she got them. When her daughter returns, you mention the marks to her. She tells you that her mother is very unsteady on her feet and had fallen down the stairs. You notice when the daughter is in the room, Mrs. Perkins no longer maintains eye contact and is reluctant to speak without looking at her daughter first. You are beginning to suspect that Mrs. Perkins has been physically mistreated.

> *Do you need any additional information to determine the validity of your suspicions?*
>
> *If abuse has occurred, what action should you take?*
>
> *Do client confidentiality concerns affect any actions you may take?*

Historically, Canada was originally inhabited by explorers and settlers from France and the United Kingdom. What is now known as the province of Quebec was governed exclusively under French civil law until the French colonies in North America were given to Great Britain from France in 1763. French civil law was based on the Roman law system. In Roman law, legal rules and principles that establish rights and responsibilities of individuals are formally written in a single document known as civil code.

With the exception of the province of Quebec, Canada's legal system is derived from English common law. The majority of **common law** was not written down or codified as statute law. Many of the essential rules and principles that govern our everyday life have been developed through precedents, which are individual sets of judges' reasons for deciding individual cases. Precedents are usually published in volumes by category, such as jurisdiction

(e.g., provincial, territorial, or federal), subject matter (e.g., criminal law, family law), or level of the court that provided the decision (e.g., Federal Court of Appeal, Supreme Court of Canada). Legal principles and rules are developed from these precedents and are then applied by judges to specific cases. This body of precedent is called case law (Keatings & Smith, 2000, pp. 52–53).

This chapter reviews how laws are enacted and implemented, and how the various types of laws affect nursing practice.

SOURCES OF LAW

The authority to make, implement, and interpret laws is generally granted in a constitution A **constitution** is a set of basic laws that specify the powers of the various segments of the government and how these segments relate to each other. Generally, it is the role of a legislative body, at the provincial, territorial, and federal levels, to enact laws. The government of Canada is made up of three branches: the judicial branch, which resolves disputes and creates common or case law; the executive branch—comprising the Queen's representative, the Governor General; the federal ministers, including the Prime Minister; and the public servants who work with the federal ministers—which crafts, administers, and enforces laws; and the legislative branch, consisting of the federal Parliament and provincial/territorial legislatures, which make statutory law (MacIvor, 2006).

PUBLIC LAW

Public law consists of constitutional law and criminal law, and defines a citizen's relationship with government.

CONSTITUTIONAL LAW

The Canadian Constitution (1982), which includes the Canadian Charter of Rights and Freedoms (1982), is the highest law in Canada. The Constitution predominantly deals with the rights and powers of the provincial, territorial, and federal governments; whereas the Charter addresses basic legal and democratic rights of Canadians. Health care is predominantly a provincial/territorial responsibility, but the federal government maintains responsibility for approximately 1 million people in certain groups, such as First Nations people living on reserves; Inuit; serving members of the Canadian Forces and the Royal Canadian Mounted Police; eligible veterans; inmates in federal penitentiaries; and refugee protection claimants.[1]

Recently, many discussions have taken place among various provincial, territorial, and federal governments related to the future of health care. The report of the Commission on the Future of Health Care in Canada

(2002), conducted by Roy Romanow, QC, is based on the five principles of the Canada Health Act (1984). In his report, Romanow recommended that the Health Council of Canada should establish a national framework for measuring and assessing the quality and safety of Canada's health care system, comparing the outcomes with other countries, and reporting regularly to Canadians (Commission on the Future of Health Care in Canada, 2002, p. 251).

Several categories of public law affect the practice of nursing. For example, nurses accommodate clients' constitutional rights to practise their religion every time they call a client's clergy as requested, follow a specific religious custom for the preparation of meals, or prepare a deceased person's remains for burial.

Controversial constitutional rights that may affect the nurse's practice include the recognized constitutional rights of a woman to have an abortion (see *R v. Morgentaler* [1993] 3 S.C.R. 463[2]) and an individual's right to die (see *Rodriguez v. British Columbia (Attorney General)*, [1993] S.C.R. 519[3]).

Nurses may not believe in either of these rights personally and may refuse to work in areas in which they would have to assist a client in exercising these rights. Nurses may not, however, interfere with another person's right to have an abortion or to forgo lifesaving measures.

CRIMINAL LAW

The Criminal Code of Canada (1985) defines criminal offences and identifies the procedures to be used in determining criminal conduct. Criminal law focuses on the actions of individuals that can intentionally do harm to others. Often the victims of such abusive actions are the very young or the very old: two categories of people that generally have a more difficult time defending themselves against physical or emotional abuse. Nurses may notice that a vulnerable client has unexplained bruises, fractures, or other injuries. Most provinces and territories have mandatory statutes that require nurses to report unexplained or suspicious injuries to the appropriate protective agency. Generally, health care institutions will have clear guidelines to follow in such a situation. Failure to report the problem as required by law can result in the nurse being fined for inaction.

Another aspect of criminal law affecting nursing practice is the provincial requirement for criminal background checks on specified categories of prospective employees who will work with the very young or the elderly in institutions such as schools and nursing homes. Again, this requirement is an attempt to protect the most vulnerable citizens from mistreatment or abuse. Failure to conduct the mandated background checks can result in the institution having to defend itself for any harm done by an employee with a past criminal conviction. The third area in which criminal law concerns affect nursing practice is the prohibition against substance abuse. Both federal and provincial/territorial laws require health care agencies to keep a strict accounting of the use and distribution of regulated drugs. Nurses routinely are expected to keep narcotic records accurate and current.

Nurses' behaviour when off duty can also affect their employment status. Abusing alcohol or drugs on one's own time, if discovered, charged, and convicted, can result in both termination from employment and restriction or revocation of registration to practise as a nurse (College of Nurses of Ontario, 2005). Frequently, regulatory nursing bodies make recommendations related to programs for the nurse with a drug or substance abuse problem; completion of such a program may be required before the nurse can resume practising. Additionally, health care facilities may conduct random drug screens on their employees to identify those who may be using illegal substances.

STATUTORY LAW

The laws made by the provincial, territorial, and federal governments are called acts or statutes. After a bill has passed through the federal Parliament and/or the provincial or territorial legislature and received Royal Assent, it is proclaimed and published. It then becomes law.

A federal statute that affects health care is the Canada Health Act (1984). This Act requires that each province and territory provide care that is publicly administered, universal, portable, accessible, and comprehensive. It also prohibits provinces and territories from charging user fees and extra billing by physicians. A

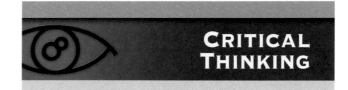

CRITICAL THINKING

One of the nurses who consistently works on your team seems to have a significant change in behaviour following her trips to the washroom. You notice that she becomes increasingly drowsy and her speech is slurred. When you used the staff washroom immediately after her, you noticed a needle and syringe discarded in the garbage. In addition, following the most recent coffee break, the nurse has returned to the unit with a fresh bandage applied to her arm.

Given this scenario what should you do as a nurse? Would you expect to find some guidance in your institution's policy and procedure manual?

penalty (i.e., a decrease in transfer payments) may be imposed by the federal government if this statute is violated.

Established in 1978, the Canadian Centre for Occupational Health and Safety (CCOHS) is a Canadian federal government agency based in Hamilton, Ontario. It reports to the Parliament of Canada through the federal minister of labour. Its vision is to eliminate all Canadian work-related illnesses and injuries. The CCOHS is governed by a council representing three key stakeholder groups: government (federal, provincial, and territorial), employers, and workers—a structure that mandates the CCOHS's impartial approach to information dissemination.[4]

Most Canadian jurisdictions have, in their occupational health and safety legislation, a "general duty provision" that requires employers to take all reasonable precautions to protect the health and safety of their employees. This provision includes protecting employees from a known risk of workplace violence. British Columbia and Saskatchewan have specific workplace violence prevention regulations; Nova Scotia has guidelines on workplace violence prevention; and Alberta has an occupational health and safety code on the prevention of workplace violence. Quebec has legislation regarding "psychological harassment," which may include forms of workplace violence. The Canada Labour Code (i.e., for federally regulated workplaces) specifies that supervisors and managers must take the prescribed steps to prevent and protect against violence in the workplace (the specific regulations are being developed). Many jurisdictions also have regulations regarding working alone, which may have implications for workplace violence prevention.[5] The province of Ontario has the Occupation Health and Safety Act.

In addition, various organizations, such as St. Michael's Hospital in downtown Toronto, have taken steps to ensure their staff's safety. In April 2006, St. Michael's Hospital hosted a conference to look at protecting everyone in the emergency room. Posters now tell patients and visitors that violence will not be tolerated, and visitor access has been limited to some areas of the emergency room. Staff are being more proactive in using the code white procedure, which calls on a team of trained individuals to respond to any dangerous situation before it escalates (Shaw, 2006).

The Registered Nurses Association of Ontario (RNAO) Healthy Work Environments Best Practice Guideline, published in November 2006, presented 21 recommendations to support the creation of healthy and safe work environments for nurses. An International Nursing Review editorial described nurses experiencing violence at a rate 16 times higher than other professions (Kingma, 2001). In addition, the International Council of Nurses revealed statistics in 2004 that found 72 percent of nurses don't feel adequately protected from assaults at work.[6]

Regulated professions, including nursing, are governed by provincial statutes and regulations. The primary mission of professional regulation is protection of the public. The regulatory bodies are given power by the provincial or territorial governments, through legislation, to set practice standards, registration requirements, entry-to-practice requirements, continuing competence requirements, quality assurance criteria, methods of handling complaints, discipline and disciplinary procedures, and development of codes of ethics. As a result, the public is assured that each professional is competent to practice. In Ontario, nurses are affected by the Regulated Health Professions Act (1991) and the regulations in the Nursing Act (1991).

CIVIL LAW

Keatings and Smith (2000) define **civil law** as a body of rules and legal principles that govern relations, rights, and obligations among individuals, corporations, or other institutions.

CONTRACT LAW

Contract law regulates certain transactions between individuals and/or legal entities, such as businesses. It also governs transactions between businesses. An agreement between two or more parties must contain the following elements to be recognized as a legal contract:

- Agreement between two or more legally competent individuals or parties stating what each must or must not do
- Mutual understanding of the terms and obligations that the contract imposes on each party to the contract
- Payment or consideration given for actions taken or not taken pursuant to the agreement

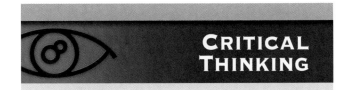

CRITICAL THINKING

You are assigned to a medical-surgical unit, working the night shift. Your supervisor calls and says that one of the registered nurses assigned to the critical care unit has called in sick and you must work that unit instead of your usual assignment. You have never worked in the critical care setting before and have received no orientation to this unit. You are now asked to work there when it is short of staff.

What should you do?

The terms of the contract may be oral or written; however, a written contract may not be legally modified by an oral agreement, which is often expressed is by the phrase *all of the terms of the contract are contained within the four corners of the document*. Therefore, if it is not written, it is not part of the agreement or contract. A contract may be express or implied. In an express contract, the terms of the contract are specified, usually in writing. In an implied contract, a relationship between parties is recognized, although the terms of the agreement are not clearly defined, such as the expectations one has for services from the dry cleaner or the grocer.

The nurse is usually a party to an employment contract. The employed nurse agrees to do the following:

■ Adhere to the policies and procedures of the employing agency
■ Fulfill the agreed-upon duties of the employer
■ Respect the rights and responsibilities of other health care providers in the workplace

In return, the employer agrees to provide the nurse with the following:

■ A specified amount of pay for services rendered
■ Adequate assistance in providing care
■ The supplies and equipment needed to fulfill the nurse's responsibilities
■ A safe environment in which to work
■ Reasonable treatment and behaviour from the other health care providers with whom the nurse must interact

This contract may be express or implied, depending on the practices of the employer. Sometimes, what is determined to be "reasonable" by the employer is not considered "reasonable" by the nurse. For instance, after 20 years of working as a nurse on the orthopedic unit, a nurse may not view it as reasonable to be assigned to the labour and delivery unit for duty. It would be prudent for the nurse to express any misgivings to the supervisor and to take assignments that are in keeping with the nurse's experience on an orthopedic unit.

TORT LAW

Keatings and Smith (2000) define **tort** as a civil wrong committed by one person against another, such that some injury or damage is caused to either person or property. A tort can be non-intentional, as occurs in negligence, or it can be intentional, as occurs in assault, when the infliction of harm is intended.

NON-INTENTIONAL TORTS

Negligence is the failure to provide the care a reasonable nurse would ordinarily provide in a similar situation. In order to win a negligence lawsuit, the person who is suing

the nurse must demonstrate that each of the following elements existed between the client and nurse:

1. A duty or obligation created by law, contract, or standard practice that is owed to the complainant by the professional
2. A breach of this duty, either by omission or commission
3. Harm, which can be physical, emotional, or financial, to the complainant (i.e., the client)
4. Proof that the breach of duty caused the harm (Morris, 1991)

When a nurse is listed as a party in a medical malpractice lawsuit, the nurse's liability is determined by provincial or federal laws, such as the Regulated Health Professions Act, the Public Hospitals Act, the standards for the practice of nursing, and the institution's policies and procedures. Therefore, if provincial or territorial laws mandate that a nurse must have a doctor's order before taking an action, then a doctor's order must be present. Problems arise when the orders are verbal, and later it is claimed that the nurse misunderstood and acted in error. Another pitfall is illegible writing, which can be misinterpreted, with a result that causes harm to the client. Many nurses who have been in practice for a long time have encountered confused doctors who write orders that are contrary to accepted medical practice. In these situations, the nurse must exercise professional judgment and follow the policies and procedures of the institution. Usually these policies require the nurse to notify the physician involved to clarify the orders.

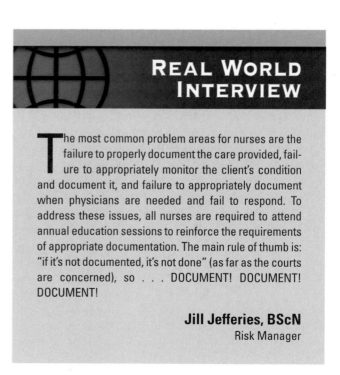

REAL WORLD INTERVIEW

The most common problem areas for nurses are the failure to properly document the care provided, failure to appropriately monitor the client's condition and document it, and failure to appropriately document when physicians are needed and fail to respond. To address these issues, all nurses are required to attend annual education sessions to reinforce the requirements of appropriate documentation. The main rule of thumb is: "if it's not documented, it's not done" (as far as the courts are concerned), so . . . DOCUMENT! DOCUMENT! DOCUMENT!

Jill Jefferies, BScN
Risk Manager

The institution's policies and procedures describe the performance expected of nurses in its employ, and a nurse deviating from these policies and procedures can be liable for negligence or malpractice. Occasionally, such failure to adhere to institutional protocol can result in the employer denying the nurse a defence in a lawsuit.

Practising nurses must also adhere to the standards of practice for the nursing profession in the community. These standards include such things as checking "the five rights" in medication administration or repositioning the bed-bound client at regular intervals. It is not uncommon for the nurses to be conflicted between an employer's expectations and the nursing standards of care, which can result either in insufficient time or lack of staff to adhere to the standards as taught in nursing school or poor evaluations for taking too long to render care. In these situations, nurses must evaluate the standards to follow to preserve their practice and protect themselves from liability. In some cases, such an evaluation will lead to a decision to change jobs.

INTENTIONAL TORTS

ASSAULT AND BATTERY   **Assault** is a threat to touch another in an offensive manner without that person's permission. An example would be if someone lunges at you in a threatening manner, but doesn't actually hit you. However, you had reason to believe that you would be harmed and threat was imminent. The aggressor would still be liable to damages for assault (Keatings & Smith, 2000). **Battery** is the touching of another person without that person's consent. An example of battery is slapping a client (i.e., direct battery) or pulling away a chair, resulting in the person falling to the ground (i.e., indirect battery). In the health care arena, complaints of battery usually pertain to whether the individual consented to the treatment administered by the health care professional. Most provinces and territories have laws that require clients to make informed decisions about their treatment.

INFORMED CONSENT

All nurses need to know the elements required for consent to treatment and the elements that constitute *informed* consent. The Ontario Health Care Consent Act, 1996, S.O. 1996, c.2, Sch. A identifies the elements required for consent:

- Consent must relate to the treatment
- Consent must be informed
- Consent must be voluntary
- Consent must not be obtained through misrepresentation or fraud.

In addition, the Act explains that a consent to treatment is *informed* only if the person received all of the information pertaining to the treatment that a reasonable person in the same circumstances would require in order to make a decision about the treatment, and the person received responses to all requests for additional information about the treatment. The nature of the treatment, the expected benefits, material risks, material side effects of the treatment, alternative courses of action, and the likely consequences of not having the treatment must be explained to the client.

Fiesta (1999) explained that informed consent laws protect the client's right to practise self-determination. The client has the right to receive sufficient information to make an informed decision about whether to consent to or refuse a procedure. The individual performing the procedure has the responsibility of explaining to the client the nature of the procedure, benefits, alternatives, and the risks and complications. The signed consent form is used to document that this explanation was completed, and it creates a presumption that the client has been advised of the appropriate risks.

Often the nurse is asked to witness a client signing a consent form for treatment. When you witness a client's signature, you are vouching for two things: the client signed the paper and the client was aware of signing a consent form (Olsen-Chavarriaga, 2000). For a consent form to be legal, in most provinces, the client must be at least 16 years old, or old enough to understand the nature of the treatment; be mentally competent; must have had the procedures, their risks, and their benefits explained in an understandable manner; must be aware of the available alternatives to the proposed treatment; and must consent voluntarily. The nurse must also be familiar with the other people who are allowed, by law, to consent to medical treatment for clients who cannot consent themselves. In Ontario, a formal hierarchy of substitute decision-makers is outlined in the Substitute Decisions Act (1992) (see Table 19-1).

A nurse may also face a charge of battery for failing to honour an advance directive, such as a power of attorney for personal care or living will. Organizations may require that a hospital ask clients, upon admission, whether they have a living will; if they do not, the hospital may ask clients whether they would like to enact one. A **living will** is a written advance directive voluntarily signed by clients that specifies the type of care they desire if and when they are in a terminal state and cannot sign a consent form or convey this information verbally. The living will can be a general statement such as "no life-sustaining measures" or specific, such as "no tube feedings or respirator."

Often, the client's family has difficulty allowing health care personnel to follow the wishes expressed in a living will, and conflicts arise. These situations should be communicated to the hospital ethics committee, the pastoral care department, the risk management department, or the hospital department responsible for handling such issues.

TABLE 19-1	HIERARCHY FOR SUBSTITUTE DECISION-MAKERS IN ONTARIO

1. Guardian appointed by the court

2. Attorney for personal care

3. Representative appointed by the Consent and Capacity Board

4. Spouse or partner of client

5. Child (at least 16 years of age) of client, parent of client, or Children's Aid Society

6. Parent of client who only has a right of access

7. Brother or sister of client

8. Any other relative of client

9. Public Guardian or Trustee

Source: Ministry of the Attorney General, "A Guide to the Substitute Decisions Act." Retrieved from http://www.attorneygeneral.jus.gov.on.ca/english/family/pgt/pgtsda.pdf, April 22, 2006.

If clients have verbalized their wishes regarding end-of-life care to the family, such difficult situations can sometimes be avoided. When possible, clients should be encouraged to discuss these issues with their family. The nurse should be familiar with the requirements for the implementation of a living will in the province or territory where the nurse practises. Figure 19-1 is an example of a living will.

DO NOT RESUSCITATE (DNR) ORDERS

There is a distinction between "no CPR" and "DNR." Keatings and Smith (2000) state that the latter is a concept that includes any treatment given to sustain life, up to and including blood transfusions, antibiotic therapy, and artificial ventilation. According to the authors, CPR is limited to the technique of compressing the client's chest without applying artificial ventilation. Therefore, it is important to document the precise wishes of the client or substitute decision-maker with respect to the request. Molloy (1992) suggests using the term *personal health care directive* to articulate one's wishes.

The attending physician may write a do not resuscitate (DNR) order on an inpatient, which directs the staff not to perform the usual cardiopulmonary resuscitation (CPR) in the event of a sudden cardiopulmonary arrest. The doctor may write such an order without evidence of a living will on the medical record, and the nurse should be familiar with the institution's policies and provincial/territorial law regarding when and how a physician can write such an order in the absence of a living will. Often, a DNR order is considered a medical decision that the doctor can make, preferably in consultation with the family, even without a living will executed by the client.

If the nurse feels such a DNR order is contrary to the client's or family's wishes, the nurse should consult the policies and procedures of the institution, which may require going up the chain of command until the nurse is satisfied with the course of action. This process may entail notifying the nursing supervisor, the medical director, the institution's chief of staff, or the chief medical officer. Often, an institution has an ethics committee that examines such issues and makes a determination of the appropriateness of the order.

FALSE IMPRISONMENT

False imprisonment is the intentional restraint of individuals who are incorrectly led to believe they cannot leave a place. False imprisonment often occurs because the nurse misinterprets the rights granted to others by legal documents, such as powers of attorney for personal care, and does not allow a client to leave a facility because the person with the power of attorney for personal care (i.e., the agent) says the client cannot leave.

A **power of attorney** for personal care is a legal document executed by an individual (the principal) granting another person (the agent) the right to perform certain activities in the principal's name. The power of attorney can be specific, such as "initiate tube feedings," or general, such as "make all health care decisions for me." In most provinces and territories, a power of attorney for personal care is voluntarily granted by individuals and does not take away clients' rights to exercise their own

Declaration made this _____ day of _____, 2006.

I,_____, being of sound mind, wilfully and voluntarily make known my desire that my dying shall not be artificially prolonged under the circumstances set forth below and do hereby declare:

If at any time I should either have a terminal and irreversible incurable injury, disease, or illness or be in a continual profound comatose state with no reasonable chance of recovery, certified by two physicians who have personally examined me, one of whom shall be my attending physician, and the physicians have determined that my death will occur whether or not life-sustaining procedures are utilized and where the application of life-sustaining procedures would serve only to prolong artificially the dying process, I direct that such procedures be withheld or withdrawn and that I be permitted to die naturally with only the administration of medication or the performance of any medical procedure deemed necessary to provide me with comfort care.

In the absence of my ability to give directions regarding the use of such life-sustaining procedures, it is my intention that this declaration shall be honoured by my family and physician(s) as the final expression of my legal right to refuse medical or surgical treatment and accept the consequences of such refusal.

I understand the full import of this declaration and I am emotionally and mentally competent to make this declaration.

Signed: _____

City, County, and Province/Territory of Residence

The declarant has been personally known to me and I believe him/her to be of sound mind.

Witness _____

Witness _____

Figure 19-1 Sample of a Living Will* Declaration.

*See provincial/territorial law requirements.

choices. Thus, if the principal (i.e., the client) disagrees with the agent's decisions, the client's wishes will prevail. If a situation occurs in which an agent, acting on a power of attorney for personal care, disagrees with your client regarding discharge plans, contact your supervisor for further assistance in deciding an action consistent with your client's wishes and best interests.

A claim of false imprisonment may be based on the inappropriate use of physical or chemical restraints. Provincial and territorial laws mandate that health care institutions employ the least restrictive method of ensuring client safety. Physical or chemical restraints are to be used only when necessary to protect the client from harm when all other methods have failed. If the nurse uses restraints on a competent person who is refusing to follow the doctor's orders, the nurse can be charged with false imprisonment or battery. If restraints are used in an emergency situation, the nurse must contact the doctor immediately after application to secure an order for the restraints. Also, the nurse must check the institution's policies regarding the type and frequency of assessments required for a client in restraints and how often it is necessary to secure a reorder for the restraints. These policies ensure the client's safety and must be consistent with provincial/territorial law.

RIGHT TO PRIVACY

In Canada, there are two federal privacy laws: the Privacy Act (1983) and the Personal Information Protection and Electronic Documents Act (2001). The Privacy Act is a code of ethics for the government handling of personal information of the citizens of Canada. The Personal Information Protection and Electronic Documents Act, which was fully implemented by 2004, addresses the collection, storage, and use of personal information by organizations in the private and public sector. In addition, the provinces and territories may have their own laws related to privacy, such as the Personal Information Protection Act in both Alberta and British Columbia, and the Personal Health Information Protection Act (2004) (PHIPA) in Ontario.

The right to privacy goes hand in hand with the right to confidentiality. These two rights affect all types of interaction with clients: from ensuring the curtains are drawn around a client's bed when bathing the client, to keeping information confidential and private when clients have told you something they don't want their family to know.

The nurse is required to respect the privacy of all clients. As a health care practitioner, the nurse may be privy to very personal information and must make every effort to keep it confidential. The need for confidentiality often necessitates policing conversations with coworkers to ensure that no client information is accidentally overheard by others.

Sometimes the protection of a client's privacy conflicts with the provincial or territorial mandatory reporting laws

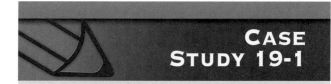

CASE STUDY 19-1

You are working the night shift. One of your client's physicians has ordered a dose of a medication that you know is too high for this client. You are unable to locate the doctor to check the order. What would you do to ensure safe care for your client?

for the occurrence of specified infectious diseases, such as syphilis or human immunodeficiency virus (HIV). The need to protect an individual's privacy may also conflict with the provincial or territorial mandatory reporting laws on suspected client abuse, discussed previously. Provincial or territorial law may also require the reporting of a client's blood alcohol level, incidences of rape and gunshot wounds, and adverse reactions to certain drugs.

Failing to strictly follow reporting laws could lead to criminal, civil, or disciplinary action and termination of employment. Nurses must consult the institution's policies and confer with its risk management department to ascertain their responsibilities and course of action. The Canadian Nurses Association (CNA) Code of Ethics for nurses states that nurses must be accountable for their practice. As a result, protection of the client and the public is required when incompetence or unethical or illegal practice compromise health care and safety. All provinces and territories have adopted this concept in their nurse practice acts. Nurses who observe unethical behaviour in a hospital should report this behaviour as directed in the institution's policies and procedures manual or by the laws of the province or territory.

LEGAL PROTECTIONS IN NURSING PRACTICE

As discussed earlier in this chapter, nursing practice is guided by provincial/territorial nurse practice acts and agency policies and procedures. Other resources for the nurse include government inquiries, Good Samaritan laws, skillful communication, and risk management programs.

GOVERNMENT INQUIRIES

Special commissions, fatality inquiries, and coroners' inquests can have immediate and direct impact on nursing and organizational practices (Hibberd & Smith, 2006, p. 275). This effect has been demonstrated time and

again in inquest and coroners' recommendations. Nurses traditionally are not aware of the numbers of coroner's recommendations that are published on an annual basis, or their content. In addition, they are not aware that these published reports are sent to health care facilities across the province and/or territory for their action. Nurses need to request these documents to ensure that recommendations are acted upon in their facility. For example, the two inquests following deaths at The Hospital for Sick Children in Toronto resulted in recommendations, some of which affected nurses directly.

The Sinclair inquiry in Winnipeg, Manitoba, found that of the 12 pediatric cardiac deaths that occurred in 1994, five were preventable, four were possibly preventable, two were uncertain, and one was likely nonpreventable (Sinclair, 2000). The central finding of the Inquest was: "the evidence suggests that, during 1994, the Pediatric Surgery Program at the Health Sciences Centre did not provide the standard of health care that it was mandated to provide and which parents believed, and had a right to expect, that their children would receive."(Sinclair, 2000, p. 465).

Some of the problems that the program faced related to the abilities of some of the individuals; however, the other problems were systemic in nature. Some issues related to the structure of the Health Sciences Centre, and specifically to policies and procedures related to staffing, leadership, teamwork, quality, communication, and decision making. Recommendations that related to the nursing division can be found in Table 19-2. It is important for nurses to pay heed to recommendations from coroner's inquests in order that the practice and the profession of nursing be strengthened.

GOOD SAMARITAN LAWS

Good Samaritan laws are laws that have been enacted to protect the health care professional from legal liability. The essential elements of commonly enacted Good Samaritan laws are as follows:

- The care is rendered in an emergency situation.
- The health care worker is rendering care without pay.
- The care provided did not recklessly or intentionally cause injury or harm to the injured party.

Note that these laws are intended to protect the volunteer who stops to render care at the scene of an accident. These laws would not protect an emergency medical technician (EMT) or other health care professionals rendering care at the scene of an accident as part of their assigned duties and for which they receive pay. In doing their duties, these paid emergency personnel would be evaluated according to the standards of their professions.

Some of Canada's provinces have passed Good Samaritan laws. Ontario has the Good Samaritan Act, 2001; Alberta

TABLE 19-2	NURSING-RELATED RECOMMENDATIONS FROM THE SINCLAIR REPORT

1. It is recommended that the HSC [Winnipeg Health Sciences Centre] establish a medical staff recruitment process for senior or specialized positions within the hospital that has as its main priority the creations of a mechanism that results in the best possible candidate being hired or appointed. The process should include the components: . . . . Personnel in related fields, such as nursing, anaesthesia and perfusion, should have input into the criteria developed for the position. . . . The recruitment process . . . should include nurses. . . .

2. It is recommended that there should be clear written lines of authority and responsibility within the Pediatric Cardiac Surgery Program. Efforts should be made to ensure that members understand these lines of authority.

3. It is recommended that there should be orientation and support for all new staff and for staff moving into new positions. This should be done even if the appointment is an Acting position.

4. It is recommended that the entire team, including those responsible for post-operative care, be prepared before the program moves to new procedures or higher-risk cases.

5. It is recommended that HSC restructure its Nursing Council to allow nurses to select its membership and to give it responsibility for nursing issues within the hospital. The Nursing Council should have representation on the hospital's governing body and be responsible for monitoring, evaluating, and making recommendations pertaining to the nursing profession within the hospital and for nursing care. The Council should also serve as a vehicle through which nurses could report incident, issues, and concerns without risk of professional reprisal.

6. It is recommended that a clear policy be established on how staff is to report concerns about risks for clients. . . . The Province of Manitoba consider passing "whistle-blowing" legislation to protect nurses and other professionals from reprisals stemming from their disclosure of information arising from a legitimately and reasonable held concern over the medical treatment of patients.

7. It is recommended that there be a patient right's handbook that would include a section on the issue of informed consent . . . as part of the consent process, that the information about a surgeon's experience in performing a particular procedure, as well as the experience of the hospital or surgical team be disclosed.

8. It is recommended that the HSC establish a clear policy on how staff is to report concerns regarding risks for clients . . . and that all staff members are made aware of their responsibility to use incident reports and fully chart problems with the process of delivery of care and any complications in the outcome of care.

Source: Adapted from Sinclair, C. M. (2000). The Report of the Manitoba Pediatric Cardiac Surgery Inquest: An Inquiry into Twelve Deaths at the Winnipeg Health Sciences Centre in 1994. Winnipeg: Provincial Court of Manitoba, pp. 467–483.

has the Emergency Medical Aid Act; British Columbia has the Good Samaritan Act; and Nova Scotia has the Volunteer Services Act. Except in Quebec, no laws oblige people to help someone in need. Quebec is unique in Canada because it imposes a duty on everyone to help a person in peril. The duty to take action stems from the Quebec Charter of Human Rights and Freedoms, enacted in 1975, and the Civil Code of Quebec, which came into force in 1994.

The Quebec Charter includes a provision that states that if assistance can be provided without serious risk to the Good Samaritan or a third person, then the Good Samaritan is obligated to provide assistance. Little precedent exists to assist in interpretation of these provisions. Under the Civil Code, every person is obligated to act as a reasonably prudent person. Failure to do so would amount to fault and lead to legal wrong.[7] Little uniformity exists among Canadian laws to protect the Good Samaritan. Some provinces' laws protect the rescuer from liability, unless evidence can prove gross negligence, but these laws do not force a person to assist. Every province except Prince Edward Island has a criminal compensation scheme to compensate Good Samaritans injured because of a criminal act. However, no common law province has established a general compensation scheme. Only five provinces and two territories have general legislation relieving a Good Samaritan from liability for negligence.[8]

SKILLFUL COMMUNICATION

The nurse must communicate accurately and completely both verbally and in writing. Often a case involving client care takes several years to come to trial; by that time, the nurse may have no memory of the incident in question and must rely on the written record from the time of the incident. This record is frequently displayed in the court-room, enlarged to billboard size for all to see. All errors are apparent and omissions stand out by their absence, especially when data should have been recorded according to institutional policy. The old adage "if it isn't written, it wasn't done" will be repeated to the jury numerous times. Thus, it is essential that the nurse chart accurately and completely. To protect themselves when charting, nurses should use the FLAT charting acronym: F—factual, L—legible, A—accurate, T—timely

F: Charting should be *factual*—what you see, not what you think happened; only your own actions

L: Charting should be *legible*, with no erasures. Corrections should be made as you have been taught, with a single line drawn through the error and initialed.

A: Charting should be *accurate* and complete, clear, and concise. What colour was the drainage and how much was present? How many times, and at what times, was the doctor notified of changes? Was the supervisor notified?

T: Charting should be *timely*, completed as soon after the occurrence as possible. "Late entries" should be avoided or kept to a minimum. Regular entries should be made in chronological order.

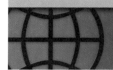

REAL WORLD INTERVIEW

The role of risk management in the health care environment is that of recognition, evaluation, and treatment of risks inherent in the organization. The goal of risk management is improving the quality of care provided by the organization while at the same time protecting its financial integrity. Risk management, while coordinated at a certain level of the organization, is not simply a one-department responsibility, but rather is the responsibility of each employee of the organization.

New graduates in nursing need to understand that in today's health care environment, each practitioner must look for ways to reduce the risks inherent in the delivery of health care. At a time when hospitals are having difficulty balancing budgets, our clients and consumers are demanding higher and higher quality of care.

Health care is at a crossroads, similar to the one that faced private industry during the 1970s. Our customers are demanding that we provide a safe environment and that we consistently strive for continuous quality improvement.

An incident report or occurrence form is a commonly used form that documents a variance from normal protocol or hospital procedures. It is not meant to place blame on an individual practitioner or department. It is used strictly to document the facts surrounding an event so the health care processes can be improved. Thus, the nurse should complete an incident report when any variance from a policy or a procedure is noticed. This assists in providing a culture of learning instead of a culture of blame.

When risk management receives the incident reports, they are logged into our database, and monthly reports are forwarded to nurse managers for follow-up and education with their staff.

Incident reports and the subsequent risk management department actions are generally reactive but we also do proactive/preventive interventions in the health care setting. These include the following:

1. Education of students completing their senior year of study in nursing

2. Participation on client safety, occupational health and safety, pharmacy, nursing, and other hospital committees, which work on proactive programs to reduce risks

3. Facilitation of the slips and falls task force to reduce our clients' fall risk

4. Education of new nurses and physicians on principles of risk management

Harriet Percy, RN
Risk Manager

FOLLOWING DOCTORS' ORDERS

In most provinces and territories, the nurse is required to follow the doctor's orders when giving care to the client unless doing so would cause the client harm. To follow this mandate, the nurse must ensure that the orders are clear and accurate. If necessary, the nurse may need to contact the physician for clarification. If the nurse is still uncomfortable following the order, the supervisor should be notified and the institution's policies followed regarding notification. Because of the opportunity for misinterpretation and misunderstanding, verbal orders are not encouraged.

RISK MANAGEMENT PROGRAMS

Risk management programs in health care organizations are designed to identify and correct system problems that contribute to errors in client care or to employee injury. The emphasis in risk management is on quality improvement and protection of the institution from financial liability. Institutions usually have reporting and tracking forms to record incidents that may lead to financial liability for the institution. Risk management will assist in identifying and correcting the underlying problem that may have led to an incident, such as faulty equipment, staffing concerns, or the need for better orientation for employees. Once a system problem has been identified, the risk management department can develop educational programs to address the problem.

The risk management department may also investigate and record information surrounding a client or employee incident that may result in a lawsuit. This investigation will help personnel to remember critical factors if called to testify at a later time. The nurse should notify the risk management department of all reportable incidents and complete all risk management and/or incident report forms as mandated by institutional policies and procedures. Note also that employee complaints of harassment or discrimination can expose the institution to significant liability and should promptly be reported to supervisors and the risk management department, human resources, or whichever department is specified in the institution's policies. See Table 19-3 for a checklist of actions to decrease the risk of nursing liability.

MALPRACTICE/ PROFESSIONAL LIABILITY INSURANCE

Nurses may need to carry their own malpractice insurance. **Malpractice** refers to a professional's wrongful

---

TABLE 19-3	ACTIONS TO DECREASE THE RISK OF LIABILITY

- Communicate with your clients by keeping them informed and listening to what they say.
- Acknowledge unfortunate incidents and express concern about these events without taking the blame, blaming others, or reacting defensively.
- Chart and time your observations immediately, while facts are still fresh in your mind.
- Take appropriate actions to meet the client's nursing needs.
- Follow the facility's policies and procedures for administering care and reporting incidents.
- Acknowledge and document the reason for any omission or deviation from agency policy, procedure, or standard.
- Maintain clinical competency and acknowledge your limitations. If you do not know how to do something, ask for help.
- Promptly report any concern regarding the quality of care, including the lack of resources with which to provide care, to a nursing administration representative.
- Use appropriate standards of care.
- Document the time of changes in conditions requiring notification of the physician and include the response of the physician.
- Delegate client care based on the documented skills of regulated and unregulated personnel.
- Treat all clients and their families with kindness and respect.

conduct in the discharge of professional duties or failure to meet standards of care for the profession that results in harm to an individual entrusted to the professional's care (Zerwekh & Claborn, 2000). Nurses often believe their actions are adequately covered by their employer's liability insurance, but this is not necessarily so. If, in giving care, the nurse fails to comply with the institution's policies and procedures, the institution may deny the nurse a defence, claiming that because of the nurse's failure to follow institutional policy, or because of the nurse working outside the scope of employment, the nurse was not acting as an employee at that time. Also, nurses are being named individually as defendants in malpractice suits more frequently than in the past. Consequently, it is advantageous for the nurse to be assured of a defence independent of that of the employer. Professional liability insurance provides that assurance and pays for an attorney to defend the nurse in a malpractice lawsuit.

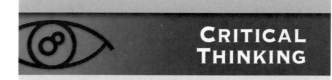

CRITICAL THINKING

You are the only registered nurse assigned to give 0900h medications on a 52-bed nursing home unit. To avoid being classified as a drug error according to the institution's policy and usual nursing practice, administration of the medications must occur within 45 minutes of the ordered time. Also, nursing practice mandates you verify the "five rights": the right drug, the right dose, the right patient, the right time, and the right route.

What are the problems with this assignment? What would you do?

KEY CONCEPTS

- Nursing practice is governed by public and private laws.

- Nurses are responsible for providing a safe environment for clients entrusted to their care.

- Nurses need to be familiar with their institution's policies and procedures in giving care and in reporting variances, illegal activities, or unexpected events.

- Nurses must have good oral and written communication skills

- Common torts include negligence, assault and battery, and false imprisonment.

- Nurses need to be familiar with their provincial or territorial nurse practice act.

- Good Samaritan laws exist in many provinces or territories.

- Risk management programs improve the quality of care and protect the financial integrity of institutions.

KEY TERMS

assault	Good Samaritan laws
battery	living will
civil law	malpractice
common law	negligence
constitution	power of attorney
contract law	public law
false imprisonment	tort

REVIEW QUESTIONS

1. Which type of law authorizes nursing regulatory bodies to enact rules that govern the practice of nursing?
   A. Provincial/Territorial law
   B. Federal law
   C. Common law
   D. Criminal law

2. If you make a threatening gesture to a client, with no contact having been made, you are liable for which of the following charges?
   A. Assault
   B. Defamation
   C. Malpractice
   D. False imprisonment

3. Battery is an example of which of the following?
   A. Intentional tort
   B. Non-intentional tort
   C. Assault
   D. Negligence

4. Which of the following is a body of law that develops through precedents over time and has the force of law?
   A. Contract law
   B. Common law
   C. Public law
   D. Civil law

REVIEW ACTIVITIES

1. Talk to the risk manager at the hospital where you have your clinical assignments. How does the risk manager

handle an incident report? Is it used for improving the hospital's care in the future? How?

2. Review the advance directive (i.e., living will) policy at the hospital where you have your clinical assignments. Notice the form that clients sign. How does it compare with the living will form on page 345?

3. Discuss how a nurse's off-duty behaviour can affect her practice as a nurse. Can the provincial or territorial regulatory body take action against the nurse's registration?

EXPLORING THE WEB

■ Go to the following sites to find malpractice information for your province or territory: *http://www.cnps.ca/joint_statement/joint_statement_e.html* and *http://www.cnps.ca/index_e.html*

■ Where can you find provincial and territorial laws regulating hospitals? *http://www.e-laws.gov.on.ca/index.html*

■ You have a client who is to be transferred to a nursing home for recuperation. Where can you suggest the family look to evaluate the local nursing homes regarding their adherence to the provincial or territorial regulations for nursing homes?
http://www.e-laws.gov.on.ca/ index.html

■ Where can you find a copy of the CNA Code of Ethics? *http://www.cna-nurses.ca/CNA/practice/ethics/code/default_e.aspx*

REFERENCES

College of Nurses of Ontario. (2005). *Legislation and regulation: Professional misconduct*. Toronto: Author. Retrieved from http://www.cno.org/docs/ih/42007_misconduct.pdf, July 29, 2007.

Commission on the Future of Health Care in Canada. (2002). *Building on values: The future of health care in Canada*. Saskatoon: Commission on the Future of Health Care in Canada. Commissioner: Roy J. Romanow.

Fiesta, J. (1999). Informed consent: What health care professionals need to know, part 2. *Nursing Management, 30*(7), 6–7.

Hibberd, J. M., & Smith, D. L. (2006). *Nursing leadership and management in Canada* (3rd Ed.). Toronto: W.B. Saunders Company.

Keatings, M., & Smith, O. B., (2000). *Ethical and legal issues in Canadian nursing* (2nd Ed.). Toronto: W.B. Saunders Company.

Kingma, M. (2001). Workplace violence in the health sector: A problem of epidemic proportion. *International Nursing Review, 48*(3), 129–130.

MacIvor, H. (2006). *Canadian politics and government in the Charter era*. Toronto: Nelson, a division of Thomson Canada Ltd.

Molloy, W., & Mepham, V. (1992). *Let me decide*. Toronto: Penguin Books.

Morris, J. (1991). *Canadian nurses and the law*. Toronto: Butterworths.

Olsen-Chavarriaga, D. (2000). Informed consent: Do you know your role? *Nursing, 30*(5), 60–61.

Shaw, J. (2006). In harm's way. *Registered Nurse Journal*. Toronto: The Journal of the Registered Nurses' Association of Ontario (RNAO).

Sinclair, C. M. (2000). *The Report of the Manitoba pediatric cardiac surgery inquest: An inquiry into twelve deaths at the Winnipeg Health Sciences Centre in 1994*. Winnipeg: Provincial Court of Manitoba.

Zerwekh, J., & Claborn, J. C. (2000). *Nursing today: Transition and trends* (2nd ed.). Philadelphia: Saunders.

SUGGESTED READINGS

Brown, S. M. (1999). Good Samaritan laws: Protection and limits. *RN, 62*(11), 65–68.

Champion, J. B. (2001). When "enough" may not be enough: Informed consent and patient communication. *Risk Management in Canadian Health Care, 2*(8), 81–88.

DeLaune, S., & Ladner, P. K. (2002). *Fundamentals of nursing* (2nd ed.). Clifton Park, NY: Delmar Learning.

Fiesta, J. (1999a). Greater need for background checks. *Nursing Management, 30*(11), 26.

Fiesta, J. (1999b). Informed consent: What health care professionals need to know, part 1. *Nursing Management, 30*(6), 8–9.

Fiesta, J. (1999c). When sexual harassment hits home. *Nursing Management, 30*(5), 16–18.

Hibberd, J. M., & Smith, D. L. (1999). *Nursing management in Canada*. Toronto: W.B. Saunders Canada.

LaDuke, S. (2000). What should you expect from your attorney? *Nursing Management, 31*(1), 10.

Mantel, D. L. (1999). Legally speaking: Off-duty doesn't mean off the hook. *RN, 62*(10), 71–74.

Martens, C. (2002). The Manitoba pediatric cardiac surgery inquest. *Risk Management in Canadian Health Care, 3*(7), 65–73.

McKee, R. (1999). Clarifying advance directives. *Nursing, 29*(5), 52–53.

Morris, M. R. (1998). Elder abuse: What the law requires. *RN, 61*(8), 52–53.

Perry, J. (2000). Legislating sharps safety. *Nursing, 30*(5), 50–51.

Report of the Review and Implementation Committee for the Report of the Manitoba Pediatric Cardiac Surgery Inquest. (2001). Winnipeg: Review and Implementation Committee for the Report of the Manitoba Cardiac Surgery Inquest.

Sheehan, J. P. (2000). Protect your staff from workplace violence. *Nursing Management, 31*(3), 24–25.

Sloan, A. J. (1999). Legally speaking: Whistleblowing: There are risks! *RN, 62*(7), 65–68.

Spencer, P. C. (2002). Developing a hospital policy re: disclosure of adverse medical events. *Risk Management in Canadian Health Care, 4*(6), 65–72.

Staten, P. A. (1999). How to cover all the bases on informed consent. *Nursing Management, 30*(9), 14.

Sullivan, G. H. (1999). Legally speaking: Minimizing your risk in patient falls. *RN, 62*(4), 69–70.

Sullivan, G. H. (2000). Legally speaking: Keep your charting on course. *RN, 63*(4), 75–79.

Ventura, M. J. (1999). Legally speaking: When information must be revealed. *RN, 62*(2), 61–62, 64.

Wilkinson, A. P. (1998). Nursing malpractice. *Nursing, 28*(6), 34–39.

CHAPTER ENDNOTES

1. Health Canada, "How Health Care Services Are Delivered." Retrieved from http://www.hc-sc.gc.ca/hcs-sss/pubs/care-soins/2005-hcs-sss/del-pres_e.html, September 21, 2006.

2. *R. v. Morgentaler*, [1993] 3 S.C.R. 463. Retrieved from http://www.canlii.org/en/ca/scc/doc/1993/1993canlii74/1993canlii74.pdf, July 29, 2007.

3. *Rodriguez v. British Columbia (Attorney General)*, [1993] 3 S.C.R. 519. Retrieved from http://www.canlii.org/en/ca/scc/doc/1993/1993canlii75/1993canlii75.pdf, July 29, 2007.

4. Canadian Centre for Occupational Health and Safety, "About CCOHS—Background." Retrieved from http://www.ccohs.ca/ccohs.html, April 28, 2006.

5. Canadian Centre for Occupational Health and Safety, "Violence in the Workplace: Is there specific workplace violence prevention legislation?" Retrieved from http://www.ccohs.ca/oshanswers/psychosocial/violence.html, April 18, 2006.

6. International Council of Nurses, "Violence: A world-wide epidemic." Retrieved from http://www.icn.ch/matters_violence.htm, July 29, 2007.

7. Canadian Association of Food Banks, "Good Samaritan Law: Obligation to Help Someone in Trouble." Retrieved from http://www.cafb-acba.ca/english/GetInvolved-GoodSamaritanLaw.html, April 22, 2007.

8. Search and Rescue Society of British Columbia, "The Risk of Rescue: The Plight of the Good Samaritan." Retrieved from http://www.sarbc.org/goodsam.html, April 22, 2007.

CHAPTER 20

Ethics and the Profession of Nursing

Nancy Walton, PhD

These virtues we acquire by first exercising them.... Whatever we learn to do, we learn by actually doing it.... By doing just acts, we come to be just ... by doing self-controlled acts, we come to be self-controlled; and by doing brave acts, we become brave. (Aristotle, Nicomachean Ethics, as cited in Burkhardt & Nathaniel, 2002)

OBJECTIVES

Upon completion of this chapter, the reader will be able to:

1. Define ethics, morality, and ethical dilemma.
2. Differentiate between bioethics and nursing ethics.
3. Demonstrate an understanding of moral distress.
4. Apply ethical principles and theories to the examination of ethical dilemmas and challenging situations.
5. Describe the foundations of ethical health care in Canada.
6. Compare the codes of ethics used in professional nursing practice and appreciate their limitations.
7. Examine and analyze four specific ethical issues commonly encountered in nursing practice: consent/autonomy, resource allocation, end-of-life care, and truth telling.
8. Examine ethical challenges for nurse leaders.
9. Examine different roles in practical ethics and ethics in practice.
10. Demonstrate an understanding of the elements of an ethical environment in nursing.
11. Examine two ethical decision-making models and evaluate their use in working through everyday ethical dilemmas found in practice.

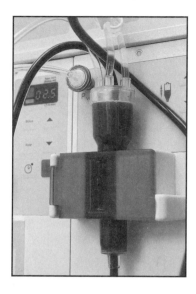

Trish, a nurse manager of a busy regional dialysis unit, received a phone call from a frantic physician, who practised out of a small community hospital in a neighbouring town. The physician told Trish that he had a 32-year-old client who was in dire need of urgent dialysis due to complications from bacterial endocarditis and septicemia. If she could receive dialysis, the client would have a good prognosis for a full recovery. Because the small community hospital did not have a dialysis unit, he was calling Trish out of desperation. He had provided care for this client throughout the course of her complicated illness and had become friendly with her husband and small children. The client was an active community member and a dedicated, well-loved teacher at the local school. She had two small children, one with cerebral palsy, who required specialized care.

Trish stated to the physician that the dialysis unit accepted clients on a first-come, first-served basis only. Frustrated and exhausted, the physician pleaded with Trish to consider removing from dialysis a client who might be older with a poorer prognosis and offer his client a chance to return to her active life and small children. Adamantly, Trish refused and reiterated that the unit treated all clients equally. Once again, the physician pleaded with Trish to use common sense and stated that his client's age, family situation, and prognosis should be considered. He also objected to what he said was a completely arbitrary method of allocation. Trish apologized and again refused, telling the physician that she would contact him if a space became available in the next few weeks. Quietly, the physician informed Trish that the client would likely not survive the next few weeks without access to dialysis.

When Trish hung up the phone, she felt terrible. On one hand, she had to abide by the unit policy of treating all clients equally, which, until now, she had felt was an effective and ethical way of allocating dialysis beds. On the other hand, she wondered if the physician could be right—that allocating by a first-come, first-served method was somehow morally arbitrary. She had always felt that the current allocation method was fair, but if it meant that some clients were refused access altogether, then how could this method be fair?

Like many nurses, Trish has been confronted with an ethical dilemma. Throughout history, nurses are faced with ethical challenges in all types of settings and, like Trish, are forced to reflect upon and examine their practices, values, and beliefs, as well as those of the institutions in which they work. Trish is confronted with a multidimensional dilemma. As a nurse manager, she occupies a "unique moral in-between position" (Storch, Rodney, & Starzomski, 2004, p. 2) because she must answer not only to the client of her unit and the larger community but to the nurses she supervises and the institution in which she practises.

As a manager, Trish is compelled to abide by the policies of her unit, put in place by the institution. However, she had no involvement in setting these policies and finds that, in practice, she is not sure of their fairness. Additionally, she feels that, as the enforcer of the admission policies on her unit, she is required to act as a gatekeeper to care for individuals and the health care providers in the community. Within this role as ad hoc gatekeeper, Trish feels she has little control over the decisions she must make and believes that some of these decisions are not what she would consider to be fair. Trish has been confronted with an ethical dilemma that has arisen out of her everyday practice. For nurses, ethical dilemmas like Trish's are a part of their daily lives in practice. These dilemmas require nurses to expend considerable energy and time devoted to serious reflection and meaningful inquiry.

ETHICS AND MORALITY

Ethics and morality are commonly used as interchangeable terms. Some agree that the two terms are very closely related, whereas others disagree, stating a difference in perception about what is understood to be *morality* and what is meant by *ethics*. **Ethics** can be defined as a way of understanding and reflecting upon social morality that encompasses moral issues, norms, and practices (Burkhardt & Nathaniel, 2002). Moral issues are those in which we find ourselves stating or reflecting that *something should happen, someone ought to act in a particular way, an action or intention is right or wrong, the consequences of an action are good or bad, there is a need to . . . , a person has a right to . . . , or we have a duty to a particular person or to act in a certain way.* Moral issues are matters that we find complicated, complex, dynamic, highly contextual, and difficult to resolve (Jameton, 1984). They are often the issues and situations that remain with nurses and other health professionals long after the clients have departed.

Morality can be defined as beliefs or traditions about what is determined to be right or wrong in terms of conduct towards ourselves and others (Beauchamp & Walters,

1999). Our ideas of morality are grounded in what we feel ought to happen, or what we believe people ought to do (Yeo & Moorhouse, 1996). Often these ideas are vague and may not provide clear guidance for approaching moral and ethical dilemmas. Additionally, many of our ideas about what is moral arise from our own values and beliefs and can differ significantly among rational, reasonable, and free-minded people. Although *morality* may provide some ideas or notions of what one ought to do, *ethics* is reflection and analysis upon the application of those ideas and notions (Yeo & Moorhouse, 1996).

Within the field of ethical inquiry, **bioethics** is relatively new, having arisen in the mid- to late 20th century in response to new technologies, choices, and concerns in matters of maintaining and intervening in the lives of human beings, such as health care, research, and the environment (Storch, Rodney, & Starzomski, 2004). Bioethics is sometimes referred to as health care ethics or biomedical ethics, although some suggest that these two terms are specific to the inquiry into issues of health care, health research, and interventions. The rise of bioethics has occurred alongside rapidly developing technological advances in health care, new frontiers in research and experimentation, and monumental advances in the dissemination of medical information via the media and the Internet. Furthermore, a noticeable change has occurred in the traditionally paternalistic model of the client–health care professional relationship, because clients and advocacy groups have challenged this model and have become empowered through knowledge of not only medicine and health care but of their rights and the rights of other individuals and groups.

A hundred years ago, a common question in health care was likely, What can we do? Now, with increased choices, alternatives, and costly interventions, the question is, What should we do? (Boetzkes & Waluchow, 2000, p. 3). Such a question constitutes an **ethical dilemma**—a situation in which the best course of action is often not clear, and strong ethical reasons exist to support each position (Beauchamp & Walter, 1999). Often, in approaching an ethical dilemma, we feel forced to choose between two or more alternatives that each seem quite plausible or morally acceptable, depending on one's viewpoint and perspective. Alternatively, we may feel forced to choose between two or more alternatives, none of which is completely fitting or without seemingly negative consequences.

Strategies and models exist to help us in approaching ethical dilemmas but the reality is that such algorithms and frameworks can provide only guidance; they do not provide instant solutions to ethical dilemmas that are complex, multifaceted, and inherently human. Positive approaches to ethical dilemmas include gathering adequate information; sorting out facts from values; seeking the perspectives of all involved stakeholders; and

problem solving and communicating with colleagues, clients, and their families.

An ethical dilemma can seem insurmountable because of lack of communication, confusion between facts and values, inadequate gathering of information, and problem solving in isolation, which can lead to moral distress. **Moral distress** results when ethical dilemmas are not acknowledged or effectively dealt with; when communication between team members, clients, and families is ineffective; or when professionals feel isolated or unsupported in their approach to solving such dilemmas. Simply put, it may be when the nurse knows the right thing to do but is unable to do it (Jameton, 1993). Moral distress involves and can lead to feelings of anxiety, frustration, and anger as well as guilt, emotional distress, and dissatisfaction with one's performance, action(s) or profession (Jameton, 1993; Keatings & Smith, 2000).

NURSING ETHICS

Bioethics is a broad field of inquiry that can relate to a variety of health care professionals and activities; however, there is agreement that nursing as a profession requires a separate field of study to examine the ethical norms, unique relationships, and sphere of nursing practice. Nursing roles are diverse in terms of responsibility, breadth, and type of everyday practice, including any number of aspects, such as provision of direct client care in an institutional, community, ambulatory, or home-care setting; supervision and management; public health and health promotion; education and welfare; multidisciplinary and independent work; and advanced practice roles, such as the nurse practitioner or nurse clinician. As the profession of nursing evolves and the scope of nursing practice grows, so do the ethical challenges and the need for reflection and examination upon these challenges.

Nursing ethics may be defined as the examination of the norms, values, and principles found in nursing practice (Yeo & Moorhouse, 1996). It focuses on the distinctive relationships found within nursing practice—such as the nurse–client relationship, the nurse–nurse relationship, and the nurse–physician relationship—and the resulting moral commitments that nurses have to others within these relationships and others (Keatings & Smith, 2000; Storch, Rodney, & Starzomski, 2004; Yeo & Moorhouse, 1996). Because nursing is situated within a relational context, it is considered by some as a "moral practice" (Gastmans, Dierckx de Casterle, & Schotsmans, 1998, p. 46).

Nursing ethics is both a field of inquiry into the norms and values in the nursing profession and a reference to the body of literature in which nursing scholars discuss, interpret, analyze, and apply these ethical norms and values. Such discussions are important to the evolution and advancement of the nursing profession, as evidenced by the existence and growth of nursing journals such as *Nursing Ethics* and *Nursing Philosophy*.

ETHICAL THEORIES

As we have noted, there are no magical solutions or easy algorithms for solving ethical dilemmas. However, systematic approaches can help us decide what is right and wrong. These are known as **ethical theories.** A rich body of theories exists as approaches to sorting through complex ethical challenges; however, we will focus here on two specific types of theories: the consequentialist, or teleological, and the deontological, or non-teleological theories.

Consequentialist theories put forth that when deciding between possible actions, the most important moral obligation is to maximize the positive consequences and minimize the negative consequences (Thomas and Waluchow, 2002). This theory, of course, requires knowledge of both the good and the negative consequences of an action. Consequentialist theories also involve reaching agreement among diverse people regarding what are positive and negative consequences. Finally, it must also be possible to prospectively evaluate and measure the goodness of actions.

Utilitarian theories, the most commonly cited type of consequentialist theories, assess the moral rightness of actions based on how much happiness they might produce. From a utilitarian perspective, deciding upon alternatives is simple and formulaic, involving three distinct steps. First, the consequences of each possible alternative must be estimated. Second, the balance of happiness and unhappiness must be calculated and compared to their alternatives. As a third step, the alternative estimated to produce the most happiness for the greatest number of people should be chosen (Yeo & Moorhouse, 2002). This apparently simple formula results in three difficulties. First, one can never be sure of the consequences of any action as one is always predicting into an unsure future. Second, what one person may consider a good consequence may not be evaluated as a good outcome by another reasonable person. Third, how do we measure good consequences or happiness?

Deontological theories posit that an action's inherent rightness never lies in its consequences but in its very adherence to a duty. Moral obligation involves determining one's moral duties or imperatives and acting consistently, according to those duties (Yeo & Moorhouse, 2002). Immanuel Kant (1724–1804) is one of the most well-known deontologists. According to Kant, the rightness of an action is never dependent on the consequences that might result from an action. Rather, an action is justified if it can meet Kant's categorical imperative, which gives no credence to possible consequences whatsoever. This imperative, as Kant describes it, compels a person to choose an action that can be universalized to all similar situations, i.e., it becomes a morally binding rule for action (Yeo & Moorhouse, 1996). Kant would ask us to imagine that every time a similar situation arose, we would will it so that everyone would always act in accordance with the duty we recognize and the subsequent action prescribed. If we could conceive that the subsequent action can be universalized, then it is the action we must take, in accordance with our duty.

Two difficulties are evident when we consider deontological theories. First, we are often not clear on what our duties are. As nurses, we might have a number of duties: to the client, to the institution that employs us, to our colleagues and profession, and to society. Moreover, we have moral duties not only in our work lives but in our personal, social, and family lives, which leads to the second difficulty. When we have conflicting duties, deontological theories offer little guidance on how to move forward and decide which duty should override.

When evaluating whether an action is ethical, the consequentialist always looks at what might happen as a result of an action. In other words, the consequentialist uses a forward-looking perspective. Meanwhile, the deontologist does not look at what might happen as a result of the action, instead using a backward-looking approach. Deontologists have little concern for the consequences of an action, only the duty lying behind it, which they must be able to articulate.

Sometimes, consequentialists and deontologists may agree on the moral rightness of an alternative; however, their justification for choosing the particular alternative might be markedly different. Consider the example in the Critical Thinking feature.

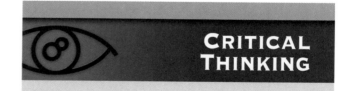

CRITICAL THINKING

Andrew is a nurse practitioner in a busy urban teaching hospital. While on his lunch break in a very crowded and busy cafeteria, he overhears his colleagues at the next table talking loudly about a particularly difficult client and family. Knowing that he is familiar with the client, his colleagues call him over to join the discussion. Andrew faces a difficult choice. Should he join the discussion with his colleagues, risking his own moral integrity and knowing that they may be easily overheard? Or should he tell his colleagues that he will not join them and that they have a professional obligation not to discuss clients and families in public places?

If we use a deontological theory to decide which action Andrew should take, we would consider the duty that we have to protect our clients' confidentiality and not discuss their cases in elevators or in cafeterias. We should refrain from doing so not out of consideration of the consequences but because we must adhere to this duty. The consequentialist might agree with this decision, but would, however, offer different reasons for not talking about clients outside of the clinical setting. The consequentialist would examine the consequences, both good and bad, of talking about clients at the cafeteria table and make a decision based on which alternative would produce the most happiness and the least unhappiness—likely ceasing the conversation. Although the deontologist and the consequentialist might agree on the preferred action in this case, they would be motivated by different factors.

PRINCIPLISM

In the 1970s, general moral philosophy and medical ethics had not yet met. Much work in academic philosophy examined ethical theories while the biomedical community focused on preventing harm and "doing good" for their clients. Little discussion of ethical principles occurred outside of individual professional codes of conduct, which were discipline-specific and not well suited to approaching complex and emerging ethical challenges. At that time, a set of basic ethical principles were articulated and formulated into a framework that is commonly referred to as **principlism** (Beauchamp & Childress, 1994). This framework for considering ethical issues includes the following guiding principles: (a) respect for autonomy, (b) beneficence, (c) nonmaleficence, and (d) justice.

Autonomy refers to the ability to self-govern and to have control over decision making concerning one's own life. **Beneficence** requires that we consider and act in the best interests of others. **Nonmaleficence** refers to the requirement that we avoid doing harm to others. Finally, **justice** is a broad principle encompassing the notion of fair distribution of benefits, resources, and risks (Beauchamp & DeGrazia, 2004).

Principlism is widely used in biomedical and health care ethics curricula as a framework for approaching ethical dilemmas. Many students in health care professions find this approach appealing because they can relate to the principles, drawn from traditional professional values, which are found in health professions, such as medicine and nursing.

Each of the ethical theories we have discussed help to answer the question, What action should I take? These theories also effectively focus the ethical issue on *action*, which may be motivated by certain factors and may be intended to abide by specific duties or to produce desired consequences. The most important consideration of these theories is the action that results from contemplation of one or more of the ethical theories.

FEMINIST ETHICS

Feminist ethics arose when scholars and philosophers recognized that, often, it is not enough to turn to a set of principles, duties, or rights when trying to resolve moral and ethical dilemmas. Moral dilemmas necessarily involve human relationships, which are inherently contextual, based on imbalances of power and involving complex understandings of priorities, stakes, and risks. The approach to moral dilemmas found in feminist ethics is affected by a perspective of the world that acknowledges the importance and influence of gender. Feminists such as Carol Gilligan posit that the differences in the social experiences and the relationships of men and women affect our moral development. In a social structure that has been traditionally male dominated, the experiences and lives of women and men are markedly different. Females, as a gender, have traditionally been oppressed and dominated within social systems (Liaschenko & Peter, 2003).

Feminism in ethics proposes that we examine ethical issues while keeping in mind conventional patterns of "discrimination, exploitation and dominance" (Sherwin, 1992, p. 4). Feminist ethics comprises a variety of approaches that are beyond the scope of this chapter; however, the common foundation of these approaches is the acknowledgment that moral dilemmas necessarily involve relationships between people at a variety of levels and within a variety of contexts. These relationships may involve power differences, politics, perceptions of imbalances of power, and diverse moral orientations, all of which may be grounded in gender. In challenging traditional approaches to ethical issues, feminist ethics strives to uncover and make explicit alternative approaches to ethical problems that openly address and incorporate considerations of these patterns and contexts (Liaschenko & Peter, 2003; Wolf, 1994).

FOUNDATIONS FOR ETHICAL CARE IN CANADA

Canada, unlike the United States, does not have a formalized bill of rights for clients. The U.S. Patient's Bill of Rights was formulated in 1973, by the American Hospital Association, with the most recent revisions made in 1992. The aim of the document is to articulate the rights and responsibilities of clients and their families, health care professionals, and the institutions in which they deliver care (American Hospital Association, 1992).

TABLE 20-1	**PRINCIPLES OF THE CANADA HEALTH ACT**
1. Public administration	Health care services must be delivered by a nonprofit, publicly administered agency.
2. Comprehensiveness	All "medically necessary" services of physicians and hospitals are provided.
3. Universality	All permanent residents of a province or territory, no matter where they live, are entitled to be insured by the publicly funded system.
4. Portability	For Canadians who move or travel within Canada or travel outside of Canada, insured services must be maintained.
5. Accessibility	All Canadians should have reasonable access to hospital and physician services, regardless of their geographic location, age, income, status, or gender.

Source: Adapted from: *Canada Health Act: Overview.* Retrieved from http://www.hc-sc.gc.ca/hcs-sss/medi-assur/overview-apercu/index_e.html, August 15, 2006.

In Canada, approaches to care are embedded in the Canadian Charter of Rights and Freedoms, a document that outlines the rights and freedoms of all citizens living in Canada. The Charter outlines particular civil, legal, social, and political rights of Canadian citizens and embodies a set of principles through articulation of and agreement on these rights. It is important, however, to note that the Charter does not explicitly identify health as a right or discuss health as a concept to which equality applies (Robinson Vollman, & Potter, 2006).

Particularly relevant to health care are two sections of the Charter: Sections 7 and 15(1). Section 7 outlines the legal rights of Canadians to life, liberty, and the security of people:

Everyone has the right to life, liberty and security of the person and the right not to be deprived thereof except in accordance with the principles of fundamental justice. (Section 7, Canadian Charter of Rights and Freedoms, 1982).

Section 15(1) outlines the equality rights of every Canadian citizen, to equality before and under the law as well as equal protection and benefit of the law, and reads as follows:

Every individual is equal before and under the law and has the right to the equal protection and equal benefit of the law without discrimination and, in particular, without discrimination based on race, national or ethnic origin, colour, religion, sex, age or mental or physical disability. (Section 15[1], Canadian Charter of Rights and Freedoms, 1982).

The emphasis on equality of people and equality of treatment of people is also embedded in another key document that guides health care in Canada, the Canada Health Act (CHA), a federal legislation for publicly funded health care insurance, which received Royal Assent in 1984. The CHA outlines specific principles that all provincial and territorial governments must abide by in the delivery of health care, as each province and territory develops, administers, and finances health care services, along with the federal contribution, the Canada Health Transfer (CHT). The CHA's five program criteria, or principles, are shown in Table 20-1.

CODES OF ETHICS IN NURSING

A professional code of ethics is not part of health law or statutory law, nor is it a set of rules. Instead, it is a code to which professionals must adhere as part of their responsibility and duty.

Professional codes of ethics define expectations of a profession. They are usually defined and shaped by members of that profession and provide guidelines and values to adhere to and to promote, in creating an ethical, accountable practice.

In 1953, the International Council of Nurses (ICN) published a code of ethics that was rewritten in 1973, as The ICN Code for Nurses—Ethical Concepts Applied to Nursing and most recently revised in 2005 (International Council of Nurses [ICN], 2006). The ICN Code of Ethics situates the ethical responsibilities of nurses in a framework that includes a number of relationships in which nurses participate, including "nurses and people," "nurses and practice," "nurses and the profession," and "nurses and co-workers" (ICN, 2006).

In its early days, the Canadian Nurses Association (CNA) adopted the ICN Code of Ethics until 1978, when the national organization decided to have its own unique code of ethics for nurses in Canada. After several drafts, the Code of Ethics for Nursing was published in 1985, and has been revised as necessary, with the most recently published version in 2002 (Canadian Nurses Association [CNA], 2002). The Code is once again under review, and its first drafts were available for external review in early 2007.

The CNA Code of Ethics situates the ethical expectation of nurses practising in Canada around eight primary values or responsibilities, which, according to the CNA, are key to the practice of nursing: safe, competent, and ethical care; health and well being; choice; dignity; confidentiality; justice; accountability; and quality practice environments. Within each of these values, explanatory responsibility statements outline specific practices, behaviours, and expectations.

A professional code of ethics doesn't guarantee that all involved in the profession will act ethically. It is a guideline and an explicit but general statement of expectations. It does not prescribe particular actions of behaviour in specific circumstances.

Alongside a code of ethics, nurses have their own values, which may evoke strong personal responses to ethical dilemmas. **Values** are personal beliefs about the truth of ideals, standards, principles, objects, and behaviours that give meaning and direction to life. Our values arise from our familial, cultural, religious, and educational experiences and can change over time as we develop our moral selves and, in doing so, become more autonomous.

The challenge of being part of a profession with a moral engagement and obligation is that we may encounter situations in which our values conflict with the values of a client, an institution, or a professional situation. Whereas much of the study of ethics deals with the values, wishes, and rights of others, as professionals, we must also focus on our own values and how they may have an effect upon our reactions, behaviours, and beliefs in professional practice. It is impossible to simply turn off our own values as we engage in our work. Instead we must take steps to acknowledge our own values and to be able to recognize situations in which we are conflicted.

In the Critical Thinking feature, June has critically examined her own values and understands that, in this case, they conflict with her ethical obligation to provide quality nursing care. In the best interests of the clients, other health care professionals, and for the sake of June's own moral integrity, June should not be forced to take part in a procedure for which she has such strong conflicting personal beliefs (Yeo & Moorhouse, 1996).

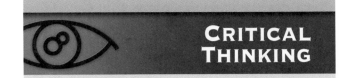

CRITICAL THINKING

June is an operating room (OR) nurse and has worked in this hospital for six years. Recently the hospital amalgamated with another institution, and the result is a great deal of changing roles and responsibilities in the OR. June has found that her day-to-day job has markedly changed as she has been asked to take part in new procedures. Today, she arrives for her shift and sees that she has been assigned to Operating Room C, in the day surgery area, an area in which she has not yet worked. When she scans the list of today's procedures, she notices a number of therapeutic abortions. June is very upset. Her personal belief is that abortion is wrong, and based on her religious and cultural beliefs, she does not consider abortion as a viable or moral option for any woman. She has never been asked to assist in a therapeutic abortion procedure, and she is worried about her ability to do her job and provide thorough, empathetic, and effective care. Additionally, she feels that she would be betraying herself and her religious beliefs by assisting with such a procedure. June approaches Sylvia, the operating room manager, explains her moral dilemma and requests to be removed from this assignment.

As the nurse manager, how should Sylvia respond? Should she honour June's request, or should she insist that June cover her assignment and fulfill her duties?

She may request to change her assignment today and move to another operating room. However, this reassignment must be done in such a way that it does not abandon or significantly disadvantage the clients. The CNA Code of Ethics clearly states that if a nurse is asked to provide care that conflicts with the nurse's personal values "the nurse must provide appropriate care until alternative care arrangements are in place" (CNA, 2002, p. 12). So, Sylvia may move June to another area with two conditions. First, Sylvia and June must find another registered nurse who has the relevant and necessary skills and experience to take June's assignment and provide competent care. Second, they must ensure that the clients are not abandoned in the interim. Once these two conditions are met, June can safely and ethically take another assignment. At a later time, it would be worthwhile for Sylvia and June to have a discussion and for June to reflect on her own reasons, beliefs, and goals related to working in this area.

PROFESSIONAL DILEMMAS

There is no end to the kinds of ethical challenges that nurses will face in their careers on a daily basis. In this section, we will examine four specific ethical issues arising in nursing practice: consent/autonomy, resource allocation, end-of-life care, and truth telling.

CONSENT/AUTONOMY

The issue of informed consent has been addressed and discussed extensively in the ethics and nursing literature. The provision of an informed consent is embedded within the notion of autonomy and allowing people the right to make informed, voluntary choices regarding their person and their care. The Code of Ethics for Registered Nurses in Canada outlines 12 specific responsibilities of registered nurses in regards to clients' choices, through respecting their autonomy, the subsequent expression of each client's health needs, and their wishes through freely given, informed choices (CNA, 2002).

Acting autonomously requires having information about the choices as well as the freedom to act. Informed consent, like autonomy, can be considered to have two important elements: the element of voluntariness and the element of cognition or ability of the person to understand the choice and aspects of the choice (Appelbaum, Lidz, & Meisel, 1987; Yeo & Moorhouse, 1996). For example, if preoperative clients receive full information regarding an optional research study they are eligible to participate in, and they are then encouraged to provide their consent by the surgeon who will be operating on them in the morning, these clients may feel implicit *coercion* to participate in the research. Alternatively, consider the client who is provided with written information on two procedures, each with similar benefits and risks, and is asked to choose which procedure is preferred. The written information is left at the client's bedside. This information is written in high-level language and has been given to a client who has limited literacy skills. The client may have been given the freedom to choose between the two procedures but cannot make a fully *informed* decision, due to lack of understanding about the procedure. Thus, an informed consent necessarily implies that the client not only understands the choices, their risks, benefits, and alternatives, but also has the ability to make a voluntary choice, free of coercion, influence, or pressure. Ontario's Health Care Consent Act states that consent is valid only if it is informed and voluntary, and it has not been obtained by misrepresentation, misinformation, or coercion (Health Care Consent Act, 1996).

A variety of issues within consent are debatable. For example, how much information is required to be informed? Who is the best person to provide consent?

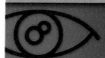

CRITICAL THINKING

Ralph is a 78-year-old man being admitted for coronary bypass surgery. The night before surgery, the surgeon visits him to obtain his informed consent. They have a quick and friendly meeting, and the surgeon leaves the room with a signed consent form on the chart.

Later that night, as the nurse does rounds, Ralph pulls her aside and expresses his trepidation at the upcoming surgery. He states that the surgeon told him that he might die, although he can't remember the "numbers" the surgeon used. He also asks her if he might get an "infection and die" or a "big stroke and never wake up." He says that he isn't sure of what the surgical team will be doing exactly but thinks that they'll be opening his heart up and "unplugging something or another." Finally, he tells her he didn't want to bother the surgeon with his worries and questions, as he seemed so busy.

Ralph goes on to tell her that at his appointments at the surgeon's office, he was too overwhelmed to understand or listen properly and depended on his son to speak for him and agree to anything. His son is out of town, returning tomorrow to be at the hospital after the surgery. Finally, Ralph says that he doesn't want the surgery if it is risky; he would rather live as he has been. He is visibly shaky, highly anxious, and unsettled.

What should the nurse do?

Should she provide comfort, some clarification of the procedure, perhaps a sleeping aid, and leave it at that?

Should she call the surgeon and have Ralph re-informed?

Do you think Ralph provided a voluntary, informed consent, earlier with the surgeon? Why or why not?

What about people with limited or fluctuating capacity? How is competence or capacity assessed? These are a few of the specific issues pertaining to consent.

For nurses, respect for autonomy and supporting people's endeavours to seek information are key elements of facilitating the provision of informed consent. Nurses can contribute to the maintenance of autonomy through informed consent by building trusting relationships with clients; providing current, complete information; ensuring understanding; respecting clients' wishes even though they may differ from the nurse's own wishes; providing opportunities for clients to make choices; respecting prior wishes communicated by an advance directive or a substitute decision-maker; and including relevant stakeholders in decision-making processes.

Nurses cannot provide care without the informed consent of the client. Doing so may constitute battery or harm to the client. Thus, any physical touch, even a slight or minor touch, done without the consent of another person may legally constitute battery (Keatings & Smith, 2000). All people have the right to provide consent for any kind of touch, be it a physical treatment or intervention, a nursing action, a medication administration, or a procedure. Although some actions such as surgeries, medical procedures, and therapies require a formal, written consent process, consent for actions such as a bed bath or a dressing change may be negotiated through less formal mechanisms. By asking the client if a nursing action is acceptable and having the client simply express agreement or expose the dressing for the nurse, usually implies consent and is, in most cases, sufficient.

Consent, although binding for the health care professional, is dynamic. That is, a client's consent is required before initiating any kind of procedure or action. However, it must be noted that because consent is a dynamic and contextual concept, clients may change their mind or withdraw their consent at any time. Clients who provide an informed consent for surgery in the morning may, upon awakening, have an additional question or clarification or may have changed their mind about the procedure. This change of status or withdrawal of consent must be respected. Similarly, if a client allows a dressing change to be done, but then, due to pain or fatigue or any other reason, decides not to have the dressing changed, this decision must be respected; the dressing change must be delayed until the client provides consent.

RESOURCE ALLOCATION

Emily and the team have a difficult decision, but not an uncommon one. Frequently, decisions are made that provide for one client while simultaneously denying another client. Every day, in busy emergency rooms and

---

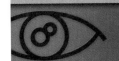

CRITICAL THINKING

Emily, a nurse clinician, works on a hectic transplant ward. Often she finds herself caring for transplant candidates for long periods of time while they await their transplant. Over these periods of time, she gets to know the clients, their families, and their lives quite well, and develops what she feels are strong therapeutic relationships. Tonight, a call comes to the unit informing them a liver is available that is a match for two of their critically ill clients awaiting an organ transplant. The decision regarding who is to receive the organ is left up to Emily and her multidisciplinary team. They must make a decision quickly. The first client, George, is a 46-year-old architect with congenital liver disease that has caused his liver to fail. George has a wife and two young children. He has been waiting eight months for a liver. The second client, Thomas, is a 53-year-old single lawyer. His liver disease resulted from excessive alcohol consumption. He has been waiting ten months for a liver.

The team must make a decision but are having difficulty with this task since both clients are an ideal match and have similarities in wait time, degree of urgency, and prognosis. Because Emily knows both clients quite well, she is asked who she feels should receive the organ. Before she answers, she realizes that, in her own view, she relates on a personal level much more to George because she also has young children. She also is conscious of the fact that she feels George is a more worthy candidate than Thomas. She realizes that she may have difficulty preventing her own personal views, values, and beliefs from taking over her decision-making process. She is puzzled, though, because she is unsure of what other criteria can be used to separate the two candidates.

Should Emily voice her distress and indecisiveness?

What criteria would you consider to be important in decision making in this case?

Is there a way to be fair to both clients in this case?

overcrowded intensive care units (ICUs), these kinds of decisions are made by triage nurses and nurse managers, who must allocate a position on a waiting list or an ICU bed to one client among many who are waiting. In allocating the emergency room time or the ICU bed to one client, however, they place others further down on a waiting list or deny others access to a necessary ICU bed. These kinds of decisions may be life and death decisions, or they may be simply perceived as inconvenient, frustrating, or unfair.

Resource allocation is an important issue to address because all health care systems operate with limited or scarce resources and their sustainability is questionable unless sensible constraints are placed on those resources. Decisions regarding resource constraints give rise to many challenging ethical issues. In Canada, we are in a period of examining and evaluating the sustainability of our health care system. Discussions of reform focus on how we should allocate resources in such a way that avoids morally arbitrary decision making but attempts to both meet society's expectations and encompass its values.

The allocation of resources is frequently a concern and responsibility of nurses. Nurse managers may find that they are forced to make staffing and retention decisions within the context and constraints of shrinking budgets. Staff nurses in hospitals undergoing cutbacks may find that their units are poorly staffed on weekends and nights and that their client assignment is markedly more difficult on those shifts. Operating room procedures may be cancelled due to nursing or support staff shortages or because of a lack of nursing staff in the recovery or intensive care area for postoperative care. Clients often find that some of their direct physical care is being provided by other health care team members, such as unregulated care providers (UCPs) or licensed practical nurses (LPNs). They may also find that their linens are no longer changed daily and that, upon discharge, only a limited amount of home care is available. All these examples are situations that involve the allocation or distribution of human and practical resources, including programs and services.

In health care, we usually discuss three levels of resource allocation. **Macro-allocation** decisions are made by governments at all levels. **Meso-allocation** decisions are those made at the institutional or program level. Finally, **micro-allocation** refers to decisions made at the bedside, regarding individual clients. All three levels are obviously linked, with each having a trickle-down effect on the others.

By virtue of the work nurses do, they often experience the end result of institutional or organizational policy changes related to resource allocation decisions. Cutbacks in nursing staff have a direct effect on client care. Additionally, cutbacks affect the remaining nurses who then need to deliver care to more clients with fewer staff. Often

nurses find themselves advocating for the best interests of their clients, armed with the knowledge that a particular client or group of clients need increased accessibility to a particular resource. Nurses also are the ones who often experience the frustration, anger, and dissatisfaction of clients who may perceive that, as a result of cutbacks or constraints on the system, they are receiving less care than they would like, are forced to do more things for themselves, or are waiting for services that are difficult to access.

There is no framework for working through ethical issues related to the allocation of resources. We tend to contemplate these issues within the broad sphere of justice, with particular relevance to theories of distributive justice. In keeping with the Canadian Charter of Rights and Freedoms, religion, ability, social status, race, or sexual orientation are examples of features considered to be irrelevant to resource allocation decision making. Criteria such as medical need, prognosis, risk, and benefit are felt to be morally relevant and objective criteria for decision making. However, even using criteria that appear to be objective and relevant can still result in ethical dilemmas and ambiguity. We may also have situations in which medical need, prognosis, and benefit may be similar—as Emily's case, in the Critical Thinking feature, on page 361, demonstrates. In these cases, how do we favour one patient over another? What kinds of criteria do we use to resolve this very practical dilemma?

Daniels addresses these thorny dilemmas as he identifies four difficult-to-resolve issues in resource allocation (Daniels, 1994):

1. **The fair chances versus best outcomes problem.** Should we always try to favour providing access to those with the best chance of a positive outcome over giving every possible client an opportunity to access resources?
2. **The priorities problem.** Should we give the most ill or disabled clients the priority to access resources?
3. **The aggregation problem.** Should we favour the situation in which we can provide moderate benefits to a larger number of people over the situation in which we can provide more significant benefits to very few?
4. **The democracy problem.** Should we focus on the process by which decisions are made, and instead rely on the fact that if we adhere to a democratic process, we will necessarily come up with fair outcomes?

Although Daniels's work was published more than a decade ago, these kinds of unresolved ethical dilemmas in resource allocation persist. With the increasing costs and capabilities of new technologies, an aging population, competing priorities at all levels of government, and increasingly knowledgeable and empowered clients, these kinds of allocation issues will surely continue to be one of the most prevailing challenges for modern health care systems.

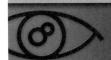

CRITICAL THINKING

Frank is a 25-year-old man with an acquired brain injury from a motor vehicle accident at age 19 that left him paralyzed and unable to care for himself. He was also severely burned in the accident. Frank lives in a long-term care institution, requiring 24-hour complete care. He has been plagued with serious and painful complications, including severe infections and persistent bedsores. He is completely and likely permanently respirator-dependent and must frequently undergo painful treatments.

Previous to his injury, Frank had been awarded a full university scholarship for football. His family and girlfriend visit once weekly. His football buddies visit once a month, but their times together are short and difficult for everyone. He looks forward to their visits but is depressed because the visits are infrequent and awkward. Last month, he told his girlfriend she should move on with her life. She is planning to take a job overseas and will leave in two months. His parents are busy caring for his two younger siblings, and they have had difficulty coping with having their son in this state. Family counselling has been ongoing but unproductive; and at Frank's request, it was discontinued. He says he stopped the counselling so that his parents "would not have to go through this anymore."

Frank is becoming more withdrawn and quiet. On her daily rounds, the nurse manager always takes time to speak with Frank. She has noted that Frank has asked vaguely, numerous times, about dying and assistance with dying. She decides to address this issue directly with Frank; when she does, he appears to be relieved. He smiles and thanks her for bringing it up so directly.

Frank goes on to say that he has a clear and accurate awareness of his future prognosis and that he considers it to be very bleak. He feels that he is a burden to his family and that he has no desire to continue his life as it is and will be. He states that he is at peace with his decision and that he has told his parents, who, although devastated, can abide by his decision.

He asks the nurse manager to talk to the team about discontinuing the respirator. The nurse manager tells Frank that she cannot support assisted suicide because it is illegal in Canada. Frank says to her in response, "You wouldn't be assisting my suicide. You would simply be abiding by the wishes of a fully competent and informed client to have a particular treatment discontinued. After all, you have done other things I have requested. This is no different!"

Is this a case of abiding by the wishes of a competent client or is it an example of assisted suicide?

If you were the nurse manager, how would you respond to Frank?

END-OF-LIFE ISSUES

End-of-life issues are extensively examined in nursing and ethics. Nurses are often the key multidisciplinary team members who can and do provide care and support throughout the entire dying process. By virtue of this intense involvement, nurses are often the ones who are engaged in the decision-making processes and the conversations and discussions about the end of life with clients and their families.

Many ethical dilemmas arise when considering death and dying. Davis and Aroskar (1983) classify three types of ethical dilemmas at the end of life: possible interventions by health professionals (i.e., resuscitation, prolonged ventilation, withdrawal of food or fluids); possible interventions by those close to the client (i.e., hastening death by various means, determining futility); and possible interventions by the client (i.e., suicide, request for assistance with suicide, use of advance directives, or refusal of interventions). This collection of ethical dilemmas, although not exhaustive, does include many important and frequent issues that arise in end-of-life care.

The need and desire for extensive examination of the dying process is a recent one. As recent as a few decades ago, dying was a more private and family process, often occurring at home and without the proliferation of assistive technologies that now function to keep dying people alive. Now, the capacity of technology to sustain life and delay death has increased, in many places becoming the norm. By virtue of this increased technological capacity, the locus of control for matters of living and dying has been transferred to specialists, and the traditional site of dying has moved from the home to the institution.

In response to these changes, two specific issues have emerged and have sparked much of the ongoing discussion and debate on end-of-life issues. The first issue is quality of life. Although it is a highly subjective and imprecise term, at the end of life, having **quality of life** may mean having some control over the process and one's final days. The other issue that leads directly from quality of life is the issue of power and control regarding decision making at the end of life.

We each have our own ideas and wishes regarding our eventual death. Many people would like to die in a place and manner of their choosing, with as much comfort and peace as possible. Overarching these ideas and wishes is the desire to have control over elements of a process that for most of us is outside of our control.

As technology became more and more a part of the dying process, a new vocabulary has developed as part of the discussions of death. One highly contentious term is **medical futility,** defined as "a medical treatment that is seen to be non-beneficial because it is believed to offer no reasonable hope of recovery or improvement of the client's condition" (CNA, 2001). This term evolved from the discussions on the high cost of technology used to keep people alive who often had poor quality of life or little hope of a meaningful recovery. The term was met with resistance from many because it defined meaningfulness using the term *utility*. For many, the use of this term implied that the measure of a worthwhile or meaningful life was limited to the degree of utility a person could contribute instead of a more holistic and subjective measure of when life is meaningful and when it has lost meaning. Futility, it was felt, should be considered in subjective and humane terms by the person most affected by the dying process—the client. Additionally, the term *medical futility* also emphasized, to many, the inappropriate focus on the economic impact of intervening in the dying process.

Resuscitation via cardiopulmonary resuscitation (CPR), medication, and ventilation is a common method of attempting to prolong life. Traditionally, when a person has a cardiac arrest or a respiratory arrest, the response is to initiate measures to take over the functions of the heart and lungs and in doing so, to save the person's life and prevent death. However, clients and their families, together with their health care providers, often decide that a *do-not-resuscitate* order is most appropriate and desired in the particular situation. Resuscitation is sometimes perceived to be too invasive, unlikely to result in appreciable improvement in condition, or likely to lead to more serious complications or distress. Specifically, resuscitation, in some cases, may lead to increased pain, discomfort, and suffering and may only serve to prolong the dying process (CNA, 1995).

The Canadian Nurses Association's Joint Statement on Resuscitative Interventions (1995) outlines important classifications regarding the efficacy of CPR in restoring function to individual people. The statement notes four categories of clients when considering whether CPR is a realistic or humane option: those who are likely to benefit from CPR, those for whom benefit is uncertain, those for whom benefit is unlikely, and those who most certainly will not benefit. This policy statement notes there is no obligation to provide or offer non-beneficial or futile treatment, which in some cases may include CPR. The futility or benefit of CPR must be "determined with reference to the person's own subjective judgement about his or her overall well-being" (p. 3).

Importantly, the CNA Joint Statement notes that the decision to withhold resuscitation by no means implies that other treatments, supportive care, or elements of palliative care should or will be withheld. It also notes the importance of communication and education of health care recipients, family members and significant others, and health care providers.

A decision to withhold resuscitation should include the client, the client's family and significant others, as noted by the client and the health care team. Key elements in the establishment of a DNR order are the clarity of roles and responsibilities, inclusion of all stakeholders, open discussions, and regular opportunities to revisit the discussion as the situation changes.

Although only physicians can write do not resuscitate (DNR) orders in Canada, because of nurses' practice and roles, they are often the health care practitioners most affected by such an order. Nurses are often present at the death of a client, and their roles, responsibilities, and feelings about their roles are affected by a DNR policy. Nurse leaders must take responsibility and be an active part of educating staff on the health care setting or unit's DNR policy and its application in everyday practice. Often, nurses must also assume a role in educating and discussing options for DNR status with families and clients. Although this responsibility is not clearly a nursing or medical role, every team member must be able to be open, approachable, and well informed about options and implications of resuscitation status for each person.

Many people, at the end of life, may not be able to voice their own wishes regarding the dying process. Nevertheless, they may have previously discussed their wishes with another person or documented their wishes as part of a living will. Living wills are documents voluntarily signed by clients that specify the type of care they desire if and when they are in a terminal state and cannot sign a consent form or convey this information verbally. Living wills can outline a client's wishes regarding specific interventions that may prolong life, such as CPR, artificial ventilation, and administration of medication, dialysis, or surgery. Now more commonly referred to as **advance directives,** these types of documents provide for two specific provisions. First, their existence aims to ensure that the wishes of a person, previously competent, are carried out when that person is no longer able to speak for him or herself. Second, an advance directive allows for the appointment of a specific person, a substitute decision-maker, who can help to carry out those wishes and ensure that they are followed (Singer, 1993). Across the country, these documents may look very different. Additionally, the adherence to these kinds of documents may vary from one setting to another. Unfortunately, unforeseen circumstances and lack of education, awareness, and information can all contribute to difficulty, hesitation, or unwillingness to identify and carry out the wishes of an advance directive.

During the dying process, nurses may be confronted with issues around easing the suffering of the dying person or facilitating the dying process. These actions may formally requested by a client or a family member, or they may be intimated through gestures, words, or implications. **Euthanasia** is defined as "a deliberate act undertaken by one person with the intention of ending the life of another person to relieve that person's suffering where the act is the cause of death" (Special Senate Committee on Euthanasia and Assisted Suicide, 1995). Examples of euthanasia may include discontinuation of respiratory assistance in a person who is ventilator-dependent, administration of a high dose of narcotic analgesia causing respiratory failure, or withdrawal of food and fluids. Euthanasia may be classified as either voluntary, involuntary, or nonvoluntary, depending on the person's competence, awareness, and known or voiced wishes (Lavery, Dickens, Boyle, & Singer, 1997).

Additionally, euthanasia is classified by some as either **passive euthanasia,** in which treatment may be ceased or withheld, and the person is thereby made more vulnerable to the underlying processes that cause death; or **active euthanasia,** in which body processes necessary to sustain life are actively interfered with or interrupted (Battin, 1994). Although these terms may provide a practical distinction, many believe that no moral or ethical distinction exists between these classifications. Active and ongoing debate continues regarding which classification is felt to be morally acceptable, whether withdrawal of treatment can be considered as morally similar or as humane as withholding of treatment and whether passive euthanasia is morally and practically inhumane. **Assisted suicide** is defined as "the act of intentionally killing oneself with the assistance of another who deliberately provides the knowledge, means, or both" (Special Senate Committee on Euthanasia and Assisted Suicide, 1995). An example of assisted suicide is the person who requests information on how much of a narcotic is necessary for an overdose and seeks to have enough of a stockpile of such medication on hand.

In Canada, euthanasia and physician-assisted suicide are illegal under the Criminal Code of Canada, regardless of the client or person's wishes (Criminal Code of Canada, Part VIII, 1985). However, as noted, nurses may play an important role in the dying process for many clients. The CNA Code of Ethics states that nurses have an obligation to assist people to achieve their optimal level of well-being in all states: health, illness, injury, or in

the dying process (CNA, 2002). The CNA position statement on end-of-life issues articulates the roles of the nurse at the end of life, as advocacy and promotion of respect and autonomy. These roles are carried out by ensuring that clients have access to and understanding of current treatments, alternatives, and options, and facilitating the expression of clients' needs, wishes, and beliefs regarding the dying process (CNA, 2000).

TRUTH TELLING

In everyday life, we encounter situations in which it is easier to not tell the entire truth, in order to avoid hurting others' feelings, causing unnecessary harm to others, or being chastised. However, the nature of the relationships that we have in everyday life varies from the nature of the relationships that we have in clinical settings. As clinicians, we have a **fiduciary obligation** to those for whom we provide care. A fiduciary obligation was originally a legal term to describe the responsibility of those entrusted to place the best interests of others above their own personal interests. By upholding the principles of beneficence (i.e., by acting in another's best interests) and nonmaleficence (i.e., by avoiding harm to another), a fiduciary relationship is one built on trust, conviction, and care. Part of this fiduciary duty is the obligation and expectation that nurses will be truthful and explicit in their communication with clients.

Traditionally, the physician has assumed the role of the clinician who provides important or difficult information to clients, such as diagnoses or prognoses. However with the expanding roles of the nurse and the increased use of advance practice nurses in health care settings, nurses are more likely to be responsible for taking part in communicating difficult messages to clients and their families. Even in more traditional or hierarchical health care settings, although physicians may still be the ones who deliver difficult news, clients often approach nurses to clarify, interpret, or advise. As a result of the physical proximity and intimate nature of nursing work, clients may turn to their nurses when they are unsure, worried, or confused. Nurses may find themselves being asked to reiterate or explain, and to offer advice or elucidation. In these types of situations, nurses need to be truthful, even in challenging circumstances or when discussing difficult or tragic outcomes and possibilities. Clients require accurate and honest information in order to make informed decisions about their health and well-being.

In some circumstances, truth telling can be especially difficult: situations of uncertainty, situations in which truth telling may be felt to be a potential source of harm to the client, or incidences of medical or nursing error (Hebert, Hoffmaster, Glass, & Singer, 1997). In these cases, the truth may be avoided in order to act beneficently, to avoid harm (i.e., nonmaleficence), or to avoid damage to the client–nurse relationship. Truth

CRITICAL THINKING

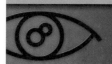

Miranda is a 28-year-old single woman, who has a history of depressive episodes and two unsuccessful suicide attempts. She lives with her parents and is with them in the outpatient unit today, undergoing a final test for her general symptoms of malaise, body aches, and night sweats.

While Miranda is dressing, the physician and the nurse manager take her parents aside to speak to them. They tell the parents that Miranda has Hodgkin's lymphoma, a malignant cancer that, in Miranda's case, will require fairly aggressive and prompt radiation therapy and chemotherapy. The therapy and preparations can begin in two days.

Her parents are very upset and ask the physician and nurse manager not to tell Miranda about her diagnosis. They feel that it would be best if they tell her and initiate treatment at some point later on. For now, they would like the physician to tell Miranda that there is nothing serious. They inform the physician that Miranda is very dependent on them and has been spiralling downwards into her recurrent depression. They are worried that news of the diagnosis would further upset her, and she would be unable to cope or make good decisions.

Furthermore, they are celebrating their 30th wedding anniversary by going on a 20-day cruise and are leaving next week. They have never been away together, having been caregivers for Miranda in addition to working full-time. It is too late to get a refund from cancelling their trip. They would like to wait until they return to tell Miranda about her diagnosis and begin treatment. While they are away, she will be staying with her brother, with whom she is not particularly close. Her parents are worried that Miranda will not have adequate supports to deal with the diagnosis while they are away.

What should Miranda be told, and why?

Who should make decisions regarding Miranda's care and treatment?

What should the role of the health care professionals involved in this case, be?

telling by all clinicians in these cases may be easier said than done, but in the long run, being honest helps to reduce resentment, increase trust, and strengthen clients' faith in the integrity of the health care team and the care they receive.

Some strategies that nurses may employ as they impart difficult news to clients include ensuring that clients and families have access to accurate, relevant, and complete information at levels they can comprehend; providing resources, supports, and follow-up services; supporting clients in their decision making; and educating clients not only on specific issues but on their rights as well as the options and alternatives available to them. The Canadian Nurses Association Code of Ethics reinforces these strategies. Although the Code of Ethics does not explicitly address truth telling, it does implicitly address it throughout the document, by stating, for example, that "nurses must admit mistake and take all necessary actions to prevent or minimize harm . . ." (CNA, 2002, p. 9). Furthermore, the Code of Ethics states that "nurses must be committed to building trusting relationships as the foundation of meaningful communication, recognizing that building this relationship takes effort" (p. 11). Finally, truth telling is referred to explicitly in a

principle under the Accountability section that states "nurses have the responsibility to conduct themselves with honesty and to protect their own integrity in all of their professional interactions" (p. 16).

The importance of **veracity,** the obligation to tell the truth, cannot be overemphasized. In a health care setting, the power imbalance created by knowledge can be overwhelming and intimidating for clients and can contribute to clients' feelings of powerlessness, confusion, and distrust. Nurses must aim to carry out their interactions in all aspects of the care they provide with integrity, honesty, and a commitment to the process of building trusting relationships over time.

LEADERSHIP ROLES AND CHALLENGES IN ETHICS

Today, nurses have many unique and rewarding opportunities to assume leadership roles in areas of ethics in a variety of settings, including hospitals, organizations, and academic institutions. Nurses may serve as members of clinical or research ethics committees in hospitals, private organizations, and academic institutions. Clinical ethics committees serve a number of purposes within health care settings, including a resource and consultation role, promotion and dissemination of research and education, and participating in policy development (Chidwick, Faith, Godkin, & Hardingham, 2004). Research ethics committees review and approve proposed and ongoing research to ensure that it meets with the guidelines for ethical research in Canada, which are outlined in the Tri-Council Policy Statement (Canadian Institutes of Health Research, National Sciences and Engineering Research Council of Canada, & Social Sciences and Humanities Research Council of Canada, 1998). Aiming for representation from a variety of professions and groups on ethics committees ensures that no one group or perspective will take precedence in decision making and deliberative processes.

Most hospitals have bioethicists on staff who serve in a variety of ways. They provide guidance, support, and advice for staff, clients, and families who face ethical challenges. The role of the bioethicist can be filled by a nurse with a completed graduate degree in bioethics. Interdisciplinary centres across Canada—such as the Joint Centre for Bioethics at the University of Toronto; the W. Maurice Young Centre for Applied Ethics at the University of British Columbia; the John Dossetor Health Ethics Centre, University of Alberta; and the Department of Bioethics, Dalhousie University—offer various graduate programs to equip nurses, physicians, and other health care professionals to assume leadership positions in ethics. A nurse with clinical expertise alongside graduate knowledge in bioethics may be an effective bioethicist and may also serve in a leadership or mentorship position for other nurses.

Leadership in terms of ethics may well be less formal, however. Nurse leaders or managers who encourage an ethical environment may also become mentors in their own practice. Encouraging open discussion of situations and issues that staff find challenging, distressing, or worrisome can lead to a more ethical environment in nursing units. Instead of an environment in which nurses are afraid to speak up, worried that they will not be supported if they do or hesitant to discuss ethical issues for fear of reprisal, an environment in which nurses are supported, listened to, and considered valuable stakeholders in ethical issues, should be facilitated and nurtured by nursing leaders.

From a practical perspective, such an environment can be achieved iteratively, through a number of relatively accessible and creative endeavours. One suggestion is to have open case conferences over lunch in which nursing staff can bring forward ethical issues from their daily practice and discuss them in a safe, confidential, and supportive environment. Another suggestion is to

address ethical issues using a prospective model. Instead of allowing situations to develop over time, becoming more complex and complicated, it is always advisable to open up discussion about particular issues early and to reopen discussions on an as required basis. Additionally, a good ethical leader can also recognize situations that may be causing distress to clinicians and should have an open-door policy for confidential discussions of such situations. This approach encourages both a level of comfort and discussion, which may, in turn, translate to a more ethically sensitive and effective group of clinicians.

Consistently involving clients and their families in discussions and decision making sets a clear example of ethical practice. Additionally, another way to prevent one group or one discipline's perspective from dominating decision-making processes is to involve a multidisciplinary team in decision making, with opportunities for all disciplines and team members to have a voice. These kinds of practices can be instituted by nurse leaders and enforced through local norms and policies.

Being involved in policymaking is one way that nurses and nurse leaders can help to create an ethical work environment. For example, if an institution were considering developing a policy for discontinuation of food and fluids for palliative clients, nurses and nurse leaders from that unit should be involved in the discussion and formation of such a policy. They could also advocate for the inclusion of laypeople who may have been involved in a similar situation with a family member or friend.

Finally, when decision making is made in a unilateral or paternalistic way by a nurse leader, it sets a tone for others that their contribution and perspective is unimportant. Nurse leaders may create an ethical environment by simply carrying out their day-to-day decision making by involving staff with a stake in those decisions, carrying out such processes in an open and transparent way, and allowing for discussion and debate over decisions without reprisal. One way to create an ethical environment might be to adapt an ethical decision-making model into the day-to-day decision-making processes of a unit, clinic, institution, or organization.

TWO MODELS FOR ETHICAL DECISION MAKING

Although ethical theories may be limited in their scope and the degree to which they can be applied in the real world, and ethical theories alone provide little guidance for actual decision making, they do provide perspectives into approaches to ethical analysis and reasoning. Furthermore, few of us can confidently say that we are consistently true deontologists or true consequentialists in all aspects of our lives and in every ethical decision-making process. Different ethical problems within a variety of contexts and with unique players often require different approaches.

So how can nurses approach ethical problems? Models for ethical decision making may not help to illuminate the right answer to a problem but they can provide direction and guidance for a systematic approach to ethical problems (Rodney 1991). Table 20-2 provides a comparative

TABLE 20-2	**COMPARISON OF TWO ETHICAL DECISION-MAKING MODELS**

A Framework for Ethical Decision Making
(Adapted from McDonald, 2001)

1. **Identify the problem and collect as much information as you can.** The key at this stage is twofold: first, be alert to ethical situations within your everyday practice. Second, be aware of what you know and what you do not know regarding the situation. It is necessary to gather as much information and as many alternative interpretations as possible, keeping in mind that there may be time constraints in real-life practice situations. Present the case with the facts you have collected and try to focus on the decision(s) that need to be made. As always, be aware of three elements: the specific and dynamic context of the situations; any potential conflicts of interest, for any involved stakeholders; and your own stake and position in the process and potential outcomes.

2. **Specify potentially feasible alternatives.** State the possible alternatives for decision making, considering the consequences, both direct and indirect, for all potentially affected persons.

3. **Use your own ethical resources to help decide what is morally relevant for each alternative.** At this stage, you likely have a number of ethical resources that you can use to help you decide between possible alternatives. These may include the stated ethical principles of your community, profession, or institution; moral mentors and trusted colleagues; policies, contexts, or relationships; formal case conferences; an ethicist; or an ethics committee.

4. **Propose and test possible resolutions.** Find the alternative resolution that you believe to be the best option, and ask yourself a number of questions: What would have to change to get me to alter the choice of this alternative? Would a good person/clinician do this? What if everyone in a similar situation did the same? Will implementing this decision have a negative impact on anyone or any trust relationships?

5. **Finally, make your choice.** Live with it and learn from it.

An Ethical Decision-Making Model for Critical Care Nursing
(Adapted from Rodney, 1991)

1. **Gather background information.** The priority is gathering relevant information in order to define and describe the problem.

2. **Identify whether the problem is an ethical issue.** Through gathering relevant information, determine whether this problem is an ethical issue, as opposed to a practical, legal, or professional issue. If it is determined that it is an ethical problem, then an ethical theory can be used to try to articulate rights, duties, principles, moral obligations, or roles.

3. **Identify key stakeholders.** In addition to identifying and articulating the problem, identify the key players; i.e., anyone who might be affected by this ethical issue or who has a stake in the outcome. As part of this stage, concepts such as responsibility, authority, professional roles, personal relationships, competence, conflicting rights, or conflicts of interest may be relevant.

4. **Identify possible courses of action.** As you identify possibilities for action, consequences must also be considered.

5. **Reconcile the facts of the case with relevant principles.** Consider alternatives in terms of their inherent value, relative to the principles that you identify as important to the case.

6. **Resolution.** Try to achieve consensus in decision making, keeping in mind that constraints may emerge, due to professional obligations, legal requirements, or social expectations. These constraints should be made explicit throughout the process.

account of two ethical decision-making models. McDonald provides us with a conceptual framework for approaching ethical problems (McDonald, 2001). He notes that this framework is not a recipe for finding solutions to ethical problems, but a guide for approaching problems. The emphasis in his framework is on examining problems from all possible perspectives and considering contexts and subtexts while ensuring that discussion and resolution is inclusive of all involved people. McDonald acknowledges that, even with a decision-making framework and the involvement of committed ethical people, it may not be possible to reach what is considered a perfect solution. It is most important to be able to learn and grow as a result of this process. Ethical decision making, if we take McDonald's model further, is not something that can be done on a sporadic basis or in isolation. It must be done regularly and vigorously as part of a team and carried out with compassion and care in a mutually supportive environment (McDonald, 2001). Rodney (1991) adapts Curtin's model of ethical

decision making to critical care nursing and the ethical challenges arising in this area. This model, although notably more concise, provides a straightforward approach to ethical decision making that can be applied in a variety of settings.

One important point to note is that most models of ethical decision making incorporate, in some way, a consideration of one's own values and beliefs, which is an important step that is often difficult to articulate or explicitly describe. Our personal values and feelings about issues are based in our own experiences, religions, cultures, and families, and thus, they cannot simply be put aside while we struggle with a value-laden problem in practice. We should not use ethical problems as opportunities to either further or promote our own personal beliefs or values to others, but we are responsible for examining our own feelings and personal values if they are relevant to a particular case or concept, as part of the initial phases of decision making.

KEY CONCEPTS

- Ethics is the branch of philosophy that concerns the distinction between right and wrong.

- A personal philosophy stems from an individual's beliefs and values. This personal philosophy will influence an individual's philosophy of nursing.

- Two ethical theories are consequentialism and deontology.

- Ethical principles and rules include beneficence, nonmaleficence, justice, and respect for autonomy.

- Ethics committees provide guidance for decision making about ethical dilemmas that arise in health care settings.

- Values clarification is an important step in the decision-making process.

- Two helpful tools are the framework for ethical decision making and the ethical decision-making model for critical care nursing.

- Today's nurses face numerous ethical issues and moral dilemmas.

- Nurse leaders who are dedicated to ethical principles can influence organizational ethics.

KEY TERMS

active euthanasia
advance directives
assisted suicide
autonomy

beneficence
bioethics
consequentialist theories
deontological theories

ethical dilemma
ethical theories
ethics
euthanasia
fiduciary obligation
justice
living will
macro-allocation
medical futility
meso-allocation
micro-allocation

moral distress
morality
nonmaleficence
nursing ethics
passive euthanasia
princi:plism
professional code of ethics
quality of life
utilitarian theories
values
veracity

REVIEW QUESTIONS

1. Mrs. Green rides the elevator to the third floor where her husband is a client. While on the elevator, Mrs. Green hears two nurses talking about Mr. Green. They are discussing the potential prognosis and whether he should be told. The nurses are violating which of the following ethical principles?
   A. Autonomy
   B. Confidentiality
   C. Beneficence
   D. Non-maleficence

2. When evaluating whether an action is ethical, which of the following approaches will the consequentialist use?
   A. Forward-looking approach
   B. Backward-looking approach
   C. Consequentialist approach
   D. Duty-oriented approach

3. Which of the following principles is not included in the framework for considering ethical issues?
   A. Principlism
   B. Beneficence
   C. Non-maleficence
   D. Justice

REVIEW ACTIVITIES

1. Review the Critical Thinking features in this chapter. As you are doing so, try to advocate from the perspective of each different person. For example, in the end-of-life Critical Thinking feature, page 363, examine and discuss the case from the perspective of Frank, the nurse manager, and Frank's family.

2. Examine a case from your own day-to-day practice. Use the ethical theories presented here to work through possible alternatives. Reflect on the effectiveness of the theories as you apply them to real-life cases.

3. Examine the Critical Thinking features found in the chapter. Using McDonald's Framework for Ethical Decision Making, work through the features using the information provided. Identify when you would have required more information, if it were a real-life case.

EXPLORING THE WEB

■ Read about codes of ethics from various nursing bodies:

International Council of Nurses: *http://www.icn.ch/ ethics.htm*

Canadian Nurses Association: *http://www.cna-nurses. ca/CNA/practice/ethics/code/default_e.aspx*

College of Nurses of Ontario: *http://www.cno.org/docs/prac/41034_Ethics.pdf*

■ Learn more about Canadian organizations dedicated to ethics:

Canadian Bioethics Society: *http://www.bioethics.ca/index-ang.html*

Alberta Provincial Health Ethics Network: *http://www.phen.ab.ca/*

■ Visit these university-based academic/clinical ethics centres:

University of Toronto Joint Centre for Bioethics: *http://www.utoronto.ca/jcb/home/main.htm*

Centre for Bioethics, Clinical Research Institute of Montreal: *http://www.ircm.qc.ca/bioethique/english/index.html*

John Dossetor Health Ethics Centre, University of Alberta: *http://www.ualberta.ca/BIOETHICS/*

W. Maurice Young Centre for Applied Ethics, University of British Columbia: http://www.ethics.ubc.ca/

Department of Bioethics, Dalhousie University: *http://bioethics.medicine.dal.ca/*

■ Other useful links for exploration and learning:

Canadian Medical Association Journal Bioethics for Clinicians series: http://www.cmaj.ca/cgi/collection/bioethics_for_ clinicians_series

Bioethics Resources on the Web (National Institutes of Health): *http://bioethics.od.nih.gov/*

A comprehensive list of links by subject, provided by the Provincial Health Ethics Network, Alberta: *http://www.phen.ab.ca/netlinks/*

REFERENCES

American Hospital Association. (1992). *A patient's bill of rights.* Chicago: Author.

Applebaum, P. S., Lidz, C. W., & Meisel, A. (1987). *Informed consent: Legal theory and clinical practice.* New York: Oxford University Press.

Battin, M. (1994). *The least worst death: Essays in Bioethics on the end of life.* New York: Oxford University Press.

Beauchamp, T. L., & Childress, J. F. (1994). *Principles of biomedical ethics* (4th ed.). New York: Oxford University Press.

Beauchamp, T. L., & DeGrazia, D. (2004). *Principles and principlism.* In G. Khushf (Ed.), *Handbook of bioethics* (pp. 55–74). Dordrecht, The Netherlands: Kluwer Academic.

Beauchamp, T. L., & Walters, L. (1999). *Contemporary issues in bioethics.* Belmont, CA: Wadsworth.

Boetzkes, S., & Waluchow, W. J. (2000). *Readings in health care ethics.* Peterborough, ON: Broadview.

Burkhardt, M. A., & Nathaniel, A. K. (2002). *Ethics and issues in contemporary nursing* (2nd ed.). New York: Delmar Thompson.

Canadian Institutes of Health Research, Natural Sciences and Engineering Research Council of Canada, Social Sciences and Humanities Resaerch Council of Canada. (1998). *Tri-Council policy statement: Ethical conduct for research involving humans* (with 2000, 2002, 2005 amendments).

Canadian Nurses Assocation. (1995). *Joint statement on resuscitative interventions.* Ottawa: Canadian Nurses Association.

Canadian Nurses Association. (2000). *Position statement: End-of-life issues.* Ottawa: Canadian Nurses Association.

Canadian Nurses Association (2001). *Futility presents many challenges for nurses. Ethics in Practice series paper.* Ottawa: Canadian Nurses Association.

Canadian Nurses Association. (2002). *Code of ethics for registered nurses.* Ottawa: Canadian Nurses Association.

Chidwick, P., Faith, K., Godkin, D., & Hardingham, L. (2004). Clinical education of ethicists: the role of a clinical ethics fellowship. *BMC Medical Ethics, 5*(6). Retrieved from http://www.biomedcentral.com/1472-6939/5/6, July 31, 2007.

Criminal Code of Canada (RS 1985, c. C-46) *Part VIII: Offences against the person and reputation.* Retrieved from http://laws.justice.gc.ca/en/C-46/, August 10, 2006.

Daniels, N. (1994). Four unsolved rationing problems: A challenge. *Hastings Center Report, 24*(4), 27–29.

Davis, A. J., & Aroskar, M. A. (1983). *Ethical dilemmas and nursing practice* (2nd ed.). Norwalk, CT: Appleton, Century, Crofts.

Gastmans, C., Dierekx de Casterle, B., & Schotsmans, P. (1998). Nursing considered as moral practice: A philosophical-ethical interpretation of nursing. *Kennedy Institute of Ethics Journal, 8*(1), 43–69.

Health Canada (2005). *Canada Health Act: Overview.* Retrieved from http://www.hc-sc.gc.ca/hcs-sss/medi-assur/overview-apercu/index_e.html, August 15, 2006.

Health Care Consent Act. (1996). S.O. 1996, c. 2. Schedule A.

Hebert, P. C., Hoffmaster, B., Glass, K. C. & Singer, P. A. (1997). Bioethics for clinicians: 7. Truth telling. *Canadian Medical Association Journal, 156*(2), 225–228.

International Council of Nurses. (2006). *The ICN Code of Ethics for Nurses.* Geneva: International Council of Nurses.

Jameton, A. (1984). *Nursing practice: The ethical issues.* New Jersey: Prentice-Hall.

Jameton, A. (1993). Dilemmas of moral distress: Moral responsibility and nursing practice. *AWHONN Clinical Issues, 3*(4), 542–551.

Keatings, M., & Smith, O. B. (2000). *Ethical and legal issues in Canadian nursing* (2nd ed.). Toronto: Elsevier.

Lavery, J. V., Dickens, B. M., Boyle, J. M., & Singer, P. A. (1997). Bioethics for clinicians: 11. Euthanasia and assisted suicide. *Canadian Medical Association Journal, 156*(10), 1405–1408.

Liaschenko, J., & Peter, E. (2003). *Feminist ethics.* In V. Tschudin, V. (Ed.), *Approaches to ethics: Nursing beyond boundaries* (pp. 33–44). New York: Butterworth.

McDonald, M. (2001). Canadian governance of health research involving human subjects: Is anyone minding the store? *Health Law Journal, 9,* 1–21.

Robinson Vollman, A., & Potter, P. A. (2006). *The Canadian health care delivery system.* In J. C. Ross-Kerr & M. J. Wood (Eds.). *Canadian fundamentals of nursing* (3rd ed., pp. 18–34). Toronto: Elsevier.

Rodney, P. A. (1991). Dealing with ethical problems: An ethical decision-making model for critical care nurses. *Canadian Critical Care Nursing Journal, 8*(2), 8–10.

Sherwin, S. (1992). *No longer patient: Feminist ethics & health care.* Philadelphia: Temple University Press.

Singer, P. A. (1993). *Living will.* Toronto: University of Toronto Joint Centre for Bioethics.

Special Senate Committee on Euthanasia and Assisted Suicide. (1995). *Of life and death.* Ottawa: Supply and Services Canada. [cat no YC2-351/1-OIE]

Storch, J. L., Rodney, P., Starzomski, R. (2004). *Toward a moral horizon: Nursing ethics for leadership and practice.* Toronto: Pearson Education Canada.

Thomas, J., & Waluchow, W. J. (2002). *Well and good: A case study approach to biomedical ethics.* Peterborough, ON: Broadview Press.

Wolf, S. M. (1994). Shifting paradigms in bioethics and health law: The rise of a new pragmatism. *American Journal of Law and Medicine, 20*(4), 395–415.

Yeo, M., & Moorhouse, A. (Eds.). (1996). *Concepts and cases in nursing ethics* (2nd ed.). Peterborough, ON: Broadview Press.

SUGGESTED READINGS

Baylis, F., Downie, J., Hoffmaster, B., & Sherwin, S. (1995). *Health care ethics in Canada.* Toronto: Harcourt Brace Canada.

Benner, P. A., Tanner, C. A., & Chesla, C. A. (1996). *Expertise in nursing practice: Caring, clinical judgment and ethics.* New York: Springer.

Birnie, L. H., & Rodriguez, S. (1994). *Uncommon will: The death and life of Sue Rodriguez.* Toronto: Macmillan.

Butts, J. B., & Rich, K. L. (2005). *Nursing ethics: Across the curriculum and into practice.* Sudbury, MA: Jones and Bartlett.

Johnstone, M.-J. (1999). *Bioethics: A nursing perspective* (3rd ed.) Philadelphia: Harcourt Saunders.

Kikuchi, J. F. (2005). Commentary on the CNA code of ethics. *Canadian Nurse, 101*(8), 16–18.

Kluge, E.-H. W. (2005). *Readings in biomedical ethics: A Canadian focus* (3rd ed.). Toronto: Pearson Prentice Hall.

Kuhl, D. (2002). *What dying people want: Lessons for living from people who are dying.* New York: Public Affairs.

McKinley, S., Rodney, P., Storch, J., & McAlpine, H. (2004). The role of ethics in nursing. *Nursing BC, 36*(1), 12–16.

Parsons, A. H., & Parsons, P. H. (1992). *Health care ethics.* Toronto: Wall & Emerson, Inc.

Storch, J. L. (2007). Enduring values in changing times: The CAN Codes of Ethics. *Canadian Nurse, 103*(4), 29–33, 37.

Tschudin, V. (2003). *Ethics in nursing: The caring relationship* (3rd ed.). New York: Butterworth-Heinemann.

CHAPTER 21

Collective Bargaining

Janice Tazbir, RN, MS, CCRN
Adapted by: Heather Crawford, BScN, MEd, CHE

Giving nurses a voice with power is our role and our continuing goal. We are the Canadian Federation of Nurses Unions.
(Canadian Federation of Nurses Unions, 2007)

OBJECTIVES

Upon completion of this chapter, the reader should be able to:

1. Review the history of collective bargaining.
2. Discuss collective action models and associated terminology.
3. Identify the steps involved in union certification.
4. Discuss professionalism in the context of unionization.
5. List the pros and cons of collective bargaining.

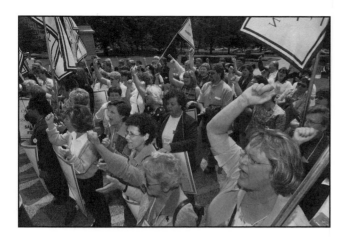

You are a new nurse on an internal medicine unit. When you have your meal break, you decide to sit in the conference room with the rest of the nurses. Two nurses are having a discussion. Sally is a registered nurse with 15 years experience, and she says, "I'm really tired of assignments that don't allow me to spend any time talking to my patients." Rose, a registered nurse with four years' experience asks, "Have you taken your concerns to our manager?" Sally responds, "Of course. I point out the number and complexity of the patients, but she says we need to cope." Rose says, "I wonder if we would have better success with these issues if we discussed them as a group, and made some suggestions to improve our satisfaction."

What are your thoughts about this situation?

What are some of the choices the nurses have?

Historically, nurses were perceived as hard-working, submissive women who did what they are told. The scope of nursing has changed so dramatically that today's nurses cannot afford to have a submissive image and do only what they are told. Clients, their illnesses, and their families are more complex than ever. Nurses are educated to advocate for their clients and themselves. Clinical situations arise in which nurses must voice their opinions and stand up for what is best for clients. To be effective in today's world, nurses must understand the tools available to deal with problems.

Collective action, or simply acting as a group with a single voice, is one method of dealing with problems. **Collective bargaining** is the practice of employees, as a collective group, bargaining with management in reference to wages, work practices, work environment, and other benefits. This chapter discusses different types of collective action models and also includes information concerning unionization, as well as professionalism in the context of unionization.

HISTORY OF NURSING UNIONIZATION IN CANADA

The Canadian Federation of Nurses Unions (CFNU) celebrated its 25th anniversary in 2003. Kathleen Connors provided an exceptional summary of the history of nursing unionization in Canada. A synopsis of the information she provided follows:

"In 1975, the then prime minister, Pierre Elliott Trudeau, announced wage and price controls in order to prevent further inflation. Shortly thereafter, Canada experienced a 42-day postal strike, which led to the federal cabinet overturning one of the first major decisions by the Anti-Inflation Board when it allowed the postal workers a 20 percent pay increase. At that time, nurses from across the country participated in a collective bargaining conference, an informal meeting that allowed senior staff of Canadian unions to share information, knowledge, and strategies. At that time, it was recognized that there was no national voice to speak on behalf of nurses, particularly in response to Trudeau's wage and price controls.

In 1978, the Canadian Nurses Association (the nurses' professional association) drafted a code of ethics, which, among other things, implied that it would be unethical for nurses to strike in Canada. Again, nurses were reminded of the importance of having a national voice for unionized nurses. At the next collective bargaining conference, nurses' unions set up a committee to examine potential structures, terms of reference, and constitutional language for a national voice. The leadership for this endeavour was provided by the Saskatchewan Union of Nurses, the Newfoundland and Labrador Nurses Union, and the Prince Edward Island Nurses Union. The founding convention was held in April 1981, and on May 1, 1981, the National Federation of Nurses Unions was created to represent unionized nurses at the national level. In 1999, the name was changed to the Canadian Federation of Nurses Unions (CFNU).

In 1987, the CFNU established a full-time office and a full-time president's position in Ottawa. The organization's focus was initially on negotiated contracts, grievances, and other labour relations issues; however, the health care system and social justice concerns soon became important issues for nurses. As a result, the Manitoba Nurses Union brought a resolution to the 1982 Special Convention that the Canadian Federation of Nurses Unions should join the Canadian Health Coalition to champion medicare and other social justice issues, which then became the focus for CFNU.

Additional provincial nursing unions gradually joined the national collective, which led to the Canadian government recognizing that CFNU was a strong and realistic voice for nurses. The British Columbia Nursing Union became a member in 1994, followed by the Staff Nurses Association of Alberta (SNAA), which affiliated in 1985. The United Nurses of Alberta affiliated in 1999, two years after amalgamating with the SNAA. In 2000, the Saskatchewan Union of Nurses, the Nova Scotia Nurses Union, and the Prince Edward Island Nurses Union reaffiliated. In November 2000, the Ontario Nurses Association became a member. The only provincial union not a member is the Fédération des Infirmiers et Infirmières du Québec (FIIQ), which does attend board meetings and conventions as an observer.

The Saskatchewan Nurses Union has a long history of firsts. In 1974, it became the first nursing union to form in Canada. In 1996, it was the first nursing union to affiliate with a provincial federation of labour, the Saskatchewan Federation of Labour. In 1997, it was the first nursing union to join the Canadian Labour Congress (CLC), and was followed by the British Columbia Nurses Union and the Manitoba Nurses Union, which joined the CLC in 1999.

A constitutional change was required for the Canadian Federation of Nurses Unions and its member organizations to affiliate with the Canadian Labour Congress, which occurred in 1997, at the CFNU convention in Vancouver. In January 1998, the CFNU became a member of the CLC, with a seat on the CLC's executive committee. The CLC membership provided the CFNU with support for collective bargaining in such areas as occupational health and safety, pensions, and other benefits.

The British Columbia Nurses Union president was an invited speaker to the Canadian Nursing Advisory Committee, which, in 2002, released its report confirming a national nursing shortage. CFNU continues to have strong advocacy efforts. It meets with premiers, participates in discussion panels, and holds press conferences. In addition, it publishes position papers regarding national nursing issues in order to keep health care on the first ministers' agendas."[1]

The United Nurses of Alberta is the only union to represent student and undergraduate nurses.

COLLECTIVE ACTION MODELS

The Canadian Federation of Nurses Unions states that its main purpose is "protecting the health of patients and our national health system, and promoting nurses and the nursing profession at the national level."[2] One of the main purposes of collective action is to advance the profession of nursing (Underwood, 1997). Many nurses belong to numerous collectives, including specialty nursing organizations, church organizations, special interest clubs, community groups, and so on. The reason most people belong to these organizations is to better themselves and their communities or to promote and support the special interests of a group. Two types of nursing collective action are discussed in this chapter: workplace advocacy and collective bargaining. Shared governance, another type of collective action, is discussed in Chapter 14.

WORKPLACE ADVOCACY

Workplace advocacy refers to activities nurses undertake to address problems in their everyday workplace setting. It is probably the most common type of collective action in nursing. An example of workplace advocacy is forming a committee to address problems, devise alternatives to achieve optimal care, and invent new ways to implement change. A supportive management will view workplace advocacy as a way to strengthen staff and promote teamwork. If the management is authoritative, however, workplace advocacy may not be encouraged, because it may be perceived as a threat to management and its policies.

COLLECTIVE BARGAINING

In collective bargaining, the group is bargaining with management for what the group desires. If the group cannot achieve its desires through informal collective bargaining with management, the group may decide to use a collective bargaining agent to form a union.

FACTORS INFLUENCING NURSES TO UNIONIZE

In general, nurses who are content in their workplace do not unionize (Hart, 1998). It is usually when nurses feel powerless that they initiate attempts to unionize. Other motivations to unionize include the desire to eliminate discrimination and favouritism, to increase an individual's power, or to increase input into organizational decision making; the need to comply with a requirement of being employed in the organization; and the belief that client outcomes and quality of care will be improved (Marquis & Huston, 2006). Research by Seago and Ash (2002) states a positive relationship between client outcomes and registered nurse unions extends beyond wages and numbers of hours and is related to staff stability, collaboration with physicians, autonomy, and increased participation in practice decisions. Nurses are also motivated to join unions when they feel the need to communicate concerns and complaints to management without fear of reprisal. Many nurses believe that they need a collective voice so that management will hear them and changes will be instituted.

Issues that are commonly the subject of collective bargaining include wage parity; staffing levels; health and safety issues; mandatory overtime; quality of care; job security; and restructuring issues, such as cross-training nurses for areas of specialty other than those in which

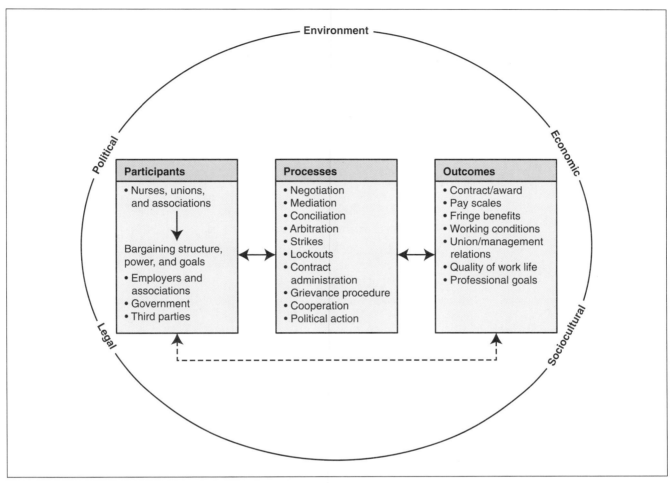

Figure 21-1 Framework for Understanding Collective Bargaining by Nurses.

Source: From Judith M. Hibberd & Donna Lynn Smith, *Nursing Leadership and Management in Canada.* 3rd Edition. (Figure 29 and page 671). Copyright © 2006 Elsevier Canada, a division of Reed Elsevier Canada, Ltd. All rights reserved. Reprinted by permission of Elsevier Canada, 2007.

they were hired to practice (American Nurses Association [ANA], n.d.). Many nurse managers believe it is best to deal quickly and effectively with issues as they arise in order to avoid collective bargaining, which usually entails an increase in costs to the hospital and limitations being placed on managers.

See Figure 21-1 to assist in understanding collective bargaining by nurses.

UNIONS

A **union** is a formal and legal group that works through a collective bargaining agent to present desires to management formally, through the legal context of labour legislation. The Canada Labour Code regulates and sets standards for government employees and interprovincial enterprises; however, each province establishes its own labour legislation. As a result, Canada has both federal and provincial labour relations systems. Because the procedures for collective bargaining are different across the provinces and territories, nurses are able to strike in some jurisdictions, but not in others.

Table 21-1 lists some collective action terminology, which is useful in understanding the collective bargaining process.

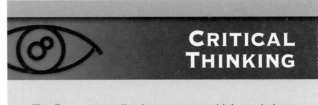

CRITICAL THINKING

Name two collective groups to which you belong. What are these collective groups able to accomplish as a whole? Are these collective groups more effective and stronger than you are, as an individual, in these interest areas? What are the downsides of belonging to a collective group?

TABLE 21-1	COLLECTIVE BARGAINING TERMINOLOGY

Term	Definition
Agency shop	Synonymous with *open shop*. Employees are not required to join the union but may join it.
Arbitration	The last step in a dispute. A non-partial third party will make the final decision. Arbitration may be voluntary or imposed by the government.
Collective agreement	A set of guidelines and rules voted and agreed upon by union members and agreed upon by representatives of management. The collective agreement, also known as a contract, states the rights and responsibilities of managers and union members and guides work practices, wages, and other benefits.
Collective bargaining	The practice of employees, as a collective, bargaining with management in reference to wages, work practices, and other benefits.
Collective bargaining agent	An agent who works with employees to formalize collective bargaining through unionization.
Fact finding	Fact finding is used in labour management disputes, or grievances, that involve government-owned companies. It is the process in which the claims of labour and management are reviewed. In the private sector, fact finding is usually performed by a board of inquiry.
Grievance	A formal complaint, or dispute, between management and a union member regarding the interpretation, application, or alleged violation of the terms of the collective agreement.
Grievance proceedings	A formal process by which a union member files a grievance to seek a settlement that is agreeable to both sides. The steps usually include (1) communication of the grievance to management, (2) mediation with a union representative and a member of management, and possibly (3) arbitration. The dispute may be settled at any step.
Lockout	An act in which management closes a place of business for the purpose of forcing employees to accept management's terms.
Mediation	A step in the grievance process in which a non-partial third party meets with management and the union to assist them in reaching an agreement. In this step, the third party, the mediator, has no actual power in decision making.
Strike	An act in which union members withhold their supply of labour for the purpose of forcing management to accept the union's terms.
Supervisor	A person with the authority to (1) impart corrective action and (2) delegate to an employee.
Union	A formal and legal group that brings forth desires to management through a collective bargaining agent and within the context of the provincial or territorial legislation.
Union dues	Money required of all union employees to support the union and its functions.
Union shop	A place of employment in which all employees are required to join the union and pay dues. *Union shop* is synonymous with the term *closed shop*.
Whistle-blowing	Whistle-blowing is the act in which an individual discloses information regarding the violation of a law, rule, or regulation, or a substantial and specific danger to public health or safety.
Work-to-rule	A job action taken to challenge terms of the contract, such as refusal to work overtime or refusal to attend meetings.

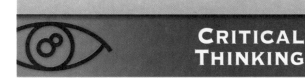

Y ou are a nurse working at an institution in which there is limited flexibility in the scheduling. You want to institute self-scheduling, with the staff nurses responsible for making and maintaining the schedule. Make a plan to present this idea to the manager. How will you elicit the support of other nurses? Now put yourself in the role of the manager. How would you respond to this request?

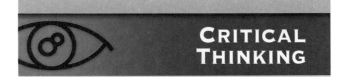

Y ou are a nurse working on a busy internal medicine unit. The union contract expired six months ago, and there has just been a strike vote. The union received an 80 percent mandate to strike.

One of the union's main issues is wages. However, the issue of greater concern to you is vacation and paid time-off provisions. In addition, you would like to see more dollars provided for an education allowance. The union is focused more on wages. You have never attended a union meeting. What is your role to ensure that the local union executive knows what the real issues are for nurses? What advice would you give to this nurse? Have you ever attended your union's meetings?

WHISTLE-BLOWING

One of the ethical dilemmas faced by individuals working in the health care field is the potential conflict between loyalty to their employers, colleagues, and professional standards, and a duty to protect their clients against incompetent, illegal, or unethical behaviour. When these conflicts arise, they are challenging in both ethical and practical terms for the individual. Nurses are often aware of errors that have been made, of actions that have been taken against an individual, but are hesitant to speak to the individuals directly involved, or to a supervisor, for fear of reprisal.

In the Report of the Review and Implementation Committee for the Report of the Manitoba Pediatric Cardiac Surgery Inquest in May 2001, **whistle-blowing** was defined as "the unauthorized internal or external disclosure of information concerning a harmful act that a superior or a colleague has committed, is allowing to occur, or is contemplating" (Report of the Review and Implementation Committee for the Report of the Manitoba Pediatric Surgery Inquest, 2001). Disclosing misconduct within an organization is usually less damaging than leaking information to external sources. Because studies suggest that whistleblowers pay a high price in terms of their careers and personal lives, stronger legal protection should be in place to protect individuals who legitimately and reasonably disclose wrongdoings. In addition, greater accountability should be demanded from leaders and the organizations that retaliate against justified complaints and reports. Ideally, organizations should develop policies and strategies to minimize the need for individuals to report on illegal behaviour or other wrongdoings.

In March 2004, the Liberal government introduced Bill C-25, the Disclosure Protection legislation commonly known as "whistleblower" legislation. The bill was introduced in response to the sponsorship scandal.[3]

THE PROCESS OF UNIONIZATION

The process of choosing a collective bargaining unit and negotiating a contract may take from three months to three years. A **collective bargaining agent** is a union representative who works with employees to formalize collective bargaining through unionization. One of the primary organizing strategies to promote union membership, as suggested by Murray (2001), is identification of issues critical to nurses, such as the amount of change in the health care system, human resource shortages, and reengineering. Several formal steps are required to legally form a union. See Table 21-2 for the steps involved in organizing a collective bargaining unit in Ontario.

THE MANAGER'S ROLE

Registered nurses have the legal authority to participate in collective bargaining in the majority of health care facilities in the country. It is important to maintain an open mind and develop collegial relationships with the potential union steward and the union membership. Equally important, listen to problems and concerns, investigate them promptly, and suggest solutions.

When a manager is flexible, fair, and open to suggestions, the chances that nurses will want to unionize may be reduced. Table 21-3 lists some ways managers can respond during a drive for unionization.

TABLE 21-2 — STEPS IN ORGANIZING A COLLECTIVE BARGAINING UNIT IN ONTARIO

Bring together a group of nurses supportive of collective bargaining.

Arrange a meeting with a representative of the provincial nurses association to discuss organizing.

Assess the feasibility of an organizing campaign at your facility.

Conduct the necessary research, such as the needs and/or complaints of the employees, to develop a plan of action.

Establish an organizing committee and subcommittees to facilitate organizing.

Complete and submit a union membership card to the union.

At least 40% of the employees must sign union membership cards for the union to submit an application for certification to the Ontario Labour Relations Board (OLRB).

The OLRB holds a secret vote at the workplace one week after applying for certification.

If 50% plus one of the employees who cast a ballot vote in favour of the union, the union is successful.

The union is then certified to represent the employee group, or bargaining unit.

The process of initiating contract negotiations for the first collective agreement is started.

Source: (Adapted from "How the Bargaining Process Works," By L. Flanagan, 1991, *American Nurse, 23*(9), 11–12 and Ontario Nurses Association, Retrieved from http://www.ona.org/home/ona/news.shtml?x=86857&AA_EX_Session=6b809baf278258c3eac4795860817273, August 29, 2006.

TABLE 21-3 — THE MANAGER'S ROLE DURING INITIATION OF UNIONIZATION

Know the law; make sure the rights of the nurses as well as the rights of management are clearly understood.

Act clearly within the law, no matter what the organization delegates to you as a manager.

Find out the reasons the nurses want collective action.

Discuss and deal with the nurses and the problems directly and effectively.

CASE STUDY 21-1

You are a nurse working in a cardiac catheterization laboratory. You notice that a certain physician routinely performs cardiac catheterizations on clients who are in their early 40s and who have no risk factors for cardiac history. The catheterizations are always negative for disease. You love your job but are troubled by this practice. You are fearful that clients will have complications. When you ask the physician why these procedures are performed on clients who do not appear to need this testing, his response is, "You don't worry about what I do; these procedures keep us all employed with healthy paycheques." You discuss this situation with your nursing manager who says, "Just do your job and let the doctor decide what is best for his clients."

You decide that whistle-blowing is your next action. What is your first step? Should you notify your manager of your whistle-blowing? What policies exist in your facility to guide the nurse when the nurse finds unprofessional activities?

TABLE 21-4	THE NURSE'S ROLE DURING INITIATION OF UNIONIZATION

Know your legal rights and the rights of the manager.

Act clearly within the law at all times.

If a manager acts unlawfully, such as firing an employee for organizing, report it to the labour relations board in your province or territory.

Keep all nurses informed by holding regular meetings close to the hospital.

Set meeting times conveniently around shift changes and assist with child care during meetings.

THE EMPLOYEE'S ROLE

Nurses desiring to choose a collective bargaining agent must ensure they carefully follow the laws pertaining to unionization. Carefully choose the collective bargaining agent, such as the Ontario Nurses Association. Research the agent and learn how nurses will be supported and where and how the union dues are spent. Talk to nurses in union settings to see how their contract is structured and whether collective bargaining has helped with the issues that led them to unionize in the first place. See Table 21-4 for a synopsis of the role of nurses during unionization.

STRIKING

Many nurses are morally opposed to unions because they believe if they are members of a union, they may be forced to strike. In reality, a collective bargaining agent cannot make the decision to strike. The decision to strike is made only if the majority of union members decide to do so. Provisions guarantee the continuation of adequate client care by requiring the union (in consultation with the organization) to provide sufficient nurses to care for the clients who were unable to be discharged to an alternate facility.

The manager should not lose sight of the fact that eventually the strike will be over! Maintain amicable, professional relationships during the strike in order that client care is not compromised and the work environment does not become poisoned. Although a strike may occur, unions are responsible and allow enough staff to work to provide essential service.

NURSING ASSOCIATIONS

The **Canadian Nurses Association (CNA)** is a federation of 11 provincial and territorial nursing associations, representing more than 129,000 Canadian registered nurses.[4] It is the national professional voice of registered nurses. The CNA is

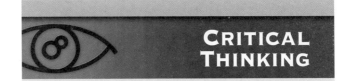

CRITICAL THINKING

You are a nurse working in a hospital that is a union shop. Nurses are concerned about unsafe staffing and being assigned to units with client populations they are not properly trained to care for. The collective bargaining agent for the union has met with management concerning these issues but nothing has been resolved. According to the rumours, these working conditions could be an issue when it is time to negotiate a new contract. Nurses may decide to strike as a result of this issue not being resolved.

What issues make people consider striking? What is your provincial or territorial association's stance on striking? What steps can be taken to avoid a strike?

politically active; advocates for healthy public policies and for a quality, publicly funded, not-for-profit health system; and supports nurses in their practice. It is not considered a union; however, in 1944, the Canadian Nurses Association approved the principle of collective bargaining for nurses.

The **Canadian Federation of Nurses Unions (CFNU)** is the body that promotes nurses and the nursing profession at the national level. The CFNU pressures the federal government to recognize the professional skills and knowledge that nurses bring to their jobs.[5] In addition, it is the national voice for nurses at the Canadian Labour Congress. Each of the provincial nurses unions, with the exception of Quebec, is a member of the CFNU.

The American Nurses Association (ANA) represents 2.6 million registered nurses in the United States through its 54 constituent state and territorial associations. The ANA's mission is to work for the improvement

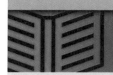

LITERATURE APPLICATION

Citation: Junor, J. (1998). What roles do unions have in preparing nursing leaders to effective change for the future? *Concern, 27*(1), 18–19.

Discussion: Nursing unions do more than serve the needs of their members. Unions empower their members, which prepares them to become nursing leaders, by formally teaching them how to be more assertive and by introducing political agendas pertinent to nursing issues. By being more assertive and politically active, nurses can realize their individual power and the power nurses have as a collective. Unions also teach nurses the skills of understanding contracts and the importance of documentation.

Implications for Practice: Nurses can grow professionally and personally from active union membership, which provides opportunities for nurses to learn skills such as assertiveness, understanding the political process, and promoting change. Nurses possessing these qualities will have the capacity to lead and the ability to make changes to better the nursing profession.

---

of health standards and availability of health care services for all people, to foster high standards for nursing, to stimulate and promote the professional development of nurses, and to advance their economic and general welfare (ANA, n.d.). The National Labor Relations Board recognizes the ANA as a collective bargaining agent. The ANA's dual role of being both a professional organization and a collective bargaining agent causes controversy. Some nurses believe that unionization is not professional and that the ANA cannot truly support nursing as a profession if it is also a collective bargaining agent. Because nurse managers are excluded from union membership, many nurse managers believe they have been left outside the organization that is supposed to represent all of nursing. Other nurse managers do not feel this separation ("The Role of Collective Bargaining and Unions," 1998).

The ANA represents the interests of nurses in collective bargaining, advances the nursing profession by fostering high standards for nursing practice, and lobbies U.S. Congress and regulatory agencies on health care issues affecting nurses and the general public. The ANA initiates many policies involving health care reform. It also publishes its position on issues ranging from whistle-blowing to patients' rights. The ANA recently launched a major campaign to mobilize nurses to address the staffing crisis, to educate and gain support from the public, and to develop and implement initiatives designed to resolve the crisis ("United American Nurses," 2001).

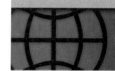

REAL WORLD INTERVIEW

I believe it is professional to be in a union because you have more opportunities to stand up for your clients and your own nursing practice. Having worked in both a union and a nonunion environment, I think being in a union allows you to speak your mind without fear of losing job security. They can't dismiss you for just any reason. There are grievance proceedings. In a nonunion environment, if they don't like you or what you say, they can punish you. But I've also seen the downside of unions. An example is when a contract comes out. The more-senior union nursing staff want to hold out from agreeing on a contract that does not address all of our concerns while the junior union nursing staff want to agree on the first contract that is presented. Holding out for what you want is why there is arbitration. The junior nurses don't realize the power of the bargaining unit in nursing. I think most nurses don't realize what we as nurses can accomplish if we stick together.

Susan Zielinski, RN
Staff Nurse

PROFESSIONALISM AND UNIONIZATION

Requirements for a vocation to be considered a profession include (1) a long period of specialized education, (2) a service orientation, and (3) the ability to be autonomous

(Jacox, 1980). Jacox (1980) defines autonomy as a characteristic of a profession in which the members of that profession are self-regulating and have control of their functions in the work situation. Nurses agree that specialized education and a service orientation are necessary to become a nurse, but many nurses disagree on the

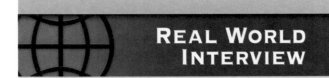

REAL WORLD INTERVIEW

I don't think it's any less professional for a physician to be in a union than any other health care provider. Doctors agree to try to help people. In return, physicians should be able to charge for that service and provide the best care they know how to deliver. Doctors should be able to bargain for better conditions and autonomy like the rest of society. More and more, the governing decision is not so much the client care as what is cost-effective. Doctors are not making those decisions and that's inherently wrong. As more and more of the medical structure becomes corporate, the workers, which doctors have become, need a means of negotiating with their employers.

Jonathan Fisher, MD
Surgical Resident

concept of autonomy. This disagreement is the central argument that divides nurses with regard to whether it is professional to be part of a union.

Many nurses believe that for nursing to be considered a profession, nurses must exercise autonomy and, like most professionals, work out issues themselves. Many argue that issues cannot be resolved without unionization. The debate about whether it is professional to be a part of a nurse's union has plagued nursing since the inception of nursing unions.

PHYSICIAN UNIONIZATION

In many provinces, student physicians are members of unions. Upon graduation, the physicians become members of provincial or territorial medical associations. These associations negotiate with provincial governments to represent the political, clinical, and economic interests of the medical profession. The Canadian Medical Association provides consultation to the provinces related to fee and benefit schedule comparisons and negotiation strategies, but does not function as a union.

UNIONIZATION OF UNIVERSITY PROFESSORS

The unionization of kindergarten through twelfth-grade teachers is well established in Canada. Now, an increasing number of professors at postsecondary institutions are

choosing to unionize. Again, wages and work environment have motivated university professors to join unions. As the average age of university faculty increases and fewer people show interest in teaching, unions may be able to protect professors from becoming overburdened and to financially reward those who enter teaching at the university level.

MANAGING IN A UNION ENVIRONMENT

Managers must work with the union to manage within the rules and context of contract agreements. In some ways, managing after a union is in place is less difficult because of the explicit language in most union contracts. Corrective actions, rules concerning allowed absences, and so on are agreed upon, voted on, and written in the contract.

GRIEVANCES

When a union member disputes management's interpretation or application of the terms of the contract, or collective agreement, this formal complaint is called a **grievance.** All union contracts specify the steps in grievance proceedings.

Grievance proceedings usually start with an employee who believes a wrongdoing has occurred on the part of management. Next, the member talks with a union representative, who helps the employee judge whether the act or condition actually justifies a formal complaint. The union representative uses knowledge of the contract, knowledge of labour legislation, and personal judgment to assist the employee. Next, the union member and the union representative meet with the manager to voice the grievance. At this step, the conflict may be resolved. If the conflict is not resolved, the next step may be to appeal management's decision and mediate with a higher-level manager. Grievance proceedings may differ from union to union.

PROS AND CONS OF COLLECTIVE BARGAINING

Nurses make a personal decision whether to support collective bargaining in the form of a union. Table 21-5 summarizes the pros and cons of collective bargaining.

TABLE 21-5　PROS AND CONS OF UNIONIZATION

Pros	Cons
The contract guides standards.	There is reduced allowance for individuality.
Members are able to be a part of the decision-making process.	Other union members may outvote your decisions.
All union members and management must conform to the terms of the contract without exception.	All union members and management must conform to the terms of the contract without exception.
A process can be instituted to question a manager's authority if a member feels something was done unjustly. More people are involved in the process.	Disputes are not handled with an individual and management only; there is less room for personal judgment.
Union dues are required to make the union work for you.	Union dues must be paid even if individuals do not support unionization.
Unions give a collective voice for employees.	Employee may not agree with the collective voice.
Employees are able to voice concerns to management without fear of reprisal.	Unions may be perceived by some as not professional.

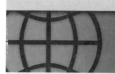

REAL WORLD INTERVIEW

The union affects my role as manager in many ways. There are so many pros and cons with it. I get frustrated as a manager when I feel like I cannot use my judgment because it may contradict the contract. For example, an employee lost a grandparent who was essentially this employee's parent, but I couldn't give this employee time off because it was not technically a parent who died. The contract also doesn't allow me to really commend employees who work hard and do their best every day. The hard-working person's pay and benefits are exactly the same as a mediocre employee. My hands are tied.

If you violate the contract, it becomes a time-consuming project for me as the manager. For example, if I had chosen to give the person time off for the grandparent who died, I would have grievances from other people because I did not give them time off for their grandparent's death. I would have to document what I did and why and would ultimately lose the grievance and have to find a way to compensate the other people for not giving them time off. I come from a pro-union family, and I understand how unions can protect employees. In general, it is good for employees to have somebody who is on their side and who treats all as equals. It's hard for me to imagine that there are managers who mistreat their employees in other institutions.

Ann Marie O'Connor, RN
Unit Manager

KEY CONCEPTS

- Nursing collective bargaining has existed in Canada since 1946.

- Workplace advocacy is a collective action model that is more informal and encompasses the everyday creativity and problem solving that occur in nursing.

- Collective bargaining through unionization is a collective action model that is formal and legally based. It uses a written contract to guide nursing and workplace issues.

- Nurses who are unhappy in the workplace because of issues such as wages and poor staffing often attempt to unionize to rectify workplace problems. Nurses who are not managers have the legal right to unionize. Employees and managers must be aware of the specific steps that must be taken during the initiation of unionization.

- The Canadian Nurses Association is a professional organization that represents the country's entire registered nurse population. Unlike the American Nurses Association, the CNA does *not* have a dual role of being a professional organization and a collective bargaining agent for nursing. The CNA is politically active and lobbies on issues affecting nursing and the general public.

- The Canadian Federation of Nurses Unions promotes nurses and nursing at the national level.

- Other professionals who do not have a tradition of unionization are opting to unionize. Physicians and university professors are joining unions for the same reasons that some nurses have chosen to join unions: to improve their wages and working conditions.

KEY TERMS

Canadian Federation of Nurses Unions (CFNU)
Canadian Nurses Association (CNA)
collective action
collective bargaining

collective bargaining agent
grievance
unions
whistle-blowing
workplace advocacy

REVIEW QUESTIONS

1. A manager should do which of the following if nurses are attempting to unionize?
   A. Nothing; most often the union attempt fails.
   B. Do not hire any registered nurses who are pro-union.
   C. Learn the reason nurses want collective action.
   D. Fire the nurse instigating unionization.

2. Workplace advocacy is best defined as
   A. a management-defined solution for the workplace.
   B. holding managers and nurses accountable.
   C. a formal structure that is voted on.
   D. activities nurses undertake to address problems in the workplace.

3. Which of the following is *not* a common reason why nurses unionize?
   A. Client care issues
   B. Wages
   C. Staffing issues
   D. Being content in the workplace

REVIEW ACTIVITIES

1. You are a new graduate nurse and have begun working on a medical unit. The nurse manager explains that the unit uses workplace advocacy. What is workplace advocacy? How will it affect your functioning as a registered nurse on the unit?

2. You are hired in a hospital that is a union shop. How does unionization differ from other collective action models, such as workplace advocacy? Give three examples of how unionization differs from workplace advocacy.

3. You are a graduate nurse, and you found out you passed the CRNE examination. As a registered nurse, you are represented by the British Columbia Nurses Union. What is the mission of the BCNU? Is the BCNU active in politics?

EXPLORING THE WEB

- What sites would you recommend to someone inquiring about collective bargaining? *http://www.hrsdc.gc.ca/en/gateways/business/cluster/category/cb.shtml*

- Go to the site for the Canadian Federation of Nurses Unions and find your provincial nursing union. What did you learn about your provincial nursing union? *http://www.nursesunions.ca/*

- What site would you access to find out the history of collective bargaining? *http://www.nursesunions.ca/content.php?doc=44*

  http://www.ona.org/faq/index.html#union_his

  http://www.law-faqs.org/nat/unions.htm

- Go to the site for the British Columbia Nurses Union: *http://www.bcnu.org/* Click on the What's New link and read some articles, then click on the Campaigns/Issues link to access the Practice Issues page. What did you learn about nursing and current events?

REFERENCES

American Nurses Association. (n.d.). "Mission statement." Retrieved from http://www.nursingworld.org, August 27, 2006.

Canadian Federation of Nurses Unions. (2007). "About us." Retrieved from http://www.nursesunions.ca/content.php?sec=1, August 1, 2007.

Flanagan, L. (1991). How the bargaining process works. *American Nurse, 23*(9), 11–12.

Hart, C. (1998). The state of the unions. *Nursing Times, 94*(15), 36–37.

Hibbard, J., & Smith, D. L.(2006). *Nursing leadership and management in Canada* (3rd ed.). Toronto: Elsevier Canada, a division of Harcourt Canada Ltd.

Jacox, A. (1980). Collective action: The basis for professionalism. *Supervisor Nurse, 11*(9), 22–24.

Junor, J. (1998). What roles do unions have in preparing nursing leaders to effective change for the future? *Concern, 27*(1), 18–19.

Kalist, D. E. (2002). The gender earnings gap in the RN labour market. *Nursing Economic$, 20*(4), 155–162.

Marquis, B. L., & Huston, C. J. (2006). *Leadership roles and management functions in nursing: Theory and application* (5th ed.). Philadelphia: Lippincott, Williams and Wilkins.

Murray, M. K. (2001). The new economy and new union organizing strategies: Union wins in healthcare. *Journal of Nursing Administration, 31*(7/8), 339–343.

Report of the Review and Implementation Committee for the Report of the Manitoba Pediatric Surgery Inquest. (2001). Winnipeg: Government of Manitoba.

The role of collective bargaining and unions in advancing the profession of nursing. (1998). *Nursing Trends & Issues, 3*(2), 1–8.

Seago, J. A., & Ash, M. (2002). Registered nurse unions and patient outcomes. *Journal of Nursing Administration, 32*(3), 143–151.

Underwood, P. (1997). Nurses need collective action to "build" profession. *Michigan Nurse, 70*(10), 3.

United American Nurses (UAN) mobilizes nurses on staffing crisis. (2001). *American Journal of Nursing, 101*(1), 65.

SUGGESTED READINGS

Aging faculty adds to RN shortage. (1999). *Nursing Spectrum (Greater Chicago/NE Illinois & NW Indiana ed.), 12*(5), 6.

Camfield, D. (2005). An Analysis of the Hospital Employees' Union Strike of 2004. *Unpublished manuscript.*

Canadian Nurses Association. (2002). *Planning for the future: Nursing human resource projections.* Ottawa, ON: Author.

Fitzpatrick, M. (2001). Collective bargaining: A vulnerability assessment. *Nursing Management, 32*(2), 40–42.

Forman, H., & Davis, G. A. (2002). The anatomy of a union campaign. *Journal of Nursing Administration, 32*(9), 444–447.

Forman, H., & Kraus, H. R. (2003). Decertification: Management's role when employees rethink unionization. *Journal of Nursing Administration, 33*(6), 313–316.

Forman, H., & Powell, T. A. (2003). Managing during an employee walkout. *Journal of Nursing Administration, 33*(9), 430–433.

Hellinghausen, A. (1999, August 9). Changes afoot. *NurseWeek,* 27–28.

Jamison, D. T., Frenk, J., & Knaul, F. (1998). International collective action in health: Objectives, functions and rationale. *Lancet, 351*(9101), 514–517.

Malott, M. (2005). From the front-line to the picket-line. *The Heart: Newsletter of the McGill School of Nursing Community/La Coeur: Communiqué de la communauté de l'École des sciences infirmières de McGill,* Issue 24: 11.

Marquis, B., & Huston, C. (1998). *Management decision making for nurses: 124 case studies* (3rd ed.). Philadelphia: Lippincott.

Meier, E. (1999). Politically speaking. *ONS News, 14*(10), 13.

Meier, E. (2000). Is unionization the answer for nurses and nursing? *Nursing Economic$, 18*(1), 36–38.

Melville, E. (1995). The history of industrial action in nursing. *Professional Nurse, 11*(2), 84–86.

National Labor Relations Act. (1994). Retrieved from http://www.nlrb.gov/about_us/overview/national_labor_relations_act.aspx, August 18, 2007.

National Labor Relations Board. (1995). *The first sixty years: The story of the National Labor Relations Board 1935–1995.* Retrieved from http://www.nlrb.gov/about_us/history/thhe_first_60_years.aspx, August 2, 2007.

Nurse staffing law may herald benchmarks. (1999). *Healthcare Benchmarks, 6*(120), 137–138.

Porter-O'Grady, T. (2001). Collective bargaining: The union as partner. *Nursing Management, 32*(6, pt. 1), 30–32.

Reffner, G. (1996). Collectively: Be prepared—each one doing our part. *Hawaii Nurse, 3*(9), 8.

Seltzer, T. M. (2001). Collective bargaining: A wake-up call—part 2. *Nursing Management, 32*(4), 35–37, 48.

Tone, B. (1999, August 9). Pulled apart: Does unionizing serve the interests of the profession? *NurseWeek,* 1–5.

Trossman, S. (1998). Doctors increasingly are looking for the union label. *American Nurse, 30*(4), 19.

Walmsley, J. (1996). Collective action brought change. *Kaitiaki: Nursing New Zealand, 9*(1), 28.

Yoder-Wise, P. (Ed.). (1999). *Leading and managing in nursing* (2nd ed.). St. Louis, MO: Mosby.

CHAPTER ENDNOTES

1. Canadian Federation of Nurses Unions, "CFNU Celebrates its 25th Anniversary". Retrieved from http://www.nursesunions.ca/cms/updir/2006-05-30-CFNU_25_years_-_history.pdf, September 1, 2006.

2. Canadian Federation of Nurses Unions, "About Us." Retrieved from http://www.nursesunions.ca/content.php?sec=1, August 1, 2007.

3. CBC News Indepth, "Whistleblower legislation Bill C-25, Disclosure Protection." Retrieved from http://www.cbc.ca/news/background/whistleblower/, September 1, 2006.

4. Canadian Nurses Association, "What is the Canadian Nurses Association?" Retrieved from http://www.cna-nurses.ca/CNA/about/who/default_e.aspx, August 3, 2007.

5. Canadian Federation of Nurses Unions, "About Us." Retrieved from http://www.nursesunions.ca/content.php?sec=1, August 2, 2007.

CHAPTER 22

Career Planning and Development: Creating Your Path to the Future

Janice Waddell, RN, PhD

Learning without thought is labour lost; thought without learning is perilous.

(Confucius)

OBJECTIVES

Upon completion of this chapter, the senior-level student should be able to:

1. Define career planning and development.

2. Describe the Donner-Wheeler Career Planning and Development Model (the Model).

3. Complete initial work in each of the five phases of the Model (Scanning Your Environment, Completing Your Self-Assessment and Reality Check, Creating Your Career Vision, Developing Your Strategic Career Plan, and Marketing Yourself) at the senior-student level.

4. Utilize the Model to choose a first job as a registered nurse.

5. Identify resources to assist with utilizing the Model to prepare for an application to graduate studies.

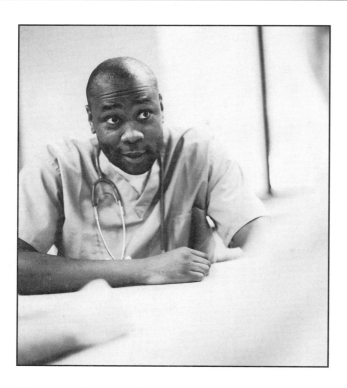

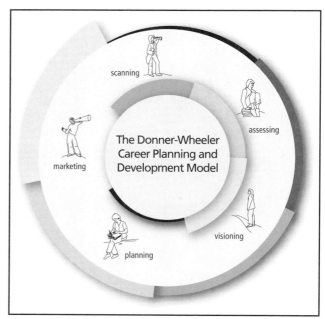

Figure 22-1 The Donner-Wheeler Career Planning and Development Model.

Source: Donner, 2004. Copyright © 2007 donnerwheeler. All rights reserved.

Alya is entering the final year of her baccalaureate nursing program. She is very excited to be so close to her dream of becoming a registered nurse but her excitement is accompanied by a sense of anxiety. She wants to ensure that she makes the best of her final year so that she is positioned for a nursing position that will help her advance toward her career goal of working with children and families in an acute care setting. She plans to stay in Canada, likely within her home province. Although some opportunities are available for fourth-year student practice experiences in acute care of children and families, due to the current health care environment, not all students who wish such a placement can be accommodated. Some questions Alya is asking include: How can I plan my career now and in the future? How can I use my educational experiences in the coming year to help me progress toward my career goal—whether or not I am able to have a practice experience focused on children and families? How can I make sure that I choose the job that is right for me? How do I market myself? Where do I start? Who can help me?

The purpose of this chapter is to introduce you to the Donner-Wheeler Career Planning and Development Model (Donner, 2004), shown in Figure 22-1, as a tool to plan your career as you complete your nursing program and move to your first job as a registered nurse! The author of this chapter has worked closely with Gail Donner, RN, PhD, and Mary Wheeler, RN, MEd, ACC, in the development and application of the Donner-Wheeler Career Planning and Development Model (the Model) to student nurses and new graduates. The Model can help you to achieve a sense of control over both your academic career and your professional practice career.

You entered your nursing program with dreams, ideas, and hopes for your future career. The career planning and development process provides a guide to help you to achieve your dreams and to create new possibilities as you build your nursing career. In this chapter, you will learn about the importance of career planning and development as you consider and plan for completing your education and the transition to the workplace. You will also learn how to use the five phases of the Model to develop your unique career goals and to guide your academic activities and your search for your first job as a registered nurse.

A career is what we choose as our profession, our path, or our life's work (Donner, 2004). You chose your path when you accepted your admission into your nursing program, and your nursing career began the day you attended your school of nursing orientation. You have now entered the final year(s) of your nursing education program. Your many classroom and practice experiences have shaped your sense of the kind of nurse you aspire to be and, perhaps, the type of nursing practice that interests you most. You are ready to take the wheel and navigate your career.

The five phases of the career planning and development model introduced in this chapter (see Table 22-1) prompt you to dedicate some time, thought, and reflection to understanding the environment in which you complete the final years of your education and the environment in which you will assume your first nursing position. Through this process, you will be assessing your strengths and the areas that require further development, creating a vision of your career, developing a realistic plan to help you progress toward your career

TABLE 22-1	THE DONNER-WHEELER CAREER PLANNING AND DEVELOPMENT MODEL

Phase One: Scanning Your Environment
What are the current realities/future trends?
Phase Two: Completing Your Self-Assessment and Reality Check
Who am I?
How do others see me?
Phase Three: Creating Your Career Vision
What do I really want to be doing?
Phase Four: Developing Your Strategic Career Plan
How can I achieve my career goals?
Phase Five: Marketing Yourself
How can I best market myself?

vision, and marketing yourself to help you to achieve your plan. In other words—this is all about you!

SCANNING YOUR ENVIRONMENT

Scanning the environment is simply taking a good look around to determine how the world around you can help you to both develop and achieve your career goals. Scanning the environment, together with knowledge of the strengths and interests you have developed to date in your nursing program, offers you information about potential nursing practice opportunities. You will also form ideas of how you can approach your classroom and practice experiences in the coming year so that your academic endeavours are in concert with your personal career goals. As a senior-level student, your scan will need to include knowledge of what is happening outside of your academic institution, including current issues within the health care sector and the nursing profession, with a particular focus on your area of interest. You have had the opportunity to complete your fundamental practice experiences across diverse settings. You have also had exposure to a range of faculty members with expertise in a number of areas of nursing scholarship and practice. Early and ongoing experiences and contacts serve as the foundation of your environmental scan.

Extending your scan to include awareness of health care issues and trends at the national and international level is also important as you contemplate potential opportunities for your first job. Knowing the realities and potentials of the current health care environment can enhance your insight regarding what is "out there" for you and the factors you will need to consider as you seek your first nursing position. Data from your scan can also assist you with your self-assessment, particularly in terms of focusing your learning activities within the context of classroom and nursing practice courses and keeping abreast of information that you will need for entry to practice. Furthermore, what you learn from your scan can be of great help when preparing for an interview and developing questions that you would like to ask of potential employers. Questions you might consider in your scan include:

- What are the key issues in health care today?
- What are some of the important social and health issues in my area of practice and location? Nationally? Internationally?
- What are significant nursing issues in my local area, nationally, and internationally that may influence my chosen practice area—and my career more broadly?
- What are global health and social issues?

Like all phases of the Model, scanning is not a one-time activity but rather a continuous process. You will scan throughout your career in order to keep on top of current and future opportunities related to your career goals. Sources for your scan can include faculty members, course readings and assignments, professional journals, professional organizations, nursing practice settings, preceptors, the Internet, news media, friends, and your fellow students.

If you are interested in a particular practice setting—in terms of a potential practice placement or future employment, a significant aspect of your scan can be researching the mission, philosophy, professional practice model, and mandate of the organization as a whole and the nursing department specifically. If you can, obtain the job descriptions of positions in your area of interest. Identifying key professional competencies required of the position informs your self-assessment and related academic and future career planning.

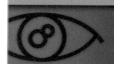

CRITICAL THINKING

Alya has a particular interest in working with children and families in an acute care setting. The third year of her nursing program focused on community health, so she has current knowledge and information related to many health and social issues faced by families within the community context. She will need to explore these issues with acute care health settings in mind—as well as related nursing issues and scopes of practice. Taking some time to review recent publications in the area of family and children's health care will also inform Alya as to the nature of practice, models of care, and current issues in the care of children and families.

Alya's scan can include the faculty members within her school of nursing. One or more faculty members have practice and/or research expertise in the area of family and children's health and can serve as excellent resources and mentors! Scanning the acute care health organizations with a department of pediatrics and obtaining nursing job descriptions can provide Alya with valuable information regarding the professional competencies required to work in this area of practice.

Alya can also access resources in her provincial professional nursing organization, including, perhaps, an interest group that focuses on family and children's health.

Alya would like to make sure that she knows as much about the role of a children's and family health nurse as possible so that she can take advantage of, and create, learning opportunities related to her career interest over the coming year.

What are other key sources of information for Alya's environmental scan? What key questions can guide her scan? How can she use her scan to develop a learning plan that would also help her develop competencies related to her career goal?

Your scan will inform and be influenced by your work in all other phases of the Model. It is always a work in progress!

YOUR SELF-ASSESSMENT AND REALITY CHECK

Your environmental scan is focused on discovering the world around you. Your **self-assessment** is about looking inside yourself (Donner, 2004). You have completed a substantial portion of your nursing education and may feel, as do many students, that you are a different person now from when you entered nursing. You have likely learned a great deal about yourself through your classroom and practice experiences and your overall involvement in your program. Your professional knowledge grows daily, and your identity as a nurse is shaped and influenced continuously. Values that you held at the time you began the program have helped you to interpret and respond to your new learning and experiences—these values may also shift or change as a result of your professional development. Self-knowledge helps you to create meaning in your learning and to recognize opportunities for further development.

Most nursing curricula include developing the skill of reflective analysis. At this point in your program, an asset in the career planning and development process is your ability to reflect on your experiences, their relevance to your professional growth, and how experiences can guide your future learning. The ability to reflect upon and articulate responses to the questions "Who am I?" and "How would I describe myself?" is a significant professional and personal strength. Who you are includes your beliefs, your values, your knowledge, your professional competencies, your interests, your accomplishments, and your hopes for the future.

A thorough self-assessment takes dedicated time. You have gathered diverse and challenging experiences that have each contributed to your unique professional identity. After each new experience, a return to your self-assessment will allow you to reflect on the contribution that experience has made to who you are as a nurse. Those experiences that have been of most meaning to you and have allowed you to live your values and beliefs most fully offer guidance and direction as you work on the remaining phases of the model. Equally informative are those experiences that were not positive or fulfilling. Reflecting on those experiences can also help you to clarify your values and articulate your interests and priorities both for your learning and for your continued development as a nurse.

You have also accomplished many things over the course of your nursing education, both curricular and extra-curricular. Remember to include these achievements in your self-assessment. Making note of your accomplishments helps you to recognize your overall personal and professional growth and development.

Your self-assessment, together with your environmental scan, serves as the foundation of your career planning and development. Neither the self-assessment nor the scan is static. The dynamic nature of your nursing education experiences and your professional career will be reflected in these and all phases of the Model.

Once you have worked through your self-assessment, ask faculty members, nursing peers, preceptors, and other involved people in your life to give you feedback regarding your strengths, unique traits, and areas for development. This aspect of your self-assessment is called the **reality check.** Oftentimes the feedback you receive will highlight strengths and attributes that you have not recognized in yourself. More often than not, the reality check is an affirming process that enhances your confidence as you begin to market your competencies, unique attributes and accomplishments.

Alya will have a great deal of information from her scan to help her in her self-assessment. She will have a better understanding of the social and health issues of children and their families, current issues and trends in family and child health nursing practice in an acute care setting, practice requirements for nurses working in this area of practice, and professional organizations available to her as a family and children's health nurse. With this information Alya can use the self-assessment process to build on her identification of values, interests, and beliefs by examining both her current strengths relative to the strengths required to practice in her area of interest and the areas in which her need for development is greatest. Asking others who know her to assess her strengths and achievements in her student experiences, both curricular and extra-curricular, will help Alya to both expand her self-assessment and feel confident about her assessment. Alya will have a more in-depth understanding of the scope of nursing practice, the areas in which she needs to focus her learning in the coming year, and her potential employment options. She is ready for the next phase of the Model—creating her career vision.

CREATING YOUR CAREER VISION

Your **career vision** describes where you want to go in your nursing career—it is a description of who and what you wish to become. Your career vision helps you to describe the kind of nurse you wish to be and can also include where you hope to focus your nursing practice. Your career vision focuses on what is possible. It makes use of your resources and has the ability to harness and direct your energy. It is a personal statement of your hopes for your career. Find a quiet spot and give yourself some time to think about your career vision. Close your eyes and answer the following questions:

- In what city/country are you working?
- In what type of organization do you work?

- What is your practice focus?
- Describe the setting.
- How do you feel when you go to work each day?
- Describe your colleagues.
- Describe your clients.
- How would your colleagues describe you?
- How would your clients describe you?

Alya's career vision may look something like this:

I am an expert pediatric nurse working in an acute care teaching hospital in a large urban setting. I am involved in direct care of children and families and serve as a resource to nursing colleagues. I feel confident in my practice and I am seen as a leader by my peers and the other health care professionals with whom I work. I am recognized for my expertise in pediatric nursing practice and my ability to work effectively with families and colleagues. I feel a sense of positive anticipation when I go to work every day, I also feel part of a team that values and respects my contributions—and I theirs. I am pursuing graduate studies to help me prepare to be an advanced practice family health nurse and the organization supports my studies both philosophically and financially.

Your vision can focus on where or how you want to practice—or both of these dimensions of your career. Either way, it can provide you with a sense of purpose, a goal, and it can help you to focus your learning in the coming year—and as you make the transition to the workplace. Your vision offers some cues as to the type of environment you desire to be satisfied in your work and ideas from which to develop interview questions.

Putting your career vision in writing makes it more accessible to you, and more real. Place it somewhere that you can see it most often (likely your computer screen!). Then, during those times when you feel overwhelmed with the work you have to do to be successful in your academic and professional work, your career vision can be a reminder of why you are doing what you are doing, and where you are going. It can also help you to focus on making your activities fit with your vision. Sharing your vision allows others to support your efforts and help keep you to keep on the path you have chosen.

At this point in your academic career, you might be quite confident that your vision will not change. However, you may have experiences in the coming year that transform your vision. Career visions are not written in stone—if your vision changes, you simply revisit all, or the most relevant, phases of the Model to help you to utilize the work you have achieved in a different way and to create new opportunities and directions. As noted earlier in the chapter, the Model is both a tool to use and a reflection of the dynamic nature of your present and future career.

Alya's vision can help her to focus on key competencies that she will need to develop in order to actualize her dream. Her vision directs her to developing confidence and competence in her knowledge, communication, leadership, and practice competencies. She can revisit her environmental scan and her self-assessment with her vision in mind to make sure that she has considered not only where she is at now but where she hopes to be in the future. Alya's vision also allows her to see that if she does not obtain a practice placement in a children's and family health acute care setting, she can still focus on the competencies that she will need to achieve her vision: communication, family-centred care, developmental care, leadership, expanding her knowledge base, and competencies that span practice specialty areas.

CREATING YOUR STRATEGIC CAREER PLAN

A **strategic career plan** requires that you take the knowledge and skills you have developed in creating learning plans and client care plans and apply it to *your* nursing career. The main difference is that you are doing this for yourself—not to fulfill course requirements, client needs, or the expectations of others. It is your action guide that is unique and personal.

Like the plans you are accustomed to, your strategic career plan should include goals, action steps, resources, timelines, and indicators of success. Setting both short- and long-term goals allows you to make realistic and achievable progress toward your vision. Your environmental scan, self-assessment, and career vision will provide you with the data you need to develop your plan. Your scan prompted you to identify opportunities and realities related to your areas of interest; your assessment has helped you to articulate your strengths, your unique attributes, and the areas you would like to further develop; and your vision shows where you are headed. Use all of this information to guide you in deciding what you need to do to meet short- and long-term goals related to your career vision. Your plan transforms your vision from fantasy to reality.

If you are ready to begin your search for the right job, your strategic career plan can focus on the short- and long-term goals you have related to your ideal job. See Table 22-2 for Alya's strategic career plan.

TABLE 22-2	EXAMPLE OF A STRATEGIC CAREER PLAN

Alya's Strategic Career Plan could look like this:

Alya's Vision: "I am an expert pediatric nurse working in an acute care teaching hospital in a large urban setting. I am involved in direct care of children and families and serve as a resource to nursing colleagues. I feel confident in my practice and I am seen as a leader by my peers and the other health care professionals with whom I work. I am recognized for my expertise in pediatric nursing practice and my ability to work effectively with families and colleagues. I feel a sense of positive anticipation when I go to work every day. I also feel part of a team that values and respects my contributions—and I theirs. I am pursuing graduate studies to help me prepare to be an advanced practice family health nurse and the organization supports my studies both philosophically and financially."

Career Goal: At the end of my undergraduate nursing education program, I will have the necessary competencies to work as a staff nurse on a pediatric unit in an acute care hospital.

Action Steps–Fall 2008	Timeline	Resources	Indicators of Success
1. Obtain job descriptions of a pediatric staff nurse position and the models of care from three acute care teaching hospitals.	September 5, 2008	Hospital websites Human resources departments Nursing education departments	I have copies of three pediatric staff nurse job descriptions and descriptions of their models of care.
2. Using the job descriptions, revise my self-assessment to identify existing strengths and areas I need	September 15, 2008	Job Descriptions of pediatric staff nurse positions, information re: my current practice placement	My self-assessment is up-to-date and reflects my strengths and areas for

(Continued)

TABLE 22-2	EXAMPLE OF A STRATEGIC CAREER PLAN (CONTINUED)

Action Steps–Fall 2008	Timeline	Resources	Indicators of Success
to work on this term to work toward competencies related to pediatric nursing and my current placement setting.		expectations and requirements, previous nursing practice evaluations, self-assessment	development related to my current placement setting and pediatric job descriptions/models of care.
3. Meet with my faculty advisor to review my self-assessment and my career vision so that I can develop learning goals that fit with both my practice setting and my career goal.	September 20, 2008	Knowledge of current practice placement expectations and requirements, self-assessment related to practice setting and pediatric staff nurse job description, practice course expectations	I will have a draft learning plan that focuses on learning goals that allow me to develop competencies that prepare me to practice competently in my practice setting and progress toward my career goal.
4. Schedule regular meetings with my mentors to help me focus on my career vision and goals for this term.	September 30, 2008	Mentors	I have regularly scheduled meetings with both of my mentors.
5. Join the provincial professional nursing association pediatric nurse interest group.	October 30, 2008	Organization website.	I am a member of the interest group
6. Attend one pediatric nursing interest group meeting in the fall and winter.	End of Fall term and End of Winter term	Interest Group meeting schedule.	I will have attended one meeting in the fall and one meeting in the winter.
7. Meet with child and family health nurse practitioner mentor to explore option of shadowing a pediatric nurse for a couple of shifts over the holiday break in December.	November 15, 2008	Mentor	I will have arranged a shadowing experience for the holiday break.

MARKETING YOURSELF

Marketing is being able to communicate your strengths, interests, and goals with confidence and clarity. You have actually been marketing yourself as a nursing student and future registered nurse throughout your program. In each encounter you have had with clients, nurses, faculty members, and other health care professionals over the course of your nursing education, you have conveyed who and what you are. Perhaps, until now, your marketing has been unintentional. As you complete your nursing education and make plans for your transition to the workplace you need to be intentional in how you communicate your values, strengths, and identity as a nurse.

Marketing yourself is much easier when your approach genuinely reflects your values, your communication style, and is true to your abilities. The work you have done in your self-assessment will be very helpful because you have already taken the time to consider and articulate your values, strengths, areas for continued development, and your unique attributes. You have the information to engage in informed and intentional self-marketing.

LITERATURE APPLICATION

Citation: Waddell, J. (2005). Choosing the right graduate program. *Canadian Nurse, 101*(5), 30–31.

Waddell, J., Donner, G. J., & Wheeler, M. M. (2004). *Building your nursing career: A guide for students* (2nd ed.). Toronto, ON: Elsevier Canada.

Discussion: Like any other career decision, the choice to pursue graduate studies should be informed, responsive to the unique needs of the individual, and congruent with one's career goals. Many excellent graduate programs are offered within and outside of Canada. Finding the right program can be a daunting and sometimes overwhelming task for an undergraduate student. Waddell, together with Donner and Wheeler, describes how students can use the Donner-Wheeler Career Planning and Development Model to plan for their application to graduate studies and position themselves to be successful in achieving admission to graduate programs that fit with their career goals. The authors describe how both beginning and graduating students can approach each of the five phases of the Model (scanning your environment, completing your self-assessment/reality check, creating your career vision, developing your strategic career plan, and marketing yourself) with a particular focus on preparing a winning application for graduate studies. The suggested activities can be initiated at any level of nursing education but have particular relevance to students in the final year(s) of their program.

Implications for Students: Engaging in graduate studies is a significant personal and financial investment. Graduate education provides nurses with the opportunity to have a dedicated focus on their area of practice/research interest and expertise. The career planning and development model provides a structure and process to guide students in their exploration and assessment of graduate programs with the goal of choosing the program that will best allow them to achieve their career goals. The broader implication is that active involvement in the career planning process can help nursing students, at any point in their academic and professional practice career, take control of their progress toward both short- and long-term career goals in their pursuit of their career vision.

This phase of the Model will help you to develop self-marketing strategies that are effective in helping you to both take advantage of and create career opportunities of significance to you. You use both personal and written resources in your marketing activities. The interview process is a significant marketing strategy as well.

PERSONAL RESOURCES

The most important personal resource you have is YOU! Knowing and having the ability to articulate who you are, your career vision, and your career goals is your best marketing strategy. A second personal resource can be a mentor. A **mentor** is a person you admire and wish to emulate. A mentor is also someone who takes a personal and professional interest in your career. This individual may practise in your area of interest and/or exemplify what you believe is the nurse you wish to become. Either way, a mentor can provide you with guidance, support, and opportunities to help you to transform your career vision to reality. You can also have more than one mentor: many students and new graduates have a number of individuals who have played significant roles in their professional development. A mentor is more than a professional role

model; being a mentor is an active role that requires time and commitment on behalf of the mentor and yourself. If you have someone in mind, don't hesitate to formally ask this person to be your mentor. Don't leave it to chance or assume that the person whom you would like to have as your mentor is aware of your feelings. It is an honour to be asked to mentor someone, and people who are able to assume the role benefit as much from the relationship as the mentee. Mentors take their role seriously and in a person who accepts to be your mentor will be making a commitment to you and to your career. Make sure that you are also in a position to make the commitment to working actively on your career with your mentor.

A third personal resource is **networking** activities. You may already be involved in student organizations, the work of your school of nursing, professional nursing organizations, and your personal and professional communities. If so, then you have already benefited from networking and can use your scan, self-assessment, and career vision to continue your professional involvement with a focus on your career vision and goals. However, if you have not been actively involved in extracurricular activities within and external to your education program, it is never too late to start!

Use your environmental scan to learn of opportunities to become involved in professional activities that fit with your interests, areas for development, and overall career goals. Strategic networking can help you to identify professional organizations with interest groups dedicated to a wide range of practice specialties. Involvement in professional groups creates opportunities for you to meet with nurses who are practising in areas of interest to you—and for you to market your interests and strengths. You can also speak with new graduates who are working in your areas of interest. New graduates offer helpful advice to help you prepare for your entry to the workforce. Your mentor can guide you in your research related to networking opportunities and can often open doors for you as you make your move into the world of professional nursing practice.

Alya has been an active member of her school of nursing since the first year of her program. She was often the spokesperson of her class when the students wished to give the school feedback regarding the curriculum, school resources, policies, and other matters. In the second year of her program, she became an active member of the Canadian Nursing Students' Association (CNSA) and was able to travel to CNSA regional and national conferences to represent the school and her student colleagues.

In her third year, Alya was elected to president of the Nursing Course Union at her university. As a result of her involvement in each of these roles, Alya developed excellent skills in leadership, lobbying, organization, and negotiation. She also was able to work with her faculty and get to know them in ways that would be difficult if she had only been exposed to them in the classroom or practice setting. The faculty were also able to observe Alya's growth in her leadership role and to learn of her career aspirations.

Alya asked two faculty members to be her mentors. One mentor exemplified the type of professional to which Alya aspired. This mentor was active in a wide range of professional organizations, was student-centred and knowledgeable with a very strong professional presence. This person introduced Alya to professional organizations that focused on the advancement of the profession at-large at local, national, and international levels. Her second mentor was a faculty member who was a nurse practitioner in child and family health. This individual helped Alya to access professional organizations relevant to her area of interest and opened the door to many opportunities for Alya to meet new graduates and experienced nurses practising child and family health in acute care settings. Networking within and external to her school of nursing helped Alya to affirm that she was heading in the right direction and to clarify and refine her strengths and career vision. After each experience she can return to phases of the Model to update and review her progress toward her vision. In her fourth year,

she plans to join the provincial professional organization's pediatric nurse interest group and the local chapter of Sigma Theta Tau International.

WRITTEN RESOURCES

Written marketing strategies include your résumé, cover letter, and business card. Because your résumé is generally the first opportunity a prospective employer has to see who you are and what you may be able to contribute to the organization, it is your most valuable written self-marketing strategy. A **résumé** is a brief summary of your background, education, and your nursing and related experiences. Generally, a résumé should not be longer than two pages, so it needs to contain concise information that clearly identifies your career objective, your strengths, accomplishments, and experiences that have contributed to your professional development. Cross-referencing your self-assessment and your résumé on an ongoing basis will ensure that your résumé is current and relevant.

A résumé should be honest and easy to read. There is no one perfect résumé style. It is agreed that an effective résumé has the following qualities: (1) attracts the employer's interest; (2) identifies the applicant's career objective, education, work experience, and other professional activities that are relevant to the position to which the applicant is applying; (3) creates a favourable first impression about you and your abilities; (4) conveys that you are someone who is a good fit for the position and the organization; and (5) is visually appealing.

If you have worked through the phases of the Model, you have completed the most difficult aspects of résumé development. Creating a customized résumé to fit the job to which you are applying should be a breeze! It is helpful to keep a generic résumé on hand that includes all of your education, nursing practice and work experiences, and extracurricular activities. You can then draw from this comprehensive résumé to create customized versions for specific positions.

Although there are two types of résumés—the chronological résumé and the functional résumé—the latter format is better suited to students and new graduates. In the functional résumé, you list your education, work experiences, and clinical practice experiences in reverse chronological order.

Three unique aspects of a new graduate's résumé are the summary of the nursing practice experience; the list of selected practice experiences, outcome competencies, and accomplishments; and documentation of past working experiences, including summer employment. Selected practice experiences are those that are most pertinent to the position to which you are applying. Limit the list of selected nursing practice placements to one or two, choosing only those experiences with responsibilities, accomplishments, and competencies that relate directly to the nursing position you are applying for.

Your résumé should include the following headings:

- Career Objective
- Education
- Selected Practice Placements—with descriptions of outcome, professional competencies and accomplishments *or*
- Summary of Practice Accomplishments per year (for third and fourth year)
- Professional Activities
  - Curricular
  - Extracurricular
- Honours/Awards
- Professional Memberships
- Professional Development
- Employment
  - Focus on professional competencies related to the position you are applying for
- Volunteer/Community Activities

Although it seems like a lot of information, being concise and using action-oriented words will enable you to include all of this information within two pages, allowing for at least 2.5-centimetre (one-inch) margins and adequate white space. Don't be alarmed if you don't have anything to put in some of the categories! Create your generic résumé with all of the headings. Gaps in your résumé can help you to plan for short- and long-term activities that fit with your career vision and contribute to the development of a comprehensive and impressive résumé. If you have a heading that remains incomplete, do not include it in your résumé, but keep working at it.

Students often find the most difficult task of writing a résumé is describing what they have accomplished using action verbs and phrases with meaning. Weigh your choice of words. Remember, you have the attention of recruiters for an average of only 30 seconds as they review your résumé. Use meaningful phrases, such as *organizational ability, ability to adapt to change, self-directed, excellent problem-solving ability, lifelong learner* when one word does not fully express a complete thought. When writing your résumé, keep in mind that it is not boasting to write about your strengths and accomplishments. If you do not write about your strengths, you may not have the opportunity to obtain an interview. See Table 22-3 for a summary of action verbs for résumé preparation.

Make sure to use a spell checker and then have someone else review your résumé for any spelling or grammatical errors. When printing a résumé for a nursing position, it is best to use white, ivory, or pale grey paper of good quality. Use a printer that prints clearly and darkly. Choose a legible, professional font, such as Times New Roman or Arial. See Figure 22-2 for Alya's résumé.

Your résumé should always be accompanied buy a one-page cover letter written on personal letterhead paper. The cover letter has three components. The introduction states the position to which you are applying and where you learned of the position. The second paragraph briefly and broadly highlights your professional strengths related to the position. The final component indicates your interest in participating in an interview and your contact information. Use personal language and focus on what you can do for the unit and organization. See Figure 22-3 for Alya's cover letter.

ELECTRONIC RÉSUMÉS

Many hiring managers and recruiters prefer to receive résumés by e-mail. Electronic résumés can be formatted as a Microsoft Word file, a text file, or a PDF file (Bookey-Bassett, 2004). If employers request an electronic résumé, be sure to send it in the requested format, or

TABLE 22-3	**LIST OF ACTION VERBS FOR RÉSUMÉ**			
accomplished	delivered	identified	operated	reorganized
achieved	demonstrated	increased	organized	revamped
administered	designed	initiated	oversaw	revised
analyzed	developed	innovated	performed	simplified
approved	directed	instituted	planned	solved
built	earned	launched	proposed	streamlined
communicated	eliminated	listed	provided	supervised
completed	established	maintained	purchased	taught
conceived	evaluated	managed	redesigned	terminated
conducted	expanded	mastered	reduced	trained
coordinated	explored	motivated	reengineered	transformed
created	generated	negotiated	reinforced	utilized

Alya Surname
123 City Street, City
Province, Postal Code
Phone, E-mail

CAREER OBJECTIVE: To contribute to holistic, comprehensive developmental and family-centred nursing care in a tertiary acute pediatric setting. To further my professional development in the care of acutely ill children and families.

EDUCATION: 2003–2007 University Name, BScN
- Expected date of completion April 2007.

AWARDS AND ACHIEVEMENTS:

2004–2006	Dean's List Standing (first, second, and third year of BScN)
May 2006	Induction to Sigma Theta Tau Nursing Honour Society
May 2006	Royal Bank Faculty of Community Services Award
Jan. 2005	Induction to Golden Key Honour Society
May 2004	Scholarship for Advocacy and Dedication

PROFESSIONAL EXPERIENCE:

Nursing Practice Experience—BScN Program

Selected Family-Centred Care Practice Experiences

Jan. 2005–April 2006   Maternal Infant Program
- Provided nursing anaesthesia consults and family-centred education regarding pain management options; prenatal care via parent groups and individual meetings for parents expecting multiples and singletons; care and counselling to young mothers, through the MIP Young Mothers Program.

Sept. 2004–Dec. 2004   Healthy Babies Healthy Children
- In collaboration with a public health nurse, conducted follow-up phone calls within the first 24 to 48 hours post-delivery to new mothers. Assessment of mother and infant conducted over the phone, with the option for additional home visit to mother and child. Pre and postnatal home visits to provide education regarding issues, such as general infant well-being and safety. Neonatal physical assessment provided in home. Developed competence in the provision of family-centred care.
- Co-facilitation of national high-risk parenting program. Empowerment of parents and teaching of parenting styles, child development, behaviour, discipline, nutrition, and stress.

Other Nursing Practice Experiences—BScN Program

Sept. 2005–Dec. 2005	"Name of Hospital" Hospital Medical Oncology
Jan. 2004–May 2004	"Name of Hospital" Nephrology/Medicine
Sept. 2003–Dec. 2003	"Name of Hospital" Alternate Level of Care Unit

LEADERSHIP ACTIVITIES:

Jan. 2005–Current   Collaborative Nursing Degree Program Evaluation Committee
- Involved in ongoing committee efforts to evaluate implementation and outcomes of Collaborative Degree Program. Active participation in the initiation of formal evaluation processes and data analysis.

May 2002–Current   University Nursing Course Union
- Two terms as president, one term as past-president (current)
- Acting on student council, under the nursing division, to coordinate social, political and educational events. Liaison between the student body and administration.

Figure 22-2 Alya's Résumé

	Sept. 2003–May 2005	University Academic Student Council-Student Member

- Acting as a student voting member on the academic council, to represent the student vote in such matters as curriculum changes and program entrance requirements.

EMPLOYMENT
EXPERIENCES: May–Aug., 2004–2006   "Name" Retirement Centre—Personal Care Assistant Summer Employment

- Provided individualized, developmental care to senior residents. Utilized positive and effective communication skills. Acknowledged for strengths in conveying compassion, sensitivity, and respect to residents and their families. Reliable and responsible.

COMMUNITY
INVOLVEMENT: Sept. 2005–May 2006   Volunteer with the Children's Wish Foundation.

REFERENCES: Available upon request.

Figure 22-2 Continued

Alya's cover letter for a new graduate position could be the following.

Alya Surname
123 City Street, City
Province, Postal Code
Phone and E-mail

Date
Name of Individual Noted on Job Posting

Title
Address

Dear "Name of Individual,"

I am writing in response to the advertisement posted in the Pediatric Nurse Interest Group April, 2007 newsletter for a staff nurse position in the General Pediatric Medical Unit of your organization.

I will be graduating from my nursing baccalaureate program in May 2007. Over the course of my education, I have focused on the development of professional competencies relevant to the care of children experiencing acute illness and their families. I am committed to the concept and practice of developmental and family-centred care, a value that is strongly supported in your organization. I would look forward to continuing my professional development in child and family health, and contributing to quality family-centred care within your program.

My enclosed résumé details how my nursing practice placements and related educational experiences have prepared me to fulfill the requirements of your staff nurse position. I would appreciate the opportunity to discuss my potential contribution to your general pediatric medical unit program. I look forward to hearing from you. Thank you for your consideration.

Sincerely,
[Signature]

Alya Surname
Enclosure: Résumé

Figure 22-3 Alya's Cover Letter

TABLE 22-4	CREATING AN ELECTRONIC RÉSUMÉ
Step 1:	In the word processing program, set margins so that 16.25 centimetres (6.5 inches) of text are displayed. This amount of text is easily viewed by the majority of e-mail programs.
Step 2:	Write the résumé using an easy-to-read font in 12-point type, such as Arial or Times New Roman.
Step 3:	Save the résumé as a text-only file with line breaks. Do not use the Tab key. Use the space bar instead. Format the text with left justification.
Step 4:	Open this new file in a text editor, such as Microsoft Notepad.
Step 5:	Review the résumé to see how the recipient will see it once it is transmitted via e-mail. Pay careful attention to unsupported formats or those formats that your word processing program may not be able to read. You may have to add ASCII-supported characters, such as asterisks, to make the résumé easier to view. Proofread!
Step 6:	Copy and paste the résumé in the body of a test e-mail message. Send it back to yourself or to a friend who uses a different e-mail program to see how the recipient views your résumé.
Step 7:	When applying for a job electronically, a cover letter should also accompany your résumé. Rather than sending both the cover letter and the résumé in the text area, or as separate attachments, the preferred approach is to send the cover letter in the text portion of the e-mail and attach the résumé.

Adapted from Smith, R. (1999). *Electronic résumés and online networking.* Franklin Lakes, NJ: Career Press, p. 72.

check with them if you are unsure which format they prefer. You need to be able to send your résumé via e-mail so that the recipient can read the résumé, regardless of the software the recipient is using. There are several ways to create an electronic résumé, including writing the résumé using standard word processing software, such as Microsoft Word or Corel WordPerfect. For tips on creating an electronic résumé, see Table 22-4.

Type the résumé using word processing software and then save it in one of three formats: ASCII plain text (.txt), rich-text (.rtf), or as hypertext (.html). ASCII text files are the most common types of data files found on the Internet. This file type allows for simplicity in reading the text but does not allow any type of text formatting, such as boldface characters, bullets, underlining, or italics. The recipient receives plain, clear text without any identifying marks, tabs, or visually appealing formatting. If you want to highlight a specific area, you can use a character such as an asterisk (*).

It is important to use keywords when sending an electronic résumé. When recruiters are looking for someone with specific skills, they often perform a search using keywords such as *pediatric nurse practitioner* or *oncology registered nurse*. Be sure to use correct grammar, spelling, and punctuation.

BUSINESS CARDS

Business cards are a way to introduce yourself to others and to provide them with your contact information in a professional manner. As you increase your networking activities at job fairs, conferences, and other professional forums, a business card is an important, and often requested, self-marketing tool. Student business cards can include your name, phone number, and e-mail address. Like your résumé and cover letter, your business card should be easy to read, printed on material that is neutral in colour and professional in appearance. You can have business cards made at stationery and business retail stores. You can also find many websites where you can create and print your own business card.

PREPARING FOR AN INTERVIEW

As you prepare for an interview, it is a good idea to scan the environment with a particular focus on the organization to which you are applying and on current issues and practices that are relevant to the position that you will be discussing in your interview. Information that you should research prior to the interview and that can be located on the organization's website includes the following:

- The specific job description
- The vision and mission statement of the organization
- The vision and mission of the department of nursing
- The professional practice model—theory adopted by the department of nursing

Also make sure that you are informed regarding the following details:

- The type of interview you can expect (e.g., individual or panel)
- The time, date, and location—particularly if the organization has more than one site

Remember that the interview is a mutual discovery process. The organization needs to make sure that you are appropriate and prepared to fulfill the requirements of the job; you need to know that the organization is a place where you can both contribute and progress toward your career vision. Prepare some questions to ask, based on your values, self-assessment, and career vision. Be ready to articulate how your skills, expertise, and accomplishments meet the position requirements. You can also anticipate the questions you may be asked (see Table 22-5) and prepare your answers to those questions. Remember to keep your responses concise and clear. It is a good idea to practise interviewing with a friend or your mentor.

On the day of the interview, plan your time well and expect to arrive early. Bring a copy of your résumé so that you can refer to it in the event that an interviewer poses specific questions related to its content. Be polite and respectful to everyone in the organization. Remember that you are marketing yourself to everyone you encounter during the interview process, including support personnel who are often your first contact.

You will also be offered the opportunity to ask questions of the interviewer, so be prepared with several questions that help you to understand how the organization can support both your practice as a new graduate and your short- and long-term career goals. Feel free to write your questions down so that you don't forget them. If your questions have been answered, then do not feel that you have to ask a question that is not of relevance to you. You can simply say that the questions that you had coming into the interview have been answered during the interview process. For samples of questions to ask during an interview, see Table 22-6.

A NOTE ABOUT REFERENCES

Your references play a key role in marketing your professional strengths to potential employers. Like your résumés, your choice of referees should be specific to the job to which you are applying. Make sure that you contact your desired referees and ask if they would be willing to provide you with a positive reference. Provide your references with

TABLE 22-5	POTENTIAL INTERVIEW QUESTIONS

- Tell us about yourself, your background, your education, and your short- and long-term career goals.
- Where do you see yourself in five years?
- What words best describe you? How would your colleagues describe you? How will your references describe you?
- Describe a difficult work situation you have had to deal with. How did you handle it?
- What are your strengths? What do you see as your areas for development?
- Why do you want to work for this organization? Why do you want this job?
- Why should we hire you?
- How can you make a difference to this organization?
- What is your philosophy of nursing? What does nursing mean to you?
- Describe a situation that demonstrates your ability to adapt to changes at work.
- Describe the best advisor/faculty member/supervisor you have ever worked with. What made them the best?

Sources: Donner, G. J., & Wheeler, M. M. (Eds.). (1994). *Taking control of your nursing career.* Toronto: Elsevier; Waddell, J., Donner, G. J., & Wheeler, M. M. (2004). *Building your nursing career: A guide for students.* Toronto: Elsevier.

TABLE 22-6	SAMPLE QUESTIONS TO ASK DURING AN INTERVIEW

- What type of orientation would I receive?
- How can I prepare myself to be a successful member of the nursing team?
- What resources will I have access to during my orientation?
- What are the ongoing opportunities for professional development?
- What other health care providers work on this team/service/program? What is the skill mix?
- What do you think will be the major challenges of this position?
- How are the working hours scheduled?
- How would you describe the ideal candidate for this position?
- How are preceptors assigned?
- How long would I work with a preceptor?
- What are the next steps in the hiring process?
- When will the hiring decision be made?

Sources: Donner, G. J., & Wheeler, M. M. (Eds.). (1994). *Taking control of your nursing career.* Toronto: Elsevier; Waddell, J., Donner, G. J., & Wheeler, M. M. (2004). *Building your nursing career: A guide for students.* Toronto: Elsevier.

an updated résumé and a description of the job for which you will be asking them to serve as a reference. Let them know the date of your interview and when they may be contacted by the employer.

If, after the interview, you are interested in pursuing the position, offer the potential employer the names and contact information for the referees you have chosen for this position. Immediately following your interview, contact your chosen referees to let them know how the interview went, and if there are any areas that you would like them to focus on in their discussion with the employment agency. Referees are often interested in whether you were successful in your interview and if you accepted the position. Send a written note offering thanks for serving as your reference and updating them on the outcome.

You are on your way! You can now use The Donner-Wheeler Career Planning and Development Model to orchestrate your final years of your program and create the path to your future—Enjoy!

KEY CONCEPTS

- Career planning and development can begin at any point in your academic or professional practice career.

- The Donner-Wheeler Career Planning and Development Model (the Model) offers students and registered nurses a structure and process to take control of their career.

- Career development is not a one-time activity and does not need to follow a step-by-step process. You can move back and forth among the phases as you gather more experiences and learn more about your self and your wishes for your career.

- The Model can be used to help you prepare for specific goals, such as applying to graduate programs and choosing your first job.

- Your career vision is your guide for reflection and action.

- A strategic career plan is your blueprint for action.

- You market yourself with every professional encounter.

- Information and insights gathered from your work in each phase of the Model informs your résumé and helps you to prepare for interviews.

- The interview is a mutual process of discovery—you are an active participant in the interview.

- You don't have to be a registered nurse to have a business card. A business card is a professional means of communication, particularly during your networking activities.

- A mentor can guide your career development and open doors for you.

KEY TERMS

career vision
marketing
mentor
networking
reality check

résumé
scanning the environment
self-assessment
strategic career plan

REVIEW ACTIVITIES

1. Write your career vision in narrative form, answering all of the questions on pages 389–390 in as much detail as possible.

2. Based on your career vision, develop a short-term career goal that you can work on in the next six months.

3. With your career goal in mind, return to your self-assessment and identify three key values, three related strengths, and three areas that you need to develop further in order to meet your stated career goal.

4. After reviewing the work you have accomplished in the previous three activities, develop four interview questions that, when answered, will help you to determine whether the position will be congruent with your values and will help you meet your career goals.

5. List three qualities you would like in a mentor.

6. Identify one potential mentor.

REVIEW QUESTIONS

1. Which of the following is the best response to the interview question, What are your strengths?
   A. "I have many. Where do you want me to begin?"
   B. "My professional and therapeutic communication skills have been acknowledged as strong. I value collaborative working relationships with clients and families. I am confident in my nursing practice and resourceful if I need further knowledge or assistance in providing a high quality of family-centered care."
   C. "I think I am well liked and get along with everyone."
   D. "Well, I am just a new nurse without many strengths right now, but I am enthusiastic and a fast learner."

2. Which of the following components are absolutely necessary to include in a résumé?

A. Identifying information, career objective, formal education, educational experiences, employment experiences, and professional/community involvement.
B. Identifying information, employment experiences, education, professional organizations, and awards and honours.
C. Identifying information, employment experiences, education, professional organizations, and references.
D. Identifying information, employment experiences, education, and professional organizations.

3. When creating an electronic résumé, which of the following is essential?
   A. Setting margins so that 17.5 centimetres (7 inches) of text are displayed in a word processing program.
   B. Using a type font in 12 point, such as Arial or Times New Roman.
   C. Saving the résumé using the right justification format.
   D. Using the bold and underline function in the résumé as a way of highlighting information.

4. What is the primary function of a cover letter?
   A. To entice the prospective employer to become interested enough to read the résumé
   B. To have a letter to include with your résumé
   C. To include references not listed on a résumé
   D. To reiterate all that is on your résumé

REFERENCES

Bookey-Bassett, S. (2004). Marketing yourself. In G. J. Donner & M. M. Wheeler (Eds.), *Taking control of your nursing career* (pp. 63–90). Toronto: Elsevier.

Donner, G. J. (2004). Taking control of your nursing career: The future is now. In G. J. Donner & M. M. Wheeler (Eds.), *Taking control of your nursing career* (pp. 3–11). Toronto: Elsevier.

Donner, G. J., and Wheeler, M. M. (Eds.). (2004). *Taking control of your nursing career.* Toronto: Elsevier.

Smith, R. (1999). *Electronic résumés and online networking.* Franklin Lakes, NJ: Career Press.

Waddell, J. (2005). Choosing the right graduate program. *Canadian Nurse, 101*(5), 30–31.

Waddell, J., Donner, G. J., & Wheeler, M. M. (2004). *Building your nursing career: A guide for students.* Toronto: Elsevier.

SUGGESTED READINGS

Bolles, R. N. (2003). *What color is your parachute? A practical manual for job-hunters and career changers.* Berkeley, CA: Ten Speed Press.

Stovall, P., & Teddlie, J. (1993). *Student guide to bias-free career planning: Opening all options.* Columbus, OH: Career, Education, and Training Associates.

Wickman, F., & Sjodin, T. (1997). *Mentoring: A success guide for mentors and protégés.* Chicago, IL: Irwin.

APPENDIX

Something unforeseen and magnificent is happening. Health care, having in our time entered its dark night of the soul, shows signs of emerging, transformed. (Barbara Dossey and Larry Dossey)

CANADIAN REGISTERED NURSE EXAMINATION

Each provincial or territorial nursing regulatory body in Canada is responsible for ensuring that the individuals it registers as nurses meet an acceptable level of competence before beginning to practise.

The level of competence of registered nurses in all provinces and territories except Quebec is measured, in part, by the Canadian Registered Nurse Examination (CRNE). The Canadian Nurses Association (CNA) develops and maintains the CRNE through its testing company, Assessment Strategies Inc., and in collaboration with the regulatory authorities. The provincial and territorial nursing regulatory authorities administer the exam and determine eligibility to write it.

The purpose of the CRNE is to protect the public by ensuring that entry-level registered nurses possess the competencies required to practise safely and effectively.

EXAMINATION LENGTH AND FORMAT

The RN Exam consists of 240 to 260 multiple-choice and short-answer questions.

ITEM PRESENTATION

The multiple-choice questions are presented either as case-based or independent questions. The short-answer questions are presented as case-based questions only. Case-based questions are presented as a set of two to five questions associated with a brief health care scenario. Independent questions each contain the information necessary to answer the questions.

For the 240 to 260 questions on the CRNE, 40 percent are presented as independent questions and 60 percent are presented within cases. Within the examination, 15 to 25 percent of the questions are short-answer questions and 75 to 85 percent are presented in a multiple-choice format.

CRNE PREPARATION TOOLS

The CNA, the developer and owner of the CRNE, offers two official tools to assist candidates studying for the exam. These two tools, the Canadian Registered Nurse Exam Prep Guide and the LeaRN™ CRNE Readiness Test, complement each other to help candidates prepare for the CRNE.

CANADIAN REGISTERED NURSE EXAM (CRNE) PREP GUIDE[1]

The CRNE Prep Guide is a study guide in print format with an accompanying CD-ROM. Available in either English or French, the prep guide offers nearly 300 practice questions, including more than 75 questions in the short-answer format. The CD-ROM allows students to study questions by format or by content category.

The guide also provides the following tools:

a) answers and explanations to help you learn;
b) a performance profile to identify your strengths and weaknesses; and
c) valuable test-taking strategies and study tips.

You may purchase the CRNE Prep Guide from your school bookstore or from CNA at http://bookstore.cna-aiic.ca or by calling 1-800-385-5881. CNA's prep guide price is $74.95 plus taxes and shipping and handling.

LeaRN CRNE READINESS TEST[2]

The LeaRN CRNE Readiness Test is the first of a series of tools and resources trademarked under the title LeaRN, which will be offered by the Canadian Nurses Association. These resources are provided to assist nurses to meet the requirements to be registered as RNs in Canada, and to integrate into the Canadian health care system.

The LeaRN CRNE Readiness Test will help to assess readiness to take the Canadian Registered Nurse Examination (CRNE). The CRNE is part of the registration requirements for nurses in all provinces or territories in Canada, with the exception of Quebec. For additional information on the Quebec exam, visit the website of Ordre des infirmières et infirmiers du Québec (www.oiiq.org).

COMPETENCY FRAMEWORK[3]

A framework was developed to identify and organize the competencies the CRNE should assess. The resulting framework reflects a primary health care nursing model. The framework and definitions of the four framework categories are presented below. The number of competencies in each category is indicated in parentheses following the category name. The number of competencies in each category does not necessarily reflect the importance of each area of competency in the practice of nursing.

PROFESSIONAL PRACTICE (44 COMPETENCIES)

Each nurse is accountable for safe, competent, and ethical nursing practice. Professional practice occurs within the context of the CNA Code of Ethics for Registered Nurses (2002) and provincial or territorial standards of practice and legislation. Nurses are expected to demonstrate professional conduct as reflected by attitudes, beliefs, and values espoused in the Code of Ethics for Registered Nurses. Professional practice in nursing involves the demonstration of teamwork, leadership attributes, basic management skills, advocacy, and political awareness. Leadership attributes, such as vision, knowledge, initiative, integrity, confidence, communication, and innovation, are necessary for the advancement of nursing practice, the nursing profession, and health care delivery systems. Entry-level management skills involve the ability to work within an organization using appropriate resources to achieve the organization's mission and vision. Professional practice includes awareness of the need for, and the ability to ensure, continued professional development. Professional development involves the capacity to perform self-assessments, seek feedback, and plan self-directed learning activities that foster professional growth. Nurses are expected to know how to locate and use results of research findings to inform and build an evidence-based practice.

NURSE-PERSON RELATIONSHIP (21 COMPETENCIES)

The nurse-person relationship is a therapeutic partnership established to promote the health of the person. This relationship is based on trust, respect, and sensitivity to diversity. An essential element involves gathering information that reflects the uniqueness of the person. It involves therapeutic use of self, communication skills, nursing knowledge, and the facilitation of empowerment to achieve collaboratively identified health goals.

NURSING PRACTICE: HEALTH AND WELLNESS (46 COMPETENCIES)

Nursing competencies in this category are focused on recognizing and valuing health and wellness as a resource. This category encompasses health promotion, illness and injury prevention, and the implementation of community or societal approaches. Practice is guided by the principles of primary health care. Nurses work in partnership with communities to influence the determinants of health, with the goal of enabling people to increase control over their health and to improve their health. Nurses partner with individuals to develop personal skills, create supportive environments for health, strengthen community action, reorient health services, and build healthy public policy. Practice reflects changes in cultural composition, demographics, health trends, and economic factors (e.g., an aging population and globalization).

NURSING PRACTICE: ALTERATIONS IN HEALTH (83 COMPETENCIES)

Nursing competencies in this category involve care across the lifespan for the person experiencing alterations in health that require acute, chronic, rehabilitative, or palliative care. Such care may be delivered across a range of institutional and community settings. Essential aspects of nursing involve critical thinking, problem solving, and decision making in providing care. Using current knowledge, nurses collaborate with the person and other health professionals to identify health priorities. In responding to and managing health issues, the aim of nursing is to promote maximal independence and to maintain optimal quality of life or ensure that individuals at the end of life experience a peaceful death.

CANADIAN PRACTICAL NURSE REGISTRATION EXAMINATION

Licensed practical nurses write a national exam, called the Canadian Practical Nurse Registration Examination (CPRNE). Two predictor tests are now available. Each predictor test comprises 100 multiple-choice questions, matching the Blueprint for Part A of the Canadian Practical Nurse Registration Examination.[4] Predictor Test 1 and Predictor Test 2 have completely different sets of questions, but are similar in difficulty. Both tests contain case-based and independent questions. Each test is available in both French and English, and students can switch freely between languages while taking the test.

The test comes equipped with a timer to simulate an actual examination environment. However, you can continue taking the test after time has "been called." If, for some reason, you have to stop the test before completing it, you will be able to return to the test later, provided you have not yet submitted your answers. Once you have completed the test and submitted your answers, you will be presented with your results. You will not be able to re-enter the test; however, if you log in again at any time after completing the test, you will be able to view the results page. The results will also be available for printing by using the link that will be sent to you by e-mail.

The predictor tests are most useful when taken under test-like conditions. You should adhere to the time limits (2.5 hours for each test), and not use any notes or textbooks when taking the tests. The prediction of readiness to take the CPRNE will only be meaningful and useful if you follow these instructions and complete the predictor tests without any assistance. The predictor tests are designed to help you focus your future studying and to help you gauge your readiness for the CPNRE. If you require a practice test, it is recommended that you consider The Canadian PN Exam Prep Guide.

A 10-question sample test is available on-line for you to try at www.asitest.ca/PN/cprne_practice_test.htm. The sample test includes Canadian trivia questions on sports, entertainment, and geography to ensure you are comfortable taking an on-line test prior to purchasing your Predictor Test.[5]

PRACTICAL NURSES CANADA[6]

On January 13, 2007, the Canadian Association of Practical Nurses announced its name change to Practical Nurse Canada (PN Canada). Incorporated in 1975, PN Canada is the national association representing provincial and territorial licensed practical nurse organizations and affiliated individuals from across Canada.

ENDNOTES

1. "Canadian Registered Nurse Exam (CRNE) Prep Guide." Retrieved from http://www.cna-aiic.ca/CNA/nursing/rnexam/preptools/default_e.aspx, August 19, 2007.

2. "LeaRN CRNE Readiness Test." Retrieved from www.cna-nurses.ca/CNA/nursing/rnexam/preptools/learn/default_e.aspx, May 21, 2007.

3. Retrieved from http://www.cna-nurses.ca/CNA/nursing/rnexam/default_e.aspx, August 19, 2007.

4. "What Does the Predictor Test Look Like?" Retrieved from http://www.asitest.ca/PN/what does the cprne.htm, May 21, 2007.

5. "CPNRE Predictor Test Practice Test." Retrieved from http://www.asitest.ca/PN/cprne_practice_test.htm, May 21, 2007.

6. "Welcome to the Official Website of Practical Nurses Canada." Retrieved from http://www.pncanada.ca/intro.shtml, May 21, 2007.

ABBREVIATIONS

AAHP	American Association of Health Plans
ACHHR	Advisory Committee on Health Human Resources
ACEN	Academy of Canadian Executive Nurses
AHRQ	Agency for Healthcare Research and Quality
AHS	Aboriginal Head Start
AIDS	Acquired Immune Deficiency Syndrome
AIM	achieving improved measurement
ALOS	average length of stay
ALS	amyotrophic lateral sclerosis
AMA	American Medical Association
AMI	acute myocardial infarction
ANA	American Nurses Association
ANCC	American Nurses Credentialing Center
ARDS	acute respiratory distress syndrome
ASA	acetylsalicylic acid
BCNU	British Columbia Nurses Union
BSN	bachelor of science in nursing
CACCN	Canadian Association of Critical Care Nurses
CADTH	Canadian Agency for Drugs and Technologies in Health
CARP	Canadian Association of Retired People
CASN	Canadian Association of Schools of Nursing
CCHSA	Canadian Council on Health Services Accreditation
CCHSE	Canadian College of Health Service Executives
CCOHS	Canadian Centre for Occupational Health and Safety
CCS	Canadian Cancer Society
CCU	coronary care unit
CDSMP	Chronic Disease Self-Management Program
CEO	chief executive officer
CERN	Conseil Européen pour la Recherche Nucléaire (European Laboratory for Particle Physics)
CEU	continuing education unit
CFNU	Canadian Federation of Nurses Unions
CHA	Canada Health Act
CHA	Canadian Healthcare Association
CHC	Community Health Centre
CHE	Certified Health Executive
CHPCA	Canadian Hospice Palliative Care Association
CHSRF	Canadian Health Services Research Foundation
CHST	Canada Health and Social Transfer
CIHI	Canadian Institute for Health Information
CIHR	Canadian Institutes of Health Research
CINAHL	Cumulative Index to Nursing and Allied Health Literature
CIPS	Canadian Information Processing Society
CIS	clinical information system
CLC	Canadian Labour Congress
CMA	Canadian Medical Association
CMG	case mix group
CNA	Canadian Nurses Association
CNAC	Canadian Nursing Advisory Committee
CNIA	Canadian Nurses Informatics Association

CNSA	Canadian Nursing Students' Association
COACH	Canadian Organization for Advancement of Computers in Health
CPHA	Canadian Public Health Association
CPHI	Canadian Population Health Initiative
CPR	cardiopulmonary resuscitation
CPRNE	Canadian Practical Nurse Registration Exam
CQI	continuous quality improvement
CRNE	Canadian Registered Nurse Examination
DER-CA	Diabetes Education Resource for Children and Adolescents
DM	disease management
DNR	Do not resuscitate
DRG	diagnosis-related group
EBP	evidence-based practice
ECE	early childhood education
ED	emergency department
EHR	electronic health record
EI	emotional intelligence
EMT	Emergency Medical Technician
ENIAC	Electronic Numerical Integrator and Computer
EPC	evidence-based practice centre
ERG	existence-relatedness-growth theory (Alderfer, 1969)
EXTRA	Executive Training for Research Application
FASD	Fetal Alcohol Spectrum Disorder
FIIQ	Federation des Infirmiers et Infirmieres du Quebec
FLAT	Factual, Legible, Accurate, Timely
FTE	full-time equivalent
GDP	gross domestic product
GRADE	Grading of Recommendations, Assessments, Development and Evalua-tion
HEAL	Health Action Lobby
HIV	human immunodeficiency virus
HPI	Human Poverty Index
ICFASD	Interdepartmental Committee on Fetal Alcohol Spectrum Disorder
ICN	International Council of Nurses
ICU	intensive care unit
IMCN	intermediate care nursery
IOM	Institute of Medicine
ISMP Canada	Institute for Safe Medication Practices Canada
JCAHO	Joint Commission on Accreditation of Healthcare Organizations
KT&E	Knowledge Transfer and Exchange
LHINs	Local Health Integration Networks
LOS	length of stay
LPI	leadership practices inventory
LPN	licensed practical nurse
MDGs	Millennium Development Goals
MEDLARS	Medical Literature Analysis and Retrieval System
MeSH	Medical Subject Headings
MIS	management information systems
MLOA	maternity leave of absence
MOHLTC	[Ontario] Ministry of Health and Long-Term Care
MRI	Magnetic Resonance Imaging
MS-HUG	Microsoft Healthcare Users Group
MSN	master's degree in nursing
NCSBN	National Council of State Boards of Nursing

NGC	National Guideline Clearinghouse
NHPPD	nursing hours per patient day
NHSRU	Nursing Health Services Research Unit
NICU	neonatal intensive care unit
NLM	National Library of Medicine
NNA	national nursing association
NWIG-AMIA	Nursing Working Informatics Group of the American Medical Informatics Association
OACHA	Ontario Advisory Committee on HIV/AIDS
OECD	Organization for Economic Cooperation and Development
OHIH	Office of Health and the Information Highway
OLRB	Ontario Labour Relations Board
OR	operating room
P3s	public-private partnerships
PAHO	Pan American Health Organization
PBMA	program budgeting and marginal analysis
PC	personal computer
PCS	patient classification system
PDCA	Plan Do Check Act
PDSA	Plan-Do-Study-Act
PERT	Program Evaluation and Review Technique
P-F-A	purpose-focus-approach
PFI	public finance initiative
PHAC	Public Health Agency of Canada
PHC	Primary Health Care
PHIPA	Personal Health Information Protection Act
PI	performance improvement
PIPEDA	Personal Information Protection and Electronic Documents Act
POSDCORB	planning, organizing, supervising, directing, coordinating, reporting, and budgeting
PRP	Participative Resolution Program
QA	quality assurance
QI	quality improvement
RIW	resource intensity weight
RN	registered nurse
RNABC	Registered Nurses Association of British Columbia
RNAO	Registered Nurses Association of Ontario
ROPs	Required Organization Practices
RPN	registered practical nurse
RPN	registered psychiatric nurse
SARS	Severe Acute Respiratory Syndrome
SNAA	Staff Nurses Association of Alberta
SPAN	Staff Planning Action Network
SRNA	Saskatchewan Association of Registered Nurses
SWOT	strengths, weaknesses, opportunities, threats
TB	tuberculosis
TQM	total quality management
UC	ubiquitous computing
UCP	Unregulated care provider
URL	uniform resource locator
UTI	urinary tract infection
VR	virtual reality
WHO	World Health Organization
WWW	World Wide Web

GLOSSARY

accommodating Satisfying the needs of others, sometimes at the expense of self.

accountability Liability for actions.

accounting An activity that nurse managers engage in to record and report financial transactions and data.

achievement Accomplishment of goals through effort.

active euthanasia A deliberate act in which body processes necessary to sustain life are actively interfered with or interrupted.

activities of daily living Tasks related to toileting, bathing, grooming, dressing, feeding, mobility, and verbal and written personal communication.

adjourning The fifth and final stage of group development, in which the group has met its objectives and the primary focus is closure activities and the termination of team relationships.

administrative principles General principles of management that are relevant to any organization.

advance directives Documents whose purpose is twofold: to ensure that a person's wishes are carried out when that person is no longer able to communicate; and to appoint a specific person, a substitute decision-maker, to ensure those wishes are carried out.

affiliation Associations and relationships with others.

altruism The unselfish concern for the welfare of others.

assault A threat of touching another in an offensive manner without that person's permission.

assisted suicide The act of intentionally killing oneself with the assistance of another who deliberately provides the knowledge, means, or both (Special Senate Committee on Euthanasia and Assisted Suicide, 1995).

attending Active listening to gain an understanding of the client's message.

auditory Pertaining to hearing.

authority A person's right to delegate, based on the provincial or territorial nursing scope of practice, and based on that person also receiving official power from an agency to delegate.

autocratic leadership A centralized decision-making style with the leader making decisions and using power to command and control others.

autonomy The ability to self-govern and to have control over decision making concerning one's own life.

avoiding Retreating.

balanced scorecard Documentation tool providing a snapshot image of pertinent information and activity reflecting a point in time.

battery The touching of another person without that person's consent.

benchmarking The continual and collaborative discipline of measuring and comparing the results of key work processes with those of the best performers.

beneficence Considering and acting in the best interests of others.

best research evidence Methodologically sound, clinically relevant research on the effectiveness and safety of nursing interventions, the accuracy and precision of nursing assessment measures, the power of prognostic markers, the strength of causal relationships, the cost-effectiveness of nursing interventions, and the meaning of illness to client experiences.

bioethics Ethical inquiry in response to new technologies, choices, and concerns in matters of maintaining and intervening in the lives of human beings, such as health care, research, and the environment; sometimes referred to as health care ethics or biomedical ethics.

blended payment schemes A payment method that combines both capitation and salary models. For example, a physician might receive both a salary and an incentive based on services provided over and above the core services.

bureaucratic organization Hierarchy with clear superior-subordinate communication and relations, based on positional authority, in which orders from the top are transmitted down through the organization via a clear chain of command.

Canadian Federation of Nurses Unions (CFNU) The organization for Canada's nursing unions that promotes nurses and the nursing profession at the national level.

Canadian Nurses Association (CAN) The professional organization representing the nation's entire registered nurse population.

capital budget The accounting of the purchases of major new or replacement equipment.

capitation Payment of a fixed dollar amount, per person, for the provision of health services to a client population for a specified period of time (e.g., one month).

case-costing A method for operationalizing activity-based costing (ABC).

care delivery model A method of organizing the work of caring for clients.

career vision A description developed in phase three of the Donner-Wheeler Career Planning and Development Model, in which individuals express where they want to go in their career—essentially a description of who and what a person wishes to become.

case management A strategy to improve client care and reduce costs through coordination of care.

case mix groups (CMGs) A Canadian client classification system used to group and describe types of clients discharged from acute-care hospitals.

change To make something different from what it was.

change agent An individual who is responsible for implementation of a change project.

civil law A body of rules and legal principles that govern relations, rights, and obligations among individuals, corporations, or other institutions.

clarifying Restating, rephrasing, or questioning a message to help make its meaning clear.

client acuity A measure of nursing workload that is generated for each client.

client-centered care A care delivery model in which care and services are brought to the client.

client-focused care A model of differentiated nursing practice that emphasizes quality, cost, and value.

client-focused clinical information system A system in which automation supports client care processes; typical applications include order entry, results reporting, clinical documentation, care planning, and clinical pathways.

clinical information system (CIS) A collection of software programs and associated hardware that supports the entry, retrieval, update, and analysis of client care information and associated clinical information related to client care.

clinical ladder A promotional model that acknowledges that staff members have varying skill sets based on their education and experience. As such, depending on skills and experience, staff members may be rewarded differently and carry differing responsibilities for client care and the governance and professional practice of the work unit.

clinical pathway A care management tool that outlines the expected clinical course and outcomes for a specific client type.

clinical practice guidelines Evidence-based statements of best practice in the prevention, diagnosis, or management of a given symptom, disease, or condition for individual clients.

collaborating Resolving conflict so that both parties are satisfied.

collective action A method of dealing with problems by acting as a group with a single voice.

collective bargaining The practice of employees, in a collective group, negotiating with management in reference to wages, work practice, and other benefits.

collective bargaining agent An individual who works with employees to formalize collective bargaining though unionization.

committee A work group with a specific task or goal to accomplish.

common law The body of law that develops from precedents set by judicial decisions that, over time, have the force of law, as distinguished from legislative enactments.

Community Health Centres Nonprofit organizations that provide primary health and health promotion programs for individuals, families, and communities.

competing Engaging in rivalry to meet a goal.

compromising Finding a middle-ground solution where each party makes a concession.

computer literacy The knowledge and understanding of computers combined with the ability to use them effectively.

conflict Disagreement about something of importance to each person involved.

confronting Working jointly with others to resolve a problem or conflict.

connection power The extent to which nurses are connected with others having power.

consensus The situation in which all group members agree to live with and support a decision, regardless of whether they totally agree.

consequentialist theories Views that state when deciding between possible actions, the most important moral obligation is to maximize the positive consequences and to minimize the negative consequences; also known as teleological theories.

consideration A focus on the employee with an emphasis on relating to and getting along with people.

constitution A set of basic laws that specify the powers of the various segments of the government and how these segments relate to each other.

construction budget The accounting of expenditures when renovation or new structures are planned.

contingency theory The view that acknowledges that other factors in the environment influence outcomes as much as leadership style and that leader effectiveness is contingent upon or depends upon something other than the leader's behaviour.

continuous quality improvement (CQI) A systematic process used to improve outcomes based on customers' needs.

contract law Rules that regulate certain transactions between individuals and/or legal entities, such as businesses.

cost centres Departmental subsections or units used for the tracking of financial data.

critical thinking A mode of thinking in which the quality of thinking is improved by skillfully taking charge of the structures inherent in thinking and imposing intellectual standards upon them.

data capture Collection and entry of data into a computer system.

decision making The cognitive process leading to the selection of a course of action among alternatives; behaviour exhibited in making a selection and implementing a course of action from alternatives.

delegation Transferring to a competent individual the authority to perform a selected nursing task in a selected situation.

delivery The method used to provide health care to the public.

Delphi technique A process that groups employ to arrive at a decision, though group members never meet face to face; questionnaires are distributed for opinions, and the responses are then summarized and disseminated to group members until consensus is achieved.

democratic leadership Style in which participation is encouraged and authority is delegated to others.

deontological theories Views that posit that an action's inherent rightness never lies in its consequences but in its very adherence to duty; also known as non-teleological theories.

departmental clinical information system A system that meets the operational needs of a particular department, such as the laboratory, radiology, pharmacy, health records, or finance.

determinants of health Social and environmental factors that strongly affect the health of a population.

direct care The provision of hands-on care to clients.

disease management Systematic, population-based approach to identify persons at risk, intervene with specific program of care, and measure clinical and other outcomes.

economics The study of how scarce resources are allocated among their possible uses.

egoism The tendency to be self-centred or to consider only oneself and one's own interests.

electronic health record (EHR) The electronic record that includes all information about an individual's lifetime health status and health care; replacement for the paper medical record as the primary source of information for health care, meeting all clinical, legal, and administrative requirements.

emotional intelligence The ability both to recognize the meaning of emotions and their relationships and to reason and solve problems on the basis of emotions.

employee-centred leadership Style with a focus on the human needs of subordinates.

empowerment Process by which we facilitate the participation of others in decision making and take action within an environment where there is an equitable distribution of power.

episodic care unit A unit that treats clients for defined episodes of care; examples include dialysis or ambulatory care units.

ethical dilemma A situation in which the best course of action is often not clear, and strong ethical reasons exist to support each position.

ethical theories Systematic approaches that can help decide what is right and wrong.

ethics The doctrine that the general welfare of society is the proper goal of an individual's actions rather than egoism; a way of understanding and reflecting upon social morality that encompasses moral issues, norms and practices.

euthanasia "A deliberate act undertaken by one person with the intention of ending the life of another person to relieve that person's suffering where the act is the cause of death" (Special Senate Committee on Euthanasia and Assisted Suicide, 1995).

evidence-based care Care based on state-of-the-art science reports and recognized by nursing, medical, health care institutions, and health care policymakers. It is a process approach to collecting, reviewing, interpreting, critiquing, and evaluating research and other relevant literature for direct application to client care.

evidence-based medicine The integration of individual clinical medical experience with external clinical evidence using a systematic research approach

evidence-based nursing practice The conscientious, explicit, and judicious use of theory-derived, research-based information in making decisions about care delivery to individuals or groups of individuals and in consideration of individual needs and preferences (Ingersoll, 2000, p. 152).

evidence-based practice The conscientious, explicit, and judicious use of current best evidence in making decisions about the care of individual clients (Sackett, et al., 1996, p. 71).

expert power Power derived from the knowledge and skills nurses possess.

false imprisonment The intentional restraint of individuals who are incorrectly led to believe they cannot leave a place.

fee-for-service A funding method in which physicians are paid separately for each service they provide.

feedback A new message that is generated by the receiver in response to the original message from the sender.

fiduciary obligation The responsibility to be truthful and explicit in communications with clients.

financing The method by which health care is paid for.

focus groups Small groups of individuals selected because of a common characteristic (e.g., a specific client population, clients in day surgery, new diabetics, and so on) who are invited to meet in a group and respond to questions about a topic in which they are expected to have an interest or expertise.

formal leadership Within an organization, the position of authority or the sanctioned role that connotes influence.

forming The first stage of group development, in which several critical phases begin: the expectation phase, the interaction phase, and the boundary formation phase.

full-time equivalent (FTE) Measure of the work commitment of a full-time employee.

functional health status The ability to care for oneself and meet one's human needs.

functional nursing A care delivery model that divides the nursing work into functional units that are then assigned to one of the team members.

funding The method by which the provincial and territorial health plans pay the provider of care.

goal The specific aim or target that an individual or a group of people wish to attain, often within a specific time span.

Good Samaritan laws Laws that have been enacted to protect the health care professional from legal liability for actions rendered in an emergency when the professional is giving service without pay.

grapevine An informal communication channel through which information moves quickly and is often inaccurate.

grievance A formal complaint in which a union member disputes management's interpretation or application of the terms of the contract, or collective agreement.

group development The five stages that a group normally progresses through as it reaches maturity: forming, storming, norming, performing, and adjourning.

Hawthorne effect The phenomenon of being observed or studied, which results in changes in behaviour.

health promotion The process of enabling people to increase control over their health and to improve their health.

health-related quality of life Those aspects of life that are influenced either positively or negatively by one's health status and health risk factors.

health risk factors Modifiable and non-modifiable variables that increase or decrease the probability of illness or death; synonymous with determinants of health.

health status The level of well-being of an individual, family, group, population, or community; the sum of existing health risk factors, level of wellness, existing diseases, functional health status, and quality of life.

horizontal integration A health care system that contains several organizations of one type, such as hospitals.

indirect care Time spent on activities that are client related but do not involve hands-on client care.

indirect costs Costs not explicitly related to client care, including utility costs and salaries of those who are not involved in direct client care.

informal leader An individual who demonstrates leadership outside the scope of a formal leadership role or as a member of a group, rather than the head or leader of the group.

information communication Interoperability of systems and linkages for exchange of data across disparate systems.

information power The authority held by a person who shares knowledge that is both accurate and useful.

initiating structure A type of leadership behaviour that involves an emphasis on the work to be done and a focus on the task and production.

inpatient unit A hospital unit that is able to provide care to clients 24 hours a day, 7 days a week.

instrumental activities of daily living (IADLs) Tasks related to food preparation and shopping; cleaning; laundry; home maintenance; verbal, written, and electronic communications; financial management; and transportation, along with activities to meet social and support needs, manage health care needs, access community services and resources, and meet spiritual needs.

integrated delivery system A network of health care organizations that provides a coordinated continuum of service to a defined population and is willing to be held clinically and fiscally accountable for the outcomes and the health status of the population served. Networks include hospitals, nursing homes, schools, public health departments, and social and community health organizations.

interdisciplinary team A group composed of members with a variety of clinical expertise.

interpersonal communication Communication between individuals.

intrapersonal communication Self-talk.

job-centred leaders Individuals whose leadership style focuses on schedules, cost, and efficiency with less attention to developing work groups and high-performance goals.

justice A broad principle encompassing the notion of fair distribution of benefits, resources, and risks.

kinesthetic Pertaining to touching.

knowledge workers Those involved in serving others through their specialized understanding of information.

laissez-faire leadership A passive and permissive style in which the leader defers decision making.

leader-member relations Feelings and attitudes of followers regarding acceptance, trust, and credibility of the leader.

leadership The process of influence whereby the person in charge influences others toward goal achievement.

legitimate power The influence derived from the position a nurse holds in a group; it indicates the nurse's degree of authority.

living will A document voluntarily signed by clients that specifies the type of care they desire if and when they are in a terminal state and are unable to either sign a consent form or convey this information verbally.

macro-allocation Resource allocation decisions that are made by governments at all levels.

maintenance or hygiene factors (Herzberg) Elements such as salary, job security, working conditions, status, quality of supervision, and relationships with others that prevent job dissatisfaction.

malpractice The wrongful conduct in the discharge of professional duties or failure to meet the standards of care for the profession, which results in harm to another individual entrusted to the professional's care.

management The process of coordinating actions and allocating resources to achieve organizational goals.

management process The function of planning, organizing, coordinating, and controlling.

marketing In the fifth and final phase of the Donner-Wheeler Career Planning and Development Model, the ability to communicate one's strengths, interests, and goals with confidence and clarity.

medical futility A medical treatment that is seen to be non-beneficial because it is believed to offer no reasonable hope of recovery or improvement of the client's condition.

MEDLARS (Medical Literature Analysis and Retrieval System) The computerized system of databases and databanks offered by the National Library of Medicine.

mentor A person who takes a personal and professional interest in your career and exemplifies the nurse you wish to become.

meso-allocation Resource allocation decisions that are made at the institutional or program level.

message A series of verbal and nonverbal stimuli that originate with a sender and are taken in by a receiver.

micro-allocation Resource allocation decisions that are made at the bedside, regarding individual clients.

mission A call to live out something that matters or is meaningful; an organization's mission reflects its purpose and direction.

mission statement A formal expression of the purpose or reason for existence of the organization.

modular nursing A team nursing care delivery system that divides a geographical space into modules of clients with each module having a team of staff led by an RN to care for them.

moral distress The result when ethical dilemmas are not acknowledged or effectively dealt with; when communication between team members, clients, and families is ineffective; or when professionals feel isolated or unsupported in their approach to solving such dilemmas.

morality Beliefs or traditions about what is determined to be right or wrong in terms of conduct towards ourselves and others.

motivation The incentive that influences our choices and creates direction, intensity, and persistence in our behaviour.

motivation factors (Herzberg) Elements such as achievement, recognition, responsibility, advancement, and the opportunity for development that contribute to job satisfaction.

negligence Failure to provide the care a reasonable person would ordinarily provide in a similar situation.

networking The continuous process of initiating and maintaining professional relationships through communication and information sharing.

nonmaleficence The principle of doing no harm.

non-unit producing Refers to indirect care activities that support the work of the direct care providers.

nonverbal communication Aspects of communication that are outside what is spoken.

norming The third stage of group development, in which people have a general understanding of the issues at hand and how to progress toward solving them. Positions in the group are established, and members have a sense both of belonging and of setting goals to meet expectations.

nursing ethics The examination of the norms, values, and principles found in nursing practice.

nursing hours per patient day (NHPPD) Standard measure that quantifies the nursing time available to each client by the available nursing staff.

objective The measurable step that must be taken to reach a goal.

operating budget The accounting of the income and expenses associated with day-to-day activity within a department or organization.

organizational change An alteration of an organization's culture, structure, technology, physical setting, or human resources.

organization evidence Information about an organization's capacity to execute tasks.

outcome elements of quality The end products of quality care that review the status of clients as a result of health care. Outcome elements ask the question, Is the client better as a result of health care?

passive euthanasia A deliberate act in which treatment is ceased or withheld, and the person is thereby made more vulnerable to the underlying processes that cause death.

payer A third-party reimburser; typically an insurance company or a government agency.

performance improvement (PI) A structured system for creating organization-wide participation and partnership in planning and implementing continuous improvement methods to understand and meet or exceed customer needs and expectations.

performing The fourth stage of group development, in which people understand their roles and work interdependently on the work needed to achieve the group's objectives.

personal change An alteration made voluntarily for one's own reasons, usually for self-improvement.

philosophy A statement of beliefs based on core values; rational investigations of the truths and principles of knowledge, reality, and human conduct.

philosophy of an organization A value statement of the principles and beliefs that direct the organization's behaviour.

political evidence Information that gives a sense of how various stakeholders may respond to policies; for example, the barriers or facilitators that may have to be managed.

political voice The stated views of individuals supporting or opposing an issue.

politics The process by which people use a variety of methods to achieve their goals.

population-based nursing practice The practice of nursing in which the focus of care is to improve the health status of vulnerable or at-risk population groups within the community by employing health promotion and disease prevention interventions across the health continuum.

population health An approach to health care that focuses on the determinants of health in order to help reduce inequities among different groups, particularly the people who are the most vulnerable; a concept that the population, or a community, as a whole has a particular state of health.

position power The degree of formal authority and influence associated with a leader.

power The ability to create, acquire, and use resources to achieve one's goals.

power of attorney A legal document executed by an individual (the principal) granting another person (the agent) the right to perform certain activities in the principal's name.

primary health care Services that emphasize the promotion of health and the prevention of illness or disability.

primary nursing A care delivery model that clearly delineates the responsibility and accountability of the RN and places the RN as the primary provider of nursing care to clients.

principlism A framework for considering ethical issues that includes four guiding principles: respect for autonomy, beneficence, nonmaleficence, and justice.

problem solving An active process that starts with a problem and ends with a solution.

process A series of actions, changes, or functions bringing about a result.

process elements of quality The nursing and health care interventions that must be in place to deliver quality, including managing the health care process, utilizing clinical practice guidelines and standards for nursing and medical interventions, administering medications, and so on.

professional change The alteration made in an individual's position or job such as obtaining education or credentials.

professional codes of ethics The guidelines and values to which members of a profession adhere to and promote in creating an ethical accountable practice; usually defined and shaped by members of the profession.

program budgeting and marginal analysis A mechanism that can link physicians to organizational decision-making processes.

public health system A system of health care that is responsible for helping to protect people from injury and disease and for helping people to stay healthy.

public law A general classification of law, consisting generally of constitutional law and criminal law. Public law defines a citizen's relationship with government.

quality assurance (QA) An inspection approach to ensure that minimum standards of care exist in health care institutions, primarily hospitals.

quality of life The level of satisfaction one has with the actual conditions of one's life, including satisfaction with socioeconomic status, education, occupation, home, family life, recreation, and the ability to enjoy life, freedom, and independence; at the end of life, having some control over the process and one's final days.

reality check The feedback, received from people involved in one's life, regarding one's strengths, unique traits, and areas for development. The reality check is part of self-assessment, the second phase of the Donner-Wheeler Career Planning and Development Model.

receiver One who takes in a message and analyzes it.

reengineering Turning an organization upside down and inside out through fundamental rethinking and radical redesign of processes to achieve dramatic improvements in critical performance.

referent power Authority derived from the degree to which others respect and like an individual, group, or organization.

reflective thinking Watching or observing ourselves as we perform a task or make a decision about a certain situation, followed by thinking about what we have done, and how we could have done it better.

regionalization An integrated health care delivery system that is structured by geographic areas.

resources The people; money; facilities; technology; and rights to properties, services, and technologies that are use to fulfill a function or achieve an end.

resource intensity weights (RIWs) Developed by the Canadian Institute for Health Information (CIHI), this relative resource methodology estimates a hospital's inpatient-specific costs for both acute care and day procedure care.

responding Verbal and nonverbal acknowledgment of a sender's message.

responsibility Reliability, dependability, and the obligation to accomplish work.

résumé Brief summary of your background, training, and experience as well as your qualifications for a position.

revenue Income generated through a variety of means (e.g., billable client services, investments, and donations to the organization).

reward/coercive power The authority to reward or punish others, as well as the ability to instill fear in others by influencing them to change their behaviour; resentment is often the result of withholding rewards or achieving a goal by causing fear.

risk adjustment The process of statistically altering client data to reflect significant client variables.

salary A payment method in which physicians are paid a lump-sum annual amount for working a specific number of hours per week.

scanning the environment The first phase of the Donner-Wheeler Career Planning and Development Model, in which individuals take a good look around to determine how the world around them can help to both develop and achieve their career goals.

secondary health care Services that emphasize detection and early intervention in illness to prevent further illness and disability.

self-assessment The second phase of the Donner-Wheeler Career Planning and Development Model, in which individuals look inside themselves to create meaning in their learning and to recognize opportunities for future development.

self-scheduling A process in which staff on a unit collectively decide and implement the monthly work schedule.

sentinel event An unexpected occurrence involving death or serious physical or psychological injury to a client.

shared governance A situation in which nurses and managers work together to define their roles and expected outcomes, holding everyone accountable for their role and expected outcomes.

situational leadership A framework that maintains that there is no one best leadership style, but rather that effective leadership lies in matching the appropriate leadership style to the individual's or group's level of motivation and task-relevant readiness.

skill mix The percentage of one type of staff to the total staff complement.

sources of power Combination of conscious and unconscious factors that allow an individual to influence others to think or act in a certain way.

staffing pattern A plan that articulates how many and what kind of staff are needed, by shift and day, to staff a unit or department.

stakeholder A provider, employer, customer, or client who may have an interest in, and may seek to influence, the decisions and actions of an organization.

stakeholders Vested interest groups.

stakeholder assessment A systematic consideration of all potential stakeholders to ensure that the needs of each of these stakeholders are incorporated in the planning phase.

storage Physical location of data in an electronic health record (EHR) system.

storming The second stage of group development, in which people begin to feel more comfortable with each other and differences among the group members may become apparent, leading to tension and conflicts.

strategic career plan A personalized action plan, developed in the fourth phase of the Donner-Wheeler Career Planning and Development Model, to help meet the short- and long-term goals of a career vision.

strategic plan The sum total or outcome of the processes by which an organization engages in environmental analysis, goal formulation, and strategy development with the purpose of organizational growth and renewal.

strategic planning A process that is designed to achieve goals in dynamic, competitive environments through the allocation of resources.

structure elements of quality The structure elements that must be in place in a health care system or health care unit to deliver quality health care, including a well-constructed hospital, quality client care standards, quality staffing policies, environmental standards, and the like.

substitutes for leadership Variables that may influence or have an effect on followers to the same extent as the leader's behaviour.

SWOT analysis A tool that is frequently used to conduct environmental assessments. SWOT stands for Strengths, Weaknesses, Opportunities, and Threats.

system An interdependent group of items, people, or processes with a common purpose.

task structure The degree to which work is defined by specific procedures, explicit directions, and measurable goals.

team Small number of people with complementary skills who are committed to a common purpose, performance goals and approach for which they hold themselves accountable (Katzenbach & Smith, 1993).

team nursing Care delivery model that assigns staff to teams that then are responsible for a group of clients.

Theory X The view that in bureaucratic organizations, employees prefer security, direction, and minimal responsibility; coercion, threats, or punishment are necessary because people do not like the work to be done.

Theory Y The view that in the context of the right conditions, people enjoy their work, they can show self-control and discipline, are able to contribute creatively and are motivated by ties to the group, the organization, and the work itself; belief that people are intrinsically motivated by their work.

Theory Z The view of collective decision making and a focus on long-term employment that involves slower promotions and less direct supervision.

tort A civil wrong committed by one person against another, such that some injury or damage is caused to either person or property.

total patient care A care delivery model in which nurses are responsible for the total care for their client assignment for the shift they are working.

transactional leader A traditional manager concerned with day-to-day operations.

transformational leader An individual who is committed to a vision that empowers others.

ubiquitous computing (UC) A term coined by Mark Weiser of Xerox PARC to describe the phase of computing in which there are many computers to one person.

union A formal, legal group that works through a collective bargaining agent and within the legal context of labour legislation to bring forth workers' requests to management.

unit producing Refers to direct care activities.

utilitarian theories The most commonly cited type of consequentialist theories; assesses the moral rightness of actions based on how much happiness they might produce.

values (organizational) The boundaries an organization will have while pursuing its vision.

values (personal) Personal beliefs about the truth of ideals, standards, principles, objects, and behaviours that give meaning and direction to life.

veracity The obligation to tell the truth.

verbal communication The aspect of communication that relies on spoken words to convey a message.

vertical integration The linking of different stages of health care that are delivered by one agency.

vision A statement that provides a clear picture of what the future will look like for an organization.

visual Pertaining to seeing.

voting block Group that represents the same political position or perspective.

vulnerable population groups Sub-groups of a community that are powerless, marginalized, or disenfranchised and are experiencing health disparities.

whistle-blowing An act in which an individual discloses information concerning a harmful act that a superior or colleague has committed, is allowing to occur, or is contemplating; a violation of a law, rule, or regulation, or a substantial and specific danger to public health or safety.

workload measurement system System for distinguishing among different clients based on their acuity, functional ability, or resource needs.

workplace advocacy Activities nurses undertake to address problems in their everyday workplace setting.

INDEX

Notes: Entries with page numbers in boldface type are key terms. Page numbers preceded by "F" reference figures; page numbers preceded by "T" reference tables.

PHOTO CREDITS